ACOG
COMPENDIUM

of Selected Publications

2009

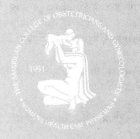

THE AMERICAN COLLEGE OF
OBSTETRICIANS AND GYNECOLOGISTS
WOMEN'S HEALTH CARE PHYSICIANS

The following resources from ACOG also contain ACOG practice guidelines and should be considered adjuncts to the documents in the *Compendium of Selected Publications 2009.*

Ethics in Obstetrics and Gynecology, Second Edition
Guidelines for Perinatal Care, Sixth Edition
Guidelines for Women's Health Care, Third Edition
Health Care for Adolescents
Special Issues in Women's Health

These documents are available online to members at www.acog.org

The *Compendium of Selected Publications* contains **only** 2007–2008 Committee Opinions, Practice Bulletins, Policy Statements, and Technology Assessments published by the American College of Obstetricians and Gynecologists (ACOG) as of December 31, 2008. The information in these documents should not be viewed as establishing standards or dictating rigid rules. The guidelines are general and intended to be adapted to many different situations, taking into account the needs and resources particular to the locality, the institution, or the type of practice. Variations and innovations that improve the quality of patient care are to be encouraged rather than restricted. The purpose of these guidelines will be well served if they provide a firm basis on which local norms may be built.

The American College of Obstetricians and Gynecologists
409 12th Street, SW
PO Box 96920
Washington, DC 20090-6920

ISBN: 978-1-934946-77-0   12345/32109

Publications can be ordered through the ACOG Distribution Center by calling toll free 800-762-2264. To receive order forms via facsimile, call (732) 885-6364 and follow the audio instructions. Publications also can be ordered from the ACOG web site at www.acog.org.

Contents

*Published in 2008

*Published in 2008
▮ Technology Assessment

*Published in 2008

PRACTICE BULLETINS — GYNECOLOGY (continued)

POLICY STATEMENTS

APPENDIX: CONTENTS FROM OTHER ACOG RESOURCES

SUBJECT INDEX

Foreword

The *2009 Compendium of Selected Publications* is a compilation of *only* 2007–2008 Committee Opinions, Practice Bulletins, Policy Statements, and Technology Assessments current as of December 31, 2008. For easy reference, this edition also includes the *Compendium of Selected Publications* CD-ROM, which includes *all* documents in these series current as of December 31, 2008:

- Committee Opinions: Brief focused documents that address clinical issues of an urgent or emergent nature or nonclinical topics such as policy, economics, and social issues that relate to obstetrics and gynecology. They are consensus statements that may or may not be based on scientific evidence.

- Practice Bulletins: Evidence-based guidelines developed to indicate a preferred method of diagnosis and management of a condition. The evidence is graded, and peer-reviewed research determines the recommendations in the document.

- Policy Statements: Position papers on key issues approved by the Executive Board.

- Technology Assessments in Obstetrics and Gynecology: Documents that describe specific technologies and their application.

These series are developed by committees of experts and reviewed by leaders in the specialty and the College. Each document is reviewed periodically and either reaffirmed, replaced, or withdrawn to ensure its continued appropriateness to practice. The contribution of the many groups and individuals who participated in the process is gratefully acknowledged.

Each section of the Compendium is devoted to a particular series, and includes those documents considered current at the time of publication. A comprehensive table of contents has been added for ease of use with titles listed numerically by committee. Those published within 2008 are indicated with an asterisk. Also provided are current Committee Opinion and Practice Bulletin lists of titles, grouped by committee in order of publication.

As the practice of medicine evolves, so do ACOG documents. As a part of the continuing process of review and revision, many documents initially published as a separate installment of a series evolve to become a part of a broader effort to educate and inform our Fellows. Books such as *Guidelines for Perinatal Care* or *Guidelines for Women's Health Care* carry equal weight as practice guidelines and should be considered adjuncts to the documents in the series. For ease of reference, the contents of these volumes are included in the appendix.

The *2009 Compendium of Selected Publications* and the *Compendium of Selected Publications* CD-ROM can be purchased by calling 800-762-2264 (2009 Compendium and CD-ROM: $226, $99 [members]; Compendium CD-ROM only: $104, $59 [members]).

Throughout the year, new documents will be published in ACOG's official journal, *Obstetrics & Gynecology*. Single copies can be obtained from the Resource Center (202-863-2518), and the series are available for sale as complete sets or subscriptions (call 800-762-2264 to order). These documents also are available to members on our web site: www.acog.org. To verify the status of documents, contact the Resource Center or check our web site.

We are making every effort to provide health professionals with current, quality information on the practice of obstetrics and gynecology. The combined *2009 Compendium of Selected Publications* and the *Compendium of Selected Publications* CD-ROM represent still another way to disseminate material designed to promote women's health.

—Ralph W. Hale, MD, Executive Vice President

The Scope of Practice of Obstetrics and Gynecology

Obstetrics and gynecology is a discipline dedicated to the broad, integrated medical and surgical care of women's health throughout their lifespan. The combined discipline of obstetrics and gynecology requires extensive study and understanding of reproductive physiology, including the physiologic, social, cultural, environmental and genetic factors that influence disease in women. This study and understanding of the reproductive physiology of women gives obstetricians and gynecologists a unique perspective in addressing gender-specific health care issues.

Preventive counseling and health education are essential and integral parts of the practice of obstetricians and gynecologists as they advance the individual and community-based health of women of all ages.

Obstetricians and gynecologists may choose a scope of practice ranging from primary ambulatory health care to concentration in a focused area of specialization.

Approved by the Executive Board
February 6, 2005

Code *of* Professional Ethics

of the American College of Obstetricians and Gynecologists

Obstetrician-gynecologists, as members of the medical profession, have ethical responsibilities not only to patients, but also to society, to other health professionals and to themselves. The following ethical foundations for professional activities in the field of obstetrics and gynecology are the supporting structures for the Code of Conduct. The Code implements many of these foundations in the form of rules of ethical conduct. Certain documents of the American College of Obstetricians and Gynecologists also provide additional ethical rules, including documents addressing the following issues: seeking and giving consultation, informed consent, sexual misconduct, patient testing, human immunodeficiency virus, relationships with industry, commercial enterprises in medical practice, and expert testimony. Noncompliance with the Code, including the above-referenced documents, may affect an individual's initial or continuing Fellowship in the American College of Obstetricians and Gynecologists. These documents may be revised or replaced periodically, and Fellows should be knowledgeable about current information.

Ethical Foundations

I. The patient–physician relationship: The welfare of the patient *(beneficence)* is central to all considerations in the patient–physician relationship. Included in this relationship is the obligation of physicians to respect the rights of patients, colleagues, and other health professionals. The respect for the right of individual patients to make their own choices about their health care *(autonomy)* is fundamental. The principle of justice requires strict avoidance of discrimination on the basis of race, color, religion, national origin, or any other basis that would constitute illegal discrimination *(justice)*.

II. Physician conduct and practice: The obstetrician–gynecologist must deal honestly with patients and colleagues *(veracity)*. This includes not misrepresenting himself or herself through any form of communication in an untruthful, misleading, or deceptive manner. Furthermore, maintenance of medical competence through study, application, and enhancement of medical knowledge and skills is an obligation of practicing physicians. Any behavior that diminishes a physician's capability to practice, such as substance abuse, must be immediately addressed and rehabilitative services instituted. The physician should modify his or her practice until the diminished capacity has been restored to an acceptable standard to avoid harm to patients *(nonmaleficence)*. All physicians are obligated to respond to evidence of questionable conduct or unethical behavior by other physicians through appropriate procedures established by the relevant organization.

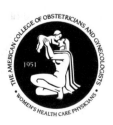

409 12th Street, SW
PO Box 96920
Washington, DC 20090-6920

III. Avoiding conflicts of interest: Potential conflicts of interest are inherent in the practice of medicine. Physicians are expected to recognize such situations and deal with them through public disclosure. Conflicts of interest should be resolved in accordance with the best interest of the patient, respecting a woman's autonomy to make health care decisions. The physician should be an advocate for the patient through public disclosure of conflicts of interest raised by health payer policies or hospital policies.

IV. Professional relations: The obstetrician–gynecologist should respect and cooperate with other physicians, nurses, and health care professionals.

V. Societal responsibilities: The obstetrician–gynecologist has a continuing responsibility to society as a whole and should support and participate in activities that enhance the community. As a member of society, the obstetrician–gynecologist should respect the laws of that society. As professionals and members of medical societies, physicians are required to uphold the dignity and honor of the profession.

Code of Conduct

I.   Patient–Physician Relationship

1. The patient–physician relationship is the central focus of all ethical concerns, and the welfare of the patient must form the basis of all medical judgments.

2. The obstetrician–gynecologist should serve as the patient's advocate and exercise all reasonable means to ensure that the most appropriate care is provided to the patient.

3. The patient–physician relationship has an ethical basis and is built on confidentiality, trust, and honesty. If no patient–physician relationship exists, a physician may refuse to provide care, except in emergencies. Once the patient–physician relationship exists, the obstetrician–gynecologist must adhere to all applicable legal or contractual constraints in dissolving the patient–physician relationship.

4. Sexual misconduct on the part of the obstetrician–gynecologist is an abuse of professional power and a violation of patient trust. Sexual contact or a romantic relationship between a physician and a current patient is always unethical.

5. The obstetrician–gynecologist has an obligation to obtain the informed consent of each patient. In obtaining informed consent for any course of medical or surgical treatment, the obstetrician–gynecologist must present to the patient, or to the person legally responsible for the patient, pertinent medical facts and recommendations consistent with good medical practice. Such information should be presented in reasonably understandable terms and include alternative modes of treatment and the objectives, risks, benefits, possible complications, and anticipated results of such treatment.

6. It is unethical to prescribe, provide, or seek compensation for therapies that are of no benefit to the patient.

7. The obstetrician–gynecologist must respect the rights and privacy of patients, colleagues, and others and safeguard patient information and confidences within the limits of the law. If during the process of providing information for consent it is known that results of a particular test or other information must be given to governmental authorities or other third parties, that must be explained to the patient.

8. The obstetrician–gynecologist must not discriminate against patients based on race, color, national origin, religion, or any other basis that would constitute illegal discrimination.

II. Physician Conduct and Practice

1. The obstetrician–gynecologist should recognize the boundaries of his or her particular competencies and expertise and must provide only those services and use only those techniques for which he or she is qualified by education, training, and experience.

2. The obstetrician–gynecologist should participate in continuing medical education activities to maintain current scientific and professional knowledge relevant to the medical services he or she renders. The obstetrician–gynecologist should provide medical care involving new therapies or techniques only after undertaking appropriate training and study.

3. In emerging areas of medical treatment where recognized medical guidelines do not exist, the obstetrician–gynecologist should exercise careful judgment and take appropriate precautions to protect patient welfare.

4. The obstetrician–gynecologist must not publicize or represent himself or herself in any untruthful, misleading, or deceptive manner to patients, colleagues, other health care professionals, or the public.

5. The obstetrician–gynecologist who has reason to believe that he or she is infected with the human immunodeficiency virus (HIV) or other serious infectious agents that might be communicated to patients should voluntarily be tested for the protection of his or her patients. In making decisions about patient-care activities, a physician infected with such an agent should adhere to the fundamental professional obligation to avoid harm to patients.

6. The obstetrician–gynecologist should not practice medicine while impaired by alcohol, drugs, or physical or mental disability. The obstetrician–gynecologist who experiences substance abuse problems or who is physically or emotionally impaired should seek appropriate assistance to address these problems and must limit his or her practice until the impairment no longer affects the quality of patient care.

III. Conflicts of Interest

1. Potential conflicts of interest are inherent in the practice of medicine. Conflicts of interest should be resolved in accordance with the best interest of the patient, respecting a woman's autonomy to make health care decisions. If there is an actual or potential conflict of interest that could be reasonably construed to affect significantly the patient's care, the physician must disclose the conflict to the patient. The physician should seek consultation with colleagues or an institutional ethics committee to determine whether there is an actual or potential conflict of interest and how to address it.

2. Commercial promotions of medical products and services may generate bias unrelated to product merit, creating or appearing to create inappropriate undue influence. The obstetrician–gynecologist should be aware of this potential conflict of interest and offer medical advice that is as accurate, balanced, complete, and devoid of bias as possible.

3. The obstetrician–gynecologist should prescribe drugs, devices, and other treatments solely on the basis of medical considerations and patient needs, regardless of any direct or indirect interests in or benefit from a pharmaceutical firm or other supplier.

4. When the obstetrician–gynecologist receives anything of substantial value, including royalties, from companies in the health care industry, such as a manufacturer of pharmaceuticals and medical devices, this fact should be disclosed to patients and colleagues when material.

5. Financial and administrative constraints may create disincentives to treatment otherwise recommended by the obstetrician–gynecologist. Any pertinent constraints should be disclosed to the patient.

IV. Professional Relations

1. The obstetrician–gynecologist's relationships with other physicians, nurses, and health care professionals should reflect fairness, honesty, and integrity, sharing a mutual respect and concern for the patient.

2. The obstetrician–gynecologist should consult, refer, or cooperate with other physicians, health care professionals, and institutions to the extent necessary to serve the best interests of their patients.

V.   Societal Responsibilities

1.   The obstetrician–gynecologist should support and participate in those health care programs, practices, and activities that contribute positively, in a meaningful and cost-effective way, to the welfare of individual patients, the health care system, or the public good.

2.   The obstetrician–gynecologist should respect all laws, uphold the dignity and honor of the profession, and accept the profession's self-imposed discipline. The professional competence and conduct of obstetrician–gynecologists are best examined by professional associations, hospital peer-review committees, and state medical and licensing boards. These groups deserve the full participation and cooperation of the obstetrician–gynecologist.

3.   The obstetrician–gynecologist should strive to address through the appropriate procedures the status of those physicians who demonstrate questionable competence, impairment, or unethical or illegal behavior. In addition, the obstetrician–gynecologist should cooperate with appropriate authorities to prevent the continuation of such behavior.

4.   The obstetrician–gynecologist must not knowingly offer testimony that is false. The obstetrician–gynecologist must testify only on matters about which he or she has knowledge and experience. The obstetrician–gynecologist must not knowingly misrepresent his or her credentials.

5.   The obstetrician–gynecologist testifying as an expert witness must have knowledge and experience about the range of the standard of care and the available scientific evidence for the condition in question during the relevant time and must respond accurately to questions about the range of the standard of care and the available scientific evidence.

6.   Before offering testimony, the obstetrician–gynecologist must thoroughly review the medical facts of the case and all available relevant information.

7.   The obstetrician–gynecologist serving as an expert witness must accept neither disproportionate compensation nor compensation that is contingent upon the outcome of the litigation.

COMMITTEE OPINIONS

COMMITTEE OPINIONS

COMMITTEE ON ADOLESCENT HEALTH CARE

COMMITTEE ON ADOLESCENT HEALTH CARE

ACOG COMMITTEE OPINION

Number 392 • December 2007

Intrauterine Device and Adolescents

Committee on Adolescent Health Care

The committee would like to thank Nicole Zidenberg, MD, Nirupama DeSilva, MD, Melissa Gilliam, MD, and Eve Espey, MD, for their contributions to the development of this document.

This document reflects emerging clinical and scientific advances as of the date issued and is subject to change. The information should not be construed as dictating an exclusive course of treatment or procedure to be followed.

ABSTRACT: The intrauterine device (IUD) is highly effective and widely used by women throughout the world. Data support the safety of IUDs for most women, including adolescents. This document addresses the major benefits of IUD use in adolescents, a population at particular risk of unintended pregnancy.

Intrauterine devices (IUDs) are used by fewer than 3% of reproductive-aged women in the United States (1). Concerns about pelvic inflammatory disease (PID), sexually transmitted diseases (STDs), infertility, and difficult insertion have limited the use of the IUD in adolescents. Data support the safety of IUDs for most women, including adolescents. The World Health Organization supports the use of intrauterine contraception in women from menarche to age 20 years, stating that the benefits of intrauterine contraception generally outweigh the risks (2).

Importance of Appropriate Contraception

Approximately 29% of ninth graders and 62% of 12th graders have engaged in intercourse (3). Sexual activity and inconsistent contraceptive use contribute to the high rate of adolescent pregnancy in the United States, which exceeds that of other industrialized countries (4, 5). Intrauterine devices offer the long-term, cost-effective, highly reliable, and effective contraception needed by women, especially adolescents (6, 7).

Common Misperceptions

The Intrauterine Device Does Not Increase an Adolescent's Risk of Pelvic Inflammatory Disease and Sexually Transmitted Diseases

Past experiences with the Dalkon Shield have perpetuated the myth that IUDs cause pelvic infections. The studies that showed a causal relationship between pelvic infection and IUDs were fraught with methodologic errors. Confounding factors included inappropriate comparison groups, overdiagnosis of salpin-

gitis in IUD users, and inability to control for the effects of sexual behavior, leading to an exaggeration of risk estimates (8). Ongoing research continues to demonstrate the safety of modern types of IUDs.

The risk of PID is increased above baseline only at the time of insertion. Among 22,908 IUD users, within the first 20 days of use, the risk of PID was 9.7 per 1,000 woman-years; from 21 days to 8 years, the incidence of PID was 1.4 per 1,000 woman-years, the same as that in the general population (9). Other multicenter randomized controlled trials confirmed these findings (8, 10). The risk of PID with IUD placement is 0–2% when no infection is present at the time of insertion and 0–5% when insertion occurred with a documented infection. The absolute risk of PID is very small in both groups (10). Case reports also have shown that women with positive chlamydia cultures identified at the time of IUD insertion are unlikely to develop PID if the infection is treated with the IUD retained (11, 12).

The levonorgestrel-releasing intrauterine system may lower the risk of PID by thickening cervical mucus and thinning the endometrium (13). Studies have demonstrated the reduced risk of PID using the levonorgestrel-releasing intrauterine system as compared with a copper IUD (14, 15).

Intrauterine Devices Do Not Affect the Fertility of Adolescents

Compared with other methods, infertility was not higher after cessation of IUD use versus cessation of other reversible methods of contraception (8). In a case–control study examining determinants of tubal infertility, the presence of chlamydial antibodies was associated with infertility in both users and

The American College of Obstetricians and Gynecologists
Women's Health Care Physicians

nonusers of IUDs (16). Fecundity rapidly returns to normal after IUD removal (17, 18).

Discontinuation

Adolescents are more likely than adult women to discontinue a range of contraceptive methods, including pills and injectable contraception. In women younger than 25 years, discontinuation of the levonorgestrel-releasing intrauterine system at 12 months was slightly higher compared with older women (19). Among copper IUD users, pain and bleeding led to discontinuation (20). The rate of amenorrhea with the levonorgestrel-releasing intrauterine system varies from 16.4% to 80% at 1 year after insertion and may alleviate bleeding concerns (21).

Expulsion

Expulsion contributes to IUD failure with a risk of 1 in 20 (22). Younger age and previous IUD expulsion may confer the greatest risk of failure (23). Prior expulsion should not be considered a contraindication for a new IUD provided that patients undergo appropriate counseling and have close follow-up (23).

Contraindications

Contraindications to IUD use include current pregnancy; PID or puerperal or postabortion sepsis that is current or within the past 3 months; current STDs; purulent cervicitis; undiagnosed abnormal vaginal bleeding; malignancy of the genital tract; known uterine anomalies or leiomyomata distorting the uterine cavity in a way incompatible with IUD insertion; or allergy to any component of the IUD or Wilson's disease (for copper-containing IUDs) (24). An asymptomatic patient may use an IUD within 3 months of a treated pelvic infection or septic abortion (2, 18).

Emergency Contraception and Menstrual Suppression

The copper IUD may be used for emergency contraception within 5 days of unprotected intercourse (24). The IUD confers the additional benefit of serving as a long-term contraceptive. One study found that 86% of parous women and 80% of nulliparous women maintained the IUD for long-term contraception after use as emergency contraception (25).

In addition to providing contraception, the levonorgestrel-releasing intrauterine system reduces menstrual blood loss by 75% at 3 months. It offers the most favorable side effect profile of the progesterone-only methods. The levonorgestrel-releasing intrauterine system offers an alternative to birth control pills for cycle control.

Confidentiality, Consent, and Counseling

Practitioners must be familiar with federal, state, and institutional guidelines governing consent by adolescents. In many states, adolescents have the right to receive confidential contraceptive services without parental permission (26). Confidential IUD insertion may be thwarted by the cost or consent issues. Preinsertion counseling about the IUD is paramount. Goals of counseling include awareness of the long-term nature of the contraceptive, side effects, risks, and benefits. Upon insertion of the IUD, self-examination to confirm the presence of strings should be taught, and condom use for STD prevention should be encouraged. It is important for adolescents using IUDs to be familiar with their anatomy and comfortable with checking for strings.

Insertion in the Nulliparous Patient

Discomfort with IUD insertion is common. In one study, 86% of adolescents reported mild to severe pain with insertion (13). Misoprostol may soften a nulliparous cervix before insertion (27). Studies of use of nonsteroidal antiinflammatory drugs for analgesia yielded mixed results but they may be used (28). Less studied methods of analgesia include paracervical blocks or preinsertion narcotics. Little data suggest that IUD insertion is technically more difficult in adolescents.

Prophylactic antibiotics are not necessary for IUD insertion (29). Because adolescents have the highest number of reported cases of chlamydia and coinfection with gonorrhea frequently occurs (30), all adolescents should be screened for gonorrhea and chlamydia before IUD insertion (27, 31). Screening at the time of insertion expedites contraceptive use. Patients with positive test results have no adverse effects if treated promptly (10–12).

Conclusion

The IUD is a highly effective method of contraception that is underused in the United States. Because adolescents contribute disproportionately to the epidemic of unintended pregnancy in this country, top tier methods of contraception, including IUDs and implants, should be considered as first-line choices for both nulliparous and parous adolescents. After thorough counseling regarding contraceptive options, health care providers should strongly encourage young women who are appropriate candidates to use this method.

References

1. Mosher WD, Martinez GM, Chandra A, Abma JC, Willson SJ. Use of contraception and use of family planning services in the United States: 1982-2002. Adv Data 2004;350:1–36.

2. World Health Organization. Intrauterine devices. In: Medical eligibility criteria for contraceptive use. 3rd ed. Geneva: WHO; 2004. p. 1–17. Available at: http://www.who.int/reproductive-health/publications/mec/7_iud.pdf. Retrieved August 16, 2007.

3. Eaton DK, Kann L, Kinchen S, Ross J, Hawkins J, Harris WA, et al. Youth risk behavior surveillance—United States, 2005. MMWR Surveill Summ 2006;55(5):1–108.

4. Zibners A, Cromer BA, Hayes J. Comparison of continuation rates for hormonal contraception among adolescents. J Pediatr Adolesc Gynecol 1999;12:90–4.

5. Guttmacher Institute. In brief: facts on American teens' sexual and reproductive health. New York (NY): GI; 2006. Available at: http://guttmacher.org/pubs/fb_ATSRH.html. Retrieved August 16, 2007.

6. Trussell J, Vaughan B. Contraceptive failure, method-related discontinuation and resumption of use: results from the 1995 National Survey of Family Growth. Fam Plann Perspect 1999;31:64–72, 93.

7. Chiou CF, Trussell J, Reyes E, Knight K, Wallace J, Udani J, et al. Economic analysis of contraceptives for women. Contraception 2003;68:3–10.

8. Grimes DA. Intrauterine device and upper-genital-tract infection. Lancet 2000;356:1013–9.

9. Farley TM, Rosenberg MJ, Rowe PJ, Chen JH, Meirik O. Intrauterine devices and pelvic inflammatory disease: an international perspective. Lancet 1992;339:785–8.

10. Mohllajee AP, Curtis KM, Peterson HB. Does insertion and use of an intrauterine device increase the risk of pelvic inflammatory disease among women with sexually transmitted infection? A systematic review. Contraception 2006;73:145–53.

11. Skjeldestad FE, Halvorsen LE, Kahn H, Nordbo SA, Saake K. IUD users in Norway are at low risk for genital C. trachomatis infection. Contraception 1996;54:209–12.

12. Faundes A, Telles E, Cristofoletti ML, Faundes D, Castro S, Hardy E. The risk of inadvertent intrauterine device insertion in women carriers of endocervical Chlamydia trachomatis. Contraception 1998;58:105–9.

13. Suhonen S, Haukkamaa M, Jakobsson T, Rauramo I. Clinical performance of a levonorgestrel-releasing intrauterine system and oral contraceptives in young nulliparous women: a comparative study. Contraception 2004;69:407–12.

14. Andersson K, Odlind V, Rybo G. Levonorgestrel-releasing and copper-releasing (Nova T) IUDs during five years of use: a randomized comparative trial. Contraception 1994; 49:56–72.

15. Toivonen J, Luukkainen T, Allonen H. Protective effect of intrauterine release of levonorgestrel on pelvic infection: three years' comparative experience of levonorgestrel- and copper-releasing intrauterine devices. Obstet Gynecol 1991;77:261–4.

16. Hubacher D, Lara-Ricalde R, Taylor DJ, Guerra-Infante F, Guzman-Rodriguez R. Use of copper intrauterine devices and the risk of tubal infertility among nulligravid women. N Engl J Med 2001;345:561–7.

17. Hov GG, Skjeldestad FE, Hilstad T. Use of IUD and subsequent fertility—follow-up after participation in a randomized clinical trial. Contraception 2007;75:88–92.

18. Penney G, Brechin S, de Souza A, Bankowska U, Belfield T, Gormley M, et al. FFPRHC Guidance (January 2004). The copper intrauterine device as long-term contraception. Faculty of Family Planning and Reproductive Health Care Clinical Effectiveness Unit [published erratum appears in J Fam Plann Reprod Health Care 2004;30:134]. J Fam Plann Reprod Health Care 2004;30:29–41; quiz 42.

19. Luukkainen T, Allonen H, Haukkamaa M, Holma P, Pyorala T, Terho J, et al. Effective contraception with the levonorgestrel-releasing intrauterine device: 12-month report of a European multicenter study. Contraception 1987;36: 169–79.

20. Rivera R, Chen-Mok M, McMullen S. Analysis of client characteristics that may affect early discontinuation of the TCu-380A IUD. Contraception 1999;60:155–60.

21. Toma A, Jamieson MA. Revisiting the intrauterine contraceptive device in adolescents. J Pediatr Adolesc Gynecol 2006;19:291–6.

22. FFPRHC Guidance (April 2004). The levonorgestrel-releasing intrauterine system (LNG-IUS) in contraception and reproductive health. Faculty of Family Planning and Reproductive Health Care Clinical Effectiveness Unit. J Fam Plann Reprod Health Care 2004;30:99–108; quiz 109.

23. Thonneau P, Almont T, de La Rochebrochard E, Maria B. Risk factors for IUD failure: results of a large multicentre case-control study. Hum Reprod 2006;21:2612–6.

24. Intrauterine device. ACOG Practice Bulletin No. 59. American College of Obstetricians and Gynecologists. Obstet Gynecol 2005;105:223–32.

25. Zhou L, Xiao B. Emergency contraception with Multiload Cu-375 SL IUD: a multicenter clinical trial. Contraception 2001;64:107–12.

26. Guttmacher Institute. State policies in brief: minors' access to contraceptive services. New York (NY): GI; 2007. Available at: http://www.guttmacher.org/statecenter/spibs/spib_MACS.pdf. Retrieved September 6, 2007.

27. McNaught J. Adolescents and IUCDs—Not a contraindication. J Pediatr Adolesc Gynecol 2006;19:303–5.

28. Grimes DA, Hubacher D, Lopez LM, Schulz KF. Non-steroidal anti-inflammatory drugs for heavy bleeding or pain associated with intrauterine-device use. Cochrane Database of Systematic Reviews 2006, Issue 4. Art. No.: CD006034. DOI: 10.1002/14651858.CD006034.pub2.

29. Grimes DA, Schulz FK. Antibiotic prophylaxis for intrauterine contraceptive device insertion. Cochrane Database of Systematic Reviews 1999, Issue 3. Art. No.: CD001327. DOI: 10.1002/14651858.CD001327.

30. Centers for Disease Control and Prevention. Sexually transmitted disease surveillance 2005. Atlanta (GA): CDC; 2006. Available at: http://www.cdc.gov/std/stats/05pdf/Surv2005.pdf. Retrieved August 16, 2007.

31. Lacy J. Clinic opinions regarding IUCD use in adolescents. J Pediatr Adolesc Gynecol 2006;19:301–3.

Intrauterine device and adolescents. ACOG Committee Opinion No. 392. American College of Obstetricians and Gynecologists. Obstet Gynecol 2007;110:1493–5.

ISSN 1074-861X

ACOG COMMITTEE OPINION

Number 415 • September 2008

Depot Medroxyprogesterone Acetate and Bone Effects

Committee on Adolescent Health Care

Committee on Gynecologic Practice

This document reflects emerging clinical and scientific advances as of the date issued and is subject to change. The information should not be construed as dictating an exclusive course of treatment or procedure to be followed.

ABSTRACT: Although depot medroxyprogesterone acetate (DMPA) is associated with bone mineral density (BMD) loss during use, current evidence suggests that partial or full recovery of BMD occurs at the spine and at least partial recovery occurs at the hip after discontinuation of DMPA. Given the efficacy of DMPA, particularly for populations such as adolescents for whom contraceptive adherence can be challenging or for those who feel they could not comply with a daily contraceptive method or a method that must be used with each act of intercourse, the possible adverse effects of DMPA must be balanced against the significant personal and public health impact of unintended pregnancy. Concerns regarding the effect of DMPA on BMD should neither prevent practitioners from prescribing DMPA nor limit its use to 2 consecutive years. Practitioners should not perform BMD monitoring solely in response to DMPA use because any observed short-term loss in BMD associated with DMPA use may be recovered and is unlikely to place a woman at risk of fracture during use or in later years.

The American College of Obstetricians and Gynecologists

Women's Health Care Physicians

Depot medroxyprogesterone acetate (DMPA) is a highly effective, long-acting contraceptive injection used by more than two million women annually in the United States, including approximately 400,000 adolescents (1). Convenient dose administration and privacy are appealing to adolescents, and the expanded use of DMPA has been credited for at least part of the decrease in adolescent pregnancy rates over the past decade (2, 3). Depot medroxyprogesterone acetate prevents pregnancy by inhibiting the secretion of pituitary gonadotropins resulting in anovulation, amenorrhea, and a decreased production of serum estrogen. Hypoestrogenism is associated with a decrease in bone mineral density (BMD). In older women, low BMD consistent with osteopenia or osteoporosis is associated with an increased risk of fracture. No studies have been conducted to examine the association between BMD and fractures in low-risk young women, including those using DMPA or those experiencing the physiologic hypoestrogenism of lactation. Although DMPA is associated with BMD loss during use, current evidence suggests that partial or full recovery of BMD occurs at the spine and at least partial recovery occurs at the hip after discontinuation of DMPA. Given the efficacy of DMPA, particularly for populations such as adolescents for whom contraceptive adherence can be challenging or for those who feel they could not comply with a daily contraceptive method or a method that must be used with each act of intercourse, the possible adverse effects of DMPA must be balanced against the significant personal and public health impact of unintended pregnancy.

Bone Mineral Density

A number of studies demonstrate the effect of DMPA on BMD. Cross-sectional and longitudinal studies using dual-energy X-ray absorptiometry (DXA) technology among current users of DMPA (ages 18–54 years) demonstrate that DMPA use results in lower BMD compared with nonusers regardless of the anatomic site measured (4–10). Longitudinal studies report BMD losses at the hip and spine of 0.5–3.5% after 1 year of DMPA use (5, 11) and a 5.7–7.5% loss in BMD after 2 years of use (8, 10).

Although few studies have examined long-term use of DMPA, it appears that the greatest BMD loss is experienced during the first few years of use (7, 10, 11). In one 3-year longitudinal study, mean change in BMD at each 6-month interval decreased as the number of cumulative months of DMPA use increased (7). Those using DMPA for 12 months or less lost BMD at a faster rate than those using DMPA for 13 months or more (7). Another recent longitudinal study with a 4-year follow-up period demonstrated that almost 75% of the BMD lost at the hip and 90% lost at the spine occurred during the first 24 months of use (9). Women who continued DMPA use beyond 24 months still lost additional bone, but the magnitude of loss was smaller with each subsequent year of use (9).

A recent prospective study of BMD monitored DMPA users and nonhormonal contraceptive users 20–25 years of age for up to 5 years of use and for up to 2 years after discontinuation. Despite BMD loss during use, total hip BMD among DMPA users had returned almost to baseline levels at 2 years after discontinuation (from -5.16% after 240 weeks of use to -0.2% at 96 weeks after discontinuation), and BMD values in the lumbar spine showed partial recovery (from -5.38% after 240 weeks of use to -1.19% at 96 weeks after discontinuation) (12). As in prior studies, the rate of BMD loss was greater in the first year of treatment than in subsequent years.

Bone loss during the reproductive years is not unique to DMPA use. Studies of adult women show a decrease in BMD of 2–8% during pregnancy and 3–5% during breastfeeding (13, 14). These losses are temporary; 6–12 months after birth or cessation of breast-feeding BMD values increase to near preconception values in most women (11). Similarly, studies suggest that at least some of the bone loss experienced as a result of DMPA use is recovered after discontinuation. However, studies differ in their assessment of the speed and completeness of this recovery (7, 9, 10, 12, 15–17). Furthermore, the degree of recovery appears to differ by site. A 3-year longitudinal study of 18–39-year-old DMPA users noted that women experienced steady gains in BMD after discontinuation, regardless of duration of DMPA use (7). Lumbar spine BMD of DMPA users was similar to that of nonusers by 30 months after discontinuation (7). Increases in BMD at the hip among those discontinuing use of DMPA also were noted, but the gain in BMD at this location was lower than that of nonusers 30 months after discontinuation. Similarly, a 4-year study of first-time users of DMPA 18–35 years of age demonstrated that the length of time required for BMD values to return to baseline levels depended on the site measured and the duration of DMPA use. Complete recovery occurred at the spine within 27–30 months among those using DMPA up to 24 months. Recovery at the hip was slower; among those women who used DMPA for 24 months or less, a return to baseline values was not observed by 30 months after discontinuation (9).

Bone mineral density normally increases during the teenaged years. Therefore, a decrease or stabilization in BMD during this period may be cause for concern. In a study of DMPA users aged 12–21 years, BMD decreased an average of 3.1% (18). In contrast, adolescents who were not using hormonal contraception gained BMD at an average rate of 9.5% over 2 years (18). Among new DMPA users aged 14–18 years, a decrease of 5% at the spine occurred after 24 months compared with an increase of 2.3% in nonusers (16). The decrease in BMD observed in these studies may be mitigated by the short-term or intermittent nature of DMPA use in many adolescents because the discontinuation rate is 50% in the first year (19). Furthermore, increases in BMD of 1–4% at the hip and spine 12 months after discontinuation of DMPA have been shown in adolescents aged 14–18 years (16).

At least two cross-sectional studies provide reassuring data that BMD in former adult DMPA users is similar to that of never users (20, 21). A World Health Organization study observed this lack of difference in BMD in an international population of former DMPA users and nonusers (20). Another study of postmenopausal women in New Zealand indicated similar BMD in former adult DMPA users compared with that of never users (21).

Fracture Risk

Although many studies have examined the intermediate outcome of decreased BMD related to DMPA, few investigations have examined the outcome of critical importance to women's health—that of fracture risk. Two studies have examined DMPA use and fracture, both in high-risk populations. A prospective, short-term study of female military recruits found that, in white women only, history of DMPA use was one of several factors associated with an increased risk of stress fractures of the calcaneus (22). This study was limited to women at high risk of fractures and is not applicable to the general population. Another recent study of developmentally delayed women suggests an increased risk of fractures in those with a history of DMPA use. This study is limited by its cross-sectional design and its use of retrospective data (23).

There are no reported studies in which the risk of osteoporosis or fractures has been examined in a low-risk population of prior DMPA users. A recent Cochrane review reveals that not a single randomized controlled trial of DMPA and fracture risk has been performed (24).

The "Black Box" Warning

Concerns over the effect of DMPA use on BMD caused the U.S. Food and Drug Administration to issue a "black box" warning in November 2004. This warning stated that prolonged use of DMPA may result in significant loss of BMD, that the loss is greater the longer the drug is used, and that the loss may not be completely reversible after discontinuation. The warning cautions that use of DMPA beyond 2 years should be considered only if other contraceptive methods are inadequate. In a letter to physicians, a manufacturer of DMPA suggested DXA monitoring after 2 years of use.

The U.S. Food and Drug Administration warning is based on intermediate effects on BMD, which may or may not be relevant to increased fracture risk. Because the evidence suggests that the rate of BMD loss may slow with longer term DMPA use, the rationale for restriction to 2 years of use or DXA monitoring is unclear. Practitioners should not perform BMD monitoring solely in response to DMPA use because any observed short-term losses in BMD may be recovered and are unlikely to place women at risk of fracture during DMPA use or in later years.

Risks of Bone Loss Versus the Benefits of Contraception

Most women and adolescents use DMPA to avoid pregnancy. The failure rate in typical users is 2–3% for DMPA (25). As a result, DMPA is widely used by women for whom successful use of a daily or partner-dependent contraceptive method is difficult. Increased use of DMPA in the past 15 years has been paralleled by a decrease in the adolescent pregnancy rate (2, 3). Although there are many factors contributing to the decrease in adolescent pregnancies, DMPA has likely played a role. It is important to weigh the theoretical risk of future fracture from decreased BMD in DMPA users against the very real risk of pregnancy if contraceptive choices are limited (26). For example, an adolescent who is at high risk for pregnancy may be best served by the use of DMPA as a contraceptive option; both pregnancy and DMPA are associated with loss of BMD. The risk–benefit ratio might differ for a noncontraceptive indication such as dysmenorrhea (23).

Counseling

Women initiating DMPA should be thoroughly counseled about the benefits and the potential risks of DMPA. Daily exercise and age-appropriate calcium and vitamin D intake should be encouraged. No studies have shown that these measures will offset loss of BMD during DMPA use, but these recommendations can benefit general health, and most adolescents do not ingest sufficient dietary calcium. Although studies of adolescents and adult women demonstrate that low-dose estrogen supplementation limits BMD loss in DMPA users (27, 28), estrogen supplementation during DMPA use is not currently recommended. Most importantly, clinicians should provide counseling regarding the side effects of DMPA, including irregular bleeding, in order to attempt to reduce the high rates of discontinuation of this method.

Conclusion

Depot medroxyprogesterone acetate is a safe and effective means of long-term contraception, which has likely contributed to a decrease in adolescent pregnancy rates over the past decade. Concerns regarding the effect of DMPA on BMD should neither prevent practitioners from prescribing DMPA nor limit its use to 2 consecutive years. Appropriate counseling with a discussion of current medical evidence should occur before the initiation of this medication and during prolonged use. Practitioners should not perform BMD monitoring solely in response to DMPA use because any observed short-term loss in BMD associated with DMPA use may be recovered and is unlikely to place a woman at risk of fracture during use or in later years. Effective long-term contraceptive methods that have no effect on BMD and have high continuation rates, such as contraceptive implants and intrauterine devices, should also be considered as first-line methods for adolescents.

References

1. Mosher WD, Martinez GM, Chandra A, Abma JC, Willson SJ. Use of contraception and use of family planning services in the United States: 1982-2002. Adv Data 2004;(350): 1–36.
2. Santelli JS, Abma J, Ventura S, Lindberg L, Morrow B, Anderson JE, et al. Can changes in sexual behaviors among high school students explain the decline in teen pregnancy rates in the 1990s? J Adolesc Health 2004;35:80–90.
3. Santelli JS, Lindberg LD, Finer LB, Singh S. Explaining recent declines in adolescent pregnancy in the United States: the contribution of abstinence and improved contraceptive use. Am J Public Health 2007;97:150–6.
4. Cundy T, Cornish J, Roberts H, Elder H, Reid IR. Spinal bone density in women using depot medroxyprogesterone contraception. Obstet Gynecol 1998;92:569–73.
5. Berenson AB, Radecki CM, Grady JJ, Rickert VI, Thomas A. A prospective, controlled study of the effects of hormonal contraception on bone mineral density. Obstet Gynecol 2001;98:576–82.
6. Wanichsetakul P, Kamudhamas A, Watanaruangkovit P, Siripakarn Y, Visutakul P. Bone mineral density at various anatomic bone sites in women receiving combined oral contraceptives and depot-medroxyprogesterone acetate for contraception. Contraception 2002;65:407–10.
7. Scholes D, LaCroix AZ, Ichikawa LE, Barlow WE, Ott SM. Injectable hormone contraception and bone density: results from a prospective study [published erratum appears in Epidemiology 2002;13:749]. Epidemiology 2002;13:581–7.
8. Berenson AB, Breitkopf CR, Grady JJ, Rickert VI, Thomas A. Effects of hormonal contraception on bone mineral density after 24 months of use. Obstet Gynecol 2004;103:899–906.
9. Clark MK, Sowers M, Levy B, Nichols S. Bone mineral density loss and recovery during 48 months in first-time users of depot medroxyprogesterone acetate. Fertil Steril 2006; 86:1466–74.
10. Clark MK, Sowers MR, Nichols S, Levy B. Bone mineral density changes over two years in first-time users of depot medroxyprogesterone acetate. Fertil Steril 2004;82:1580–6.
11. Ulrich CM, Georgiou CC, Snow-Harter CM, Gillis DE. Bone mineral density in mother-daughter pairs: relations to lifetime exercise, lifetime milk consumption, and calcium supplements. Am J Clin Nutr 1996;63:72–9.
12. Kaunitz AM, Miller PD, Rice VM, Ross D, McClung MR. Bone mineral density in women aged 25-35 years receiving depot medroxyprogesterone acetate: recovery following discontinuation. Contraception 2006;74:90–9.

13. Karlsson C, Obrant KJ, Karlsson M. Pregnancy and lactation confer reversible bone loss in humans. Osteoporos Int 2001;12:828–34.

14. Sowers M, Corton G, Shapiro B, Jannausch ML, Crutchfield M, Smith ML, et al. Changes in bone density with lactation. JAMA 1993;269:3130–5.

15. Cundy T, Cornish J, Evans MC, Roberts H, Reid IR. Recovery of bone density in women who stop using medroxyprogesterone acetate. BMJ 1994;308:247–8.

16. Scholes D, LaCroix AZ, Ichikawa LE, Barlow WE, Ott SM. Change in bone mineral density among adolescent women using and discontinuing depot medroxyprogesterone acetate contraception. Arch Pediatr Adolesc Med 2005; 159:139–44.

17. Johnson CC, Burkman RT, Gold MA, Brown RT, Harel Z, Bruner A, et al. Longitudinal study of depot medroxyprogesterone acetate (Depo-Provera) effects on bone health in adolescents: study design, population characteristics and baseline bone mineral density. Contraception 2008;77: 239–48.

18. Cromer BA, Stager M, Bonny A, Lazebnik R, Rome E, Ziegler J, et al. Depot medroxyprogesterone acetate, oral contraceptives and bone mineral density in a cohort of adolescent girls. J Adolesc Health 2004;35:434–41.

19. Zibners A, Cromer BA, Hayes J. Comparison of continuation rates for hormonal contraception among adolescents. J Pediatr Adolesc Gynecol 1999;12:90–4.

20. Petitti DB, Piaggio G, Mehta S, Cravioto MC, Meirik O. Steroid hormone contraception and bone mineral density: a cross-sectional study in an international population. The WHO Study of Hormonal Contraception and Bone Health. Obstet Gynecol 2000;95:736–44.

21. Orr-Walker BJ, Evans MC, Ames RW, Clearwater JM, Cundy T, Reid IR. The effect of past use of the injectable contraceptive depot medroxyprogesterone acetate on bone mineral density in normal post-menopausal women. Clin Endocrinol 1998;49:615–8.

22. Lappe JM, Stegman MR, Recker RR. The impact of lifestyle factors on stress fractures in female Army recruits. Osteoporos Int 2001;12:35–42.

23. Watson KC, Lentz MJ, Cain KC. Associations between fracture incidence and use of depot medroxyprogesterone acetate and anti-epileptic drugs in women with developmental disabilities. Womens Health Issues 2006;16:346–52.

24. Lopez LM, Grimes DA, Schulz KF, Curtis KM. Steroidal contraceptives: effect on bone fractures in women. Cochrane Database of Systematic Reviews 2006, Issue 4. Art. No.: CD006033. DOI: 10.1002/14651858.CD006033

25. Trussell J. Contraceptive failure in the United States. Contraception 2004;70:89–96.

26. Cromer BA, Scholes D, Berenson A, Cundy T, Clark MK, Kaunitz AM, et al. Depot medroxyprogesterone acetate and bone mineral density in adolescents—the Black Box Warning: a Position Paper of the Society for Adolescent Medicine. Society for Adolescent Medicine. J Adolesc Health 2006;39:296–301.

27. Cundy T, Ames R, Horne A, Clearwater J, Roberts H, Gamble G, et al. A randomized controlled trial of estrogen replacement therapy in long-term users of depot medroxyprogesterone acetate. J Clin Endocrinol Metab 2003;88: 78–81.

28. Cromer BA, Lazebnik R, Rome E, Stager M, Bonny A, Ziegler J, et al. Double-blinded randomized controlled trial of estrogen supplementation in adolescent girls who receive depot medroxyprogesterone acetate for contraception. Am J Obstet Gynecol 2005;192:42–7.

Depot medroxyprogesterone acetate and bone effects. ACOG Committee Opinion No. 415. American College of Obstetricians and Gynecologists. Obstet Gynecol 2008;112:727–30.

ISSN 1074-861X

ACOG COMMITTEE OPINION

Number 417 • September 2008

Addressing Health Risks of Noncoital Sexual Activity

Committee on
Adolescent Health
Care

Committee on
Gynecologic
Practice

This document reflects
emerging clinical and scientific advances as of the
date issued and is subject
to change. The informa-
tion should not be con-
strued as dictating an
exclusive course of treatment or procedure to be
followed.

ABSTRACT: Noncoital sexual behaviors, which include mutual masturbation, oral sex, and anal sex, are common expressions of human sexuality. Couples may engage in noncoital sexual activity instead of penile–vaginal intercourse hoping to reduce the risk of sexually transmitted diseases and unintended pregnancy. Although these behaviors carry little or no risk of pregnancy, women engaging in noncoital behaviors may be at risk of acquiring sexually transmitted diseases. Practitioners can assist by assessing patient risk and providing risk reduction counseling for those participating in noncoital sexual activities.

**The American College
of Obstetricians
and Gynecologists**
*Women's Health Care
Physicians*

Noncoital sexual activities are common in both adults and adolescents. The 2002 National Survey of Family Growth found that 88% of females and 90% of males aged 25–44 years, and 55% of males and 54% of females aged 15–19 years, have had oral sex with an opposite-sex partner (1). Anal sex is less common than oral or vaginal sex and is commonly initiated at a later age; 35% of females and 40% of males aged 25–44 years and 11% of male and female adolescents aged 15–19 years reported anal sex with an opposite-sex partner (1). Comparison of data on oral sex from the 2002 National Survey of Family Growth with data from three national surveys from the early and mid 1990s (the 1991 National Survey of Men, the 1992 National Health and Social Life Survey, and the 1995 National Survey of Adolescent Men) provides no evidence for a recent increase in oral sex prevalence among adolescents and young adults despite concerns expressed in the popular media (1).

Noncoital behaviors commonly co-occur with coital behaviors. Both oral sex and anal sex are much more common among adolescents who have already had vaginal intercourse as compared with those who have not (2). Likewise, the prevalence of oral sex among adolescents jumps dramatically in the first 6 months after initiation of vaginal intercourse, suggesting that both are often initiated at the same time and with the same partner. Initiation of anal sex before

initiation of coitus is rare, and the prevalence of anal sex increases slowly after initiation of coitus.

When engaging in oral sex, most individuals, including adolescents, are unlikely to use barrier protection for a variety of reasons, including a greater perceived safety of noncoital sexual activity compared with vaginal sex (3, 4). In the 2002 National Survey of Family Growth, only 11% of females and 15% of males aged 15–17 years who had ever engaged in oral sex reported using a condom the most recent time that they had engaged in oral sex (5).

Some sexually transmitted diseases (STDs) may be transmitted during noncoital sexual activity. Infections can be spread through saliva, blood, vaginal secretions, semen, and fecal material. Preexisting infections, open sores, abrasions, or any compromise of the epithelial tissue can increase the risk of transmission. Transmission of STDs is organism specific, with certain infections commonly infecting the oral or rectal cavity, and many rarely doing so or causing infection without sequelae.

Human Immunodeficiency Virus

Human immunodeficiency virus (HIV) transmission is highly correlated with the HIV viral load of the infected partner. In addition, the risk of acquiring HIV varies dramatically according to the specific sexual behavior, especially whether it is insertive or receptive. The U.S. Centers for Disease Control and Prevention (CDC) estimates a 100-fold increase in risk from the safest to the least safe behavior (Table 1). Human immunodeficiency virus is most readily transmitted through anal sex. Receptive anal sex with a partner who is infected with HIV is the sexual behavior associated with the greatest risk of HIV transmission. Condom use reduces HIV transmission by approximately 80% in HIV-serodiscordant couples (6). Although saliva appears to have components that inactivate HIV, there are case reports of HIV acquisition in men who engaged only in oral sex with other men (7).

Herpes Simplex Virus

Herpes infection is commonly transmitted through kissing and via oral, vaginal, and anal sex. Typically, herpes simplex virus type 1 (HSV-1) is associated with oral lesions, whereas herpes simplex virus type 2 (HSV-2) is associated with genital lesions. However, both HSV-1 and HSV-2 are capable of infecting oral, anal, and genital sites. A study of university students seeking treatment for herpes found the percentage of HSV-1 genital herpes infections increased from 31% in 1993 to 78% in 2001 (8). Therefore, older studies that based their results solely on the presence of HSV-2 have underestimated the prevalence of genital herpes infections (9, 10).

Human Papillomavirus

Human papillomavirus (HPV) is a very common sexually transmitted virus that causes anogenital and oral cancers as well as the benign genital warts. There are more than 100 strains of HPV, 40 of which selectively infect the anogenital and oral areas. More than 90% of the HPV infections resolve spontaneously without sequelae; however, persistent infection in the anogenital area or oral cavity may cause cancer. Although the most efficient means of transmission appear to be penile–vaginal sex or penile–anal sex, oral transmission appears to occur as well. However, data currently suggest that transmission is

Table 1. Risk of Human Immunodeficiency Virus Transmission According to Sexual Behavior

Sex Act	Relative Risk*
Insertive fellatio	1
Receptive fellatio	2
Insertive vaginal sex	10
Insertive anal sex	13
Receptive vaginal sex	20
Receptive anal sex	100

*Refers to relative risk of acquiring human immunodeficiency virus (HIV) infection among persons without HIV infection.

Varghese B, Maher JE, Peterman TA, Branson BM, Steketee RW. Reducing the risk of sexual HIV transmission: quantifying the per-act risk for HIV on the basis of choice of partner, sex act, and condom use. Sex Transm Dis 2002;29:38–43.

less efficient to the oral cavity than to the genital area. The digital spread of HPV is theoretically possible because genital HPV DNA has been detected on the hand. However, because this is only detection of DNA, it is not proved that this DNA is infectious.

Hepatitis Viruses

Hepatitis B virus can be found in semen, saliva, and feces and is commonly spread through sexual contact. Hepatitis A is transmitted from fecal contamination of the oral cavity, thus explaining the higher incidence of infection in homosexual men who engage in oral–anal contact. Sexual transmission of hepatitis C is uncommon but has been associated with both preexisting hepatitis B and HIV infection and with oral–genital contact (7).

Nonviral Sexually Transmitted Diseases

A substantial number of recent primary and secondary cases of syphilis reported in Chicago were attributable to oral sex, with 86 of 627 (13.7%) individuals with syphilis reporting oral sex as the only sexual exposure that could account for their infection (11).

Most gonorrheal infections are sexually transmitted and involve the urethra, cervix, rectum, or mouth (12). Disseminated disease after oral–genital contact has been documented. Although only 10% of isolated pharyngeal gonorrheal infections are symptomatic, pharyngitis, with or without fever or lymphadenopathy, should raise suspicion for gonorrheal infection when all other etiologies have been ruled out.

Chlamydia has been isolated from throat cultures in both men and women. In women, pharyngeal infection is associated with performing oral sex on men (12, 13). Chancroid, shigellosis, salmonellosis, and other enteric infections have been linked to oral–genital or oral–anal sex in a few case reports but appear to be relatively uncommon. The role of noncoital sexual activity in the transmission of other nonviral infections, such as vulvovaginal candidiasis, bacterial vaginosis, and trichomoniasis remains unclear (12).

Patient Counseling

Noncoital sexual activity is not necessarily "safe sex." Because people define sexuality in a variety of ways, it is important that practitioners ask direct questions regarding sexual activity, including questions about oral or anal sex and mutual masturbation, and questions about sexual partners, including whether the patient has sex with men, women, or both men and women.

A positive response to these questions indicates the need for counseling regarding infection prevention strategies specific to noncoital sexual activity. To individualize counseling, the clinician must consider the woman's infection risk from partner factors (number of sexual partners and her partners' sexual behaviors, particularly multiple sexual partnerships) and the community prevalence of

STDs. Because most women who engage in noncoital sexual activity also are engaging in penile–vaginal intercourse, the clinician needs to consider whether noncoital behaviors add any additional risks to those already posed by sexual intercourse. When a young person engages in only oral or anal sex, the likelihood of encountering a partner infected with an STD should be considered. Correct and consistent condom use should be encouraged, especially for anal sex and vaginal sex. Practitioners also should consider the patient's history of STDs and patterns of barrier method use with each partner. In brief, practitioners need to consider the totality of the patient's STD risk.

Counseling should focus on reducing STD risk factors such as multiple partners. This may be more effective than discouraging oral or anal sex. Risk-reduction strategies may include engaging in safer behaviors (eg, oral sex often is safer than vaginal intercourse, anal sex often is riskier than penile–vaginal sex), abstinence, mutual monogamy, limiting the number of partners, STD testing before engaging in sexual activity with a new partner, and correct and consistent use of condoms, particularly for vaginal and anal sex. Sex toys should be cleaned between uses. Couples counseling may be helpful for STD-serodiscordant couples.

Routine screening for chlamydia is recommended annually for all sexually active women aged 25 years or younger, and routine screening for gonorrhea is recommended for all sexually active adolescents. Although the 2006 CDC STD Treatment Guidelines recommend behavioral screening for anal and oral sex, they do not make specific recommendations for routine oral or anal STD laboratory screening (14). Selected laboratory testing for oral and anal STDs should be based on clinical symptoms and behavioral risks.

Lesbians and bisexual women should be screened for STDs based on the same risk factors as other women. Because most lesbians have been sexually active with men at some point in their lives and because some STDs also can be transmitted by sexual activity exclusively among lesbians, it should not be assumed that STD screening is unnecessary.

Conclusion

Great efforts are needed to educate health care practitioners and the public regarding the potential health risks of noncoital sexual activities and the importance of risk reduction and barrier methods of protection. Practitioners can assist by assessing patient risk and providing risk reduction counseling for those participating in noncoital sexual activities. Ultimately, additional research is needed to determine the full impact of noncoital sexual activity on the health of patients.

References

1. Mosher WD, Chandra A, Jones J. Sexual behavior and selected health measures: men and women 15–44 years of age, United States, 2002. Adv Data 2005;(362):1–55.

2. Lindberg LD, Jones R, Santelli JS. Non-coital sexual activities among adolescents. J Adolesc Health 2008;42(suppl 1): 44–5.

3. Prinstein MJ, Meade CS, Cohen GL. Adolescent oral sex, peer popularity, and perceptions of best friends' sexual behavior. J Pediatr Psychol 2003;28:243–9.

4. Halpern-Felsher BL, Cornell JL, Kropp RY, Tschann JM. Oral versus vaginal sex among adolescents: perceptions, attitudes, and behavior. Pediatrics 2005;115:845–51.

5. Terry-Humen E, Manlove J, Cottingham S. Trends and recent estimates: sexual activity among U.S. teens. Child Trends Research Brief No. 2006–08. Washington, DC: Child Trends; 2006. Available at: http://childtrends.org/files/sexualactivityrb.pdf. Retrieved April 23, 2008.

6. Weller SC, Davis-Beaty K. Condom effectiveness in reducing heterosexual HIV transmission. Cochrane Database of Systematic Reviews 2002, Issue 1. Art. No.: CD003255. DOI: 10.1002/14651858.CD003255.

7. Edwards S, Carne C. Oral sex and the transmission of viral STIs. Sex Transm Infect 1998;74:6–10.

8. Roberts CM, Pfister JR, Spear SJ. Increasing proportion of herpes simplex virus type 1 as a cause of genital herpes infection in college students. Sex Transm Dis 2003;30:797–800.

9. Cherpes TL, Meyn LA, Hillier SL. Cunnilingus and vaginal intercourse are risk factors for herpes simplex virus type 1 acquisition in women. Sex Transm Dis 2005;32:84–9.

10. Lafferty WE, Downey L, Celum C, Wald A. Herpes simplex virus type 1 as a cause of genital herpes: impact on surveillance and prevention. J Infect Dis 2000;181:1454–7.

11. Centers for Disease Control and Prevention (CDC). Transmission of primary and secondary syphilis by oral sex—Chicago, Illinois, 1998-2002. MMWR Morb Mortal Wkly Rep 2004;53:966–8.

12. Edwards S, Carne C. Oral sex and transmission of non-viral STIs. Sex Transm Infect 1998;74:95–100.

13. Jones RB, Rabinovitch RA, Katz BP, Batteiger BE, Quinn TS, Terho P, et al. Chlamydia trachomatis in the pharynx and rectum of heterosexual patients at risk for genital infection. Ann Intern Med 1985;102:757–62.

14. Workowski KA, Berman SM. Sexually transmitted diseases treatment guidelines, 2006. Centers for Disease Control and Prevention [published erratum appears in: MMWR Morb Mortal Wkly Rep 2006;55:997]. MMWR Recomm Rep 2006;55:1–94.

Addressing health risks of noncoital sexual activity. ACOG Committee Opinion No. 417. American College of Obstetricians and Gynecologists. Obstet Gynecol 2008;112:735–7.

ISSN 1074-861X

COMMITTEE ON ETHICS

COMMITTEE ON ETHICS

ACOG COMMITTEE OPINION

Number 358 • January 2007

Professional Responsibilities in Obstetric–Gynecologic Education*

Committee on Ethics

ABSTRACT: Physicians must learn new skills in a manner consistent with their ethical obligations to benefit the patient, to do no harm, and to respect a patient's right to make informed decisions. Patients should be given the opportunity to consent to or refuse treatment by students. Students must hold in confidence any information they learn about patients. The relationship between teacher and student involves an imbalance of power and the risk of exploitation of a student for the benefit of the teacher. Students should not be placed in situations where they must provide care or perform procedures for which they are not qualified and not adequately supervised. Students have the obligation to be honest, conscientious, and respectful in their relationships with their teachers. They should act in ways that preserve the dignity of patients and do not undermine relationships between patients and their physicians. If a student observes unethical behavior or incompetent conduct by a teacher, the appropriate institutional authority should be informed. Institutions have an obligation to provide a work environment that enhances professional competence by ensuring that students and residents work reasonable hours, helping them balance education and patient care responsibilities; providing adequate support services; and, in the case of residents, providing reasonable salaries and benefits. With increasing numbers of women in education programs, special attention must be given to the parallel demands of pregnancy and career goals.

Education of health care professionals is essential to maintain standards of competent and beneficial practice. Inherent in the education of health professionals is the problem of disparity in power and authority, including the power of teachers over students and the power of practitioners over patients[†] (1). It is therefore important to clarify both the professional responsibilities to those patients whose care provides educational opportunities and the responsibilities of teachers and students toward one another. Students in the context of this Committee Opinion include both medical students and residents. However, residents have a dual responsibility as teacher and student and must be aware of that in understanding their ethical responsibilities to the students they teach and the patients they care for.

Ethical Responsibilities Toward Patients in Educational Settings

At the turn of the 20th century, some medical educators were concerned about the needs of

The American College of Obstetricians and Gynecologists
Women's Health Care Physicians

---

*Update of "Obstetric–Gynecologic Education," in *Ethics in Obstetrics and Gynecology,* Second Edition, 2004.

[†]As commonly categorized by medical schools, residencies, and postgraduate fellowships, the learning and teaching roles of "student" and "teacher" represent a hierarchical approach to learning that does not reflect the reality of lifelong learning and teaching. The line between students

and teachers in medicine is fluid and nonlinear. All clinicians learn from and teach each other at each point in the development of their profession. In this statement, the ethical obligations of teachers apply to all of those in the teaching role, wherever they may be in the educational continuum, and the obligations of students apply to all of those in the learning role.

patients in "teaching hospitals," and they took steps to ensure that patients' rights would be protected. However, the prevailing opinion was more aptly characterized by a medical school faculty member: "Patients must clearly understand from the beginning that they are admitted for teaching purposes and that they are to be willing to submit to this when pronounced physically fit" (2). Unfortunately, this sentiment persists as an unstated presumption in some contemporary education programs. If the power inherent in the role of medical practitioner is misused in the educational setting, this misuse is likely to carry over into attitudes and relationships with future patients as well.

If health care professionals are to benefit society, they must be well educated and experienced. Acquisition of knowledge and skills in the educational process entails both benefits and risks. The benefits of health care to society provide the justification for exposure of patients to risks associated with education in clinical medicine. Although the benefits generally accrue to society at large, the burdens fall primarily on individual patients, especially the economically disadvantaged. These burdens are inherent in situations in which patients interact with students, for example, during medical history taking, physical examinations, and diagnostic and surgical procedures.

Physicians must learn new skills and techniques in a manner consistent with the ethical obligations to benefit the patient, to do no harm, and to respect a patient's right to make informed decisions about health matters. These obligations must not be unjustifiably subordinated to the need and desire to learn new skills. In consideration of society's interest in the education of physicians, all patients should be considered "teaching patients." Race or socioeconomic status should not be the basis for selection of patients for teaching.

Although patients are given the opportunity to consent to or refuse treatment by students, the obligations of the profession, the institution, and patients should be made more uniform and explicit. Professional obligations include disclosure of the risks and benefits inherent in the teaching setting and provision of adequate supervision at all levels of training. The patient should be encouraged to participate in the teaching process to contribute her fair share to the development of a new generation of health care providers. A situation may arise in which a patient refuses, for whatever reason, to have a student involved in her health care. Such refusals should initiate discussion and counseling. Patient choice, however, must be handled with compassion and respect.

Some procedures, such as pelvic examinations, require specific consent (3). If any pelvic examination planned for an anesthetized woman undergoing surgery offers her no personal benefit and is performed solely for teaching purposes, it should be performed only with her specific informed consent, obtained when she has full decision-making capacity.

Participation by anesthetized women in teaching exercises may be less common today than in the past. Alternatives to this training method exist that do not raise the challenges of securing informed consent. Today, many medical schools employ surrogates for patients to teach students how to perform pelvic examinations. These surrogates are variously referred to as gynecology teaching associates, professional patients, patient surrogates, standardized patients, or patient simulators. It is acknowledged, however, that in women preparing for surgery, the administration of anesthesia results in increased relaxation of the pelvic muscles, which may be beneficial in some educational contexts. Improvements in technology continue to allow for increased training in the virtual setting for residents and medical students. Specifically, technology has allowed surgical training using laparoscopic and hysteroscopic surgery simulation and has improved resident education in these areas.

Finally, students as well as residents must hold in confidence any information about patients learned in the context of a professional relationship. They should discuss specific patient care matters only in appropriate settings, such as teaching conferences or patient care rounds. Conversations in public places, such as hospital corridors or elevators, involving comments about patients, their families, or the care they are receiving are inappropriate (4). Furthermore, as medical records are increasingly kept in electronic form, it is important to ensure patient privacy and security of information in accordance with the Health Insurance Portability and Accountability Act of 1996 (HIPAA) regulations.

Ethical Responsibilities of Teachers to Students

The relationship between teacher and student in medical education inevitably involves the problem of imbalance of power and the risk of exploitation of a student for the benefit of the teacher (1). The teacher–student relationship exists at multiple levels among faculty members, medical students, attending physicians, fellows, and residents. Complex as it may be, there is a fundamental ethical responsibility at all levels for the teacher to impart wisdom, experience, and skill for the benefit of the student, without expectation of personal service by or reward from the student. Because so much of medicine is learned in a preceptor–student relationship, great care must be taken that the teacher does not exploit the student. An example is the teacher who expects a student to spend time that is out of proportion to the educational value involved on a research project, but gives little or no credit for such a contribution. In this regard, the behavior of teachers toward students is a powerful example of ethics in action. Students are likely to model their behavior on that of their teachers (5).

The relationship of a teacher to a student involves not only trust and confidence but also power and dependency. It is the role of the teacher to foster independence in the student while nurturing the student in the learning process. This is a complex relationship, the boundaries of which can become obscured in the intense setting of a clinical preceptorship (6). For example, the long hours spent by teachers and students in relatively arduous and isolated circumstances may foster amorous relationships. Regardless of the situation, the power imbalance makes a romantic or sexual relationship between a teacher and student ethically suspect. Amorous relationships between teachers and their current students are never appropriate.

Students should not be placed in situations where they must provide care or perform procedures for which they are not qualified and not adequately supervised. To do otherwise violates an ethical responsibility to the student as well as to the patient. A healthy relationship between teachers and students allows students to request assistance or supervision without fear of humiliation or retribution. Teaching should take place in an atmosphere that fosters mutual respect.

Conduct and Responsibilities of Students Toward Their Teachers

Students have the obligation to be honest, conscientious, and respectful in their relationships with their teachers. They should act in ways that preserve the dignity of patients and do not undermine relationships between patients and their physicians. It is the student's responsibility to ask for assistance and supervision when it is needed. Unfettered communication between student and teacher is essential in fostering an atmosphere that will allow, even encourage, students to request help. When such communication does not occur, both education and patient care suffer.

Inherent in the teacher–student relationship is the vulnerability of the student in dealing with perceived unethical behavior or incompetent conduct of a teacher. If a student observes such behavior or conduct, the matter should be brought to the attention of the appropriate institutional authority. Mechanisms that are nonjudgmental and without penalty should be clearly defined to encourage an open dialogue about these observed behaviors.

Institutional Responsibilities

Institutions have ethical obligations to students, patients, and teachers, including an obligation to provide a work environment that enhances professional competence. The health care system often has exploited students at all levels of education. Students may be viewed as a source of cheap labor, especially in busy hospitals on a teaching service. Students often provide long hours of service, and the resultant neglect of the student's physical and mental health must be balanced against the provision of an effective clinical experience. Lack of sleep, heavy workloads, and increasing amounts of responsibility without commensurate levels of authority are sources of great stress in

medical education, especially during residency (7–9). The potentially negative impact of such an educational experience on the student's developing attitude toward patients and the profession should be considered. The obligation to provide a good work environment includes ensuring that students and residents work reasonable hours, establishing a balance between medical education and responsibility for patient care, providing adequate ancillary and administrative support services, and, in the case of residents, providing reasonable salaries and benefits (10).

A source of substantial stress for some students and residents is the conflict between family responsibilities and the demands of medical education (11). For many students, sleep deprivation caused by long work hours results in fatigue, irritability, and anxiety. The inability to relate with consideration or affection to a partner or spouse or to participate in any effective way with child care or other domestic responsibilities may seriously impair family relationships. Also, with increasing numbers of women in education programs, special attention must be given to the parallel demands of pregnancy (including the postpartum period) and career goals. Providing ample time for all residents to sustain family relationships without adversely affecting the educational experience or imposing excessive burdens on colleagues is a daunting task, but one that must be confronted. Shared positions and more flexible timelines for completing educational requirements can be helpful in solving such problems.

Institutions should maintain a well-established reporting and review process for investigating allegations of unethical behavior or incompetent conduct. Access to such a process can facilitate fair and just relationships between students and teachers in these precarious situations.

As concerns about cost containment increase, education could become a low priority. The process of medical education may reduce the efficiency of patient care and increase costs. It is the responsibility of all physicians and institutions involved in the education of health care professionals to ensure that cost-reduction efforts do not diminish the opportunities for education in clinical medicine. Institutions have an ethical responsibility to develop policy statements and guidelines for the inclusion of students in patient care in ways that ensure sound medical education and high-quality medical care.

Summary

The effective education of students, residents, interns, fellows, and other professionals is essential if the health care professions are to benefit society. The power and authority inherent in relationships between students and patients as well as between teachers and students are important ethical concerns. Power and authority should be exercised responsibly to protect patients' dignity and welfare and to enhance the educational process.

Respect for autonomy requires that patients be informed about the extent to which students at any level are involved in their care and that patients' concerns be addressed. Students should provide only that level of care for which they are qualified and adequately supervised. Working conditions and work schedules should reflect sensitivity for student welfare in its broadest terms. This attention to ethics will promote attitudes conducive to the compassionate and skilled treatment of patients. This emphasis also should serve as a model for the next generation of teachers.

References

1. Brody H. Medical ethics and power. In: The healer's power. New Haven (CT): Yale University Press; 1992. p. 12–25.

2. Ludmerer KM. The rise of the teaching hospital. In: Learning to heal: the development of American medical education. New York (NY): Basic Books Inc; 1985. p. 219–33.

3. Ubel PA, Jepson C, Silver-Isenstadt A. Don't ask, don't tell: a change in medical student attitudes after obstetrics/gynecology clerkships toward seeking consent for pelvic examinations on an anesthetized patient. Am J Obstet Gynecol 2003;188:575–9.

4. Ubel PA, Zell MM, Miller DJ, Fischer GS, Peters-Stefani D, Arnold RM. Elevator talk: observational study of inappropriate comments in a public space. Am J Med 1995;99: 190–4.

5. Bosk CL. Forgive and remember: managing medical failure. 2nd ed. Chicago (IL): University of Chicago Press; 2003.

6. Plaut SM. Boundary issues in teacher-student relationships. J Sex Marital Ther 1993;19:210–9.

7. Butterfield PS. The stress of residency. A review of the literature. Arch Intern Med 1988;148:1428–35.

8. Stress and impairment during residency training: strategies for reduction, identification, and management. Resident Services Committee, Association of Program Directors in Internal Medicine. Ann Intern Med 1988;109:154–61.

9. McCall TB. The impact of long working hours on resident physicians. N Engl J Med 1988;318:775–8.

10. Asch DA, Parker RM. The Libby Zion case. One step forward or two steps backward? N Engl J Med 1988;318: 771–5.

11. Green MJ. What (if anything) is wrong with residency overwork? Ann Intern Med 1995;123:512–7.

Bibliography

American Medical Association. Medical student involvement in patient care. In: Code of medical ethics: current opinions with annotations. Chicago (IL): AMA; 2006. p. 234.

American Medical Association. Resident physicians' involvement in patient care. In: Code of medical ethics: current opinions with annotations. Chicago (IL): AMA; 2006. p. 235.

Professional responsibilities in obstetric–gynecologic education. ACOG Committee Opinion No. 358. American College of Obstetricians and Gynecologists. Obstet Gynecol 2007;109:239–42.

ISSN 1074-861X

ACOG COMMITTEE OPINION

Number 359 • January 2007

Commercial Enterprises in Medical Practice*

Committee on Ethics

Reaffirmed 2008

ABSTRACT: Increasing numbers of physicians sell and promote both medical and nonmedical products as part of their practices. Physicians always have rendered advice and treatment for a fee, and this practice is appropriate. It is unethical under most circumstances, however, for physicians to sell or promote medical or nonmedical products or services for their financial benefit. The following activities are considered unethical: sale of prescription drugs to be used at home, sale or promotion of nonprescription medicine, sale or promotion of presumptively therapeutic agents that generally are not accepted as part of standard medical practice, sale or promotion of non–health-related items, recruitment of patients or other health care professionals into multilevel marketing arrangements, and sale or promotion of any product in whose sale the physician has a significant financial interest. It is ethical and appropriate, however, to sell products to patients as follows: sale of devices or drugs that require professional administration in the office setting; sale of therapeutic agents, when no other facilities can provide them at reasonable convenience and at reasonable cost; sale of products that clearly are external to the patient–physician relationship, when such a sale would be considered appropriate in an external relationship; and sale of low-cost products for the benefit of community organizations. A rationale is provided for both the prohibited activities and exceptions.

The American College of Obstetricians and Gynecologists
Women's Health Care Physicians

Increasing financial pressures and the pervasiveness of entrepreneurial values in our society have led to an increase in the scope of activities for which physicians have sought reimbursement. As a result, increasing numbers of physicians sell and promote both medical and nonmedical products as part of their practices.

Physicians always have rendered advice and treatment for a fee, and this practice is appropriate; however, the sale and promotion of products for financial benefit is qualitatively different from these traditional activities. It is unethical under most circumstances for physicians to sell or promote medical or nonmedical products or services for their financial benefit. In this Committee Opinion, the American College of Obste-

tricians and Gynecologists' Committee on Ethics examines the following issues:

- The scope of the inappropriate activities
- The reasons for their unacceptability
- The limited circumstances under which they may be acceptable

Recommendations

Sale or promotion of products by physicians to their patients is unethical, with some exceptions, in either clinical sites or other places. This is true whether the sale is conducted in person, by telephone, or by written solicitation. The following activities are considered unethical, subject to the exceptions outlined later in the discussion:

- Sale of prescription drugs to be used at home (For example, some commercial drug repackagers prepare these medi-

*Update of "Commercial Enterprises in Medical Practice," in *Ethics in Obstetrics and Gynecology*, Second Edition, 2004.

cines in standard doses and provide them to physicians, who then resell them to patients [1].)

- Sale or promotion of nonprescription medicine
- Sale or promotion of presumptively therapeutic agents that generally are not accepted as part of standard medical practice
- Sale or promotion of non–health-related items, such as household supplies (2)
- Recruitment of patients or other health care professionals into multilevel marketing arrangements (These are enterprises in which individuals recruit other individuals to sell products and receive a commission on sales by their recruits. These recruits, in turn, can recruit a third generation of marketers, whose commissions are shared with participants of earlier generations.)
- Sale or promotion of any product in whose sale the physician has a significant financial interest, even if the sale would otherwise be appropriate (Such financial interest includes, among other things, sale for a direct profit or sale of a product when the physician holds a substantial equity interest in the product's manufacturer or wholesaler [3].)

Exceptions

It is ethical and appropriate for physicians to sell products to patients in the following circumstances:

- Sale of devices or drugs that require professional administration in the office setting (Under these circumstances, the charge for the product should not exceed the costs, which may include both the direct cost of the product and the overhead incurred in obtaining, storing, and administering it.)
- Sale of therapeutic agents, when no other facilities can provide them at reasonable convenience and at reasonable cost (This circumstance might occur in a thinly populated area or in a locality in which certain forms of reproductive control are unpopular. If physicians sell such products, the price charged should not exceed the cost of the product, including both direct and overhead costs.)
- Sale of products that clearly are external to the patient–physician relationship, when such a sale ordinarily would be considered appropriate in the context of an external relationship (An example of such a transaction is a brokered house sale at a fair market price.)
- Sale of low-cost products for the benefit of community organizations (An example of such a product is Girl Scout cookies. These products must be sold without pressure, and the physician must not derive a profit from such sales.)

Rationale

There have been arguments given to support the sale in physicians' offices of drugs and other products related to the treatment of patients (1). One is convenience—a busy patient need not go to a pharmacy. Another, although not borne out by empirical studies, is that increasing the number of dispensers of drugs reduces the cost of drugs (1). Finally, it is possible that adherence to treatment is improved if the patient purchases the drug from the physician.

Under most circumstances, however, the sale of products by physicians violates several generally accepted principles of medical ethics. First, and most important, the practice of physician sales to patients creates a potential conflict of interest with the physician's fiduciary responsibility to provide "a right and good healing action taken in the interests of a particular patient" (4). This principle of fidelity is defined as the obligation of physicians to put the interests of patients above their own.

Physicians must not engage in actions that violate or call into question their fiduciary relationship with patients. The term *conflict of interest* refers to circumstances in which this commitment to the fiduciary relationship is compromised. Conflict of interest contains two elements: "1) an individual with an obligation, fiduciary or otherwise, and 2) the presence of conflicting interests that may undermine fulfillment of the obligation" (5).

The American Medical Association and other professional societies have long opposed practices that result in conflicts of interest. The association's Council on Ethical and Judicial Affairs (CEJA) states that "as professionals, physicians are expected to devote their energy, attention and loyalty fully to the service of their patients" (6). Many statements issued by CEJA and other American Medical Association bodies have condemned various practices resulting in conflict of interest. These related improper commercial practices include fee splitting (payment by or to a physician solely for the referral of a patient), physician self-referral, physician ownership of pharmacies, and selling medical products (7). They have condemned physician ownership of stock in laboratories that pay physicians in proportion to the amount of work they refer and have disapproved of rebates from optical or medical instrumentation companies (5, 8).

Referral by physicians to health care facilities, such as laboratories, in which they do not engage in professional activities but in which they have a financial interest is called *self-referral*. This practice is analogous to product sales in that physicians are deriving a profit from goods (eg, laboratory tests or drugs) that they did not produce. Both of these practices create a clear conflict of interest because referring physicians accept money from vendors to direct patients to use their products or services instead of alternative products or services (including the option of no treatment at all). The conflict, therefore, is between the financial advantage that accrues from physicians' sales or referrals and physicians' obligation to arrange the best possible ancillary and consultative services for their patients. For example, CEJA states that self-referral to outside facilities is ethical only "if there is a demonstrated need in the community for the facility and alternative financing is not available" (6). In these circumstances, the practice is considered ethical only if referring physicians meet certain requirements designed to ensure that they receive no more financial consideration than would an ordinary investor and that certain safeguards are taken to avoid exploitation of patients.

Several other cardinal principles are violated by the practice of sales by physicians. The principle of truthfulness is violated if a conflict of interest related to the sale exists and is not communicated to the patient.

The principle of nonmaleficence is violated when there is a potential for injury to patients, which could occur in several ways. Physicians may be tempted to sell to patients items that they do not need. Even if its use is appropriate, the product in question may not be the most suitable for given patients. For example, joint ventures in radiation oncology (ie, those in which referring physicians had a financial interest) were found to provide more frequent and more intense use of radiation therapy than did freestanding facilities, without increased benefit (9).

Another principle that may be violated by this practice is that of respect for autonomy. A patient might prefer comparing various alternatives when purchasing products. If the product is offered by the physician on whom she depends for advice and treatment, she could feel constrained to accept the physician's product. She may feel coercion to comply with treatments with which she does not agree. If the product is not health related, patients might feel constrained to purchase goods they do not want (8).

Finally, this practice violates the principles of professionalism and professional solidarity by weakening public trust in the profession. As CEJA has stated, "The medical profession's ability to preserve autonomy and the nature of the physician–patient relationship during periods of transformation have succeeded in large part due to the profession's lack of tolerance for 'commercialism' in medicine" (6).

Conclusion

The sale or promotion of products by physicians to their patients rarely is ethical. Exceptions have been described in this Committee Opinion. Practitioners of obstetrics and gynecology should not engage in commercial arrangements that result in real, apparent, or potential conflicts of interest.

References

1. James DN. Selling drugs in the physician's office: a problem of medical ethics. Bus Prof Ethics J 1992;11:73–88.

2. Rice B. What's a doctor doing selling Amway? Med Econ 1997;74(13):79–82, 85–6, 88.

3. Responsibility of applicants for promoting objectivity in research for which PHS funding is sought. 42 C.F.R. §50 Subpart F (2005).

4. Pellegrino ED, Thomasma DC. A philosophical reconstruction of medical morality. In: A philosophical basis of medical practice: toward a philosophy and ethic of the healing professions. New York (NY): Oxford University Press; 1981. p. 192–220.

5. Rodwin MA. The organized American medical profession's response to financial conflicts of interest: 1890–1992. Milbank Q 1992;70:703–41.

6. Conflicts of interest. Physician ownership of medical facilities. Council on Ethical and Judicial Affairs, American Medical Association. JAMA 1992;267:2366–9.

7. American Medical Association. Sale of health-related products from physicians' offices. In: Code of medical ethics of the American Medical Association: current opinions with annotations. Chicago (IL): AMA; 2006. p. 225–6.

8. Sale of non-health-related goods from physicians' offices. Council on Ethical and Judicial Affairs, American Medical Association. JAMA 1998;280:563.

9. Mitchell JM, Sunshine JH. Consequences of physicians' ownership of health care facilities—joint ventures in radiation therapy. N Engl J Med 1992;327:1497–501.

Commercial enterprises in medical practice. ACOG Committee Opinion No. 359. American College of Obstetricians and Gynecologists. Obstet Gynecol 2007;109:243–5.

ISSN 1074-861X

ACOG COMMITTEE OPINION

Number 360 • February 2007

Sex Selection*

Committee on Ethics

Reaffirmed 2008

ABSTRACT: In this Committee Opinion, the American College of Obstetricians and Gynecologists' Committee on Ethics presents various ethical considerations and arguments relevant to both prefertilization and postfertilization techniques for sex selection. The principal medical indication for sex selection is known or suspected risk of sex-linked genetic disorders. Other reasons sex selection is requested are personal, social, or cultural in nature. The Committee on Ethics supports the practice of offering patients procedures for the purpose of preventing serious sex-linked genetic diseases. However, the committee opposes meeting requests for sex selection for personal and family reasons, including family balancing, because of the concern that such requests may ultimately support sexist practices. Because a patient is entitled to obtain personal medical information, including information about the sex of her fetus, it will sometimes be impossible for health care professionals to avoid unwitting participation in sex selection.

The American College of Obstetricians and Gynecologists

Women's Health Care Physicians

Sex selection is the practice of using medical techniques to choose the sex of offspring. Patients may request sex selection for a number of reasons. Medical indications include the prevention of sex-linked genetic disorders. In addition, there are a variety of social, economic, cultural, and personal reasons for selecting the sex of children. In cultures in which males are more highly valued than females, sex selection has been practiced to ensure that offspring will be male. A couple who has one or more children of one sex may request sex selection for "family balancing," that is, to have a child of the other sex.

Currently, reliable techniques for selecting sex are limited to postfertilization methods. Postfertilization methods include techniques used during pregnancy as well as techniques used in assisted reproduction before the transfer of embryos created in vitro. Attention also has focused on preconception techniques, particularly flow cytometry separation of X-bearing and Y-bearing spermatozoa before intrauterine insemination or in vitro fertilization (IVF).

*Update of "Sex Selection," in *Ethics in Obstetrics and Gynecology*, Second Edition, 2004.

In this Committee Opinion, the American College of Obstetricians and Gynecologists' Committee on Ethics presents various ethical considerations and arguments relevant to both prefertilization and postfertilization techniques for sex selection. It also provides recommendations for health care professionals who may be asked to participate in sex selection.

Indications

The principal medical indication for sex selection is known or suspected risk of sex-linked genetic disorders. For example, 50% of males born to women who carry the gene for hemophilia will have this condition. By identifying the sex of the preimplantation embryo or fetus, a woman can learn whether or not the 50% risk of hemophilia applies, and she can receive appropriate prenatal counseling. To ensure that surviving offspring will not have this condition, some women at risk for transmitting hemophilia choose to abort male fetuses or choose not to transfer male embryos. Where the marker or gene for a sex-linked genetic disorder is known, selection on the basis of direct identification of affected embryos or fetuses, rather than on the basis of sex, is possible. Direct identification has the advantage of avoiding the possibility of aborting an unaffected fetus or deciding not to transfer unaffected embryos. Despite the increased ability to identify genes and markers, in certain situations, sex determination is the only current method of identifying embryos or fetuses potentially affected with sex-linked disorders.

Inevitably, identification of sex occurs whenever karyotyping is performed. When medical indications for genetic karyotyping do not require information about sex chromosomes, the prospective parent(s) may elect not to be told the sex of the fetus.

Other reasons sex selection is requested are personal, social, or cultural in nature. For example, the prospective parent(s) may prefer that an only or first-born child be of a certain sex or may desire a balance of sexes in the completed family.

Methods

A variety of techniques are available for sex identification and selection. These include techniques used before fertilization, after fertilization but before embryo transfer and, most frequently, after implantation.

Prefertilization

Techniques for sex selection before fertilization include timing sexual intercourse and using various methods for separating X-bearing and Y-bearing sperm (1–5). No current technique for prefertilization sex selection has been shown to be reliable. Recent attention, however, has focused on flow cytometry separation of X-bearing and Y-bearing spermatozoa as a method of enriching sperm populations for insemination. This technique allows heavier X-bearing sperm to be separated; therefore, selection of females alone may be achieved with increased probability (3). More research is needed to determine whether any of these techniques can be endorsed in terms of reliability or safety.

Postfertilization and Pretransfer

Assisted reproductive technologies, such as IVF, make possible biopsy of one or more cells from a developing embryo at the cleavage or blastocyst stage (6). Fluorescence in situ hybridization can be used for analysis of chromosomes and sex selection. Embryos of the undesired sex can be discarded or frozen.

Postimplantation

After implantation of a fertilized egg, karyotyping of fetal cells will provide information about fetal sex. This presents patients with the option of terminating pregnancies for the purpose of sex selection.

Ethical Positions of Other Organizations

Many organizations have issued statements concerning the ethics of health care provider participation in sex selection. The ethics committee of the American Society for Reproductive Medicine maintains that the use of preconception sex selection by preimplantation genetic diagnosis for nonmedical reasons is ethically problematic and "should be discouraged" (7). However, it issued a statement in 2001 that if prefertilization techniques, particularly flow cytometry for sperm sorting, were demonstrated to be safe and efficacious, these techniques would be ethically permissible for family balancing (8). Because a preimplantation genetic diagnosis is physically more burdensome and necessarily involves the destruction and discarding of embryos, it was not considered similarly permissible for family balancing (9).

The Programme of Action adopted by the United Nations International Conference on Population and Development opposed the use of sex selection techniques for any nonmedical reason (10). The United Nations urges governments of all nations "to take necessary measures to prevent . . . prenatal sex selection."

The International Federation of Gynecology and Obstetrics rejects sex selection when it is used as a tool for sex discrimination. It supports preconception sex selection when it is used to avoid sex-linked genetic disorders (11).

The United Kingdom's Human Fertilisation and Embryology Authority Code of Practice on preimplantation genetic diagnosis states that "centres may not use any information derived from tests on an embryo, or any material removed from it or from the gametes that produced it, to select embryos of a particular sex for nonmedical reasons" (12).

Discussion

Medical Testing Not Expressly for the Purpose of Sex Selection

Health care providers may participate unknowingly in sex selection when information about the sex of a fetus results from a medical procedure performed for some other purpose. For example, when a procedure is done to rule out medical disorders in the fetus, the sex of a fetus may become known and may be used for sex selection without the health care provider's knowledge.

The American College of Obstetricians and Gynecologists' Committee on Ethics maintains that when a medical procedure is done for a purpose other than obtaining information about the sex of a fetus but will reveal the fetus's sex, this information should not be withheld from the pregnant woman who requests it. This is because this information legally and ethically belongs to the patient. As a consequence, it might be difficult for health care providers to avoid the possibility of unwittingly participating in sex selection. To minimize the possibility that they will unknowingly participate in sex selection, physicians should foster open communication with patients aimed at clarifying patients' goals. Although health care providers may not ethically withhold medical information from patients who request it, they are not obligated to perform an abortion, or other medical procedure, to select fetal sex.

Medical Testing Expressly for the Purpose of Sex Selection

With regard to medical procedures performed for the express purpose of selecting the sex of a fetus, the following four potential ethical positions are outlined to facilitate discussion:

Position 1: Never participate in sex selection. Health care providers may never choose to perform medical procedures with the intended purpose of sex selection.

Position 2: Participate in sex selection when medically indicated. Health care providers may choose to perform medical procedures with the intended purpose of preventing sex-linked genetic disorders.

Position 3: Participate in sex selection for medical indications and for the purpose of family balancing. Health care providers may choose to perform medical procedures for sex selection when the patient has at least one child and desires a child of the other sex.

Position 4: Participate in sex selection whenever requested. Health care providers may choose to perform medical procedures for the purpose of sex selection whenever the patient requests such procedures.

The committee shares the concern expressed by the United Nations and the International Federation of Gynecology and Obstetrics that sex selection can be motivated by and reinforce the devaluation of women. The committee supports the ethical principle of equality between the sexes.

The committee rejects, as too restrictive, the position that sex selection techniques are always unethical (position 1). The committee supports, as ethically permissible, the practice of sex selection to prevent serious sex-linked genetic disorders (position 2). However, the increasing availability of testing for specific gene mutations is likely to make selection based on sex alone unnecessary in many of these cases. For example, it supports offering patients using assisted reproductive techniques the option of preimplantation genetic diagnosis for identification of male sex chromosomes if patients are at risk for transmitting Duchenne's muscular dystrophy. This position is consistent with the stance of equality between the sexes because it does not imply that the sex of a child itself makes that child more or less valuable.

Some argue that sex selection techniques can be ethically justified when used to achieve a "balance" in a family in which all current children are the same sex and a child of the opposite sex is desired (position 3). To achieve this goal, couples may request 1) sperm sorting by flow cytometry to enhance the probability of achieving a pregnancy of a particular sex, although these techniques are considered experimental; 2) transferring only embryos of one sex in assisted reproduction after embryo biopsy and preimplantation genetic diagnosis; 3) reducing, on the basis of sex, the number of fetuses in a multifetal pregnancy; or 4) aborting fetuses that are not of the desired sex. In these situations, individual parents may consistently judge sex selection to be an important personal or family goal and, at the same time, reject the idea that children of one sex are inherently more valuable than children of another sex.

Although this stance is, in principle, consistent with the principle of equality between the sexes, it nonetheless raises ethical concerns. First, it often is impossible to ascertain patients' true motives for requesting sex selection procedures. For example, patients who want to abort female fetuses because they value male offspring more than female offspring would be unlikely to espouse such beliefs openly if they thought this would lead physicians to deny their requests. Second, even when sex selection is requested for nonsexist reasons, the very idea of preferring a child of a particular sex may be interpreted as condoning sexist values and, hence, create a climate in which sex discrimination can more easily flourish. Even preconception techniques of sex selection may encourage such a climate. The use of flow cytometry is experimental, and preliminary reports indicate that achievement of a female fetus is not guaranteed. Misconception about the accuracy of this evolving technology coupled with a strong preference for a child of a particular sex may lead couples to terminate a pregnancy of the "undesired" sex.

The committee concludes that use of sex selection techniques for family balancing violates the norm of equality between the sexes; moreover, this ethical objection arises regardless of the timing of selection (ie, preconception or postconception) or the stage of development of the embryo or fetus.

The committee rejects the position that sex selection should be performed on demand (position 4) because this position may reflect and encourage sex discrimination. In most societies where sex selection is widely practiced, families prefer male offspring. Although this preference sometimes has an economic rationale, such as the financial support or physical labor male offspring traditionally provide or the financial liability associated with female offspring, it also reflects the belief that males are inherently more valuable than females. Where systematic preferences for a particular sex dominate (13, 14), there is a need to address underlying inequalities between the sexes.

Summary

The committee has sought to assist physicians and other health care providers facing requests from patients for sex selection by calling attention to relevant ethical considerations, affirming the value of equality between the sexes, and emphasizing that individual health care providers are never ethically required to participate in sex selection. The committee accepts, as ethically permissible, the practice of sex selection to prevent sex-linked genetic disorders. The committee opposes meeting other requests for sex selection, such as the belief that offspring of a certain sex are inherently more valuable. The committee opposes meeting requests for sex selection for personal and family reasons, including family balancing, because of the concern that such requests may ultimately support sexist practices.

Medical techniques intended for other purposes have the potential for being used by patients for sex selection without the health care provider's knowledge or consent. Because a patient is entitled to obtain personal medical information, including information about the sex of her fetus, it will sometimes be impossible for health care professionals to avoid unwitting participation in sex selection.

References

1. Gray RH. Natural family planning and sex selection: fact or fiction? Am J Obstet Gynecol 1991;165:1982–4.

2. Check JH, Kastoff D. A prospective study to evaluate the efficacy of modified swim-up preparation for male sex selection. Hum Reprod 1993;8:211–4.

3. Fugger EF, Black SH, Keyvanfar K, Schulman JD. Births of normal daughters after MicroSort sperm separation and intrauterine insemination, in-vitro fertilization, or intracytoplasmic sperm injection. Hum Reprod 1998;13:2367–70.

4. Michelmann HW, Gratz G, Hinney B. X-Y sperm selection: fact or fiction? Hum Reprod Genet Ethics 2000; 6:32–8.

5. Schulman JD, Karabinus DS. Scientific aspects of preconception gender selection. Reprod Biomed Online 2005;10 (suppl 1):111–5.

6. Sermon K, Van Steirteghem A, Liebaers I. Preimplantation genetic diagnosis. Lancet 2004;363:1633–41.

7. Sex selection and preimplantation genetic diagnosis. Ethics Committee of the American Society for Reproductive Medicine. Fertil Steril 2004;82 (suppl):S245–8.

8. Preconception gender selection for nonmedical reasons. Ethics Committee of the American Society for Reproductive Medicine. Fertil Steril 2004;82(suppl):S232–5.

9. Robertson J. Sex selection: final word from the ASRM Ethics Committee on the use of PGD [news]. Hastings Cent Rep 2002;32(2):6.

10. United Nations. Gender equality, equity and empowerment of women. In: Population and development: programme of action adopted at the International Conference on Population and Development, Cairo, 5–13 September 1994. New York (NY): UN; 1995. p. 17–21.

11. Ethical guidelines on sex selection for non-medical purposes. FIGO Committee for the Ethical Aspects of Human Reproduction and Women's Health. Int J Gynaecol Obstet 2006;92:329–30.

12. Human Fertilisation and Embryology Authority. Code of practice. 6th ed. London: HFEA; 2003.

13. Jha P, Kumar R, Vasa P, Dhingra N, Thiruchelvam D, Moinedin R. Low female [corrected]-to-male [corrected] sex ratio of children born in India: national survey of 1.1 million households [published erratum appears in Lancet 2006;367:1730]. Lancet 2006;367:211–8.

14. Hesketh T, Lu L, Xing ZW. The effect of China's one-child family policy after 25 years. N Engl J Med 2005;353:1171–6.

Sex selection. ACOG Committee Opinion No. 360. American College of Obstetricians and Gynecologists. Obstet Gynecol 2007;109:475–8.

ISSN 1074-861X

ACOG COMMITTEE OPINION

Number 362 • March 2007

Medical Futility*

Committee on Ethics

Reaffirmed 2008

ABSTRACT: The construct of medical futility has been used to justify a physician's unilateral refusal to provide treatment requested or demanded by a patient or the family of a patient. It is important that physicians and their institutions develop a process for dealing with conflict surrounding the construct of medical futility. Prospective policies on medical futility are preferable to unilateral decision making by individual physicians. When there is disagreement, patient and family values regarding treatment options and the default position of maintaining life ordinarily should take priority.

The American College of Obstetricians and Gynecologists

Women's Health Care Physicians

A proliferation in medical technology has dramatically increased the number of diagnostic and therapeutic options available in patient care. Health care costs also have increased as a byproduct of this technologic expansion. Simultaneously, medical ethics has undergone a rapid metamorphosis from a beneficence-focused ethic to one in which autonomy dominates: that is, from an ethic in which the physician attempted to determine what was in the patient's best interest and then acted on behalf of the patient to an ethic in which alternatives are presented to the patient and the patient makes the ultimate decision. Thus, both the physician and the patient may face the daunting task of selecting from among myriad highly technologic and expensive health care choices.

These choices, among other factors, have created situations in which patients or families have sometimes demanded care that physicians may deem futile, or incapable of producing a desired result. The construct of medical futility has been used to justify a physician's unilateral refusal to provide treatment requested or demanded by a patient or the family of a patient. Such decisions may be based on the physician's perception of the inability of treatment to achieve a physiologic goal, to attain other

*Update of "Medical Futility," in *Ethics in Obstetrics and Gynecology*, Second Edition, 2004.

goals of the patient or family, or to achieve a reasonable quality of life.

Although there is general agreement with the notion that physicians are not obligated to provide futile care (1), there is vigorous debate and little agreement on the definition of futile care, the appropriate determinants of each component of the definition, and on whose values should determine the definition of futility. Proposed definitions of medical futility include one or more of the following elements:

- The patient has a lethal diagnosis or prognosis of imminent death.

- Evidence exists that the suggested therapy cannot achieve its physiologic goal.

- Evidence exists that the suggested therapy will not or cannot achieve the patient's or family's stated goals.

- Evidence exists that the suggested therapy will not or cannot extend the patient's life span.

- Evidence exists that the suggested therapy will not or cannot enhance the patient's quality of life.

The following questions need to be addressed concerning each of the previously identified elements:

- What is imminent death? Is it death that is expected within hours or days, or would it include death expected at any time up to 6 months or longer?

- At what point can a therapy be defined as unable to achieve a physiologic goal? Is futility reached when the goal could never be achieved or when the goal could be achieved in less than 1% of the cases, in 5% of the cases, or within some other established limit?
- What defines when a therapy can no longer achieve the patient's or family's goals, and who should decide this?
- What constitutes an enhanced life span—1 day, 1 week, 1 month?
- How is quality of life measured, and who should determine what constitutes a satisfactory quality of life for a given patient?

What these definitions have in common is an assessment of whether a particular therapy will be effective (ie, that it might alter the course of the disease or symptoms of the patient), whether it offers any benefit to the patient, and whether it adds to the burdens suffered by the patient (2). It is important to note that the concept of futility does not apply exclusively to situations in which a patient has a terminal illness, but can apply to any clinical situation in which a proposed treatment offers virtually no chance of achieving a desired result. For example, futility would be a sufficient reason to refuse in vitro fertilization treatments to a couple who wishes to use their own gametes when the female partner is older than 50 years and has a markedly elevated follicle-stimulating hormone level (3).

Disagreements will sometimes occur between stakeholders in the decision about whether a therapy will be considered futile or not. These disagreements may concern the definition of futility or whether the conditions to establish futility have been met. These differences frequently arise because one party places a different value on one possible outcome of the therapy than the other party.

For example, a patient may judge that even one more day of life is worth a therapeutic attempt or that living in a coma is more desirable than death, while a physician caring for that patient may feel differently. Physicians or society may be less willing to provide the requested care as they balance the use of resources and their individual or collective view of the potential for and degree of benefit. Patients may not include the use of resources in their equation at all but simply balance negative side effects and risks against the likelihood and degree of a beneficial outcome. Society may be more likely to accede to patient wishes when the use of resources is minimal than when it is significant, regardless of the likelihood of achieving physiologic goals, increasing life span, or achieving patient goals. Reasonableness and equity in the distribution of resources may play a role in determining whether societal and institutional values should prevail in contested decisions. When resource distribution is an issue, however, the values of the patient and the preservation of life ordinarily take priority and are ethical default positions.

Ultimately, these are differences of value, with individuals placing different values on the likelihood of a good outcome, different assessments of what would constitute an acceptable outcome, and different views about how much effort and expense can be justified in the pursuit of an unlikely outcome. Consensus is most likely in situations where the likelihood of achieving an outcome that anyone would consider valuable is very low. One suggestion has been that most physicians could agree that something was futile if it had not worked in the previous 100 similar cases (4).

Litigation also has generally resulted in courts supporting the views of patient or family in cases in which patient and caregiver disagree regarding withholding care, at least when withholding or withdrawing a medical treatment would likely result in the death of the patient (5–9). Commentators have observed that court decisions in favor of patient or family wishes appear to be based on one of the following factors:

- Medicine's inability to quantify the likelihood of futility with certainty
- The lack of a prospective and clearly stated process for determining medical futility
- The courts' current bias toward autonomy
- A desire to be consistent in upholding the patient's rights whether the patient is refusing or requesting treatment
- Recognition that withdrawal of life-sustaining care would likely result in the death of the patient

Need for a Medical Futility Policy

Inability to achieve a physiologic goal—strict physiologic futility—is an appropriate basis for a physician to refuse to provide requested therapeutic intervention. However, the ability to declare strict physiologic futility with certainty exists in only a limited number of clinical situations in which there are conflicts about whether to continue a therapy.

Other interpretations of medical futility are too subjective to form the basis for unilateral physician decisions. Therefore, in the absence of strict physiologic futility, the construct of medical futility should be applied only according to a prospective organizational policy that provides a process rather than a rule for resolving conflict.

The preferred approach for resolving all disputes about whether a particular therapy should be offered or continued should first be communication between the patient and the physician. This conversation should focus on reasonable goals of treatment, with emphasis on whether the therapy in question can, in fact, achieve the therapeutic goals set by the patient and physician (10). The discussion should focus on specific clinical problems, goals, and therapies rather than on whether the family wants "everything done," which represents a meaningless and misleading request or offer. If resolution cannot be achieved through provider–patient communication, an ethics consultant or ethics committee should be involved to assist in the resolution of the dispute.

A policy can be valuable in those situations in which the probability of reaching a physiologic goal or the potential for enhancement of life's duration or quality is remote and there is disparity in the subjective interpretations by patient (family), physician, institution, and society regarding the cost (economic, physical, emotional) versus benefit ratio. A medical futility policy should emphasize communication and negotiation rather than unilateral physician decision making.

Designing a Medical Futility Policy

A medical futility policy should be built on the following foundations:

- It should be designed to enhance discussion among the parties.
- The responsible physician should be encouraged to involve all appropriate members of the treatment team (eg, house staff, nurses, and social workers) to help reach an agreement between the patient (or surrogate), the physician, and other members of the health care team.
- It should be designed to seek input from other individuals or groups with expertise in the relevant medical discipline or medical ethics (including clergy, attorneys, and ethics committees).
- It should include some formal institutional mechanism for conflict resolution, such as ethics consultation or an ethics committee that ensures a thorough review of the institution and provides a fair hearing for all stakeholders.
- It should allow a patient to select another caregiver whose view is more consistent with her own and facilitate transfer of care, without prejudice, by the original physician.
- If transfer of care is arranged, all ongoing, life-sustaining treatment and interventions must be continued while the transfer is awaited.
- If no conciliation of views or patient transfer occurs, or if no other caregiver or facility is willing to provide the desired treatment, the caregivers are not required to provide care that they regard as medically futile.
- There must be some process of appeal as the situation comes closer to action by the physician or facility that is still contested by the patient or family.
- When caregivers refuse to provide a futile intervention or abrogate a certain aspect of treatment on the basis of its futility, their obligation to provide care is undiminished. Providing comfort care and palliative care and maximizing quality of life at the end of life remain fundamental obligations of the physician responsible for a patient's care.

- The policy should require documentation that includes the following information:
  —Probable diagnoses
  —Probable prognosis
  —Physician-recommended alternatives
  —Patient-desired pathway
  —Process of decision making that was followed, including notes from relevant meetings

An example of a policy that provides a process for decision making in medical futility is outlined in the American Medical Association Council on Ethical and Judicial Affairs report, "Medical Futility in End-of-Life Care" (1) (see http://jama.ama-assn.org/cgi/reprint/281/10/937 for a decision tree). Other institutions have published their policies (11), and at least one state (Texas) provides a law that outlines the conditions under which a treatment team or institution can unilaterally withhold or withdraw a therapy that has been deemed futile. These conditions include 1) notifying the patient or the person responsible for the health care decisions of the patient in writing about the hospital's policy on ethics consultation, 2) providing the patient or responsible person with 48-hour notice of consultation and inviting him or her to participate in the consultation, and 3) providing the patient or responsible person with a written report of the ethics review process.

Under Texas law, when the ethics consultation process fails to resolve the dispute, the hospital must work with the patient or responsible person to try to arrange transfer to an institution or physician that will provide the disputed therapy. If no provider can be found after 10 days, the therapy can be unilaterally withheld or withdrawn. A judicial appeal for an extension beyond 10 days can be made by the patient or responsible person, but it can be granted only if the judge determines there is a reasonable likelihood of finding a provider willing to provide the disputed treatment. When these conditions are met, the treatment team and institution receive immunity from civil or criminal prosecution (12).

Summary

It is difficult to define medical futility prospectively and objectively. Nonetheless, as technology continues to advance and use more resources, it is important that physicians and their institutions develop a process for dealing with conflict surrounding the construct of medical futility.

Prospective policies on medical futility are preferable to unilateral decision making by individual physicians. Such a medical futility policy should provide a systematic process for dealing with disagreements, for ensuring that all parties have received a fair hearing, and for reaching a fair resolution, as outlined previously. When there is disagreement, patient and family values regarding treatment options and the default position of maintaining life ordinarily should take priority. However, situations may occur in which claims of reasonableness and equity in the distribution of resources are so powerful that the views of caregivers, the institution, and society will prevail.

References

1. Medical futility in end-of-life care: report of the Council on Ethical and Judicial Affairs. JAMA 1999;281:937–41.

2. Pellegrino ED. Decisions at the end of life—the abuse of the concept of futility. Pract Bioethics 2005;1(3):3–6.

3. Fertility treatment when the prognosis is very poor or futile. Ethics Committee of the American Society for Reproductive Medicine. Fertil Steril 2004;82:806–10.

4. Schneiderman LJ, Jecker NS, Jonsen AR. Medical futility: its meaning and ethical implications. Ann Intern Med 1990;112:949–54.

5. Capron AM. In re Helga Wanglie. Hastings Cent Rep 1991; 21(5):26–8.

6. Capron AM. Abandoning a waning life. Hastings Cent Rep 1995;25(4):24–6.

7. Angell M. The case of Helga Wanglie. A new kind of "right to die" case [editorial]. N Engl J Med 1991;325:511–2.

8. Miles SH. Informed demand for "non-beneficial" medical treatment. N Engl J Med 1991;325:512–5.

9. Diekema DS. What is left of futility? The convergence of anencephaly and the Emergency Medical Treatment and Active Labor Act. Arch Pediatr Adolesc Med 1995; 149:1156–9.

10. Berg JW, Appelbaum PS, Lidz CW, Parker LS. The role of informed consent in medical decision making. In: Informed consent: legal theory and clinical practice. 2nd ed. New York (NY): Oxford University Press; 2001. p. 167–87.

11. Singer PA, Barker G, Bowman KW, Harrison C, Kernerman P, Kopelow J, et al. Hospital policy on appropriate use of life-sustaining treatment. University of Toronto Joint Centre for Bioethics/Critical Care Medicine Program Task Force. Crit Care Med 2001;29:187–91.

12. Advance Directives Act. Tex. Health and Safety. §166 (1999). Available at: www.capitol.state.tx.us/statutes/docs/HS/content/htm/hs.002.00.000166.00.htm. Retrieved July 28, 2006.

Medical futility. ACOG Committee Opinion No. 362. American College of Obstetricians and Gynecologists. Obstet Gynecol 2007;109:791–4.

ISSN 1074-861X

ACOG COMMITTEE OPINION

Number 363 • April 2007

Patient Testing: Ethical Issues in Selection and Counseling*

Committee on Ethics

ABSTRACT: Recommendations to patients about testing should be based on current medical knowledge, a concern for the patient's best interests, and mutual consultation. In addition to establishing a diagnosis, testing provides opportunities to educate, inform, and advise. The ethical principles of respect for autonomy (patient choice) and beneficence (concern for the patient's best interests) should guide the testing, counseling, and reporting process. Clear and ample communication fosters trust, facilitates access to services, and improves the quality of medical care.

The American College of Obstetricians and Gynecologists

Women's Health Care Physicians

In the practice of medicine, clinical evaluation is enhanced by a broad range of tests. Recommendations to patients about testing should be based on current medical knowledge, a concern for the patient's best interests, and mutual consultation. Patient testing embodies many scientific and human ideals. From an ethical perspective, the most important principles involve a trusting patient–physician relationship emphasizing beneficence (the benefits the patient may derive from testing) and respect for autonomy (an appreciation that patients make choices about their medical care). Issues of nonmaleficence (using tests when the consequences of the test are uncertain) and justice (applying tests to low-risk groups) also may be important (1).

Rapid technologic development and the need to consider legal and sociocultural factors as well as medical knowledge have increased the complexity of the decision-making process. The physician often is in the position of ordering tests—for human immunodeficiency virus (HIV) or genetic markers, for example—that may, unlike a urinalysis or a hemogram, have a profound effect on the patient, her partner, her fam-

ily, and society in general. This new level of complexity requires the specification of both medical and ethical guidelines for decisions about patient testing. This Committee Opinion provides ethical guidance for decisions about ordering tests, counseling patients, and reporting results.

Ordering Tests

- *The physician and the patient have a shared responsibility.* The quality of medical care improves when there is clear communication and mutual understanding between physician and patient. It is the responsibility of the obstetrician–gynecologist to communicate effectively and to develop skills that promote a patient–physician relationship that is characterized by trust and honesty. Similarly, it is the responsibility of the patient to provide accurate information about her lifestyle, health habits, sexual practices, and religious and cultural beliefs when these factors may affect medical judgment. In decisions about testing, physicians should be guided by scientific knowledge. Care must be taken to avoid subjective assumptions based on bias that could affect the appropriateness of testing (2).

---

*Update of "Patient Testing," in *Ethics in Obstetrics and Gynecology*, Second Edition, 2004.

- *Testing should be performed primarily for the benefit of the patient.* Testing at the request of third parties—partners, health care providers, members of the patient's extended family, employers, or health insurers—is justifiable only when the patient or her valid proxy understands the potential risks and benefits and gives consent (3). Examples of this type of testing include genetic tests to assist family members with reproductive decisions, HIV tests to fulfill conditions for the purchase of life insurance, and requests for patient testing after the occupational exposure of health care workers.

- *The decision to offer or to withhold a test should not be made solely on the basis of a physician's assumptions about the patient's expected response to test results (4).* Prejudgments about a patient's wishes regarding fetal abnormalities, for example, should not preclude her being offered prenatal testing. The patient should join with the physician in deciding the amount of diagnostic information that is appropriate for making intelligent choices about preventive care and treatment options. The physician is not, however, ethically obligated to perform every test a patient requests, particularly if disease prevalence and risk factors are low, generating a high false-positive risk.

- *The patient must be informed prospectively about policies regarding use of information and legal requirements.* The patient must be told what will be communicated, to whom, and the potential implications of reporting the information. If, for example, a patient is concerned about posting HIV test results in the medical record and who may have access to the results, she may choose instead to use an anonymous testing procedure available through another laboratory. In some situations, reporting of results is mandated by law. Physicians should be familiar with the laws regarding mandatory testing and reporting requirements in their own jurisdictions.

- *The physician and patient should discuss concerns about cost containment and reimbursement.* The mutual goal of physician and patient should be to avoid both undertesting and overtesting. Contemporary focus on the economics of health care has created worries for both physician and patient about access to care, limitations to testing, appropriateness of use, and the impact of financial constraints on quality of care. Testing done with low probability of improving patient diagnosis or testing solely for the sake of professional liability concerns should be avoided. Open communication about cost concerns and perceived benefit is the best way to alleviate suspicion and to promote trust.

Pretest and Posttest Counseling

- *Testing that may have multiple medical or psychosocial consequences requires specific counseling.* The extent of counseling beneficial to each patient will vary depending on the individual and on the implications inherent in the potential test results. With simple tests like urinalysis, it is sufficient to provide information about the nature and purpose of the test and how the results will guide management. Tests that may have multiple medical or psychosocial ramifications require comprehensive explanation of the process, the goals, and the implications (4). Counseling can be appropriate for genetic testing and maternal toxicology assays, for example, because of the potential for psychologic, social, and economic effects. Tests with low positive predictive value, such as cervical cytology and mammography, can generate the need for additional and more extensive testing. Testing for HIV or inherited breast cancer mutations may limit future insurance coverage.

- *In some cases, the potential benefits—including societal benefits—of certain tests may lead some to recommend alternative schemes for counseling and consent in order to maximize the rate of testing.* The U.S. Centers for Disease Control and Prevention, ACOG, and the American Academy of Pediatrics have endorsed an "opt-out" protocol with patient notification for prenatal HIV testing (5–7). The use of patient notification provides women the opportunity to decline testing but eliminates the requirement to obtain specific informed consent.

- *Autonomy of the individual in shared decision making should always be respected.* It is essential in the informed consent process that subsequent election of the patient to forgo a recommended intervention (informed refusal) be carefully documented in the patient's medical record along with the patient's reason for refusal. Both pretest and posttest counseling facilitate women's access to appropriate health care. Pretest counseling includes both medical considerations and issues such as the availability of emotional support while waiting for test results. Posttest counseling offers an opportunity to provide access to resource networks and community-based services.

- *Referral may be needed for comprehensive counseling.* If time constraints or lack of technical expertise make it difficult to offer comprehensive counseling in a particular practice, appropriate options include either 1) referral to a specialized center for both counseling and testing, or 2) referral for counseling only, with return to the original physician for testing and medical follow-up.

Confidentiality and the Reporting of Test Results

• *Information ordinarily may not be revealed without the patient's express consent.* Physicians have an obligation to be familiar with federal privacy protection legislation (Health Insurance Portability and Accountability Act) (8). Guidance is provided here for the ethical duty to maintain confidentiality. Maintaining confidentiality is intrinsic to respect for patient autonomy and permits the free exchange of information that is relevant to medical decision making. Situations may arise, however, in which a physician has competing obligations: protecting the patient's confidentiality or disclosing test results to prevent harm to a third party. In these situations, every avenue of communication should be explored first in discussions with the patient about rights and responsibilities. Consultation with an institutional ethics committee or a medical ethics specialist may be helpful in weighing benefits and harms of disclosure. Legal advice may be prudent.

• *A violation of confidentiality may be ethically justified as a last resort.* A violation of confidentiality may be justifiable only when legally required or when all of the following conditions have been met: 1) there is a high probability of harm to a third party, 2) the potential harm is a serious one, 3) the information communicated can be used to prevent harm, and 4) greater good will result from breaking confidentiality than from maintaining it. Case law has not yet been developed to address the grey area where, on rare occasions, legal obligations to protect patient confidentiality and ethical and professional obligations to act for the benefit of the patient may conflict.

Conclusion

In addition to establishing a diagnosis, testing provides opportunities to educate, inform, and advise. The ethical principles of respect for autonomy (patient choice) and beneficence (concern for the patient's best interests) should guide the testing, counseling, and reporting process. Clear and ample communication fosters trust, facilitates access to services, and improves the quality of medical care.

References

1. Beauchamp TL, Childress JF. Priniciples of biomedical ethics. 5th ed. New York (NY): Oxford University Press; 2001.

2. Malm HM. Medical screening and the value of early detection. When unwarranted faith leads to unethical recommendations. Hastings Cent Rep 1999;29:26–37.

3. Offit K, Groeger E, Turner S, Wadsworth EA, Weiser MA. The "duty to warn" a patient's family members about hereditary disease risks. JAMA 2004;292:1469–73.

4. McGowan R. Beyond the disorder: one parent's reflection on genetic counselling. J Med Ethics 1999;25:195–9.

5. Prenatal and perinatal human immunodeficiency virus testing: expanded recommendations. ACOG Committee Opinion No. 304. American College of Obstetricians and Gynecologists. Obstet Gynecol 2004;104:1119–24.

6. Revised recommendations for HIV screening of pregnant women. Centers for Disease Control and Prevention. MMWR Recomm Rep 2001;50(RR-19):63–85; quiz CE1-19a2–CE6-19a2.

7. American Academy of Pediatrics, American College of Obstetricians and Gynecologists. Joint statement on human immunodeficiency virus screening. ACOG Statement of Policy 75. Elk Grove Village (IL): AAP; 2005; Washington, DC: ACOG; 2006.

8. American College of Obstetricians and Gynecologists. HIPAA privacy manual. 2nd ed. Washington, DC: ACOG; 2003.

Patient testing: ethical issues in selection and counseling. ACOG Committee Opinion No. 363. American College of Obstetricians and Gynecologists. Obstet Gynecol 2007;109:1021–3.

ISSN 1074-861X

ACOG COMMITTEE OPINION

Number 364 • May 2007

Patents, Medicine, and the Interests of Patients*

Committees on Ethics and Genetics

This document reflects emerging scientific advances as of the date issued and is subject to change. The information should not be construed as dictating an exclusive course of treatment or procedure to be followed.

ABSTRACT: Many basic scientists and clinicians support the right to obtain and enforce patents on drugs, diagnostic tests, medical devices, and most recently, genes. Although those who develop useful drugs, diagnostic and screening tests, and medical technologies have the right to expect a fair return for their efforts and risks, current interpretations of patent law have the potential to impede rather than promote scientific and medical advances. Policies regarding the patenting of scientific inventions, discoveries, and improvements must balance the need for the open exchange and use of information with the need to make the pursuit of such knowledge financially rewarding.

New technologies and the translation of research discoveries into clinical medicine are essential for improvements in patient care. The increasing commercialization of medical discoveries, however, may hamper the dissemination of new knowledge and the ability of physicians and patients to benefit from applications of this knowledge. Many basic scientists and clinicians support the right to obtain and enforce patents on drugs, diagnostic tests, medical devices, and most recently, genes. Some primarily are concerned with recovering the costs they incur in developing new treatments and technologies. Others see patents in medicine as a legitimate means, within a society based on the principle of free enterprise, of protecting and enhancing intellectual capital.

Such patent protections may be regarded as necessary incentives for the development of new tests and treatments. Also, they may limit the ability of clinicians, patients, and researchers to obtain the right to use these discoveries commercially under reasonable conditions and at an affordable price. Furthermore, the issue of gene patenting

poses unique challenges to knowledge development and academic collaboration because a gene sequence, unlike previous technical advances, is both a tool for pursuing scientific knowledge and the basis for any diagnostic or therapeutic application.

Patent Protections

The U.S. Patent and Trademark Office (PTO) is guided by federal statutes, regulations, and case law in granting patents. Patent protection is intended to promote research and discovery and to act as a stimulus to progress in science and the useful arts. The PTO evaluates an application for a U.S. patent to determine whether the claimed invention satisfies the following three conditions: the invention is a 1) "new" and 2) "useful" discovery or improvement that is 3) "not obvious" to individuals with ordinary skill in the art (1, 2). In evaluating patent applications, the PTO also assesses whether the specification adequately describes the invention and enables the skilled artisan to make and use it. A patent is granted for an invention that meets the three conditions and other requirements, such as being patentable subject matter. For example, "products of nature" can be patented if they are in an isolated form that does not occur in nature.

The American College of Obstetricians and Gynecologists
Women's Health Care Physicians

---

*Update of "Patents, Medicine, and the Interests of Patients" in *Ethics in Obstetrics and Gynecology*, Second Edition, 2004.

Patents that may affect the practice of medicine fall into four categories: 1) patents on medical and surgical procedures, 2) patents on surgical or diagnostic instruments, 3) patents on drugs, and 4) patents on genes and gene-based diagnostic or predictive tests. All of these types of patents raise ethical issues and may create conflicts of interest for physicians who contribute to the development of new products through research. The commercial potential of medical discoveries may motivate physicians to increase their own incomes in ways that may jeopardize the care of patients. Academic and research physicians may be offered incentives by their institutions to maximize the institution's extramural revenues through patent arrangements that restrict use by other researchers and, thus, act as barriers to further research discoveries.

Patenting Medical and Surgical Procedures

Historically, physicians have taught and shared medical information without regarding this knowledge as trade secrets to be protected from others. Physicians have a fundamental obligation to provide advice to their patients about the most appropriate care, without being influenced by any profit they might gain through associated commercial ventures. Open communication of information gained from research and experience with medical and surgical procedures is essential if safety and efficacy are to be validated or refuted by colleagues. It is through further scientific work by one's peers that diagnostic methodologies and medical procedures are either validated, refined, and improved or discarded as ineffective or unhelpful.

Some corporate or individual business arrangements—including the patenting and licensing of medical and surgical procedures—can be adverse to the welfare of patients. These arrangements present barriers to the availability of the protected procedures to other physicians and patients. Moreover, they may inhibit new research that might otherwise be stimulated by open access to information about the procedures. Investigational use of patented procedures is permitted under the "experimental use doctrine," which allows a patented invention to be used in a manner that does not interfere with the economic interests of the patent holder (ie, used with no commercial intentions).

For these reasons, the enforceability of patents covering medical and surgical procedures has been challenged, both ethically and legally. The American Medical Association asserts that it is unethical for physicians "to seek, secure or enforce patents on medical procedures" because such practices may limit the availability of new procedures to patients (3). In the 1996 case *Pallin v Singer*, Dr. Pallin was prohibited from enforcing his patent claims on a particular type of incision used in cataract surgery (4). As a result of this case, Congress enacted a 1996 statute making patents of medical or surgical procedures unenforceable (5). In the United States, medical and sur-

gical procedures are still patentable, but patent claims are not enforceable against a medical practitioner unless the practitioner uses a patented pharmaceutical, medical device, or biotechnology process. Thus, the U.S. legal system provides some support for the traditional ethic of physicians to share their knowledge and the use of advances in medical and surgical procedures. Other countries view the patentability of medical procedures differently than the United States. For instance, the European Union and Great Britain consider medical procedures to be nonpatentable subject matter.

Patenting Surgical and Diagnostic Instruments

The U.S. patent system also permits medical and surgical devices to be patented, including surgical and diagnostic instruments. The U.S. patent protection permits the patent holder to exclude other individuals or entities from making, using, or selling the patented invention in the United States for a period of 20 years, thus providing market exclusivity to the patent holder. Both ethically and legally, physicians may obtain patents on surgical or diagnostic instruments that they have invented (6). However, out of concern for the welfare of patients, the patent holder should make the instrument available at a fair and reasonable cost.

Patenting Drugs

The granting of patents to pharmaceutical companies for drugs that they have developed may appear to be relatively uncontroversial. Drug makers have successfully argued the need for patent protection to recoup the cost of their investment in drug research and to gain a profit before the makers of generic equivalent drugs are permitted to enter the market.

However, some techniques used by pharmaceutical companies to extend the terms of their patents and their products' market exclusivities have recently come under criticism. For example, companies have paid manufacturers of generic drugs to drop a legal challenge to a patent or to postpone the manufacture of a generic equivalent, they have developed minimally altered formulations or dosages that become eligible for new patents, and they have lobbied Congress for statutory and legislative patent extensions on highly profitable drugs. These techniques may allow the patent holder to continue to charge prices that are far higher than would be the case in a competitive market and to extend the government-sanctioned market exclusivity long beyond when the original patent term would have expired. As a result, the cost to consumers or patients may be inflated beyond providing a reasonable return on research investments and may, in fact, prevent some patients from using drugs that would be beneficial to them. As patients bear an increasing share of the cost of their prescribed drugs, the issue of drug pricing and extended market exclusivities should be of concern to physicians. Cost may influence patient compliance with physician recommendations.

The Patenting of Genes

Patent and Trademark Office Guidance

The PTO maintains that genes and gene sequences are patentable subject matter under existing U.S. federal statutes and case law. Since 1980, more than 20,000 patents on genes or other gene-related molecules have been granted, but this total includes gene patents for all organisms, not only humans. More than 25,000 applications for patents on genes or related molecules are pending (7).

Because of continuing controversy over the granting of patents on genes and gene sequences, the PTO has attempted to clarify its standards for granting such patents in its final guidelines on the written description and utility requirements of patents. The guidelines were issued after consideration of public comments on interim guidelines, and they are pertinent to gene patents. The PTO guidelines confirm that an isolated and purified gene (a chemical entity modified from its natural state) is not a naturally occurring substance. Substances as they occur in nature in an unisolated form are not patentable.

Under U.S. patent law, the PTO regards a newly isolated gene or modified gene sequence to be a "composition of matter." This is subject matter that is eligible for a product patent as long as the product satisfies all the statutory conditions for a patent. These conditions require that the patent specification describe an invention that is a new discovery or improvement (novel), that is not obvious to those with ordinary skill in the art (inventive), and that has utility (is useful) (1, 2). Product patents may be enforced broadly against a variety of uses of the claimed product. For example, a product patent claiming an isolated gene sequence can be used to exclude others from using the sequence for commercial purposes (ie, both the isolated gene sequence and the methods of using it in tests and treatments).

If the gene sequence is not new, it may nonetheless be eligible for a use patent (ie, a patent having claims directed to the product's use). The enforcement of a use patent is narrower, being limited to the patented use. Although a use patent restricts the right to use a patented method using a product or composition, it does not restrict access to the product or composition itself.

A patent claiming an isolated gene covers the isolated gene but does not apply to the gene as it occurs in nature. Genes as they occur in the body are not patentable because they do not exist in an isolated and purified form. Therefore, individuals who possess such genes in their bodies would not infringe the patent.

In its final guidelines on the utility requirement for patentability, the PTO requires that the utility be "specific, substantial, and credible" (8). To satisfy this requirement, the inventor must disclose at least one way in which the purified gene, isolated from its natural state, may be used or applied, for example, for diagnostic or predictive genetic testing. However, if the applicant does not explicitly identify a specific utility for the isolated gene sequence, the guidelines permit the utility requirement to be satisfied if the examiner believes that an individual with ordinary skill in the art would recognize that the gene or sequence has a readily apparent "well-established utility." Some commentators have suggested that this well-established utility may be simply a comparison with a structurally analogous gene or sequence that is known to have utility.

In the view of some commentators, the PTO guidelines do not set a high enough standard for establishing the usefulness of a gene or gene sequence and, therefore, may deem a product useful and allow a patent to be issued covering a gene or gene sequence before the applicant is able to identify a specific practical application (9). Allowing patents on genes and sequences to be issued before their function and purpose are adequately identified could create barriers to other researchers pursuing such studies or could lessen the incentive for them to do so. Moreover, researchers warn against relying too heavily on structural analogues to predict utility because minor changes in a gene sequence "may produce profound changes in biological activity" (10).

Gene Patents and the Interests of Patients

Those who support the granting of broad patents believe that patent protection encourages rather than impedes research. It was the intent of Congress that the disclosure required to secure a patent and the limited exclusivity provided by the patent would stimulate progress in science and the useful arts. As the PTO notes, a patent application requires complete public disclosure of the invention, discovery, or improvement and, therefore, may promote dissemination of knowledge rather than secrecy. In the PTO's view, gene patents foster scientific progress because other inventors are encouraged to discover new uses beyond the one specified in the patent application (8). Inventors who develop new and nonobvious uses for a patented gene may patent these inventions, according to the PTO, thereby rewarding researchers who develop the genetic information to the endpoint of a useful method or product (11, 12).

Opponents of broad gene patenting fear that the welfare of the patient, the traditional role of the physician, and the public trust are compromised by gene patents. According to opponents of gene patenting, the patenting of genes can impinge on the interests of patients in at least four ways:

1. By retarding the transmission of knowledge (possible if researchers choose to delay the announcement or the publication of their findings until after a patent application is filed)

2. By inhibiting other researchers from pursuing further investigation on the patented product (developing a subsequent invention often is difficult, complicated, or unprofitable because of the need to coordinate licensing with the original patent holder)

3. By establishing a monopoly on all diagnostic and predictive tests based on a patented gene (such action would limit the ability of practitioners and researchers to improve genetic testing by adding new mutations, devising new testing techniques, and developing national quality assurance programs [13])

4. By infringing on the interests of groups of patients who have provided the original genetic material on which the discovery of a gene or sequence is based (they may feel that their concerns are disregarded because of restrictions on access to tests and treatments made possible by their contribution of biologic material)

European challenges to the patent on the breast cancer gene *BRCA1* illustrate problems that arise when a patent holder claims that a patent on a gene precludes other researchers or organizations from developing their own tests for gene mutations. French researchers, supported by the European parliament, argue that such a monopoly could impede or even prevent the development and use of cheaper and more effective tests for *BRCA1* mutations, such as tests that cover a broader range of mutations (14, 15).

Similarly, in the clinical setting, experience has shown that patent holders may in effect deprive patients and physicians of reasonable access (eg, to a genetic test) by placing significant hurdles to its use. These hurdles can include substantial royalties or licensing fees and restrictions on the licensing of clinics or on the number of tests allowed, such as the conditions placed on prenatal and carrier testing for some autosomal recessive diseases (16).

Responses to the problem of restricted access to patented genes have led to several proposed solutions. One proposed solution is to develop a system similar to the music licensing system, where gene patent holders would be required to grant nonexclusive licenses for a reasonable set fee (17). Another proposed solution is that genes and genetic sequences should not be granted composition-of-matter patents because the market exclusivity of their patents extends beyond the use identified by the patent applicant and covers uses of the substance that may be discovered later. Instead, a patent would be granted to an applicant who identifies a specific function of a gene, but the patent would cover only the use or utility identified, such as a particular genetic test. Then researchers who later discovered additional applications for the gene would be able to patent these new discoveries (18).

Response to the issue of access to genetic tests has led some patient advocacy groups to take a proactive stance at the time that patients provide tissue samples to researchers. To ensure that any genetic tests that result from their participation will be inexpensive and widely available, these groups are seeking patents held jointly by the patient group and the researchers (19). Therefore, rather than objecting to the patenting of genes and genetic tests, these patients are seeking to use the patent system to protect their own interests.

Recommendations

Practitioners and researchers need to be aware of public policies that may jeopardize their ability to advance medical knowledge and provide the best tests and treatments to patients. Although those who develop useful drugs, diagnostic and screening tests, and medical technologies have the right to expect a fair return for their efforts and risks, current interpretations of patent law have the potential to impede rather than promote scientific and medical advances. Because the purpose of the patent system is to promote the public welfare, practices that are inimical to the public good and overly protective of commercial monopolies should be altered (18).

Policies regarding the patenting of scientific inventions, discoveries, and improvements must balance the need for the open exchange and use of information with the need to make the pursuit of such knowledge financially rewarding. Therefore, the Committee on Ethics and the Committee on Genetics of the American College of Obstetricians and Gynecologists suggest the following recommendations regarding the patenting of medical and surgical procedures, medical devices, genes, DNA sequences, screening and diagnostic tests, and gene-based therapies:

1. Patents on medical or surgical procedures are ethically unacceptable, and some are legally unenforceable. Physicians may obtain patents on surgical and diagnostic instruments that they have developed. However, the patent holders should make these instruments available at a fair and reasonable cost for the benefit of patients.

2. Because a patent claiming a gene as a composition of matter enables a patent holder to control future applications of the patented gene or sequence, such patents should not be granted. A patent should be granted only for the specified use or application of the gene or sequence (a "use" patent), thus enabling others to develop additional applications (18). Because case law and the PTO interpret a gene as being a patentable chemical composition of matter, such a limitation would require congressional intervention. The Committee on Ethics and the Committee on Genetics support legislation that would make composition-of-matter patents on genes unenforceable.

3. If composition-of-matter patents on genes continue to be enforceable, such patents on genes with clinical applications should be subject to federal regulation and oversight to ensure reasonable availability of the genes and their products for research and clinical use. Such regulation should include requirements on licensing arrangements to ensure access for the public good, including both the advancement of knowl-

edge and the clinical care of patients. Specifically, licensing agreements should permit reasonable but not excessive royalties and should allow unlimited access to tests by qualified laboratories, precluding exclusionary arrangements and quotas on the number of tests that may be offered.

References

1. Patentability of inventions, 35 U.S.C. §101–103 (2004).

2. Application for patent, 35 U.S.C. §112 (2004).

3. American Medical Association. Patenting of medical procedures. In: Code of medical ethics of the American Medical Association: current opinions with annotations. 2006–2007 ed. Chicago (IL): AMA; 2006. p. 292–3.

4. *Pallin v Singer* 1995 U.S. Dist. LEXIS 20824, 36 U.S.P.Q.2d (BNA) 1050 (D.Vt. May 1 1995).

5. Remedies for infringement of patent and other actions, 35 U.S.C. §281–297 (2004).

6. American Medical Association. Patent for surgical or diagnostic instrument. In: Code of medical ethics of the American Medical Association: current opinions with annotations. 2006–2007 ed. Chicago (IL): AMA; 2006. p. 291–2.

7. Doll JJ. Talking gene patents. Sci Am 2001;285:28.

8. Utility examination guidelines. United States Patent and Trademark Office. Fed Regist 2001;66:1092–9.

9. United States Patent and Trademark Office. Public comments on the United States Patent and Trademark Office "revised interim utility examination guidelines." Alexandria (VA): USPTO; 2000. Available at: http://www.uspto.gov/web/offices/com/sol/comments/utilguide/index.html. Retrieved January 5, 2007.

10. Spiegel J. Comment 44. In: United States Patent and Trademark Office. Public comments on the United States Patent and Trademark Office "revised interim utility examination guidelines." Alexandria (VA): USPTO; 2000. Available at: http://www.uspto.gov/web/offices/com/sol/comments/utilguide/nih2.pdf. Retrieved January 5, 2007.

11. Doll JJ. The patenting of DNA. Science 1998;280:689–90.

12. Wheeler DL. Will DNA patents hinder research? Lawyers say not to worry. Chron High Educ 1999 July 16; 46:A19.

13. American College of Medical Genetics. Position statement on gene patents and accessibility of gene testing. Bethesda (MD):ACMG;1999. Available at http://genetics.faseb.org/genetics/acmg/pol-34.htm. Retrieved December 13, 2006.

14. Dorozynski A. France challenges patent for genetic screening of breast cancer. BMJ 2001;323:589.

15. Watson R. MEPs add their voice to protest at patent for breast cancer gene. BMJ 2001;323:888.

16. Marshall E. Genetic testing. Families sue hospital, scientist for control of Canavan gene. Science 2000;290:1062.

17. Heller MA, Eisenberg RS. Can patents deter innovation? The anticommons in biomedical research. Science 1998; 280:698–701.

18. Williamson AR. Gene patents: socially acceptable monopolies or an unnecessary hindrance to research? Trends Genet 2001;17:670–3.

19. Smaglik P. Tissue donors use their influence in deal over gene patent terms. Nature 2000;407:821.

Suggested Reading

U.S. Department of Energy Office of Science. Genetics and patenting. Washington, DC: USDOE; 2002. Available at: http://www.ornl.gov/hgmis/elsi/patents.html. Retrieved December 13, 2006.

United States Patent and Trademark Office. General information concerning patents. Alexandria (VA): USPTO; 2002. Available at: http://www.uspto.gov/web/offices/pac/doc/general/index.html. Retrieved December 13, 2006.

Patents, medicine, and the interests of patients. ACOG Committee Opinion No. 364. American College of Obstetricians and Gynecologists. Obstet Gynecol 2007;109:1249–53.

ISSN 1074-861X

ACOG COMMITTEE OPINION

Number 365 • May 2007

Seeking and Giving Consultation*

**Committee on
Ethics**

ABSTRACT: Consultations usually are sought when practitioners with primary clinical responsibility recognize conditions or situations that are beyond their level of expertise or available resources. One way to maximize prompt, effective consultation and collegial relationships is to have a formal consultation protocol. The level of consultation should be established by the referring practitioner and the consultant. The referring practitioner should request timely consultation, explain the consultation process to the patient, provide the consultant with pertinent information, and continue to coordinate overall care for the patient unless primary clinical responsibility is transferred. The consultant should provide timely consultation, communicate findings and recommendations to the referring practitioner, and discuss continuing care options with the referring practitioner.

Physicians have a long history of working together and with other health care professionals to provide efficient and comprehensive care for the patients they serve. Achieving these goals sometimes requires that physicians or other care providers seek consultation from or provide consultation to their colleagues (1). The basic principles of consultation for obstetrician–gynecologists are summarized in the "Code of Professional Ethics of the American College of Obstetricians and Gynecologists" as follows (2):

- "The obstetrician–gynecologist's relationships with other physicians, nurses, and health care professionals should reflect fairness, honesty, and integrity, sharing a mutual respect and concern for the patient."

- "The obstetrician–gynecologist should consult, refer, or cooperate with other physicians, health care professionals, and institutions to the extent necessary to serve the best interests of their patients."

Often, these relationships among clinicians lead to professional dialogue. In professional dialogue, clinicians share their

opinions and knowledge with the aim of improving their ability to provide the best care to their patients. Such dialogue may be part of a clinician's overall efforts to maintain current scientific and professional knowledge or may arise in response to the needs of a particular patient.

In professional dialogue, a second clinician is typically asked a simple question and he or she does not talk with or examine the patient. For example, questions might be asked regarding the significance of an irregular blood antibody or the follow-up interval for an abnormal cervical cytology result. The second clinician does not make an entry in the patient's medical record or charge a fee, and the first clinician should not attribute an opinion to the second clinician.

Professional dialogue does not constitute a formal consultation or establish a patient–consultant relationship. Sometimes, however, professional dialogue does lead to a formal request for consultation. If, for example, a physician is asked to provide an opinion regarding a patient's care and believes an examination of the patient or her medical record is necessary to answer the question appropriately, he or she should ask to see the patient for a formal consultation.

**The American College
of Obstetricians
and Gynecologists**

*Women's Health Care
Physicians*

---

*Update of "Seeking and Giving Consultation" in *Ethics in Obstetrics and Gynecology*, Second Edition, 2004.

Although consultation usually is requested in an efficient manner that expedites patient care, situations occur in which the relationship between practitioners or between institutions and practitioners results in an inefficient, less-than-collegial consultative process that may not be in the best interest of the patient. For example, a patient and a consultant may be put at serious disadvantage when consultation is requested late in the process of care or is not accompanied by sufficient background information or the reason for consultation is not clearly stated. Conversely, those seeking consultation may be denied assistance on arbitrary grounds.

This Committee Opinion outlines the purpose of consultation and referral, states the underlying ethical foundations that govern consultation and referral, and elaborates specifically the responsibilities of those who seek and those who provide consultation. The Committee Opinion is directed to physicians but it should be recognized that nonphysician practitioners also may be involved in consultation.

The Purpose of Consultation and Referral

Typically, a patient first seeks care from her primary caregiver, who should be aware that the patient's needs may go beyond his or her education, training, or experience (2–4). Various levels of consultation may be needed to make correct diagnoses, provide technical expertise, and recommend a course of action (see the box). Occasionally, consultation or referral may be indicated when a patient's request for care is in conflict with her primary caregiver's recommendations or preferences. Finally, a patient may seek consultation with another caregiver to obtain a second opinion or explore other options for care (5). In all of these types of consultation, the interests of the patient should remain paramount (3).

Ethical Foundations

Ethical principles require that the consultative process be guided by the following concepts (2, 6):

- The welfare of the patient should be central to the consultant–patient relationship (beneficence).
- The patient should be fully informed about the need for consultation and participate in the selection of the consultant (respect for autonomy).
- The patient should have access to adequate consultation regardless of her medical condition, social status, or financial situation (justice).
- Practitioners must disclose to patients any pertinent actual or potential conflict of interest that is involved in a consultation relationship, including financial incentives or penalties or restrictive guidelines (truth-telling).

In addition, both practitioners with primary clinical responsibility and consultants must respect the rights of

---

Definitions: Levels of Consultation

Consultation is the act of seeking assistance from another physician(s) or health care professional(s) for diagnostic studies, therapeutic interventions, or other services that may benefit the patient. There are several levels of consultation: single-visit consultations, continuing collaborative care, and transfer of primary clinical responsibility. Their descriptions are as follows:

- **A single-visit consultation** involves examination of the patient or the patient's medical record and performance of diagnostic tests or therapeutic procedures. The findings, procedures, and recommendations of the consultant are recorded in the patient's medical record or provided to the practitioner with the primary clinical responsibility for the patient in a written report or letter, and a fee may be charged. The subsequent care of the patient continues to be provided by the referring practitioner. Examples of such consultations are confirming the findings of a pelvic examination, performing a specific urodynamic procedure on a patient with urinary stress incontinence, and interpreting an electronic fetal monitoring tracing or imaging studies. In the latter two cases, the tracing or other output can be transmitted electronically, allowing for the performance of a single-visit consultation without personal contact between the patient and consultant.

- **Continuing collaborative care** describes a relationship in which the consultant provides ongoing care in conjunction with the referring practitioner. Thus, the consultant assumes at least partial responsibility for the patient's care. An example is a high-risk obstetric patient with a medical complication of pregnancy who is periodically assessed by the consultant, whereas the referring practitioner is responsible for the day-to-day management of the patient.

- **Transfer of primary clinical responsibility** to the consultant may be appropriate for the management of problems outside the scope of the referring practitioner's education, training, and experience or in cases in which the patient must be transferred to another facility. Examples are the transfer of care of a patient in preterm labor from a birth center to a consultant in a perinatal center or referral of a patient with ovarian cancer to a gynecologic oncologist. In many of these situations, patients will eventually return to the care of the referring practitioner when the problem for which the consultation was sought is resolved.

---

the patient and also the rights of their respective professional colleagues.

Responsibilities Associated With Consultation

Seeking Consultation and Requesting Referral

Consultations usually are sought when practitioners with primary clinical responsibility recognize conditions or situations that are beyond their level of expertise or available resources. Historically, these practitioners acted as independent agents who decided when consultation was appropriate, determined the level of consultation, and were free to choose particular consultants. More recently, as a result of recognition of the importance of respect for patient autonomy, practitioners now inform patients of the need for consultation and discuss options with them. The quality of the consultation often is improved by this collaborative relationship between practitioners and patients.

Today, this practitioner–patient partnership operates under new conditions that may affect the process of consultation. Health care guidelines and protocols used by certain types of managed care arrangements may limit the freedom of the practitioner to provide complete care or to request consultation (7). These guidelines may include instructions about specific situations or medical conditions in which consultation, second opinion, or referral is mandated (8). Examples include abnormal labor that may require operative delivery or chronic uterine bleeding that may require hysterectomy. Other guidelines may require that practitioners seek consultation when patients develop signs and symptoms of severe preeclampsia or if ovarian cancer is discovered. Such arrangements and guidelines may be designed to ensure a high level of care for patients by requiring that consultants be involved appropriately in certain clinical problems.

Conversely, practitioners may find themselves in situations that create disincentives to medically appropriate consultation or that mandate the use of a consultant panel that is not adequate to support appropriate patient care. The policies that lead to such situations involve potential conflicts of interest (9) and may have a negative effect on the patient's medical needs, thus limiting her autonomy and her right to informed choice. Under all conditions of practice—solo or group, fee for service, or managed care contract—consultation and referral should be carried out in the patient's best interest and obtained with the patient's consent after full disclosure of limitations and potential conflicts of interest.

It is in everyone's best interest—practitioners with primary clinical responsibility, consultants, patients, and health care plans—that the criteria for consultation be mutually agreed on in advance and stated clearly in writing. Financial incentives or penalties for consultation and referral that exist either overtly or covertly under many managed care contracts are sources of serious conflicts of interest. Practitioners must be free to inform patients of the best medical practice or options of care, even when the mandate of directed referrals under contracted care does not include these alternatives. Ethical responsibility for patients' best interests demands that practitioners disclose any proscriptions to serving as patients' advocates. Practitioners have a responsibility to provide patients with their best medical judgment and serve as advocates for patients if recommended care is denied. It then becomes the patients' responsibility to decide whether to abide by insurance plan restrictions, challenge them, or seek care outside the scope of coverage.

Giving Consultation and Accepting Referral

Physicians generally provide consultations or accept referred patients in the interest of providing excellent care for patients and promoting good relationships among colleagues. Open communication and established professional relationships facilitate effective consultation and referral. However, at times a consultant may be called on unexpectedly, inconveniently, and sometimes inappropriately to be involved in or to assume the care of a patient. In these situations, a physician is only ethically obligated to provide consultation or assume the care of the patient if there is a contractual agreement or a preexisting patient–physician relationship or if there is a severe medical emergency, in which there is no reasonably available alternative caregiver (10). Hospital or departmental guidelines for consultation and referral may prevent such confrontations.

Practical Recommendations

Providing optimal care demands a good working relationship with a number of other physicians and health care professionals. Consultation may be needed by the practitioner with primary clinical responsibility regardless of specialty designation or level of training. Ideally, the referring practitioner–consultant relationship has been established before the need for consultation or referral arises, and the referring practitioner–consultant relationship should be ongoing.

One way to maximize prompt, effective consultation and collegial relationships is to have a formal consultation protocol. This may be especially advantageous for family physicians who provide obstetric or gynecologic care and for collaborative practice between obstetrician–gynecologists and nurse practitioners, certified nurse–midwives, and other health care professionals. Such protocols create pathways that anticipate difficult or complex situations. The level of consultation should be established by a dialogue between the referring practitioner and the consultant that results in mutual agreement (see the box on the previous page).

Electronic means of communication, such as e-mail, may be used as long as the consultant and referring physician agree to use such media and have established systems to confirm receipt and transfer of reports to the medical chart. Electronic communication must be done in a manner that protects patient confidentiality.

Responsibilities of the Referring Practitioner

The responsibilities of the referring practitioner can be outlined as follows:

1. The referring practitioner should request consultation in a timely manner, whenever possible before an emergency arises. A good working relationship

between the referring practitioner and the consultant requires shared concern for the patient's needs and a commitment to timely and clear-cut communication.

2. The referring practitioner is responsible for preparing the patient with an explanation of the reasons for consultation, the steps involved, and the names of qualified consultants.

3. The referring practitioner should provide a summary of the history, results of the physical examination, laboratory findings, and any other information that may facilitate the consultant's evaluation and recommendations (11).

4. Whenever possible, the referring practitioner should document in the medical record the indications for the consultation and specific issues to be addressed by the consultant.

5. The referring practitioner should discuss the consultant's report with the patient and give his or her own recommendation based on all available data in order to serve the best interest of the patient.

6. A complex clinical situation may call for multiple consultations. Unless authority has been transferred elsewhere, the responsibility for the patient's care should rest with the referring practitioner (3). This practitioner should remain in charge of communication with the patient and coordinate the overall care on the basis of information derived from the consultants. This will ensure a coordinated effort that remains in the patient's best interest.

Responsibilities of the Consultant

The responsibilities of the consultant can be outlined as follows:

1. Consultants should recognize their individual boundaries of expertise and provide only those medically accepted services and technical procedures for which they are qualified by education, training, and experience.

2. When asked to provide consultation, the consultant should do so in a timely manner and without regard to the specialty designation or qualifications of the referring practitioner.

3. The consultant should effectively communicate findings, procedures performed, and recommendations to the referring practitioner at the earliest opportunity (12).

4. A summary of the consultation should be included in the medical record or sent in writing to the referring practitioner.

5. The extent to which the consultant will be involved in the ongoing care of the patient should be clearly established by mutual agreement of the consultant, the referring practitioner, and the patient. At times it

may be appropriate for the consultant to assume primary clinical responsibility for the patient. Even if this is only a temporary circumstance, the consultant should obtain the referring practitioner's cooperation and assent, whenever possible.

6. When the consultant does not have primary clinical responsibility for the patient, he or she should try to obtain concurrence for major procedures or additional consultants from the referring practitioner.

7. In all that is done, the consultant must respect the relationship between the patient and the referring practitioner, being careful not to diminish inappropriately the patient's confidence in her other caregivers (3).

8. The consultant should be cognizant of the referring practitioner's abilities, and the consultant and referring practitioner should discuss who can best provide the agreed-upon care. Reliance on the referring practitioner's abilities may increase convenience to the patient, limit transportation needs, and ultimately result in more cost-effective care. In other cases, however, it may not be possible for the consultant's recommendations to be addressed adequately by the referring practitioner.

9. If the consultant believes that the referring practitioner is not qualified to provide an appropriate level of continuing care, the consultant should recommend to the referring practitioner and, if necessary, to the patient that the referring practitioner transfer care of the patient.

References

1. American Medical Association. Referral of patients. In: Code of medical ethics of the American Medical Association: current opinions with annotations. 2006–2007 ed. Chicago (IL): AMA; 2006. p. 116–8.

2. American College of Obstetricians and Gynecologists. Code of professional ethics of the American College of Obstetricians and Gynecologists. Washington, DC: ACOG; 2004. Available at: http://www.acog.org/from_home/acogcode.pdf. Retrieved January 10, 2007.

3. Snyder L, Leffler C. Ethics manual: fifth edition. Ethics and Human Rights Committee, American College of Physicians. Ann Intern Med 2005;142:560–82.

4. American College of Obstetricians and Gynecologists. Physicians working with physicians. In: The assistant: information for improved risk management. Washington, DC: ACOG; 2001. p. 19–20.

5. American Medical Association. Second opinions. In: Code of medical ethics of the American Medical Association: current opinions with annotations. 2006–2007 ed. Chicago (IL): AMA; 2006. p. 198–9.

6. Beauchamp TL, Childress JF. Principles of biomedical ethics. 5th ed. New York (NY): Oxford University Press; 2001.

7. Wallach EE, Fox HE, Gordon T, Faden R. Symposium: managed care and ethics. Contemp Ob Gyn 1998;43:162–76.

8. Chervenak FA, McCullough LB, Chez RA. Responding to the ethical challenges posed by the business tools of managed care in the practice of obstetrics and gynecology. Am J Obstet Gynecol 1996;175:523–7.

9. Cain JM, Jonsen AR. Specialists and generalists in obstetrics and gynecology: conflicts of interest in referral and an ethical alternative. Womens Health Issues 1992;2:137–45.

10. American Medical Association. Free choice. In: Code of medical ethics of the American Medical Association: current opinions with annotations. 2006–2007 ed. Chicago (IL): AMA; 2006. p. 282–4.

11. Role of the obstetrician–gynecologist in the screening and diagnosis of breast masses. ACOG Committee Opinion No. 334. American College of Obstetricians and Gynecologists. Obstet Gynecol 2006;107:1213–4.

12. American Medical Association. Consultation. In: Code of medical ethics of the American Medical Association: current opinions with annotations. 2006–2007 ed. Chicago (IL): AMA; 2006. p. 198.

Seeking and giving consultation. ACOG Committee Opinion No. 365. American College of Obstetricians and Gynecologists. Obstet Gynecol 2007;109:1255–9.

ISSN 1074-861X

ACOG COMMITTEE OPINION

Number 368 • June 2007

Adoption*

Committee on Ethics

ABSTRACT: Obstetrician–gynecologists may find themselves at the center of adoption issues because of their expertise in the assessment and management of infertility, pregnancy, and childbirth. Physicians have a responsibility to provide information about adoption to all patients with unwanted pregnancies, to all patients with infertility concerns, and to same-sex partners seeking information on parenting. Unless physicians are truly expert in the field of adoption, they should guard against advocating for a particular action. Physicians should not serve as brokers in independent adoptions. When authorized by patients to fill out forms for adoption agencies, physicians should do so truthfully, with full disclosure to patients of what they intend to say.

Adoption is a commonly used alternative strategy for family building. Although adoption is not a medical event per se, obstetrician–gynecologists may find themselves at the center of adoption issues because of their expertise in the assessment and management of infertility, pregnancy, and childbirth. There are several specific roles that the obstetrician–gynecologist may be asked to assume regarding adoption. Physicians commonly provide information, advice, and counsel, and they refer birth parents and prospective adoptive parents to adoption agencies. They also may be asked to link or match pregnant women with families desiring adoption. Frequently, they are asked to provide information about prospective parents to adoption agencies. In each of these roles, it is important that obstetrician–gynecologists consider the rights, responsibilities, and safety of all concerned parties: the child, the birth parents, the prospective adoptive parents, and themselves.

Six principles have historically guided adoption practices (1):

1. Consent of the birth mother was a necessary precondition for adoption, whereas presumed waiver of consent by absent birth fathers has been routine.

2. The purpose of adoption was to serve the child's best interests by placement with suitable adoptive parents.

3. Adoption practices were based on the principle of gratuitous transfer, and financial transactions suggestive of purchase of a child were prohibited.

4. Relationships with adoptive parents were expected to substitute entirely for relationships with biologic parents.

5. Relinquishing birth mothers and adopting parents were assured that their confidentiality and anonymity would be protected.

6. Adoptive relationships were presumed to be permanent once they were finalized in court.

These principles currently are undergoing redefinition and reconsideration. Physicians should be aware of the following new trends in adoption practices:

1. There is increased emphasis on the rights of biologic fathers and reluctance to use a waiver process to release a child for adoption when the biologic father cannot be located.

2. Concepts of suitability of adoptive parents and the best interests of the child are undergoing reconsideration.

3. The present environment of competition for adoptive infants may lead to inducements in the form of subsidies for medical care and other support, making the gratuitous nature of adoption less clear and free of financial conflict.

The American College of Obstetricians and Gynecologists

Women's Health Care Physicians

---

*Update of "Adoption" in *Ethics in Obstetrics and Gynecology*, Second Edition, 2004.

4. Proponents of openness in adoption argue that adoption should include complementary relationships with birth parents. Even in a closed adoption, proponents argue that the adopted child and adoptive parents need to have access to relevant genetic and medical information about the biologic parents.

5. It is no longer possible to guarantee absolute confidentiality to either birth or adoptive parents. Many states have laws that give adopted individuals access to their birth records.

6. Adoption can no longer be considered to be permanent in every case because situations have arisen in which adoptive relationships were terminated by adoptive parents, biologic parents, or adopted children after a final adoption decree had been granted.

The resulting lack of clarity about both ethical issues and legal consequences may create a potentially hazardous situation for physicians. In the following sections, the different roles that the obstetrician–gynecologist may be asked to play in adoption are described. Ethical concerns are discussed, and safeguards are proposed.

Education

The physician's role in education is to ensure that adoption is introduced into the description of alternatives for women with unwanted pregnancies and for potential adoptive parents. Physicians have a responsibility to provide information about adoption to all patients with unwanted pregnancies, to all patients with infertility concerns, and to same-sex partners seeking information on parenting (2, 3). Fact sheets are available to support this educational role (4). Physicians have an obligation to present alternatives fairly, regardless of personal values and beliefs. They should not advocate for or against relinquishment or adoption. Nor should they avoid discussing these issues when they are appropriate to the patient's situation. This position is consistent with the right of adults to the information required to make fully informed decisions. It also is consistent with the ethical obligation to promote what is good for the patient. These obligations can be met, for some patients, by placing literature about adoption in the reception area, thereby validating adoption as a legitimate, respected choice. A lengthy counseling session, in which the risks and benefits of adoption are weighed against other alternatives, may be indicated for other patients.

Physicians may have both positive and negative personal biases about adoption for various reasons. For example, physicians who have chosen the adoption alternative as their own method of family building may present this option either positively or negatively, depending on their individual experiences. Physicians would do well to disclose their potential sources of bias and take special care to uphold the principle of respect for patient autonomy.

Physicians also should ensure that financial incentives do not bias the presentation of information about adoption. For example, physicians must be especially careful to offer information about adoption to patients with established infertility because gynecologists have the potential to benefit financially from the treatment of infertile patients, and these fees may cease with a decision to adopt rather than pursue further treatment.

Advice and Counseling

The physician's role in advising and counseling patients is to assist those for whom adoption may be appropriate in making a decision that is right for them. Patients often turn to their physicians and say, "Doctor, what do you think I should do?" Women experiencing unwanted pregnancy or infertility are vulnerable, facing confusing and painful situations. The physician is a caregiver, trained to solve problems and help patients feel better. The temptation to advocate for a specific position can be great. It may seem to the physician that the obvious solution for a young woman who is unemployed is to relinquish her child or for an infertile couple who are reasonable candidates for in vitro fertilization to pursue that option before considering adoption.

It is appropriate for physicians to give advice on medical matters. This is an essential part of the physician–patient relationship and an expert role for which physicians are trained. Patients count on the guidance of physicians for medical decisions. Adoption, however, is only tangentially a medical matter, and few physicians are expert in this field. Furthermore, for the physician, the particular encounter with an individual patient or couple, no matter how compelling, occurs only during a finite point in time. The patients will be living with the lifelong consequences of these decisions. Therefore, physicians who provide advice and counsel, unless they are truly expert in the field of adoption, should guard against advocating for a particular action. The best counsel will permit the involved parties to explore their options fully and make a decision that arises out of their own beliefs, values, needs, and circumstances.

Referrals

The physician's role in referrals is to identify appropriate resources. Physicians often may best fulfill their obligations to patients through referral to other professionals who have the appropriate skills and expertise to address the difficult issues raised by adoption. For example, referral to a mental health professional for short-term counseling provides an opportunity for both birth and prospective adoptive parents to explore their emotional reactions and the ways that different alternatives may affect their lives. Some patients may feel more comfortable having a discussion of this type with someone who is not involved with their ongoing medical care.

When an obstetrician–gynecologist makes a medical referral, there is an ethical obligation to investigate the skills and credentials of the consultant. The same responsibility for protecting the patient's best interests pertains to psychologic and social referral resources. As a starting point, there are many sources of information available to assist physicians in developing their own lists of referral alternatives (see "Resources" at the end of this Committee Opinion). In addition, local hospitals maintain referral rosters.

Screening

When authorized by patients, the physician's role in screening is to provide appropriate information to screening agencies regarding patients' qualifications as prospective parents for an adoptive child. Physicians often are asked by patients to fill out forms requesting information about their mental, psychologic, and medical suitability as prospective adoptive parents. Physicians are bound by ethical precepts to be truthful, to act in their patients' best interests, and to protect their patients' confidentiality. Adoption agencies, however, give precedence to the needs and interests of adoptive children.

Difficult situations may arise. A patient may request, for example, that a physician not reveal to the agency the extent of her chronic illness and its potential effect on her life expectancy. Although a physician may wish to advocate for a patient, there is an obligation to be truthful and to let patients know what can and cannot be said.

Many agency forms request the treating physician to certify that the individual or couple is fit to parent. If the physician of record believes that he or she does not have enough information to make a judgment, the agency may count that as evidence against the couple. The physician must be honest and speak accurately to the information that is available. The best approach is for the physician to disclose to the patient what will be written in the report, followed by frank discussion with the patient of the potential impact of the report.

Limits to the Physician's Role

Physicians should not serve as brokers in independent adoptions. If asked to do so, they should refer the patient to an appropriate agency or adoption resource. Among all the roles that physicians may be asked to play in adoption, that of a broker is perhaps the most hazardous because of ethical issues related to undue influence, competing obligations, and lack of expertise.

Although both birth parents and prospective adoptive parents generally view the adoption agreement as a binding promise, patients may find themselves unable or unwilling to fulfill that promise after delivery of the child. The pregnant woman who agreed to relinquish her child may have done so in good faith with the best knowledge available to her at that time. She may not know what that promise really means or if she can really do what she agreed to until she has given birth to this child, held it, and experienced the extent of loss. The couple who agreed to accept a child may regret that decision and feel unable to keep their part of the agreement if, for example, the child is born with serious medical problems. For these and similar reasons, no adoption agreement is legally binding before the birth of the child.

If a physician has acted as a broker and the adoption agreement falls through, he or she will be aware of the loss experienced by the other party, may feel responsible, and may be tempted to use the power of the patient–physician relationship to influence the patient to fulfill the original promise. The physician's ability to provide current or future medical care for this patient may be compromised by these events.

Brokering adoptions is properly the role of an independent authority or agency, which is in a position to protect the interests of all involved parties—the child, the birth parents, and the adoptive parents. For these reasons, many hospitals have bylaws prohibiting staff physicians from direct involvement as adoption brokers. Physicians should avoid matching prospective adoptive parents with women who have unwanted pregnancies and should instead refer patients to agencies or other adoption resources, when available. Physicians should receive only the usual compensation for medical and counseling services. Referral fees and other arrangements for financial gain beyond usual fees for clinical services are inappropriate.

When physicians also are prospective adoptive parents, there may be a temptation to adopt an infant from one of their own patients. This arrangement is unethical. It contravenes principles of fairness to other potential parents and takes advantage of patients' highly vulnerable situations.

Summary

The adoption field is evolving, and the issues are complex. Obstetrician–gynecologists can play helpful and effective roles in adoption as educators and advisers. Adoption should be presented fairly, along with other options, to all those who might benefit. Physicians can be excellent sources of information, can assist in weighing risks and benefits, and can provide emotional support. When authorized by patients to fill out forms for adoption agencies, physicians should do so truthfully, with full disclosure to patients of what they intend to say.

Physicians should involve themselves in counseling and screening roles with great care because potential exists for unintended misuse of the physician–patient relationship. Patient confidentiality, patient autonomy, and the principle of the patient's best interest may be compromised by subtle or blatant conflicts of interest. Physicians are advised to delegate to an independent authority all responsibility for matching pregnant women with prospective adoptive parents.

References

1. Hollinger JH. Adoption law. Future Child 1993;3:43–61.
2. Kaunitz AM, Grimes DA, Kaunitz KK. A physician's guide to adoption. JAMA 1987;258:3537–41.

3. American College of Obstetricians and Gynecologists. Special issues in women's health. Washington, DC: ACOG; 2005.

4. American Society for Reproductive Medicine. Patient's fact sheet: adoption. Birmingham (AL): ASRM; 2003. Available at: http://www.asrm.org/Patients/FactSheets/Adoption-Fact.pdf. Retrieved January 10, 2007.

Resources

Arcus D. Adoption. In: Strickland B, editor. The Gale encyclopedia of psychology. 2nd ed. Detroit (MI): Gale Group; 2001. p. 15–9.

Child Welfare Information Gateway (Children's Bureau/ACYF, 1250 Maryland Avenue, SW, Eighth Floor, Washington, DC 20024; telephone: (703) 385-7565 or (800) 394-3366; http://www.childwelfare.gov), a comprehensive resource on all aspects of adoption, is a service of the U.S. Department of Health and Human Services.

Perspectives Press (PO Box 90318, Indianapolis, IN 46290; telephone: (317) 872-3055; http://www.perspectivespress.com) concentrates on issues related to adoption.

Resolve (7910 Woodmont Avenue, Suite 1350, Bethesda, MD 20814; telephone: (301) 652-8585; http://www.resolve.org), the organization for infertile couples, maintains a directory of nationally and locally recognized and accredited organizations and individuals who provide adoption support.

Adoption. ACOG Committee Opinion No. 368. American College of Obstetricians and Gynecologists. Obstet Gynecol 2007;109:1507–10.

ISSN 1074-861X

ACOG COMMITTEE OPINION

Number 369 • June 2007

Multifetal Pregnancy Reduction*

Committee on Ethics

ABSTRACT: Counseling for treatment of infertility should include a discussion of the risks of multifetal pregnancy, and multifetal pregnancy reduction should be discussed with patients before the initiation of any treatment that could increase the risk of multifetal pregnancy. In almost all cases, it is preferable to terminate an ovulation induction cycle or limit the number of embryos to be transferred to prevent a situation in which fetal reduction will have to be considered. The best interests of the patient and the future child or children should be at the center of the risk–benefit equation. Although no physicians need to perform fetal reductions if they believe that such procedures are morally unacceptable, all obstetricians and gynecologists should be aware of the medical and ethical issues in these complex situations and be prepared to respond in a professional, ethical manner.

The ethical issues surrounding the use and consequences of reproductive technologies are highly complex, and no one position reflects the variety of opinions within the membership of the American College of Obstetricians and Gynecologists. The purpose of this Committee Opinion is to review the ethical issues involved in multifetal pregnancy reduction. For the purposes of this document, multifetal pregnancy reduction is defined as a first-trimester or early second-trimester procedure for termination of one or more fetuses in a multifetal pregnancy, to increase the chances of survival of the remaining fetuses and decrease long-term morbidity for the delivered infants (1).

To many, the ethical issues involved in multifetal pregnancy reduction are somewhat different from the issues involved in abortion, as discussed in the "Analysis" section. Although no physicians need to perform multifetal pregnancy reductions if they believe that such procedures are morally unacceptable, all physicians should be aware of the medical and ethical issues in these complex situations and be prepared to respond in a professional, ethical manner to patient requests for information and procedures.

The American College of Obstetricians and Gynecologists
Women's Health Care Physicians

*Update of "Multifetal Pregnancy Reduction" in *Ethics in Obstetrics and Gynecology,* Second Edition, 2004.

Background

Spontaneous occurrences of multifetal pregnancies always have been a medical problem. More recently, increased use of potent ovulation-induction drugs and assisted reproductive technology (ART), such as in vitro fertilization (IVF), have been effective in the treatment of infertility but subsequently also have increased the risk of multifetal pregnancy (2). Thousands of patients previously unable to have children have been assisted to achieve conception. In a small percentage of these patients, the resultant pregnancy has involved more than two fetuses, thereby creating potentially serious problems (2–6). There is widespread agreement that the risks of perinatal morbidity and mortality and maternal morbidity increase with the number of fetuses. Recent reports have shown improving outcomes with multifetal pregnancies, but the risks are still significant (6).

Prevention

The first approach to this problem is or should be prevention. It might be argued that the problem is best remedied by discontinuing technologic assistance to reproduction. On the one hand, this approach discounts the major benefits that ART offers to patients and suggests an unwarranted coercive restriction on parental choice and autonomy. On the other hand, the association of an increased rate of multifetal pregnancies with infertility treatment deserves serious attention. Some multifetal pregnancies will inevitably occur despite the best of intentions, knowledge, skill, and equipment, but it is essential that those providing infertility treatment exercise a high degree of diligence to minimize the problem.

Both ovulation induction alone and IVF contribute to high-order multiple births (more than two). In 1977, 43.3% of all births of triplets or greater were the result of ART (ie, IVF) and 38.2% were the result of the use of ovulation drugs (5). In 1996, the order was reversed; 40.4% of births of triplets or greater were the result of ovulation drugs, whereas 38.7% were the result of ART (5). According to the Centers for Disease Control and Prevention, 3,390 infants were born in triplet or higher-order multiple deliveries after ART treatment in 2003, accounting for 44% of all infants born in triplet or higher-order multiple deliveries (7). Similar data are not available for ovulation induction cycles.

Ovulation induction with gonadotropin cycles in which ultrasound imaging demonstrates the presence of many mature follicles, each capable of releasing an ovum, presents a difficult decision on whether to give human chorionic gonadotropin (hCG) to induce ovulation. If an hCG injection is withheld, the patient will have spent considerable time and emotional and financial resources for a nonovulatory cycle. Yet, if hCG is given to trigger ovulation, a high-order multifetal pregnancy may result. Attempts have been made to develop criteria for withholding hCG (eg, more than six large follicles or estradiol levels greater than 1,500 pg/mL). However, a large study showed that the occurrence of high-order multifetal pregnancies after gonadotropin therapy increases with higher estradiol levels but cannot be reliably predicted by the number of mature follicles on ultrasound examination (8). The authors concluded that adherence to criteria for withholding hCG will not prevent high-order multiple births and that better criteria cannot easily be established. They suggest that the use of treatment protocols with less-intensive stimulation of the ovaries may reduce the incidence of high-order multifetal pregnancies, but only to a limited extent and at the expense of pregnancy rates. When many follicles are present, alternative approaches would be conversion of the gonadotropin cycle to an IVF cycle or selective aspiration of the supernumerary follicles (9).

In ART, there may be pressure to be successful because of both prospective parents' and programs' interests. Direct costs for IVF cycles are many times higher than those for ovulation induction alone with gonadotropins. Ovulation induction with gonadotropins may be more likely to be covered by insurance. Patients who choose to undergo IVF may be paying for treatment out of pocket, and this may add pressure to achieve pregnancy on the first attempt. In addition, IVF programs face public scrutiny not faced by programs that offer only ovulation induction. Although success rates for individual IVF programs are public information, published by the Centers for Disease Control and Prevention, similar reporting is not done for ovulation induction alone (2). As the number of embryos transferred increases, program success rates may increase, but so does the risk of a multifetal pregnancy (2).

The physician who makes decisions about the circumstances for triggering ovulation or guidelines for embryo transfer must, as in any medical situation, place the best interests of the patient and the future child or children at the center of the risk–benefit equation. In some countries, such as England, where ART is centrally regulated, limitations are placed on the number of embryos that can be transferred, and subsequently fewer multifetal pregnancies result.

In the United States, the decision is left to individual physicians and programs. In almost all cases, it is preferable to terminate a gonadotropin cycle used for ovulation induction alone or limit the number of embryos to be transferred in IVF to prevent a situation in which patients and physicians will have to consider fetal reduction. The Practice Committee of the American Society for Reproductive Medicine (ASRM) has issued a report suggesting prognosis-dependent guidelines for limiting the number of embryos to be transferred. These guidelines limit risk while allowing individualization of patient care for optimal results (10). Multifetal pregnancy reduction should be viewed as a response to a consequence of ovulation induction that cannot always be avoided; it should not be a routinely accepted treatment for an iatrogenic problem.

The ultimate goal in prevention is to significantly reduce the likelihood that any multifetal pregnancy will occur, including twins. This will require patients, physicians, and payers to support a culture in which IVF may replace gonadotropin-only therapy in treatment algorithms. When IVF is performed, the eventual goal in the future may be to transfer only the embryo with the greatest chance for growth and implantation; currently ASRM recommends that consideration be given to transferring only a single embryo for patients with the most favorable prognosis (10). Nonetheless, data from the Centers for Disease Control and Prevention indicate that approximately 56% of embryo transfers that used fresh nondonor eggs in 2003 involved the transfer of three or more embryos (2).

Another strategy under study is transfer of blastocysts instead of cleavage-stage embryos, hoping that higher pregnancy rates would allow fewer embryos to be transferred. Yet, although some randomized trials have found higher pregnancy or live-birth rates with the transfer of a single blastocyst-stage embryo over a single cleavage-stage embryo (11, 12), the transfer of blastocyst-stage embryos has not been supported by others (13). The current position of ASRM is that either blastocyst transfer or cleavage stage-embryo transfer may be performed (10).

Counseling

As with all medical care, counseling for treatment of infertility should incorporate discussions of risks, benefits, and treatment alternatives, including the option for no treatment. Counseling should be considered an ongoing process, beginning before treatment decisions are made and continuing throughout the patient's care. The risks of certain treatments of infertility include, but are not limited to, the occurrence of multifetal pregnancy, with its associated risks of spontaneous abortion, preterm labor and delivery, and neonatal morbidity and mortality. The informed consent process must include information about the potential for multifetal pregnancy and associated maternal risks, such as prolonged hospitalization, antepartum bleeding, postpartum hemorrhage, hypertensive diseases of pregnancy, and an increased rate of cesarean delivery. Whether patients decide to maintain or to reduce high-order multiple pregnancies, they should be assured that they will receive the best available care (14).

It also is the responsibility of the physician to inform the patient that fetal reduction as a response to multifetal pregnancy has inherent medical risks to the remaining fetuses. Pregnancy loss rates of approximately 4–6% have been reported for triplet-to-twin reduction in large samples (15–17), but higher rates also have been reported (18). Reports of lower birth weights for twins reduced from triplets also are of concern (19–20), although more recent reports have suggested that reduction from triplets or quadruplets to twins is associated with an outcome as good as with an unreduced twin gestation (15, 22–26). Nonetheless, patients should not be given the impression that multifetal pregnancies are without problems because fetal reduction is available.

Patients struggle with the ethical and emotional issues of fetal reduction. In a postdelivery informational survey of couples who had undergone multifetal pregnancy reduction, few of the small sample of respondents reported that they understood the procedure or its consequences fully at the time of fetal reduction (27). In semi-structured interviews of 10 women who had undergone multifetal pregnancy reduction, one third reported still feeling guilt 1 year after the procedure (28). Many infertility patients have unrealistic ideas about the outcomes for high-order multifetal pregnancies that leave them unprepared for feelings of loss and grief at the time of a reduction procedure (29, 30). However, in studies that used standard psychologic tests to assess the emotional state of patients after multifetal pregnancy reduction, serious long-term psychologic sequelae were not identified. Among women who underwent multifetal pregnancy reduction and subsequently miscarried the entire pregnancy, depression scores were similar to scores for a control group of women who did not undergo fetal reduction and subsequently miscarried the entire pregnancy (31).

A report that 93% of patients who decided to proceed with fetal reduction would make that decision again despite their experience of stress and sadness is somewhat reassuring, but the number of patients studied was quite small (n = 91) (32). The ethical issues that this option involves should be discussed with patients before the initiation of any treatment that could increase the risk of multifetal pregnancy. Although patients should be encouraged to examine their feelings about these risks and options at the onset, the counseling process should encourage them to continue this assessment at appropriate points in the treatment process (33).

Options

In the presence of an already established multifetal pregnancy, the options are inevitably difficult. No choice is without potential consequences, and the potential benefits must be carefully weighed against the potential harms. There are three options in multifetal pregnancies:

1. Abort the entire pregnancy (all of the fetuses).

2. Continue the pregnancy (all of the fetuses).

3. Perform multifetal pregnancy reduction on one or more of the fetuses.

The first option involves aborting the entire multifetal pregnancy. However, for some patients, aborting the pregnancy is not an acceptable option. For other patients who may have achieved pregnancy after infertility treatment, this option may be considered the least desirable.

The second option is attempting to carry the multifetal pregnancy to term. However, the risks of perinatal and maternal morbidity and mortality increase directly with the number of fetuses (8). These risks include losing all of the fetuses or having some survive with permanent impairment as a consequence of extreme preterm birth. The assessment of what constitutes "significant risk" varies among patients and physicians and, therefore, is not amenable to uniform definition. Physicians should respect their patients' conclusions about which risks are acceptable and which are too high.

The third option in multifetal pregnancies is multifetal pregnancy reduction. The technique brings about the demise of one or more fetuses with the intent to allow continuation of the pregnancy, resulting in the delivery of fewer infants with lower risks of preterm birth, morbidity, and mortality. Although this procedure is successful in most cases, it may raise some unsettling ethical concerns. There is a complex interrelationship between the intention to reduce the morbidity of a smaller number of surviving fetuses and the intentional sacrifice of others that demands an ethical as well as medical assessment of the relative benefits and risks of multifetal pregnancy reduction. What follows is an attempt to outline such an assessment, with the understanding that each case ultimately must be examined on its own merits.

Analysis

Many would argue that there are differences between the ethical analyses involved in multifetal pregnancy reduction and elective abortion because the intent is different. A woman has an elective abortion because, for many complex and varied reasons, she does not wish or feels unable to have a child. In contrast, an infertility patient who has a multifetal pregnancy undergoes fetal reduction precisely because she does wish to bear a child. The patient and her physician may conclude that fetal reduction is the preferred way to continue her pregnancy. For some individuals, the primary intention justifying fetal reduction may be the life and well-being of the fetuses that do survive and continue to develop. For others, it is unethical to terminate an apparently healthy fetus, even for the sake of the survival or well-being of other fetuses in the pregnancy.

Some individuals who believe that abortion is generally unacceptable find multifetal pregnancy reduction to be justified ethically when the risks of carrying the pregnancy are considerable and could be reduced if the number of fetuses were fewer. Individual patients will evaluate varying degrees of risk differently. As advances in maternal–fetal and neonatal medicine continue, the risk of extreme preterm birth is expected to decrease. The issues of patient choice and physician participation and consultation need to be analyzed on a case-by-case basis.

Summary

Although physicians may choose not to participate in multifetal pregnancy reduction, they should be knowledgeable about this procedure and be prepared to react in a professional and ethical manner to patient requests for information or services or both. The first approach to the problem of multifetal pregnancies should be prevention. Although fetal reduction will be ethically acceptable to many as a response to an unforeseen and unavoidable contingency, in almost all cases, it is preferable to terminate a gonadotropin cycle or limit the number of embryos to be transferred to prevent a situation in which the patient and physician need to consider fetal reduction. Counseling for treatment of infertility should include a discussion of the risks of multifetal pregnancy, and the ethical issues surrounding fetal reduction should be discussed with patients before the initiation of any treatment that could increase the risk of multifetal pregnancy.

References

1. Berkowitz RL, Lynch L. Selective reduction: an unfortunate misnomer. Obstet Gynecol 1990;75:873–4.

2. Centers for Disease Control and Prevention. 2004 Assisted reproductive technology success rates: national summary and fertility clinic reports. Atlanta (GA): CDC; 2006. Available at: http://ftp.cdc.gov/pub/Publications/art/2004 ART508.pdf. Retrieved January 11, 2007.

3. Multiple gestation: complicated twin, triplet, and high-order multifetal pregnancy. ACOG Practice Bulletin No. 56. American College of Obstetricians and Gynecologists. Obstet Gynecol 2004;104:869–83.

4. Perinatal risks associated with assisted reproductive technology. ACOG Committee Opinion No. 324. American College of Obstetricians and Gynecologists. Obstet Gynecol 2005;106:1143–6.

5. Contribution of assisted reproductive technology and ovulation-inducing drugs to triplet and higher-order multiple births—United States, 1980–1997. Centers for Disease Control and Prevention (CDC). MMWR Morb Mortal Wkly Rep 2000;49:535–8.

6. Jones HW, Schnorr JA. Multiple pregnancies: a call for action. Fertil Steril 2001;75:11–3.

7. Wright VC, Chang J, Jeng G, Macaluso M. Assisted reproductive technology surveillance—United States, 2003. MMWR Surveill Summ 2006;55(SS-4):1–22.

8. Gleicher N, Oleske DM, Tur-Kaspa I, Vidali A, Karande V. Reducing the risk of high-order multiple pregnancy after ovarian stimulation with gonadotropins. N Engl J Med 2000;343:2–7.

9. Ethical issues related to multiple pregnancies in medically assisted procreation. ESHRE Task Force on Ethics and Law. Hum Reprod 2003;18:1976–9.

10. Guidelines on number of embryos transferred. The Practice Committee of the Society for Assisted Reproductive Technology and the Practice Committee of the American Society for Reproductive Medicine. Fertil Steril 2006; 86(suppl 5):S51–2.

11. Papanikolaou EG, Camus M, Kolibianakis EM, Van Landuyt L, Van Steirteghem A, Devroey P. In vitro fertilization with single blastocyst-stage versus single cleavage-stage embryos. N Engl J Med 2006;354:1139–46.

12. Gardner DK, Surrey E, Minjarez D, Leitz A, Stevens J, Schoolcraft WB. Single blastocyst transfer: a prospective randomized trial. Fertil Steril 2004;81:551–5.

13. Blake DA, Proctor M, Johnson NP. The merits of blastocyst versus cleavage stage embryo transfer: a Cochrane review [published erratum appears in Hum Reprod 2004;19:2174]. Hum Reprod 2004;19:795–807.

14. Ethical recommendations on multiple pregnancy and multifetal reduction. FIGO Committee for the Ethical Aspects of Human Reproduction and Women's Health. Int J Gynaecol Obstet 2006;92:331–2.

15. Evans MI, Berkowitz RL, Wapner RJ, Carpenter RJ, Goldberg JD, Ayoub MA, et al. Improvement in outcomes of multifetal pregnancy reduction with increased experience. Am J Obstet Gynecol 2001;184:97–103.

16. Timor-Tritsch IE, Bashiri A, Monteagudo A, Rebarber A, Arslan AA. Two hundred ninety consecutive cases of multifetal pregnancy reduction: comparison of the transabdominal versus the transvaginal approach. Am J Obstet Gynecol 2004;191:2085–9.

17. Stone J, Eddleman K, Lynch L, Berkowitz RL. A single center experience with 1000 consecutive cases of multifetal pregnancy reduction. Am J Obstet Gynecol 2002;187: 1163–7.

18. Antsaklis A, Souka AP, Daskalakis G, Papantoniou N, Koutra P, Kavalakis Y, et al. Embryo reduction versus expectant management in triplet pregnancies. J Matern Fetal Neonatal Med 2004;16:219–22.

19. Silver RK, Helfand BT, Russell TL, Ragin A, Sholl JS, MacGregor SN. Multifetal reduction increases the risk of preterm delivery and fetal growth restriction in twins: a case-control study. Fertil Steril 1997;67:30–3.

20. Groutz A, Yovel I, Amit A, Yaron Y, Azem F, Lessing JB. Pregnancy outcome after multifetal pregnancy reduction to twins compared with spontaneously conceived twins. Hum Reprod 1996;11:1334–6.

21. Depp R, Macones GA, Rosenn MF, Turzo E, Wapner RJ, Weinblatt VJ. Multifetal pregnancy reduction: evaluation of fetal growth in the remaining twins. Am J Obstet Gynecol 1996;174:1233–8; discussion 1238–40.

22. Papageorghiou AT, Liao AW, Skentou C, Sebire NJ, Nicolaides KH. Trichorionic triplet pregnancies at 10–14 weeks: outcome after embryo reduction compared to expectant management. J Matern Fetal Neonatal Med 2002;11:307–12.

23. Miller VL, Ransom SB, Shalhoub A, Sokol RJ, Evans MI. Multifetal pregnancy reduction: perinatal and fiscal outcomes. Am J Obstet Gynecol 2000;182:1575–80.

24. Yaron Y, Bryant-Greenwood PK, Dave N, Moldenhauer JS, Kramer RL, Johnson MP, et al. Multifetal pregnancy reductions of triplets to twins: comparison with nonreduced triplets and twins. Am J Obstet Gynecol 1999;180:1268–71.

25. Torok O, Lapinski R, Salafia CM, Bernasko J, Berkowitz RL. Multifetal pregnancy reduction is not associated with an increased risk of intrauterine growth restriction, except for very-high-order multiples. Am J Obstet Gynecol 1998; 179:221–5.

26. Dodd J, Crowther C. Multifetal pregnancy reduction of triplet and higher-order multiple pregnancies to twins. Fertil Steril 2004;81:1420–1.

27. Vauthier-Brouzes D, Lefebvre G. Selective reduction in multifetal pregnancies: technical and psychological aspects. Fertil Steril 1992;57:1012–6.

28. Garel M, Stark C, Blondel B, Lefebvre G, Vauthier-Brouzes D, Zorn JR. Psychological reactions after multifetal pregnancy reduction: a 2-year follow-up study. Hum Reprod 1997;12:617–22.

29. Goldfarb J, Kinzer DJ, Boyle M, Kurit D. Attitudes of in vitro fertilization and intrauterine insemination couples toward multiple gestation pregnancy and multifetal pregnancy reduction. Fertil Steril 1996;65:815–20.

30. Baor L, Blickstein I. En route to an "instant family": psychosocial considerations. Obstet Gynecol Clin North Am 2005;32:127–39, x.

31. McKinney M, Leary K. Integrating quantitative and qualitative methods to study multifetal pregnancy reduction. J Womens Health 1999;8:259–68.

32. Schreiner-Engel P, Walther VN, Mindes J, Lynch L, Berkowitz RL. First-trimester multifetal pregnancy reduction: acute and persistent psychologic reactions. Am J Obstet Gynecol 1995;172:541–7.

33. Zaner RM, Boehm FH, Hill GA. Selective termination in multiple pregnancies: ethical considerations. Fertil Steril 1990;54:203–5.

Multifetal pregnancy reduction. ACOG Committee Opinion No. 369. American College of Obstetricians and Gynecologists. Obstet Gynecol 2007;109:1511–5.

ISSN 1074-861X

ACOG COMMITTEE OPINION

Number 370 • July 2007

Institutional Responsibility to Provide Legal Representation*

Committee on Ethics

ABSTRACT: Hospitals, academic institutions, professional corporations, and other health care organizations should have policies and procedures by which alleged violations of professional behavior can be reported and investigated. These institutions should adopt policies on legal representation and indemnification to protect those whose responsibilities in managing such investigations may expose them to potentially costly legal actions. The American College of Obstetricians and Gynecologists' Committee on Ethics supports the position of the American Association of University Professors regarding institutional responsibility for legal demands on faculty.

The "Code of Professional Ethics of the American College of Obstetricians and Gynecologists" states, "The obstetrician–gynecologist should strive to address through the appropriate procedures the status of those physicians who demonstrate questionable competence, impairment, or unethical or illegal behavior. In addition, the obstetrician–gynecologist should cooperate with appropriate authorities to prevent the continuation of such behavior" (1). The Code also identifies those "appropriate procedures" and "appropriate authorities": "The obstetrician–gynecologist should respect all laws, uphold the dignity and honor of the profession, and accept the profession's self-imposed discipline. The professional competence and conduct of obstetrician–gynecologists are best examined by professional associations, hospital peer-review committees, and state medical and licensing boards. These groups deserve the full cooperation of the obstetrician–gynecologist" (1).

Academic institutions, professional corporations, hospitals, and other health care organizations should have policies and procedures by which alleged violations of professional behavior can be reported and investigated. Also, it is necessary for these institutions to adopt policies on legal representation and indemnification for their employees or others acting in an official capacity who, in discharging their obligations relative to unethical or illegal behavior of individuals, are exposed to potentially costly legal actions.

The American College of Obstetricians and Gynecologists agrees with the position of the American Association of University Professors in its 1998 statement, "Institutional Responsibility for Legal Demands on Faculty," that institutions should "ensure effective legal and other necessary representation and full indemnification in the first instance for any faculty member named or included in lawsuits or other extra-institutional legal proceedings arising from an act or omission in the discharge of institutional or related professional duties or in the defense of academic freedom at the institution" (2).

Reference

1. American College of Obstetricians and Gynecologists. Code of professional ethics of the American College of Obstetricians and Gynecologists. Washington, DC: ACOG; 2004. Available at: http://www.acog.org/from_home/acogcode.pdf. Retrieved January 11, 2007.

2. Institutional responsibility for legal demands on faculty. American Association of University Professors. Academe 1999;85 (1):52.

The American College of Obstetricians and Gynecologists
Women's Health Care Physicians

*Update of "Institutional Responsibility to Provide Legal Representation" in *Ethics in Obstetrics and Gynecology,* Second Edition, 2004.

Institutional responsibility to provide legal representation. ACOG Committee Opinion No. 370. American College of Obstetricians and Gynecologists. Obstet Gynecol 2007;110:215–6.

ISSN 1074-861X

ACOG COMMITTEE OPINION

Number 371 • July 2007

Sterilization of Women, Including Those With Mental Disabilities*

Committee on Ethics

ABSTRACT: Sterilization, like any other surgical procedure, must be carried out under the general ethical principles of respect for autonomy, beneficence, and justice. Women requesting sterilization should be encouraged to discuss their decision and associated issues with their husbands or other appropriate intimate partners. The physician who objects to a patient's request for sterilization solely as a matter of conscience has the obligation to inform the patient that sterilization services may be available elsewhere and should refer the patient to another caregiver. The presence of a mental disability does not, in itself, justify either sterilization or its denial. When a patient's mental capacity is limited and sterilization is considered, the physician must consult with the patient's family, agents, and other caregivers in an effort to adopt a plan that protects what the consulted group believes to be the patient's best interests while, at the same time, preserving, to the maximum extent possible, the patient's autonomy.

Sterilization, like any other surgical procedure, must be carried out under the general ethical principles of respect for autonomy, beneficence, and justice. Special ethical considerations are imposed by the unique attributes of sterilization. The procedure usually is done not for medical indications but electively for family planning. It may have a significant impact on individuals other than the patient, especially her partner. It is intended to be permanent, although techniques are available to attempt reversal or circumvent sterility. Finally, sterilization affects procreation and, therefore, may conflict with the moral beliefs of the patient, her family, or the physician. When the patient has diminished mental abilities or chronic mental illness, even more stringent ethical constraints apply.

General Ethical Principles

Under the principle of respect for autonomy, patients have the right to seek, accept, or refuse care. Respecting the patient's autonomy means that the physician cannot impose treatments. It does not mean that the physician must provide treatment, especially if the physician considers it inappropriate or harm-

*Update of "Sterilization of Women, Including Those With Mental Disabilities" in *Ethics in Obstetrics and Gynecology*, Second Edition, 2004.

ful (eg, an 18-year-old patient who asks to undergo sterilization).

Sterilization is for many a social choice rather than purely a medical issue, but all patient-related activities engaged in by physicians are subject to the same ethical guidelines. Patients sometimes request a physician's counsel in deciding whether to request sterilization. Physicians should be cautious in giving advice and making recommendations that go beyond health-related issues, even though nonmedical factors might be the most compelling for the patient. It may be difficult for the physician to address nonmedical issues without bias. Also, the physician may not have a full understanding of the patient's situation. However, it is entirely appropriate for the physician to assist the patient in exploring and articulating the reasons for her decision.

Although a woman's request for sterilization may conflict with the physician's medical judgment or moral beliefs, the patient's values and request cannot be dismissed or ignored. In such cases, the physician has an obligation to inform the patient of his or her professional recommendation and the medical reasons for it. The physician remains responsible for his or her actions and generally is not obligated to act in violation of

The American College of Obstetricians and Gynecologists
Women's Health Care Physicians

personal principles of conscience, but the patient should be informed when personal principles limit action or treatment. If the patient still desires sterilization, the physician who objects solely as a matter of conscience has the obligation to inform her that sterilization services may be available elsewhere and should refer her to another caregiver. The physician's values; sense of societal goals; and racial, ethnic, or socioeconomic issues should not be the basis of a recommendation to undergo sterilization.

Sterilization requires the patient's informed consent for ethical and medical–legal reasons. The physician performing the procedure has the responsibility of ensuring that the patient is properly counseled concerning the risks and benefits of sterilization. The patient should receive comprehensive and individualized counseling on reversible alternatives to sterilization (1). The procedure's intended permanence should be stressed, as well as the possibility of future regret. An estimate of the procedure's failure rate and risk of ectopic pregnancy should be provided. A variety of patient education materials are available to assist in preoperative counseling, but it is essential for the patient to be given the opportunity to discuss all relevant issues with her physician and to ask questions.

The physician should be familiar with any laws and regulations that may constrain sterilization, such as limitations on the patient's age and requirements for the consent process. The physician should inform the patient that insurance coverage for sterilization is variable so that she can discuss this issue with her insurer.

Specific Ethical Issues

Because sterilization may have important effects on individuals other than the patient, women requesting sterilization should be encouraged to discuss the issues with their husbands or other appropriate intimate partners. In many cases, it is preferable for the male partner to be sterilized. It may be helpful for the physician to counsel the partner directly, with the patient's consent.

Hysterectomy solely for the purpose of sterilization is inappropriate. The risks and cost of the procedure are disproportionate to the benefit, given the available alternatives. In disabled women with limited functional capability, indications for major surgical procedures remain the same as in other patients. In all cases, indications for surgery must meet standard criteria, and the benefits of the procedure must exceed known procedural risks. Disabled women with limited functional capacity may sometimes be physically unable to care for their menstrual hygiene and are profoundly disturbed by their menses. On occasion, such women's caretakers have sought hysterectomy for these indications. Hysterectomy for the purpose of cessation of normal menses may be considered only after other reasonable alternatives have been attempted.

Women may be vulnerable to various forms of coercion in their medical decision making. For example, the withholding of other medical care by linking it to the patient's consent to undergo sterilization is ethically unacceptable. Laws, regulations, and reimbursement restrictions concerning sterilization have been created to protect vulnerable individuals, including those with mental disabilities, from abuse. However, sterilization should not be denied to individuals simply because they also may be vulnerable to coercion. Physicians caring for patients who request or require procedures that result in sterilization may find themselves in a dilemma when legal and reimbursement restrictions interfere with a patient's choice of treatment. Rigid timing and age requirements can restrict access to good health care and result in unnecessary risk (2). Physicians are encouraged to seek legal or ethical consultation or both whenever necessary in their efforts to provide care that is most appropriate in individual situations.

At a public policy level, medical professionals have an opportunity to be a voice of reason and compassion by pointing out when legislative and regulatory measures intended to be safeguards interfere with patient choice and appropriate medical care.

Special Considerations Concerning Patients With Mental Disabilities

As used in this Committee Opinion, the term "women with mental disabilities" refers to individuals whose ability to participate in the informed consent process is, or might be, limited and whose autonomy is, or might be, thereby impaired. Such individuals constitute a heterogeneous group, including those with varying degrees of presumably irreversible "mental retardation" as well as those with varying types and degrees of "chronic mental illness." Some of these illnesses are reversible to varying degrees and for varying periods. The concept of "chronically and variably impaired autonomy" has been proposed to describe such situations (3).

Physicians who perform sterilizations must be aware of widely differing federal, state, and local laws and regulations, which have arisen in reaction to a long and unhappy history of sterilization of "unfit" individuals in the United States and elsewhere. The potential remains for serious abuses and injustices. Individuals who are capable of reproducing and parenting without a presumptive risk of child neglect or abuse may be deprived of their procreative rights simply because they carry a label, such as mild retardation, that suggests an inherent unfitness to parent. The implications of this labeling process for reproductive rights should be examined as thoroughly and objectively as possible before making a decision about sterilization.

Conversely, individuals for whom pregnancy is a serious burden or harm may be denied the opportunity for a full range of contraceptive options. For example, federal funds may not be used for the sterilization of "mentally incompetent" or "institutionalized" individuals (2). Physicians always should have the maximum respect for patient autonomy, and the presence of a mental disability does not, in itself, justify either sterilization or its denial.

Determination of Ability to Give Informed Consent

Before carrying out any surgical procedure, the physician has the important responsibility of ascertaining the patient's capacity to provide informed consent. It may be difficult to be sure that patients with normal intellectual function understand the complexities of some situations; when the patient has a mental disability, the task is more difficult and the responsibility is more challenging.

Evaluating a mentally impaired patient's ability to provide informed consent is seldom straightforward (4). For example, although degrees of mental retardation have been defined according to intelligence quotient, there is no direct relationship between such diagnostic categories and the capacity to consent. Among the issues that may need to be considered in the assessment are the patient's language and culture, the quality of information provided (clarity, completeness, and lack of bias), the setting of counseling (privacy and comfort), and possible fluctuations in the patient's comprehension. Such fluctuations may result from various stressors and medications. Multiple interviews over an adequate period may be required. Obtaining the assistance of professionals trained in communicating with mentally disabled individuals is essential. These professionals may include special educators, psychologists, nurses, attorneys familiar with disability law, and physicians accustomed to working with mentally disabled patients.

The process of evaluating a patient's ability to give informed consent may be set forth in laws of the jurisdiction involved, and legal requirements for the determination of competence vary greatly. The concept of legal competence is quite complex. Standards for the definition of competence may vary with the specific purpose (eg, marriage; making a will; consenting to or refusing life-saving treatment; or, as in the case of sterilization, consenting to elective surgery).

Court approval of sterilization may be required by law or may be necessary in difficult cases because of disagreement among the patient's caregivers and consultants. In most jurisdictions, court action is not required to carry out a sterilization procedure if there is agreement among these consultants that a nonminor is capable of consenting. Certain jurisdictions may not recognize guardian consent for sterilization of minors with mental disabilities under any circumstances. Whether or not recourse to the courts is necessary, every effort should be made to conduct the determination of competence fairly and to preserve autonomy.

Ethical Issues When the Patient Cannot Give Informed Consent

When the patient has been determined to be irreversibly incapable of participating in all or part of the informed consent process, others must make beneficence-based decisions regarding medical treatment. Such a determination is relatively uncommon. Even in these situations, it often is possible and highly desirable to obtain at least the patient's assent. The initial premise should be that non-voluntary sterilization generally is not ethically acceptable because of the violation of privacy, bodily integrity, and reproductive rights that it may represent.

Physicians and other caregivers should avoid paternalistic decisions in all cases in which the individual may be capable of participating to some degree in decisions regarding her care. The following recommendations are based in part on those of McCullough et al (3). They do not apply to mentally impaired individuals who can participate in the consent process.

For patients with chronically and variably impaired autonomy, initial efforts should be directed toward restoring decision-making ability by such means as adjustment of medication and avoidance of stressors. This may allow the patient to exercise full autonomy. For cases in which these efforts fail, the following guidelines are recommended:

- Efforts should be made to conform to the patient's expressed values and beliefs regarding reproduction. Such information may be available from interviewing the patient, her family, caregivers, and others in her environment. If possible, alternatives (including no action) consistent with her beliefs, medical condition, and social situation should be presented to decision makers.

- Physicians should be aware of the possibility of undue pressure from family members whose interests, no matter how legitimate, may not be the same as the patient's. When appropriate, the patient should have the opportunity to be interviewed without family members present.

- Noninvasive modalities designed to assist family members and other caregivers with setting behavioral limits should be considered as alternatives to sterilization. These resources may include socialization training, sexual abuse avoidance training, supportive family therapy, and sexuality education.

- Consideration should be given to the degree of certainty of various adverse outcomes. For example, given the patient's living circumstances, how likely is it that she might be sexually exploited? Given available knowledge concerning her reproductive potential (ovulatory status and tubal patency), how likely is it that she will become pregnant? How likely are adverse medical or social consequences from a pregnancy? Because it is uncommon for such risks to be reliably predicted, it may be preferable to recommend a reversible long-term form of contraception, such as an intrauterine device, long-term injectable progestin, or long-acting subdermal progestin implants (if available), instead of sterilization. In most cases, the chosen method of contraception should be the least restrictive in preserving future reproductive options. This is especially true when a major factor in the request for sterilization is concern about burdens for others. At the same time, risks and inconveniences of contraception over a long period, as compared with a single, relatively simple, and definitive surgical procedure, should not be ignored.

- The well-being of a child potentially conceived also should receive consideration.

Summary

Sterilization is an elective procedure with permanent and far-reaching consequences. Physicians who perform sterilization have ethical responsibilities of the highest order to counsel patients fully and without bias. Physicians must assess thoroughly the capacity of patients with impaired mental abilities to participate fully in the informed consent process. When this capacity is limited, the physician must consult with the patient's other caregivers in reaching a decision, which is based on the patient's best interests and preserves her autonomy to the maximum extent possible. In difficult cases, a hospital ethics committee may provide useful perspectives.

References

1. Benefits and risks of sterilization. ACOG Practice Bulletin No. 46. American College of Obstetricians and Gynecologists. Obstet Gynecol 2003;102:647–58.

2. Sterilization of persons in federally assisted family planning projects. 42 C.F.R. § 50 Subpart B (2006).

3. McCullough LB, Coverdale J, Bayer T, Chervenak FA. Ethically justified guidelines for family planning interventions to prevent pregnancy in female patients with chronic mental illness. Am J Obstet Gynecol 1992;167:19–25.

4. Appelbaum PS, Grisso T. Assessing patients' capacities to consent to treatment [published erratum appears in N Engl J Med 1989;320:748]. N Engl J Med 1988;319:1635–8.

Sterilization of women, including those with mental disabilities. ACOG Committee Opinion No. 371. American College of Obstetricians and Gynecologists. Obstet Gynecol 2007;110:217–20.

ISSN 1074-861X

ACOG COMMITTEE OPINION

Number 373 • August 2007

Sexual Misconduct*

Committee on Ethics

ABSTRACT: The physician–patient relationship is damaged when there is either confusion regarding professional roles and behavior or clear lack of integrity that allows sexual exploitation and harm. Sexual contact or a romantic relationship between a physician and a current patient is always unethical, and sexual contact or a romantic relationship between a physician and a former patient also may be unethical. The request by either a patient or a physician to have a chaperone present during a physical examination should be accommodated regardless of the physician's sex. If a chaperone is present during the physical examination, the physician should provide a separate opportunity for private conversation. Physicians aware of instances of sexual misconduct have an obligation to report such situations to appropriate authorities.

**The American College
of Obstetricians
and Gynecologists**

*Women's Health Care
Physicians*

The privilege of caring for patients, often over a long period, can yield considerable professional satisfaction. The obstetrician–gynecologist may fill many roles for patients, including primary physician, technology expert, prevention specialist, counselor, and confidante. Privy to both birth and death, obstetrician–gynecologists assist women as they pass through adolescence; grow into maturity; make choices about sexuality, partnership, and family; experience the sorrows of reproductive loss, infertility, and illness; and adapt to the transitions of midlife and aging. The practice of obstetrics and gynecology includes interaction at times of intense emotion and vulnerability for the patient and involves both sensitive physical examinations and medically necessary disclosure of especially private information about symptoms and experiences. The relationship between the physician and patient, therefore, requires a high level of trust and professional responsibility.

Trust of this sort cannot be maintained without a basic understanding of the limits and responsibilities of the professional's role. Physician sexual misconduct is an example of abuse of limits and failure of responsibility. The valued human experience of the physician–patient relationship is damaged when there is either confusion regarding profes-

sional roles and behavior or clear lack of integrity that allows sexual exploitation and harm.

Sexual misconduct is of particular concern in today's environment of shifting roles for women and men, greater sexual freedom, and critical evaluation of power relations in society (1–4). Prohibitions against sexual contact between patient and physician are not new; they can be found in the earliest guidelines in western antiquity. From the beginning, physicians were enjoined to "do no harm" and specifically avoid sexual contact with patients (5). In the intervening centuries, as the study of medical ethics has evolved, attention has been focused on respect for individual rights, the problem of unequal power in relationships between professionals and patients, and the potential for abuse of that power (6).

In this context, the American Medical Association's Council on Ethical and Judicial Affairs developed a report, "Sexual Misconduct in the Practice of Medicine," condemning sexual relations between physicians and current patients (7). It raises serious questions about the ethics of romantic relationships with former patients. It is summarized as follows (8):

> Sexual contact that occurs concurrent with the physician–patient relationship constitutes sexual misconduct. Sexual or romantic interactions between physi-

---

*Update of "Sexual Misconduct" in *Ethics in Obstetrics and Gynecology,* Second Edition, 2004.

cians and patients detract from the goals of the physician–patient relationship, may exploit the vulnerability of the patient, may obscure the physician's objective judgment concerning the patient's health care, and ultimately may be detrimental to the patient's well-being.

If a physician has reason to believe that non-sexual contact with a patient may be perceived as or may lead to sexual contact, then he or she should avoid the non-sexual contact. At a minimum, a physician's ethical duties include terminating the physician–patient relationship before initiating a dating, romantic, or sexual relationship with a patient.

Sexual or romantic relationships between a physician and a former patient may be unduly influenced by the previous physician–patient relationship. Sexual or romantic relationships with former patients are unethical if the physician uses or exploits trust, knowledge, emotions, or influence derived from the previous professional relationship.

The Council provides clear guidelines (7):

- Mere mutual consent is rejected as a justification for sexual relations with patients because the disparity in power, status, vulnerability, and need make it difficult for a patient to give meaningful consent to sexual contact or sexual relations.
- Sexual contact or a romantic relationship concurrent with the physician–patient relationship is unethical.
- Sexual contact or a romantic relationship with a former patient may be unethical under certain circumstances (9). The relevant standard is the potential for misuse of physician power and exploitation of patient emotions derived from the former relationship.
- Education on ethical issues involved in sexual misconduct should be included throughout all levels of medical training (10–13).
- Physicians have a responsibility to report offending colleagues to disciplinary boards.

The Society of Obstetricians and Gynaecologists of Canada has adopted a similar statement that "acknowledges and deplores the fact that incidents of physicians abusing patients do occur" and finds that "these incidents include 'sexual impropriety' due to poor clinical skills, chauvinism, or abuse of the power relationship, and outright systematic sexual abuse" (14). The Society also supports the right to "informed, safe, and gender-sensitive" care and the right of victims of abuse to receive "prompt treatment." "Identification, discipline, and, where possible, rehabilitation of the perpetrators" is recommended.

Although much discussion of sexual misconduct by health care professionals has centered around the particular vulnerability that exists within the relationship a woman has with her mental health care professional (15, 16), sexual contact between patients and obstetrician–gynecologists also has been documented (3, 4). Physicians themselves acknowledge that there is a problem, but the extent of the problem is difficult to determine because information relies on self-reporting, which carries the potential for bias in response.

The Committee on Ethics of the American College of Obstetricians and Gynecologists endorses the ethical principles expressed by the American Medical Association and the Society of Obstetricians and Gynaecologists of Canada and affirms the following statements:

- Sexual contact or a romantic relationship between a physician and a current patient is always unethical.
- Sexual contact or a romantic relationship between a physician and a former patient also may be unethical. Potential risks to both parties should be considered carefully. Such risks may stem from length of time and intensity of the previous professional relationship; age differences; the length of time since cessation of the professional relationship; the former patient's residual feelings of dependency, obligation, or gratitude; the former patient's vulnerability to manipulation as a result of private information disclosed during treatment; or physician vulnerability if a relationship initiated with a former patient breaks down.
- Physicians should be careful not to mix roles that are ordinarily in conflict. For example, they should not perform breast or pelvic examinations on their own minor children unless an urgent indication exists. Children and adolescents are particularly vulnerable to emotional conflict and damage to their developing sense of identity and sexuality when roles and role boundaries with trusted adults are confused. It is essential to ensure the young individual's privacy and prevent subtly coercive violations from occurring.
- The request by either a patient or a physician to have a chaperone present during a physical examination should be accommodated regardless of the physician's sex. Local practices and expectations differ with regard to the use of chaperones, but the presence of a third party in the examination room can confer benefits for both patient and physician, regardless of the sex of the chaperone. Chaperones can provide reassurance to the patient about the professional context and content of the examination and the intention of the physician and offer witness to the actual events taking place should there be any misunderstanding. The presence of a third party in the room may, however, cause some embarrassment to the patient and limit her willingness to talk openly with the physician because of concerns about confidentiality. If a chaperone is present, the physician should provide a separate opportunity for private

conversation. If the chaperone is an employee of the practice, the physician must establish clear rules about respect for privacy and confidentiality. In addition, some patients (especially, but not limited to, adolescents) may consider the presence of a family member as an intrusion. Family members should not be used as chaperones unless specifically requested by the patient and then only in the presence of an additional chaperone who is not a family member.

- Examinations should be performed with only the necessary amount of physical contact required to obtain data for diagnosis and treatment. Appropriate explanation should accompany all examination procedures.

- Physicians should avoid sexual innuendo and sexually provocative remarks.

- When physicians have questions and concerns about their sexual feelings and behavior, they should seek advice from mentors or appropriate professional organizations (16, 17).

- It is important for physicians to self-monitor for any early indications that the barrier between normal sexual feelings and inappropriate behavior is not being maintained (4, 16, 18). These indicators might include special scheduling, seeing a patient outside normal office hours or outside the office, driving a patient home, or making sexually explicit comments about patients.

- Physicians involved in medical education should actively work to include as part of the basic curriculum information about both physician and patient vulnerability, avoidance of sexually offensive or denigrating language, risk factors for sexual misconduct, and procedures for reporting and rehabilitation.

- Physicians aware of instances of sexual misconduct on the part of any health professional have an obligation to report such situations to appropriate authorities, such as institutional committee chairs, department chairs, peer review organizations, supervisors, or professional licensing boards.

- Physicians with administrative responsibilities in hospitals, other medical institutions, and licensing boards should develop clear and public guidelines for reporting instances of sexual misconduct, prompt investigation of all complaints, and appropriate disciplinary and remedial action (19).

Sexual misconduct on the part of physicians is an abuse of professional power and a violation of patient trust. It jeopardizes the well-being of patients and carries an immense potential for harm. The ethical prohibition against physician sexual misconduct is ancient and forceful, and its application to contemporary medical practice is essential.

References

1. Gabbard GO, Nadelson C. Professional boundaries in the physician-patient relationship [published erratum appears in JAMA 1995;274:1346]. JAMA 1995;273:1445–9.

2. Gawande A. Naked. N Engl J Med 2005;353:645–8.

3. Dehlendorf CE, Wolfe SM. Physicians disciplined for sex-related offenses. JAMA 1998;279:1883–8.

4. Enbom JA, Parshley P, Kollath J. A follow-up evaluation of sexual misconduct complaints: the Oregon Board of Medical Examiners, 1998 through 2002. Am J Obstet Gynecol 2004;190:1642–50; discussion 1650–3; 6A.

5. Campbell ML. The Oath: an investigation of the injunction prohibiting physician–patient sexual relations. Perspect Biol Med 1989;32:300–8.

6. Beauchamp TL, Childress JF. Principles of biomedical ethics. 5th ed. New York (NY): Oxford University Press; 2001.

7. Sexual misconduct in the practice of medicine. Council on Ethical and Judicial Affairs, American Medical Association. JAMA 1991;266:2741–5.

8. American Medical Association. Sexual misconduct in the practice of medicine. In: Code of medical ethics of the American Medical Association: current opinions with annotations. 2006–2007 ed. Chicago (IL): AMA; 2006. p. 255–8.

9. Hall KH. Sexualization of the doctor-patient relationship: is it ever ethically permissible? Fam Pract 2001;18:511–5.

10. Goldie J, Schwartz L, Morrison J. Sex and the surgery: students' attitudes and potential behaviour as they pass through a modern medical curriculum. J Med Ethics 2004; 30:480–6.

11. White GE. Setting and maintaining professional role boundaries: an educational strategy. Med Educ 2004;38: 903–10.

12. White GE. Medical students' learning needs about setting and maintaining social and sexual boundaries: a report. Med Educ 2003;37:1017–9.

13. Spickard A, Swiggart WH, Manley G, Dodd D. A continuing education course for physicians who cross sexual boundaries. Sex Addict Compulsivity 2002;9:33–42.

14. Sexual abuse by physicians. SOGC Policy Statement No. 134. Society of Obstetricians and Gynaecologists of Canada. J Obstet Gynaecol Can 2003;25:862.

15. Gabbard GO, editor. Sexual exploitation in professional relationships. Washington, DC: American Psychiatric Press; 1989.

16. Simon RI. Therapist–patient sex. From boundary violations to sexual misconduct. Psychiatr Clin North Am 1999; 22:31–47.

17. Crausman RS. Sexual boundary violations in the physician-patient relationship. Med Health R I 2004;87:255–6.

18. Searight HR, Campbell DC. Physician–patient sexual contact: ethical and legal issues and clinical guidelines. J Fam Pract 1993;36:647–53.

19. Federation of State Medical Boards. Addressing sexual boundaries: guidelines for state medical boards. Dallas (TX): FSMB; 2006. Available at: http://www.fsmb.org/pdf/ GRPOL _Sexual%20Boundaries.pdf. Retrieved January 23, 2007.

Sexual misconduct. ACOG Committee Opinion No. 373. American College of Obstetricians and Gynecologists. Obstet Gynecol 2007; 110:441–4.

ISSN 1074-861X

ACOG COMMITTEE OPINION

Number 374 • August 2007

Expert Testimony*

Committee on Ethics

ABSTRACT: It is the duty of obstetricians and gynecologists who testify as expert witnesses on behalf of defendants, the government, or plaintiffs to do so solely in accordance with their judgment on the merits of the case. Obstetrician–gynecologists must limit testimony to their sphere of medical expertise and must be prepared adequately. They must make a clear distinction between medical malpractice and medical maloccurrence. The acceptance of fees that are greatly disproportionate to those customary for professional services can be construed as influencing testimony given by the witness, and it is unethical to accept compensation that is contingent on the outcome of litigation.

The American College of Obstetricians and Gynecologists (ACOG) recognizes that it is the duty of obstetricians and gynecologists who testify as expert witnesses on behalf of defendants, the government, or plaintiffs to do so solely in accordance with their judgment on the merits of the case. Furthermore, ACOG cannot condone the participation of physicians in legal actions where their testimony will impugn performance that falls within accepted standards of practice or, conversely, will support obviously deficient practice. Because the experts articulate the standards in a given case, care must be exercised to ensure that such standards do not narrowly reflect the experts' views to the exclusion of other choices deemed acceptable by the profession. The American College of Obstetricians and Gynecologists considers unethical any expert testimony that is misleading because the witness does not have appropriate knowledge of the standard of care for the particular condition at the relevant time or because the witness knowingly misrepresents the standard of care relevant to the case.

The Problem of Professional Liability—Reality and Perceptions

The American College of Obstetricians and Gynecologists recognizes its responsibility, and that of its Fellows, to continue efforts to

advance health care for women through every available method of quality assessment and improvement. The American College of Obstetricians and Gynecologists also recognizes, however, that many claims of professional liability represent the response of a litigation-oriented society to a technologically advanced form of health care that has fostered unrealistic expectations. As technology becomes more complex, associated benefits and risks may increase, making the complication-free practice of medicine less possible.

It therefore becomes important to distinguish between medical "maloccurrence" and medical "malpractice." *Medical maloccurrence* is defined as a bad or undesirable outcome that is unrelated to the quality of care provided. In some cases, specific medical or surgical complications may be anticipated but are felt by the patient and the health care provider to be offset by the balance of benefits from the planned intervention and, therefore, represent unavoidable risks of appropriate medical care. There are other types of complications that cannot be anticipated and in their unpredictability are similarly unavoidable. Still other complications occur as a result of decisions that have been made carefully by patients and physicians with fully informed consent but appear, in retrospect, to have been a less optimal choice among several options. Each of these situations represents a type of maloccurrence, rather than an example of malpractice, and is the result of the uncertainty inherent in all of medicine. *Malpractice*, in contrast, requires a

The American College of Obstetricians and Gynecologists
Women's Health Care Physicians

---

*Update of "Expert Testimony" in *Ethics in Obstetrics and Gynecology,* Second Edition, 2004.

demonstration of negligence (ie, substandard practice that causes harm). The potential for personal, professional, and financial rewards from expert testimony may encourage testimony that undermines the distinction between unavoidable maloccurrence and actual medical malpractice. It is unethical to distort or to represent a maloccurrence as an example of medical malpractice or, conversely, represent malpractice as a case of maloccurrence.

The American College of Obstetricians and Gynecologists supports the concept of appropriate and prompt compensation to patients for medically related injuries. Any such response, however, also should reflect the distinction between medical maloccurrence, for which all of society should perhaps bear financial responsibility, and medical malpractice, for which health care providers should be held responsible.

Responsibility of Individual Physicians

The moral and legal duty of physicians who testify before a court of law is to do so in accordance with their expertise. This duty implies adherence to the strictest personal and professional ethics. Truthfulness is essential. Misrepresentation of one's personal clinical opinion as absolute right or wrong may be harmful to individual parties and to the profession at large. The obstetrician–gynecologist who is an expert witness must limit testimony to his or her sphere of medical expertise and must be prepared adequately. Witnesses who testify as experts must have knowledge and experience that are relevant to obstetric and gynecologic practice at the time of the occurrence and to the specific areas of clinical medicine they are discussing. The acceptance of fees that are greatly disproportionate to those customary for professional services can be construed as influencing testimony given by the witness. It is unethical for a physician to accept compensation that is contingent on the outcome of litigation (1, 2).

The American College of Obstetricians and Gynecologists encourages the development of policies and standards for expert testimony. Such policies should address safeguards to promote truth-telling and to encourage openness of the testimony to peer review. These policies also would encourage testimony that does not assume an advocacy or partisan role in the legal proceeding.

The following principles are offered as guidelines for the physician who assumes the role of an expert witness:

1. The physician must have experience and knowledge in the areas of clinical medicine that enable him or her to testify about the standards of care that applied at the time of the occurrence that is the subject of the legal action.

2. The physician's review of medical facts must be thorough, fair, and impartial and must not exclude any relevant information. It must not be biased to create a view favoring the plaintiff, the government, or the defendant. The goal of a physician testifying in any judicial proceeding should be to provide testimony that is complete, objective, and helpful to a just resolution of the proceeding.

3. The physician's testimony must reflect an evaluation of performance in light of generally accepted standards, neither condemning performance that falls within generally accepted practice standards nor endorsing or condoning performance that falls below these standards. Experts and their testimony should recognize that medical decisions often must be made in the absence of diagnostic and prognostic certainty.

4. The physician must make a clear distinction between medical malpractice and medical maloccurrence.

5. The physician must make every effort to assess the relationship of the alleged substandard practice to the outcome. Deviation from a practice standard is not always substandard care or causally related to a bad outcome.

6. The physician must be prepared to have testimony given in any judicial proceeding subjected to peer review by an institution or professional organization to which he or she belongs.

References

1. American Medical Association. Medical testimony. In: Code of medical ethics of the American Medical Association: current opinions with annotations. 2006–2007 ed. Chicago (IL): AMA; 2006. p. 286–9.

2. American Bar Association. Rule 3.4. Fairness to opposing party and counsel. In: Annotated model rules of professional conduct. 5th ed. Chicago (IL): ABA; 2003. p. 347–58.

Expert testimony. ACOG Committee Opinion No. 374. American College of Obstetricians and Gynecologists. Obstet Gynecol 2007; 110:445–6.

ISSN 1074-861X

ACOG COMMITTEE OPINION

Number 377 • September 2007

Research Involving Women*

**Committee on
Ethics**

ABSTRACT: All women should be presumed to be eligible for participation in clinical studies. The potential for pregnancy should not automatically exclude a woman from participating in a clinical study, although the use of contraception may be required for participation. Research objectives should not interfere with appropriate clinical management. If a conflict arises between medically appropriate patient care and research objectives, patient care should prevail. Consent of the pregnant woman alone is sufficient for most research. Pregnant women considering participation in a research study should determine the extent to which the father is to be involved in the process of informed consent and the decision.

Attitudes concerning inclusion of women in research trials have changed dramatically over the past four decades. In the 1970s and 1980s, women were systematically excluded from participating in research trials either because of the fear that unrecognized pregnancy might place an embryo at risk or because a uniform all-male sample would simplify analysis of data. In addition, pregnant women were excluded from most research trials because they were viewed as a vulnerable population requiring special protection, and there was concern that trial participation would result in harm to the fetus. Another fear was that participation of pregnant women in research trials would result in increased liability risk for researchers. In the 1990s, there was a dramatic policy shift toward wide-scale inclusion of women in research trials. This policy shift is a direct result of a conscious effort by government agencies to expand participation of women in research in order to obtain valid, evidence-based information about health and disease in this population (1).

This Committee Opinion is designed to provide reasonable guidelines for research involving women. The American College of Obstetricians and Gynecologists' Committee on Ethics affirms both the need for women to serve as participants in research and the obligation for researchers, institutional review boards (IRBs), and others reviewing clinical research to evaluate the potential effect of proposed research on women of childbearing potential, pregnant women, and the developing fetus.

Rationale for Including Women in Research

All women should be presumed to be eligible for participation in clinical studies. The potential for pregnancy should not automatically exclude a woman from participating in a clinical study, although the use of contraception may be required for participation. Inclusion of women in clinical studies is necessary for valid inferences about health and disease in women. The generalization to women of results from trials conducted in men may yield erroneous conclusions that fail to account for the biologic differences between men and women.

The rationale for conducting research in women is to advance knowledge in the following areas:

* Medical conditions in women (eg, cardiovascular disease)
* Physiology of women
* Sex differences in responses to drugs (eg, antiretroviral agents)
* Sex differences in drug toxicities
* Sex differences in responses to disease (eg, mental disorders)

**The American College
of Obstetricians
and Gynecologists**
*Women's Health Care
Physicians*

*Update of "Research Involving Women," in Ethics in
Obstetrics and Gynecology, *Second Edition, 2004.*

- Effects of hormonal contraceptives on response to other therapies (eg, seizure medication)
- Variations in response to therapy at different stages of the menstrual cycle and the life cycle

The rationale for conducting research in pregnant and postpartum women is to advance knowledge in the following areas:

- Medical conditions (eg, human immunodeficiency virus [HIV]) in women who become pregnant
- Medical conditions unique to pregnancy (eg, preeclampsia)
- Conditions that threaten the successful course of pregnancy (eg, preterm labor)
- Prenatal conditions that might threaten the health of the fetus (eg, diaphragmatic hernia)
- Physiologic changes that accompany pregnancy and lactation
- Medical conditions related to pregnancy that might affect the future health of women (eg, gestational diabetes)
- Safety of medication during pregnancy and breastfeeding

Human experimentation is a necessary and important part of biomedical research because certain information can be obtained in no other way. Guidelines for protection of research participants have been established and are applicable to women of childbearing potential as well as to pregnant women (2–4). Additional protections have been established for pregnant women (5, 6). Participants in research should expect full disclosure of the known burdens and benefits of the research study and should understand the potential risks as well as benefits. Investigators must use research design methods that aim to maximize safety and minimize risk. A fully informed consent process and review of study protocols by IRBs help to ensure that efforts to increase access to and participation of women in clinical trials will not result in procedural shortcuts that violate basic ethical standards.

Involvement in research protocols should not diminish a woman's expectation that she will receive appropriate medical care during the study and in the future. Health care professionals have a responsibility to provide the most appropriate clinical management, whether or not a woman is a participant in research. Research objectives should not affect clinical management. If a conflict arises between medically appropriate patient care and research objectives, patient care should prevail. For example, it is inappropriate to attempt to delay a medically indicated induction of labor solely to meet gestational age criteria for participation in a research project. The welfare of the patient and, in the case of pregnancy, the patient and her fetus is always the primary concern.

The Ethical Context

Ethical Requirements for Research

To be considered ethically justified, research on human participants must satisfy several conditions. These include a reasonable prospect that the investigation will produce the knowledge that is being sought, a favorable balance of benefits over risks, a proven necessity to use human participants, a system for independent monitoring of outcomes and protection of human participants, and a fair allocation of the burdens and benefits of the research among potential groups of participants (7). These principles should not be weakened by attempts to increase participation of women in research trials.

Although it is important to try to distinguish ethical problems involving patient care from ethical issues related to research, a definitive line cannot always be drawn between the two areas. The dual role that physicians often assume as research scientists and clinical practitioners may result in conflict of interest because each role has different goals and priorities. For example, the primary goal of the investigator is to generate knowledge that has the potential to benefit patients in the future, whereas clinicians are expected to act in the best interests of their current patients. Researchers need to recognize potential conflicts, strive to resolve them before beginning specific research projects, and inform patients about potential conflicts as they seek consent for research participation.

The potential for role conflict becomes readily apparent when innovative therapies are introduced (8). In the context of maternal–fetal surgery, for example, innovative surgical procedures have been conducted, but the long-term impact on both the woman and the fetus is unclear. In this context, it is important to conduct rigorous scientific evaluation of maternal–fetal surgery before these innovative therapies are offered as routine care.

Ethical Principles Supporting the Inclusion of Women

The recent movement to enroll more women in clinical research can be justified by ethical principles: beneficence, nonmaleficence, respect for autonomy, and justice. Because disease processes may have different characteristics in women and men and because women and men may respond differently to treatments and interventions, women need to be included as participants in clinical research. For women to benefit from the results of research (beneficence), the research must be designed to provide a valid analysis as to whether women are affected differently than men (1). Such differential analysis is necessary not only to benefit women, but also to prevent harm; if data from studies with men are inappropriately extrapolated to women, women may actually suffer harm (nonmaleficence).

Arguments previously advanced to defend the exclusion of women from research often cited the possibility of harm to women of reproductive potential or to pregnant women and their fetuses, harm that did not apply to men. However, the risk of such harm can be minimized and, in itself, does not justify the exclusion of women from research that is needed to make valid inferences about the medical treatment of women.

Women have frequently been regarded as a vulnerable population that needs to be protected. Today, however, both civil society and medical ethics recognize the right and the capacity of women to make decisions regarding their own lives and their medical care (respect for autonomy). Similarly, women have the right and the capacity to weigh the risks and potential benefits of participation in research and to decide for themselves whether to consent to participate. This autonomy right is limited, however, by the responsibility of investigators and IRBs to take precautions to limit the risk for research participants, including pregnant women and their fetuses.

Systematic exclusion of women from research violates the ethical principle of justice, which first requires that persons be given what is due them. If the medical treatment of women is invalidly based on studies that excluded women, then women are not receiving fair treatment. Justice requires that women be included in clinical studies in sufficient numbers to determine whether their responses are different from those of men.

In the research setting, justice requires that the benefits of scientific advancement be shared fairly between men and women. Both women and men should be encouraged to participate in research. Researchers should specifically address those obstacles to participation that are experienced disproportionately by women—for example, problems obtaining and paying for adequate child care during time spent as a research participant.

Because of a history of systematic exclusion of women from research, in 1993 Congress directed that women were to be included in all federally funded research projects (9). Consequently, the National Institutes of Health (NIH) now require that women be included in all NIH-funded clinical research, unless a clear and compelling rationale establishes that such involvement would be inappropriate or unsafe (1). Particular focus on the health needs of women is justifiable at this time in view of a history of neglect of such studies.

Informed Consent

Appropriate and adequately informed consent by the potential participant or another authorized person and an independent review of the risks and benefits of research by appropriate institutions or agencies (or both) are fundamental to the formulation of any research protocol (10). The informed consent process should not be weakened to benefit the researcher. The consent document should be understandable and written in simple language. In situations in which English is not the primary language of the potential study participant, an interpreter should be used for the consent process to verify the participant's level of understanding of the issues related to risk and benefit. The statement of informed consent may need to be translated into the participant's native language. Researchers should be familiar with federal and state laws and regulations for informed consent in settings where pregnant minors and adolescents may be recruited as participants (11).

The researcher has an obligation to disclose to the woman and discuss with her all material risks affecting her; in the case of a pregnant woman, this includes all material risks to the woman and her fetus (12). Disclosure should include risks that are likely to affect the patient's decision to participate or not to participate in the research. Because the process of informed consent cannot anticipate all conceivable risks, women who develop unanticipated complications should be instructed to contact the researcher or a representative of the IRB immediately. Pregnant women who enroll in a research trial and experience a research-related injury should be informed about their therapeutic options, including those related to the pregnancy.

The potential participant should be encouraged to consult her physician independently before deciding to participate in a research study (13). At the woman's request, the researcher should provide information about the study to her physician. If relevant, this information may include the requirements of the study and its possible outcomes and complications.

Both the researcher and the primary caregiver should guard against inflating the patient's perception of the therapeutic benefit expected from participating in the study. Studies have shown that research participants tend to believe, despite careful explanation of research protocols, that they will always benefit from participation or that the level of actual benefit will be greater than stated in the consent process (14). This risk of "therapeutic misconception" may be increased when the patient's own physician is involved in the consent process, especially when one physician serves as both researcher and clinician.

Consent of the pregnant woman alone is sufficient for most research. When research has the prospect of direct benefit to the fetus alone, paternal consent also may be required (see Table 1). Federal regulations that call for involvement of the father in the consent process for research intended to benefit the fetus are controversial and have generated vigorous debate. Proponents of paternal consent endorse this requirement because they believe that the requirement is consistent with recognition of and respect for the rights of the father in protecting the welfare of his unborn child. They believe that this represents a reasonable compromise between acknowledging paternal rights and reducing barriers to participation in research by pregnant women.

The Committee on Ethics, however, does not support recognition of distinct paternal rights before the birth of a child. Recognition of paternal rights during pregnancy may infringe on and weaken maternal autonomy—the right of a woman, when pregnant, to independent action

Table 1. Selected Federal Regulations on Informed Consent for Participants in Human Research*

Issue	Citation	Regulation
Maternal consent	45 C.F.R. §46.204(d)	If the research holds out the prospect of direct benefit to the pregnant woman, the prospect of a direct benefit both to the pregnant woman and the fetus, or no prospect of benefit for the woman nor the fetus when risk to the fetus is not greater than minimal and the purpose of the research is the development of important biomedical knowledge that cannot be obtained by any other means, her consent is obtained in accord with the informed consent provisions of subpart A† of this part;
Paternal consent	45 C.F.R. §46.204(e)	If the research holds out the prospect of direct benefit solely to the fetus then the consent of the pregnant woman and the father is obtained in accord with the informed consent provisions of subpart A† of this part, except that the father's consent need not be obtained if he is unable to consent because of unavailability, incompetence, or temporary incapacity or the pregnancy resulted from rape or incest.

*Federal regulations on protection of human research participants are found in the Code of Federal Regulations in Title 45, Part 46. Selected sections of the regulations dealing with informed consent are reprinted here; the complete, current version may be found at http://www.hhs.gov/ohrp/ humansubjects/guidance/45cfr46.htm.

†Basic HHS policy for protection of human research subjects. 45 C.F.R. §46.101–124 Subpart A (2006).

in decisions that affect her body and her health. As in clinical situations, the pregnant woman's consent should be sufficient for research interventions that affect her or her fetus. To further complicate matters, the interpretation as to whether research is intended for the benefit of the pregnant woman, the fetus, or both may be subjective. Two researchers conducting identical studies may reach different conclusions as to whether benefits of the research apply to the pregnant woman, the fetus, or both (eg, maternal–fetal surgery for spina bifida).

Informed consent means that women have the right to choose not to participate in a research protocol and the right to withdraw from a study at any time. The participation of a woman in a research study is based on the expectation that she will consider carefully her own interests. The participation of a pregnant woman in a research study is based on the expectation that she will consider carefully her own interests as well as those of her fetus. Typically, pregnant women are quite willing to take personal risks for the benefit of their fetuses; combined with society's expectation that they will do so, women may find themselves under pressure to participate in research that carries risk to them. Such pressure actually may interfere with the ability of the pregnant woman to give fully free consent. In these situations, special care should be taken to ensure that a woman's consent is truly voluntary.

Research Related to Diagnosis and Therapy

Research that consists of observation and recording without clinical intervention (descriptive research) is of ethical concern primarily to the extent that it requires informed consent and the preservation of confidentiality. In research trials where clinical intervention is a compo-

nent, the benefits and burdens of the trial must be clearly articulated to the participant by the researcher (12). In research studies conducted in pregnant women, both the potential benefit to the woman, the fetus, and society as a whole and the level of risk that may be incurred as a result of participation in the study should be considered. The involvement of the participant's obstetrician ordinarily is appropriate. All parties concerned need to strive for clear communication with regard to the following questions:

- Does the research involve intervention or diagnosis that might affect the woman's or the fetus's well-being, or is the goal of the study to produce scientific results that will be likely to be useful to future patients but offer no demonstrable benefit to current participants?

- Can the prospective participant expect any explicit benefit as a result of participating in the study? If not, she must be apprised of this fact. Those studies that search for general information and are not associated with diagnostic or treatment modalities would be less likely to create the impression that the research will result in direct benefit to the participant. The researcher is still obligated to verify that the participant has understood this aspect of the study correctly.

- Is there more than "minimal risk" to the fetus generated by the research?

According to applicable federal regulations, "minimal risk means that the probability and magnitude of harm or discomfort anticipated in the research are not greater in and of themselves than those ordinarily encountered in daily life or during the performance of routine physical or psychological examinations or tests" (15). It has been questioned whether the "daily life" used for comparison should be that of the general population or that of the participant. Using the participant's daily life as the standard might make a higher level of risk acceptable; therefore, the general population standard is advised (10). Anything beyond minimal risk must be weighed carefully against the potential benefits to the woman and the fetus when the advisability of participation is considered. When a pregnancy has been exposed to risk in the conduct of research, the woman should be strongly encouraged to participate in follow-up evaluations to assess the impact on her and her fetus or child.

It is appropriate for investigators and sponsors, with the approval of the IRB, to require a negative pregnancy test result as a criterion for participation in research when the research may pose more than minimal risk to the fetus. For an adolescent, the process of informed consent should include a discussion about pregnancy testing and the management of pregnancy test results, including whether the results will be shared with her parents or guardian.

Similarly, it is reasonable for investigators and research sponsors, with the IRB's approval, to require the use of effective birth control measures for women of reproductive capacity as an inclusion criterion for participation in research that may entail more than minimal risk to the fetus. Consultation with an obstetrician–gynecologist or other knowledgeable professional is encouraged if questions arise about efficacy and risk of contraceptive measures.

Some study protocols mandate use of a specific contraceptive method, such as oral contraceptives or an intrauterine device. These mandates are inappropriate based on the principles of respect for autonomy, beneficence, and justice. A woman should be allowed to choose a birth control method, including abstinence, according to her needs and values (16). Requiring birth control use by women who are not sexually active violates a commitment to respect them as persons. Hormonal contraceptive methods that could interfere with study results may be excluded on scientific grounds, but additional restrictions are inappropriate.

After informed discussion about the research trial, some women will decline to participate. Researchers should respect this decision and not allow patient refusal to affect subsequent clinical care. Reasonable compensation for a woman's time, effort, and expense as a participant in a research study is both acceptable and desired, but researchers should not offer inducements, financial or otherwise, to influence participation in research beyond reasonable compensation for the woman's time, effort, and expense.

Recommendations of the Committee on Ethics

Federal and state laws and regulations governing research involving women should be observed (2, 5, 11). In addi-

tion, the Committee on Ethics makes the following recommendations for research involving women:

1. Women should be presumed to be eligible for participation in all clinical studies except for those addressing health concerns solely relevant to men.
2. Women should be included in research in sufficient numbers to ensure that inferences from a clinical trial apply validly to both sexes.
3. All research on women should be conducted in a manner consistent with the following ethical principles:
   —Research should conform to general scientific standards for valid research.
   —Research may be conducted only with the informed consent of the woman.
   —Researchers should not offer inducements, financial or otherwise, to influence participation in research beyond reasonable compensation for the woman's time, effort, and expense.
   —Conscientious efforts should be made to avoid any conflicts between appropriate health care and research objectives. Health care needs of the individual woman should take precedence over research interests in all situations affecting clinical management.
4. Research involving pregnant women should conform to the following recommendations:
   —Research may be conducted only with the informed consent of the woman. Pregnant women considering participation in a research study should determine the extent to which the father is to be involved in the process of informed consent and the decision.
   —Informed consent of the father must be obtained when federal regulations require it for research that has the prospect of direct benefit to the fetus alone.
   —Research protocols should be evaluated for their potential impact on both the woman and the fetus, and that evaluation should be made as part of the process of informed consent.

In this Committee Opinion, an attempt has been made to take into account protection of human participants, the eligibility of women to participate in research, and the benefits that society could derive from participation of women in research. These potential benefits include reduction in morbidity and mortality from sex-specific disease processes, as well as reduction in fetal, infant, and maternal morbidity and mortality.

References

1. National Institutes of Health. NIH policy and guidelines on the inclusion of women and minorities as subjects in clinical research – Amended, October, 2001. Bethesda (MD): NIH; 2001. Available at http://grants.nih.gov/grants/funding/women_min/guidelines_amended_10_2001.htm. Retrieved May 1, 2007.

2. Protection of human subjects. 45 C.F.R. §46 (2006).

3. National Commission for the Protection of Human Subjects of Biomedical and Behavioral Research (US). The Belmont Report: ethical principles and guidelines for the protection of human subjects of research. Washington, DC: U.S. Government Printing Office; 1979. Available at: http://www.hhs.gov/ohrp/humansubjects/guidance/belmont.htm. Retrieved May 1, 2007.

4. World Medical Association. Declaration of Helsinki: Ethical principles for medical research involving human subjects. Ferney-Voltaire (France): WMA; 2004. Available at: http://www.wma.net/e/policy/pdf/17c.pdf. Retrieved May 1, 2007.

5. Additional protections for pregnant women, human fetuses and neonates involved in research. 45 C.F.R. §§46.201-207 Subpart B (2006).

6. Research on transplantation of fetal tissue. Informed consent of donor. 42 U.S.C. §289g-1(b) (2000).

7. Beauchamp TL. The intersection of research and practice. In: Goldworth A, Silverman W, Stevenson DK, Young EW, Rivers R. Ethics and perinatology. New York (NY): Oxford University Press; 1995. p. 231–44.

8. Innovative practice: ethical guidelines. ACOG Committee Opinion No. 352. American College of Obstetricians and Gynecologists. Obstet Gynecol 2006;108:1589–95.

9. NIH Revitalization Act of 1993, Pub. L. No. 103-43 (1993).

10. National Bioethics Advisory Commission. Ethical and policy issues in research involving human participants. Bethesda (MD): NBAC; 2001. Available at: http://www.georgetown.edu/research/nrcbl/nbac/human/overvol1.pdf. Retrieved May 1, 2007.

11. Additional protections for children involved as subjects in research. 45 C.F.R. §§46.401–409 Subpart D (2006).

12. General requirements for informed consent. 45 CFR §46.116 (2006).

13. Institute of Medicine (US). Women and health research: ethical and legal issues of including women in clinical studies. Vol. 1. Washington, DC: National Academy Press; 1994.

14. Appelbaum PS, Roth LH, Lidz CW, Benson P, Winslade W. False hopes and best data: consent to research and the therapeutic misconception. Hastings Cent Rep 1987;17(2):20–4.

15. Definitions. 45 C.F.R. §46.102 (2006).

16. Anderson JR, Schonfeld TL, Kelso TK, Prentice ED. Women in early phase trials: an IRB's deliberations. IRB 2003;25 (4):7–11.

Research involving women. ACOG Committee Opinion No. 377. American College of Obstetricians and Gynecologists. Obstet Gynecol 2007;110:731–6.

ISSN 1074-861X

ACOG COMMITTEE OPINION

Number 385 • November 2007

The Limits of Conscientious Refusal in Reproductive Medicine

Committee on Ethics

ABSTRACT: Health care providers occasionally may find that providing indicated, even standard, care would present for them a personal moral problem—a conflict of conscience—particularly in the field of reproductive medicine. Although respect for conscience is important, conscientious refusals should be limited if they constitute an imposition of religious or moral beliefs on patients, negatively affect a patient's health, are based on scientific misinformation, or create or reinforce racial or socioeconomic inequalities. Conscientious refusals that conflict with patient well-being should be accommodated only if the primary duty to the patient can be fulfilled. All health care providers must provide accurate and unbiased information so that patients can make informed decisions. Where conscience implores physicians to deviate from standard practices, they must provide potential patients with accurate and prior notice of their personal moral commitments. Physicians and other health care providers have the duty to refer patients in a timely manner to other providers if they do not feel that they can in conscience provide the standard reproductive services that patients request. In resource-poor areas, access to safe and legal reproductive services should be maintained. Providers with moral or religious objections should either practice in proximity to individuals who do not share their views or ensure that referral processes are in place. In an emergency in which referral is not possible or might negatively have an impact on a patient's physical or mental health, providers have an obligation to provide medically indicated and requested care.

The American College of Obstetricians and Gynecologists
Women's Health Care Physicians

Physicians and other providers may not always agree with the decisions patients make about their own health and health care. Such differences are expected—and, indeed, underlie the American model of informed consent and respect for patient autonomy. Occasionally, however, providers anticipate that providing indicated, even standard, care would present for them a personal moral problem—a conflict of conscience. In such cases, some providers claim a right to refuse to provide certain services, refuse to refer patients to another provider for these services, or even decline to inform patients of their existing options (1).

Conscientious refusals have been particularly widespread in the arena of reproductive medicine, in which there are deep divisions regarding the moral acceptability of pregnancy termination and contraception. In Texas, for example, a pharmacist rejected a rape victim's prescription for emergency contraception, arguing that dispensing the medication was a "violation of morals" (2). In Virginia, a 42-year-old mother of two was refused a prescription for emergency contraception, became pregnant, and ultimately underwent an abortion she tried to prevent by requesting emergency contraception (3). In California, a physician refused to perform intrauterine insemination for a lesbian couple, prompted by religious beliefs and disapproval of lesbians having children (4). In Nebraska, a 19-year-old woman with a life-threatening pulmonary embolism at 10 weeks of gestation was refused a first-trimester pregnancy termination when admitted to a religiously affiliated hospital and was ultimately transferred by ambulance to another facility to undergo the procedure (5). At the heart of each of these examples of refusal is a claim of conscience—a claim that to provide certain services would compromise the moral integrity of a provider or institution.

In this opinion, the American College of Obstetricians and Gynecologists (ACOG) Committee on Ethics considers the issues raised by conscientious refusals in reproductive medicine and outlines a framework for defining the ethically appropriate limits of conscientious refusal in reproductive health contexts. The committee begins by offering a definition of conscience and describing what might constitute an authentic claim of conscience. Next, it discusses the limits of conscientious refusals, describing how claims of conscience should be weighed in the context of other values critical to the ethical provision of health care. It then outlines options for public policy regarding conscientious refusals in reproductive medicine. Finally, the committee proposes a series of recommendations that maximize accommodation of an individual's religious or moral beliefs while avoiding imposition of these beliefs on others or interfering with the safe, timely, and financially feasible access to reproductive health care that all women deserve.

Defining Conscience

In this effort to reconcile the sometimes competing demands of religious or moral freedom and reproductive rights, it is important to characterize what is meant by conscience. *Conscience* has been defined as the private, constant, ethically attuned part of the human character. It operates as an internal sanction that comes into play through critical reflection about a certain action or inaction (6). An appeal to conscience would express a sentiment such as "If I were to do 'x,' I could not live with myself/I would hate myself/I wouldn't be able to sleep at night." According to this definition, not to act in accordance with one's conscience is to betray oneself—to risk personal wholeness or identity. Thus, what is taken seriously and is the specific focus of this document is not simply a broad claim to provider autonomy (7), but rather the particular claim to a provider's right to protect his or her *moral integrity*—to uphold the "soundness, reliability, wholeness and integration of [one's] moral character" (8).

Personal conscience, so conceived, is not merely a source of potential conflict. Rather, it has a critical and useful place in the practice of medicine. In many cases, it can foster thoughtful, effective, and humane care. Ethical decision making in medicine often touches on individuals' deepest identity-conferring beliefs about the nature and meaning of creating and sustaining life (9). Yet, conscience also may conflict with professional and ethical standards and result in inefficiency, adverse outcomes, violation of patients' rights, and erosion of trust if, for example, one's conscience limits the information or care provided to a patient. Finding a balance between respect for conscience and other important values is critical to the ethical practice of medicine.

In some circumstances, respect for conscience must be weighed against respect for particular social values. Challenges to a health care professional's integrity may occur when a practitioner feels that actions required by an external authority violate the goals of medicine and his or her fiduciary obligations to the patient. Established clinical norms may come into conflict with guidelines imposed by law, regulation, or public policy. For example, policies that mandate physician reporting of undocumented patients to immigration authorities conflict with norms such as privacy and confidentiality and the primary principle of nonmaleficence that govern the provider–patient relationship (10). Such challenges to integrity can result in considerable moral distress for providers and are best met through organized advocacy on the part of professional organizations (11, 12). When threats to patient well-being and the health care professional's integrity are at issue, some individual providers find a conscience-based refusal to comply with policies and acceptance of any associated professional and personal consequences to be the only morally tenable course of action (10).

Claims of conscience are not always genuine. They may mask distaste for certain procedures, discriminatory attitudes, or other self-interested motives (13). Providers who decide not to perform abortions primarily because they find the procedure unpleasant or because they fear criticism from those in society who advocate against it do not have a genuine claim of conscience. Nor do providers who refuse to provide care for individuals because of fear of disease transmission to themselves or other patients. Positions that are merely self-protective do not constitute the basis for a genuine claim of conscience. Furthermore, the logic of conscience, as a form of self-reflection on and judgment about whether one's own acts are obligatory or prohibited, means that it would be odd or absurd to say "I would have a guilty conscience if she did 'x.'" Although some have raised concerns about complicity in the context of referral to another provider for requested medical care, the logic of conscience entails that to act in accordance with conscience, the provider need not rebuke other providers or obstruct them from performing an act (8). Finally, referral to another provider need not be conceptualized as a repudiation or compromise of one's own values, but instead can be seen as an acknowledgment of both the widespread and thoughtful disagreement among physicians and society at large and the moral sincerity of others with whom one disagrees (14).

The authenticity of conscience can be assessed through inquiry into 1) the extent to which the underlying values asserted constitute a core component of a provider's identity, 2) the depth of the provider's reflection on the issue at hand, and 3) the likelihood that the provider will experience guilt, shame, or loss of self-respect by performing the act in question (9). It is the genuine claim of conscience that is considered next, in the context of the values that guide ethical health care.

Defining Limits for Conscientious Refusal

Even when appeals to conscience are genuine, when a provider's moral integrity is truly at stake, there are clearly limits to the degree to which appeals to conscience may justifiably guide decision making. Although respect for conscience is a value, it is only a prima facie value, which means it can and should be overridden in the interest of other moral obligations that outweigh it in a given circumstance. Professional ethics requires that health be delivered in a way that is respectful of patient autonomy, timely and effective, evidence based, and nondiscriminatory. By virtue of entering the profession of medicine, physicians accept a set of moral values—and duties—that are central to medical practice (15). Thus, with professional privileges come professional responsibilities to patients, which must precede a provider's personal interests (16). When conscientious refusals conflict with moral obligations that are central to the ethical practice of medicine, ethical care requires either that the physician provide care despite reservations or that there be resources in place to allow the patient to gain access to care in the presence of conscientious refusal. In the following sections, four criteria are highlighted as important in determining appropriate limits for conscientious refusal in reproductive health contexts.

1. Potential for Imposition

The first important consideration in defining limits for conscientious refusal is the degree to which a refusal constitutes an imposition on patients who do not share the objector's beliefs. One of the guiding principles in the practice of medicine is respect for patient autonomy, a principle that holds that persons should be free to choose and act without controlling constraints imposed by others. To respect a patient's autonomy is to respect her capacities and perspectives, including her right to hold certain views, make certain choices, and take certain actions based on personal values and beliefs (17). Respect involves acknowledging decision-making rights and acting in a way that enables patients to make choices for themselves. Respect for autonomy has particular importance in reproductive decision making, which involves private, personal, often pivotal decisions about sexuality and childbearing.

It is not uncommon for conscientious refusals to result in imposition of religious or moral beliefs on a patient who may not share these beliefs, which may undermine respect for patient autonomy. Women's informed requests for contraception or sterilization, for example, are an important expression of autonomous choice regarding reproductive decision making. Refusals to dispense contraception may constitute a failure to respect women's capacity to decide for themselves whether and under what circumstances to become pregnant.

Similar issues arise when patients are unable to obtain medication that has been prescribed by a physician. Although pharmacist conduct is beyond the scope of this document, refusals by other professionals can have an important impact on a physician's efforts to provide appropriate reproductive health care. Providing complete, scientifically accurate information about options for reproductive health, including contraception, sterilization, and abortion, is fundamental to respect for patient autonomy and forms the basis of informed decision making in reproductive medicine. Providers refusing to provide such information on the grounds of moral or religious objection fail in their fundamental duty to enable patients to make decisions for themselves. When the potential for imposition and breach of autonomy is high due either to controlling constraints on medication or procedures or to the provider's withholding of information critical to reproductive decision making, conscientious refusal cannot be justified.

2. Effect on Patient Health

A second important consideration in evaluating conscientious refusal is the impact such a refusal might have on well-being as the patient perceives it—in particular, the potential for harm. For the purpose of this discussion, harm refers to significant bodily harm, such as pain, disability, or death or a patient's conception of well-being. Those who choose the profession of medicine (like those who choose the profession of law or who are trustees) are bound by special *fiduciary duties*, which oblige physicians to act in good faith to protect patients' health—particularly to the extent that patients' health interests conflict with physicians' personal or self-interest (16). Although conscientious refusals stem in part from the commitment to "first, do no harm," their result can be just the opposite. For example, religiously based refusals to perform tubal sterilization at the time of cesarean delivery can place a woman in harm's way—either by putting her at risk for an undesired or unsafe pregnancy or by necessitating an additional, separate sterilization procedure with its attendant and additional risks.

Some experts have argued that in the context of pregnancy, a moral obligation to promote fetal well-being also should justifiably guide care. But even though views about the moral status of the fetus and the obligations that status confers differ widely, support of such moral pluralism does not justify an erosion of clinicians' basic obligations to protect the safety of women who are, primarily and unarguably, their patients. Indeed, in the vast majority of cases, the interests of the pregnant woman and fetus converge. For situations in which their interests diverge, the pregnant woman's autonomous decisions should be respected (18). Furthermore, in situations "in which maternal competence for medical decision making is impaired, health care providers should act in the best interests of the woman first and her fetus second" (19).

3. Scientific Integrity

The third criterion for evaluating authentic conscientious refusal is the scientific integrity of the facts supporting the objector's claim. Core to the practice of medicine is a commitment to science and evidence-based practice.

Patients rightly expect care guided by best evidence as well as information based on rigorous science. When conscientious refusals reflect a misunderstanding or mistrust of science, limits to conscientious refusal should be defined, in part, by the strength or weakness of the science on which refusals are based. In other words, claims of conscientious refusal should be considered invalid when the rationale for a refusal contradicts the body of scientific evidence.

The broad debate about refusals to dispense emergency contraception, for example, has been complicated by misinformation and a prevalent belief that emergency contraception acts primarily by preventing implantation (20). However, a large body of published evidence supports a different primary mechanism of action, namely the prevention of fertilization. A review of the literature indicates that Plan B can interfere with sperm migration and that preovulatory use of Plan B suppresses the luteinizing hormone surge, which prevents ovulation or leads to the release of ova that are resistant to fertilization. Studies do not support a major postfertilization mechanism of action (21). Although even a slight possibility of postfertilization events may be relevant to some women's decisions about whether to use contraception, provider refusals to dispense emergency contraception based on unsupported beliefs about its primary mechanism of action should not be justified.

In the context of the morally difficult and highly contentious debate about pregnancy termination, scientific integrity is one of several important considerations. For example, some have argued against providing access to abortion based on claims that induced abortion is associated with an increase in breast cancer risk; however, a 2003 U.S. National Cancer Institute panel concluded that there is well-established epidemiologic evidence that induced abortion and breast cancer are not associated (22). Refusals to provide abortion should not be justified on the basis of unsubstantiated health risks to women.

Scientific integrity is particularly important at the level of public policy, where unsound appeals to science may have masked an agenda based on religious beliefs. Delays in granting over-the-counter status for emergency contraception are one such example. Critics of the U.S. Food and Drug Administration's delay cited deep flaws in the science and evidence used to justify the delay, flaws these critics argued were indicative of unspoken and misplaced value judgments (23). Thus, the scientific integrity of a claim of refusal is an important metric in determining the acceptability of conscience-based practices or policies.

4. Potential for Discrimination

Finally, conscientious refusals should be evaluated on the basis of their potential for discrimination. Justice is a complex and important concept that requires medical professionals and policy makers to treat individuals fairly and to provide medical services in a nondiscriminatory manner. One conception of justice, sometimes referred to as the *distributive paradigm*, calls for fair allocation of society's benefits and burdens. Persons intending conscientious refusal should consider the degree to which they create or reinforce an unfair distribution of the benefits of reproductive technology. For instance, refusal to dispense contraception may place a disproportionate burden on disenfranchised women in resource-poor areas. Whereas a single, affluent professional might experience such a refusal as inconvenient and seek out another physician, a young mother of three depending on public transportation might find such a refusal to be an insurmountable barrier to medication because other options are not realistically available to her. She thus may experience loss of control of her reproductive fate and quality of life for herself and her children. Refusals that unduly burden the most vulnerable of society violate the core commitment to justice in the distribution of health resources.

Another conception of justice is concerned with matters of oppression as well as distribution (24). Thus, the impact of conscientious refusals on oppression of certain groups of people should guide limits for claims of conscience as well. Consider, for instance, refusals to provide infertility services to same-sex couples. It is likely that such couples would be able to obtain infertility services from another provider and would not have their health jeopardized, per se. Nevertheless, allowing physicians to discriminate on the basis of sexual orientation would constitute a deeper insult, namely reinforcing the scientifically unfounded idea that fitness to parent is based on sexual orientation, and, thus, reinforcing the oppressed status of same-sex couples. The concept of oppression raises the implications of all conscientious refusals for gender justice in general. Legitimizing refusals in reproductive contexts may reinforce the tendency to value women primarily with regard to their capacity for reproduction while ignoring their interests and rights as people more generally. As the place of conscience in reproductive medicine is considered, the impact of permissive policies toward conscientious refusals on the status of women must be considered seriously as well.

Some might say that it is not the job of a physician to "fix" social inequities. However, it is the responsibility, whenever possible, of physicians as advocates for patients' needs and rights not to create or reinforce racial or socioeconomic inequalities in society. Thus, refusals that create or reinforce such inequalities should raise significant caution.

Institutional and Organizational Responsibilities

Given these limits, individual practitioners may face difficult decisions about adherence to conscience in the context of professional responsibilities. Some have offered, however, that "accepting a collective obligation does not mean that all members of the profession are forced to violate their own consciences" (1). Rather, institutions and professional organizations should work to create and maintain organizational structures that ensure nondiscriminatory access to all professional services and minimize the need for individual practitioners to act in opposition to their deeply held beliefs. This requires at the very least that systems be in place for counseling and referral, particularly in resource-poor areas where conscientious refusals have significant potential to limit patient choice, and that individuals and institutions "act affirmatively to protect patients from unexpected and disruptive denials of service" (13). Individuals and institutions should support staffing that does not place practitioners or facilities in situations in which the harms and thus conflicts from conscientious refusals are likely to arise. For example, those who feel it improper to prescribe emergency contraception should not staff sites, such as emergency rooms, in which such requests are likely to arise, and prompt disposition of emergency contraception is required and often integral to professional practice. Similarly, institutions that uphold doctrinal objections should not position themselves as primary providers of emergency care for victims of sexual assault; when such patients do present for care, they should be given prophylaxis. Institutions should work toward structures that reduce the impact on patients of professionals' refusals to provide standard reproductive services.

Recommendations

Respect for conscience is one of many values important to the ethical practice of reproductive medicine. Given this framework for analysis, the ACOG Committee on Ethics proposes the following recommendations, which it believes maximize respect for health care professionals' consciences without compromising the health and well-being of the women they serve.

1. In the provision of reproductive services, the patient's well-being must be paramount. Any conscientious refusal that conflicts with a patient's well-being should be accommodated only if the primary duty to the patient can be fulfilled.

2. Health care providers must impart accurate and unbiased information so that patients can make informed decisions about their health care. They must disclose scientifically accurate and professionally accepted characterizations of reproductive health services.

3. Where conscience implores physicians to deviate from standard practices, including abortion, sterilization, and provision of contraceptives, they must provide potential patients with accurate and prior notice of their personal moral commitments. In the process of providing prior notice, physicians should not use their professional authority to argue or advocate these positions.

4. Physicians and other health care professionals have the duty to refer patients in a timely manner to other providers if they do not feel that they can in con-

science provide the standard reproductive services that their patients request.

5. In an emergency in which referral is not possible or might negatively affect a patient's physical or mental health, providers have an obligation to provide medically indicated and requested care regardless of the provider's personal moral objections.

6. In resource-poor areas, access to safe and legal reproductive services should be maintained. Conscientious refusals that undermine access should raise significant caution. Providers with moral or religious objections should either practice in proximity to individuals who do not share their views or ensure that referral processes are in place so that patients have access to the service that the physician does not wish to provide. Rights to withdraw from caring for an individual should not be a pretext for interfering with patients' rights to health care services.

7. Lawmakers should advance policies that balance protection of providers' consciences with the critical goal of ensuring timely, effective, evidence-based, and safe access to all women seeking reproductive services.

References

1. Charo RA. The celestial fire of conscience—refusing to deliver medical care. N Engl J Med 2005;352:2471–3.

2. Denial of rape victim's pills raises debate: moral, legal questions surround emergency contraception. New York (NY): Associated Press; 2004. Available at: http://www.msnbc.msn.com/id/4359430. Retrieved July 10, 2007.

3. L D. What happens when there is no plan B? Washington Post; June 4, 2006. p. B1. Available at: http://www.washingtonpost.com/wp-dyn/content/article/2006/06/02/AR2006060201405.html. Retrieved July 10, 2007.

4. Weil E. Breeder reaction: does everyone now have a right to bear children? Mother Jones 2006;31(4):33–7. Available at: http://www.motherjones.com/news/feature/2006/07/breeder_reaction.html. Retrieved July 10, 2007.

5. American Civil Liberties Union. Religious refusals and reproductive rights: ACLU Reproductive Freedom Project. New York (NY): ACLU; 2002. Available at: http://www.aclu.org/FilesPDFs/ACF911.pdf. Retrieved July 10, 2007.

6. Childress JF. Appeals to conscience. Ethics 1979;89:315–35.

7. Wicclair MR. Conscientious objection in medicine. Bioethics 2000;14:205–27.

8. Beauchamp TL, Childress JF. Principles of biomedical ethics. 5th ed. New York (NY): Oxford University Press; 2001.

9. Benjamin M. Conscience. In: Reich WT, editor. Encyclopedia of bioethics. New York (NY): Simon & Schuster Macmillan; 1995. p. 469–73.

10. Ziv TA, Lo B. Denial of care to illegal immigrants. Proposition 187 in California. N Engl J Med 1995;332:1095–8.

11. American College of Obstetricians and Gynecologists. Code of professional ethics of the American College of Obste-

tricians and Gynecologists. Washington, DC: ACOG; 2004. Available at: http://www.acog.org/from_home/acogcode.pdf. Retrieved July 10, 2007.

12. American Medical Association. Principles of medical ethics. In: Code of medical ethics of the American Medical Association: current opinions with annotations. 2006–2007 ed. Chicago (IL): AMA; 2006. p. xv.

13. Dresser R. Professionals, conformity, and conscience. Hastings Cent Rep 2005;35:9–10.

14. Blustein J. Doing what the patient orders: maintaining integrity in the doctor-patient relationship. Bioethics 1993;7:290–314.

15. Brody H, Miller FG. The internal morality of medicine: explication and application to managed care. J Med Philos 1998;23:384–410.

16. Dickens BM, Cook RJ. Conflict of interest: legal and ethical aspects. Int J Gynaecol Obstet 2006;92:192–7.

17. Faden RR, Beauchamp TL. A history and theory of informed consent. New York (NY): Oxford University Press; 1986.

18. Maternal decision making, ethics, and the law. ACOG Committee Opinion No. 321. American College of Obstetricians and Gynecologists. Obstet Gynecol 2005;106:1127–37.

19. International Federation of Gynecology and Obstetrics. Ethical guidelines regarding interventions for fetal well being. In: Ethical issues in obstetrics and gynecology. London (UK): FIGO; 2006. p. 56–7. Available at: http://www.figo.org/docs/Ethics%20Guidelines.pdf. Retrieved July 10, 2007.

20. Cantor J, Baum K. The limits of conscientious objection—may pharmacists refuse to fill prescriptions for emergency contraception? N Engl J Med 2004;351:2008–12.

21. Davidoff F, Trussell J. Plan B and the politics of doubt. JAMA 2006;296:1775–8.

22. Induced abortion and breast cancer risk. ACOG Committee Opinion No. 285. American College of Obstetricians and Gynecologists. Obstet Gynecol 2003;102:433–5.

23. Grimes DA. Emergency contraception: politics trumps science at the U.S. Food and Drug Administration. Obstet Gynecol 2004;104:220–1.

24. Young IM. Justice and the politics of difference. Princeton (NJ): Princeton University Press; 1990.

The limits of conscientious refusal in reproductive medicine. ACOG Committee Opinion No. 385. American College of Obstetricians and Gynecologists. Obstet Gynecol 2007;110:1203–8.

ISSN 1074-861X

ACOG COMMITTEE OPINION

Number 389 • December 2007

Human Immunodeficiency Virus*

Committee on Ethics

ABSTRACT: Because human immunodeficiency virus (HIV) infection often is detected through prenatal and sexually transmitted disease testing, an obstetrician–gynecologist may be the first health professional to provide care for a woman infected with HIV. Universal testing with patient notification and right of refusal ("opt-out" testing) is recommended by most national organizations and federal agencies. Although opt-out and "opt-in" testing (but not mandatory testing) are both ethically acceptable, the former approach may identify more women who are eligible for therapy and may have public health advantages. It is unethical for an obstetrician–gynecologist to refuse to accept a patient or to refuse to continue providing health care for a patient solely because she is, or is thought to be, seropositive for HIV. Health care professionals who are infected with HIV should adhere to the fundamental professional obligation to avoid harm to patients. Physicians who believe that they have been at significant risk of being infected should be tested voluntarily for HIV.

Between 1 million and 1.2 million individuals in the United States are estimated to be living with human immunodeficiency virus (HIV) or acquired immunodeficiency syndrome (AIDS) (1). Women represent the fastest-growing group of individuals with new HIV infections (2). Many women who are infected with HIV are not aware of their serostatus (3).

Human immunodeficiency virus often is diagnosed in women during prenatal antibody screening or in conjunction with screening for sexually transmitted diseases (STDs). Because many women initially identified as infected with HIV are not aware that they have been exposed to HIV and do not consider themselves to be at risk, universal testing with patient notification is more effective than targeted, risk-based testing in identifying those who are infected with HIV (4). The tension between competing goals for HIV testing—testing broadly in order to treat the maximum number of women infected with HIV and, if pregnant, to protect their newborns, and counseling thoroughly in order to maximally protect a woman's autonomy and right to participate in decision making—has sparked considerable debate.

Because HIV infection often is detected through prenatal and STD screening, it is not uncommon for an obstetrician–gynecologist to be the first health professional to provide care for an infected woman. This Committee Opinion is designed to provide guidance to obstetrician–gynecologists regarding ethical issues associated with HIV testing, including the use of newly developed rapid HIV tests and disclosure of positive test results. It also outlines responsibilities related to patient care for women who are infected with HIV, access for affected couples to assisted reproductive technology, and the health care professional who is infected with HIV.

Human Immunodeficiency Virus Counseling and Testing

The major ethical principles that must be considered when formulating policies for HIV counseling and testing include respect for autonomy, confidentiality, justice, protection of vulnerable individuals, and beneficence to both the woman tested and, if she is pregnant, to her newborn as well. Individuals offering testing need to be mindful not only of the benefits of testing but also its potential risks because, if a woman's test result is positive, she faces the possibility of being ostra-

The American College of Obstetricians and Gynecologists
Women's Health Care Physicians

---

*Update of "Human Immunodeficiency Virus" in *Ethics in Obstetrics and Gynecology*, Second Edition, 2004.

cized by her family, friends, and community or being subjected to intimate partner violence. In addition, although the overt stigma of HIV infection has been reduced over the past 20 years, the potential for job discrimination, loss of health insurance, and loss of housing still exists.

Over time, three potential strategies for HIV testing have been considered by public health and public policy officials: 1) universal testing with patient notification and right of refusal, also called "opt-out" testing; 2) voluntary testing with pretest counseling regarding risks and benefits, also called "opt-in" testing; and 3) mandatory testing with no right of refusal. In order to understand their ethical merits, each is considered briefly in the sections that follow. Increasingly, national organizations and federal agencies have recommended opt-out testing in preference to other strategies.

Universal Testing With Patient Notification and Right of Refusal—Opt-Out Testing

Opt-out testing removes the requirement for pretest counseling and detailed, testing-related informed consent. Under the opt-out strategy, physicians must inform patients that routine blood work will include HIV testing and that they have the right to refuse this test. The goal of this strategy is to make HIV testing less cumbersome and more likely to be performed by incorporating it into the routine battery of tests (eg, the first-trimester prenatal panel or blood counts and cholesterol screening for annual examinations). In theory, if testing barriers are reduced, more physicians may offer testing, which may lead to the identification and treatment of more women who are infected with HIV and, if pregnant, to the prevention of mother-to-infant transmission of HIV. This testing strategy aims to balance competing ethical considerations. On the one hand, personal freedom (autonomy) is diminished. On the other hand, there are medical and social benefits for the woman and, if she is pregnant, her newborn from identifying HIV infection. Although many welcome the now widely endorsed opt-out testing policy for the potential benefits it confers, others have raised concerns about the possibility that the requirement for notification before testing will be ignored, particularly in today's busy practice environment. Indeed, the opt-out strategy is an ethically acceptable testing strategy only if the patient is given the option to refuse testing. In the absence of that notification, this approach is merely mandatory testing in disguise. If opt-out testing is elected as a testing strategy, a clinician must notify the patient that HIV testing is to be performed. Refusal of testing should not have an adverse effect on the care the patient receives or lead to denial of health care. This guarantee of a right to refuse testing ensures that respect for a woman's autonomy is not completely abridged in the quest to achieve a difficult-to-reach public health goal.

Voluntary Testing With Pretest Counseling Regarding Risks and Benefits—Opt-In Testing

Voluntary testing with counseling is the strategy most consistent with respect for patient autonomy. Under this option, physicians provide both pretest and posttest counseling. Some physicians may perform such counseling themselves, whereas others may prefer to refer the patient for counseling and testing. (Such specialized HIV counseling was more widely available in previous years but has become less available as more health care professionals have become more comfortable treating patients with HIV and as the opt-out approach to testing—an approach that places less emphasis on pretest counseling—has become more common.) In addition to medical information, such counseling could include information regarding potential uses of test information and legal requirements pertaining to the release of information. Patients should be told what information will be communicated and to whom and the possible implications of reporting the information. This approach to testing maintains HIV's status as being in a class by itself (sui generis), even as many ethicists have acknowledged the end to the exceptionalism that marked this disease in the early years of the epidemic (5).

Mandatory Testing With No Right of Refusal

Mandatory testing strategies are problematic because they abridge a woman's autonomy. In addition, during pregnancy, the public health objective of this strategy, identification of women who are infected with HIV who will benefit from treatment, has been accomplished in certain populations by other ethically sound testing strategies noted previously (6). Some see mandatory testing as a more efficient way of achieving universal testing. Advocates support this strategy, believing it provides the greatest good for the greatest number and that the potential benefit to the woman and, if pregnant, her newborn justifies abridging a woman's autonomy. However, because of the limits it places on autonomy, the Committee on Ethics believes that mandatory HIV screening without informing those screened and offering them the option of refusal is inappropriate. Mandatory prenatal testing is difficult to defend ethically and has few precedents in modern medicine, although HIV testing of newborns is now required in New York, Connecticut, and Illinois (There are provisions, however, that permit refusal in a few defined circumstances.) (7, 8). Importantly, mandatory testing may compromise the ability to form an effective physician–patient relationship at the very time when this relationship is critical to the success of treatment.

Selecting a Testing Strategy

Among these three strategies, the opt-out approach is now recommended by most national organizations and federal agencies. For prenatal HIV testing, universal testing with patient notification and right of refusal was recommended by the Institute of Medicine to address clinicians' concerns that pretest counseling and informed consent mandates for routine voluntary testing in pregnancy were too time consuming and, thus, reduced the likelihood of testing being offered (9). The Centers for Disease Control and Prevention, the American Academy of Pediatrics, and the American College of Obstetricians and Gynecologists (ACOG) endorse this approach (10, 11). Evidence suggests that this strategy may be acceptable to many pregnant women (12, 13). "To expand the gains made in diagnosing HIV infection among pregnant women," the Centers for Disease Control and Prevention (14) has recently released, and ACOG (15) has adopted, recommendations to make HIV testing a "routine part of medical care" using a similar opt-out approach for all women at the time of routine health care visits.

In recommending the opt-out approach for prenatal HIV testing, ACOG encouraged Fellows to include counseling as a routine part of care but not as a prerequisite for, or barrier to, prenatal HIV testing (11). Similarly, the American Medical Association, in recommending that universal HIV testing of all pregnant women with patient notification of the right of refusal be a routine component of prenatal care, indicated that basic counseling on HIV prevention and treatment also should be provided to the patient, consistent with the principles of informed consent (16). Accordingly, if adopting this option, physicians should be prepared to provide both pretest and posttest counseling. Broad implementation of an opt-out strategy, however, will require changing laws in states that require detailed and specific counseling and consent before testing. Physicians should be aware of the laws in their states that affect HIV testing. The National HIV/AIDS Clinicians' Consultation Center at the University of California—San Francisco maintains an online compendium of state HIV testing laws that can be a useful resource (see http://www.ucsf.edu/hivcntr/).

The benefits of identifying those with HIV infection will be limited if necessary treatments are unavailable or not covered by appropriate insurance. Where access to HIV treatment is limited, Fellows should advocate for changes in existing policies to broaden access.

Special Issues Involved With Rapid Human Immunodeficiency Virus Testing

Technologies have recently become available that allow for testing with rapid results (eg, turnaround less than 1 hour). The advantage of these tools is that patients can be informed of their results at the same visit at which the testing occurs. In that manner, it is possible to lower the rate of loss to follow-up associated with the traditional two-stage testing and notification approach. Nothing about rapid testing precludes the need for a patient to opt-in or to be offered the opportunity to opt-out of testing (depending on which strategy is adopted). Rapid testing should not be implemented either as mandatory

testing or testing performed without informing the patient that she will be tested.

In communities with a relatively low prevalence of HIV, rapid testing can present certain logistic difficulties. With the traditional approach, testing would occur during an initial visit, and results would be provided during a follow-up encounter. That would give the health care professional an opportunity to arrange for an individual with expertise in posttest counseling to be available in a circumstance in which the health care professional knew that a patient was returning to receive a positive result. A program of testing and notification at the same visit does not allow the health care professional the luxury of notifying a counselor before a patient who is infected with HIV returns for a visit or of steering an individual who is infected with HIV to a certain session at which the counselor is routinely available. However, the obligation to make sure that appropriate counseling and support services are available still holds. Health care professionals should develop links with individuals who can provide those services on an emergent basis or train their own staff to handle the initial encounter and thereafter transition infected individuals to professionals who can serve as ongoing resources to them.

Human Immunodeficiency Virus Reporting and Partner Notification

The clinician providing care for a woman who is infected with HIV has important responsibilities concerning disclosure of the patient's serostatus. Clinicians providing health care should be aware of and respect legal requirements regarding confidentiality and disclosure of HIV-related clinical information.

In considering disclosure, clinicians may have competing obligations: protecting the patient's confidentiality, on the one hand, and disclosing test results to prevent substantial harm to a third party, on the other. In some jurisdictions, a breach of confidentiality may be required by mandatory reporting regulations. Even absent legal requirements, in some situations the need to protect potentially exposed third parties may seem compelling. In these situations, the clinician first should educate the patient about her rights and responsibilities and encourage her to inform any third parties involved. If she remains reluctant to voluntarily share information regarding her infection, consultation with an institutional ethics committee, a medical ethics specialist, or an attorney may be helpful in deciding whether to disclose her HIV status. In general, a breach of confidentiality may be ethically justified for purposes of partner notification when all of the following four conditions are met:

1. There is a high probability of harm to the partner.
2. The potential harm is serious.
3. The information communicated can be used to prevent harm.

4. Greater good will result from breaking confidentiality rather than maintaining it.

Indeed, many if not all of these conditions are likely met for intimate partners of women and men who are infected with HIV. Nevertheless, when a breach of confidence is contemplated, practitioners should weigh the potential harm to the patient and to society at large. Negative consequences of breaking confidentiality may include the following situations:

- Personal risks to the individual whose confidence is breached, such as serious implications for the patient's relationship with family and friends, the threat of discrimination in employment and housing, intimate partner violence, and the impact on family members
- Loss of patient trust, which may reduce the physician's ability to communicate effectively and provide services
- A ripple effect among cohorts of women that may deter other women at risk from accepting testing and have a serious negative impact on the educational efforts that lie at the heart of attempts to reduce the spread of disease

If, on balance, a breach of confidence is deemed necessary, practitioners should work in advance to anticipate and manage potentially negative consequences (ie, reactions of intimate partners, family). As well, practitioners should consider whether the goal of maintaining patient privacy would be better served by personal communication with the individual placed at risk by the patient's seropositivity or by notification of local public health authorities. In some areas, anonymous notification of sexual contacts is possible through local or state departments of health. As a practical matter, because disclosure is only possible when the index case freely identifies at-risk partners, superseding an individual's refusal to disclose should be a rare occurrence.

Confidentiality should not be breached solely because of perceived risk to health care workers. Health care workers should rely on strict observance of standard precautions rather than obtaining information about a patient's serostatus to minimize risk. Even in the setting of an accidental needle-stick or other exposure, the patient's consent for release of serostatus (or for testing) should be obtained. Efforts to protect patient confidentiality should not prevent other health care professionals caring for the patient from learning her serostatus, information they need to ensure optimal medical management.

Health Care Professionals' Obligation to Provide Care

It is unethical for an obstetrician–gynecologist to refuse to accept a patient or to refuse to continue providing health care for a patient solely because she is, or is thought to be, seropositive for HIV. Refusing to provide care to women who are infected with HIV for fear of contracting HIV infection or simply as a practice preference is unreasonable, unscientific, and unethical.

Epidemiologic studies have shown that the risk of HIV transmission from patient to health care professional is exceedingly low and is related to needle stick or intraoperative injury or to potentially infectious fluid that comes in contact with a mucous membrane (17). Most contacts between health care professionals and women who are infected with HIV occur, however, during routine obstetric and gynecologic care. Health care practitioners should observe standard precautions with all patients to minimize skin, mucous membrane, and percutaneous exposure to blood and body fluids to protect against a variety of pathogens, including HIV.

Health care professionals who fail to provide care to women who are infected with HIV because of personal practice preferences violate professional ethical standards. The public appropriately expects that health care practitioners will not discriminate based on diagnosis, provided that the patient's care falls within their scope of practice. Physicians should demonstrate integrity, compassion, honesty, and empathy. Failure to provide health care to a woman solely because she is infected with HIV violates these fundamental characteristics. As with any other patient, it is acceptable, however, to refer women who are infected with HIV for care that the physician is not competent to provide or if care elsewhere would be more convenient or associated with decreased financial burden to the patient.

Assisted Reproductive Technology

There is an emerging consensus that indications for assisted reproductive technology use should not vary with HIV serostatus; therefore, assisted reproductive technology should be offered to couples in which one or both partners are infected with HIV. This approach is consistent with the principles of respect for autonomy and beneficence (18, 19). In addition, those who advocate providing these services cite three clinical arguments to support their position:

1. Therapeutic improvements in the management of HIV infection have enhanced both quality and length of life for individuals who are seropositive for HIV.
2. Advances in prenatal therapy have substantially reduced the risk of mother-to-infant HIV transmission.
3. Current assisted reproductive technology methods may reduce transmission of HIV from an infected partner to an uninfected partner relative to natural means of conception.

The Ethics Committee of the American Society for Reproductive Medicine has said, "Health care workers who are willing to provide reproductive assistance to couples whose offspring are irreducibly at risk for a serious genetic disease should find it ethically acceptable to treat HIV-positive individuals or couples who are willing to take reasonable steps to minimize the risks of transmission." (20).

Those who oppose offering these technologies to couples who are infected with HIV cite two major objections:

1. Uncertain long-term parental prognosis
2. The continuing risk of mother-to-infant HIV transmission

The ethical underpinning of this opposition is that it is not felt to be in the best interest of the child to be born to a parent who may not be available for continued child-rearing. In addition, the risk of mother-to-infant transmission places the infant at risk of acquiring a highly debilitating illness. Yet as stated previously, HIV infection currently is a manageable chronic illness with a life-expectancy equivalent to that with many other chronic diseases for which assisted reproductive technology is not routinely precluded. Further, interventions, such as antiretroviral therapy or cesarean delivery or both, reduce the absolute risk of transmission to a level comparable, again, to risks significantly lower than those tolerated among couples choosing assisted reproductive technology (eg, parents who are carriers of autosomal recessive conditions) or risks often assumed as part of assisted reproductive technology (eg, risks of prematurity from multiple pregnancies).

Health Care Professionals Who Are Infected With Human Immunodeficiency Virus

In making decisions about patient care, health care professionals who are infected with HIV should adhere to the fundamental professional obligation to avoid harm to patients. Physicians who have reason to believe that they have been at significant risk of being infected should be tested voluntarily for HIV for the protection of their patients as well as for their own benefit. The physician as a patient is entitled to the same rights to privacy and confidentiality as any other patient.

Although the risk of clinician-to-patient transmission is extremely low, all infected physicians must make a decision as to which procedures they can continue to perform safely. This decision primarily will depend on the particular surgical technique involved and also on the physician's level of expertise and medical condition, including mental status. The clinician's decision should be made in consultation with a personal physician and may possibly involve such other responsible individuals as the chief of the department, the hospital's director of infectious diseases, the chief of the medical staff, or a specialized advisory panel. If physicians avoid procedures that place patients at risk of harm, they have no obligation

to inform the patient of their positive HIV serostatus. Physicians who are infected with HIV should follow standard precautions, including the appropriate use of hand-washing, protective barriers, and care in the use and disposal of needles and other sharp instruments.

Recommendations

The Committee on Ethics makes the following recommendations:

- All women, pregnant or not, should have the opportunity to learn their HIV serostatus.
- Women should, at a minimum, be told that they are being tested and that they may refuse such tests.
- Although opt-out and opt-in testing are both ethically acceptable, the former approach may identify more women who are eligible for therapy and may have public health advantages.
- Rapid testing carries the same ethical responsibilities as "standard" testing.
- It is unethical for an obstetrician–gynecologist to refuse to accept a patient or to discontinue providing health care for a patient solely because she is, or is thought to be, seropositive for HIV.
- Seropositivity for HIV per se should not be used as a reason to refuse to provide assisted reproductive technology to a family.

References

1. Epidemiology of HIV/AIDS—United States, 1981–2005. MMWR Morb Mortal Wkly Rep 2006;55:589–92.

2. Chou R, Smits AK, Huffman LH, Fu R, Korthuis PT. Prenatal screening for HIV: a review of the evidence for the U.S. Preventive Services Task Force. U.S. Preventive Services Task Force. Ann Intern Med 2005;143:38–54.

3. Gwinn M, Wortley PM. Epidemiology of HIV infection in women and newborns. Clin Obstet Gynecol 1996;39: 292–304.

4. Revised recommendations for HIV screening of pregnant women. MMWR Recomm Rep 2001;50(RR–19):63–85; quiz CE1–19a2–CE6–19a2.

5. Bayer R, Fairchild AL. Changing the paradigm for HIV testing—the end of exceptionalism. N Engl J Med 2006;355: 647–9.

6. Prenatal discussion of HIV testing and maternal HIV testing—14 states, 1996–1997. MMWR Morb Mortal Wkly Rep 1999;48:401–4.

7. HIV testing among pregnant women—United States and Canada, 1998–2001. MMWR Morb Mortal Wkly Rep 2002; 51:1013–6.

8. Perinatal HIV Prevention Act. 410 ILCS § 335 (2006).

9. Institute of Medicine (US). Reducing the odds: preventing perinatal transmission of HIV in the United States. Washington, DC: National Academy Press; 1999.

10. Prenatal and perinatal human immunodeficiency virus testing: expanded recommendations. ACOG Committee

Opinion No. 304. American College of Obstetricians and Gynecologists. Obstet Gynecol 2004;104:1119–24.

11. American Academy of Pediatrics, American College of Obstetricians and Gynecologists. Joint statement on human immunodeficiency virus screening. Elk Grove Village (IL): AAP; Washington, DC: ACOG; 2006. Available at: http://www.acog.org/publications/policy_statements/sop9905.cfm. Retrieved July 10, 2007.

12. Stringer EM, Stringer JS, Cliver SP, Goldenberg RL, Goepfert AR. Evaluation of a new testing policy for human immunodeficiency virus to improve screening rates. Obstet Gynecol 2001;98:1104–8.

13. Jayaraman GC, Preiksaitis JK, Larke B. Mandatory reporting of HIV infection and opt-out prenatal screening for HIV infection: effect on testing rates. CMAJ 2003;168: 679–82.

14. Branson BM, Handsfield HH, Lampe MA, Janssen RS, Taylor AW, Lyss SB, et al. Revised recommendations for HIV testing of adults, adolescents, and pregnant women in health-care settings. MMWR Recomm Rep 2006;55 (RR–14):1–17; quiz CE1–4.

15. Primary and preventive care: periodic assessments. ACOG Committee Opinion No. 357. American College of Obstetricians and Gynecologists. Obstet Gynecol 2006;108: 1615–22.

16. American Medical Association. Universal, routine screening of pregnant women for HIV infection. CSA Report I–01. Council on Scientific Affairs. Chicago (IL): AMA; 2001. Available at: http://www.ama-assn.org/ama/pub/category/13548.html. Retrieved July 10, 2007.

17. Updated U.S. Public Health Service guidelines for the management of occupational exposures to HBV, HCV, and HIV and recommendations for postexposure prophylaxis. MMWR Recomm Rep 2001;50(RR–11):1–52.

18. Anderson DJ. Assisted reproduction for couples infected with the human immunodeficiency virus type 1. Fertil Steril 1999;72:592–4.

19. Minkoff H, Santoro N. Ethical considerations in the treatment of infertility in women with human immunodeficiency virus infection. N Engl J Med 2000;342:1748–50.

20. Human immunodeficiency virus and infertility treatment. Ethics Committee of the American Society for Reproductive Medicine. Fertil Steril 2002;77:218–22.

Human immunodeficiency virus. ACOG Committee Opinion No. 389. American College of Obstetricians and Gynecologists. Obstet Gynecol 2007;110:1473–8.

ISSN 1074-861X

ACOG COMMITTEE OPINION

Number 390 • December 2007

Ethical Decision Making in Obstetrics and Gynecology*

Committee on Ethics

ABSTRACT: Physicians vary widely in their familiarity with ethical theories and methods and their sensitivity toward ethical issues. It is important for physicians to improve their skills in addressing ethical questions. Obstetrician–gynecologists who are familiar with the concepts of medical ethics will be better able to approach complex ethical situations in a clear and structured way. By considering the ethical frameworks involving principles, virtues, care and feminist perspectives, concern for community, and case precedents, they can enhance their ability to make ethically justifiable clinical decisions. Guidelines, consisting of several logical steps, are offered to aid the practitioner in analyzing and resolving ethical problems.

The importance of ethics in the practice of medicine was manifested at least 2,500 years ago in the Hippocratic tradition, which emphasized the virtues that were expected to characterize and guide the behavior of physicians. Over the past 50 years, medical technology expanded exponentially, so that obstetrician–gynecologists have had to face complex ethical questions regarding assisted reproductive technologies, prenatal diagnosis and selective abortion, medical care at the beginning and end of life, the use of genetic information, and the like. Medical knowledge alone is not sufficient to solve these problems. Instead, responsible decisions in these areas depend on a thoughtful consideration of the values, interests, goals, rights, and obligations of those involved. All of these are the concern of medical ethics. The formal discipline of biomedical ethics and structured ethical analysis can help physicians resolve ethical dilemmas.

Physicians vary widely in their familiarity with ethical theories and methods and their sensitivity toward ethical issues. It is important for physicians to improve their skills in addressing ethical questions through formal undergraduate and graduate medical education, organized continuing education,

or personal experience and reading as well as discussion with others.

Ethical Frameworks and Perspectives

Principle-Based Ethics

In recent decades, medical ethics has been dominated by principle-based ethics (1–3). In this approach, four principles offer a systematic and relatively objective way to identify, analyze, and address ethical issues, problems, and dilemmas: 1) respect for patient autonomy, 2) beneficence, 3) nonmaleficence, and 4) justice. (These four principles will be discussed in some detail in subsequent sections.) However, critics claim that a principle-based approach cannot adequately resolve or even helpfully evaluate many difficult clinical problems. As a result, several other perspectives and frameworks have emerged: virtue-based ethics, an ethic of care, feminist ethics, communitarian ethics, and case-based reasoning, all of which have merit as well as limitations (2–8). As this discussion will stress, these different perspectives and frameworks are not necessarily mutually exclusive. They often are complementary because each emphasizes some important features of moral reasoning, agents, situations, actions, or relationships. Perspectives such as an ethic of care or feminist ethics also may change the lens through which to view both principles

The American College of Obstetricians and Gynecologists
Women's Health Care Physicians

*Update of "Ethical Decision Making in Obstetrics and Gynecology" in *Ethics in Obstetrics and Gynecology*, Second Edition, 2004.

and particular situations in which decisions have to be made.

Virtue Ethics

A virtue-based approach relies on qualities of character that dispose health professionals to make choices and decisions that achieve the well-being of patients, respect their autonomous choices, and the like (8, 9). These qualities of character include trustworthiness, prudence, fairness, fortitude, temperance, integrity, self-effacement, and compassion. Virtues need not replace principles as a basis for ethical decision making or conduct. Indeed, some virtues correlate with principles and dispose people to act according to those principles—for instance, the virtue of benevolence disposes agents to act beneficently. Virtues also can complement and enhance the principles of medical ethics. Interpreting the principles, applying them in concrete situations, and setting priorities among them require the judgment of morally sensitive professionals with good moral character and the relevant virtues. Furthermore, in deliberating what to do, a physician may find helpful guidance by asking, "What would a good, that is, morally virtuous, physician do in these circumstances?" Ethical insight may come from imagining which actions would be compatible with, for instance, being a compassionate or honest or trustworthy physician.

Care-Based Ethics

Care-based ethics, also called "the ethic of care," directs attention to dimensions of moral experience often excluded from or neglected by traditional ethical theories (10). It is concerned primarily with responsibilities that arise from attachment to others rather than with impartial principles so emphasized in many ethical theories. The moral foundations of an ethic of care are located not in rights and duties, but rather in commitment, empathy, compassion, caring, and love (11). This perspective also pays closer attention to context and particularity than to abstract principles and rules. It suggests that good ethical decisions both result from personal caring in relationships, and should consider the impact of different possible actions on those relationships. An ethic of care overlaps with a virtue ethic, in emphasizing the caregiver's orientation and qualities. In this ethical approach, care represents the fundamental orientation of obstetrics and gynecology as well as much of medicine and health care, and it indicates the direction and rationale of the relationship between professionals and those who seek their care. An ethic of care also joins case-based approaches in focusing on particular contexts of decision making.

Feminist Ethics

Feminist ethics uses the tools of feminist theory to examine ethical issues in at least three distinctive ways (12). First, it indicates how conceptions of sex often distort people's view of the world and, more specifically, how gendered conceptions constrain and restrict women. For instance, feminist theory shows how human society tends to be androcentric, or male centered, so that man becomes the generic representative for what it means to be human, and woman is viewed as different or deviant. Thus, feminist ethics can expose forms of androcentric reasoning in ethics of clinical care and public policy, calling into question, for example, the rationale for excluding women from participation in clinical research. Second, feminist ethics indicates how gendered thinking has distorted the tools that philosophers and bioethicists use to examine ethical issues. Historically entrenched associations between man and reason, woman and emotion—dubious in and of themselves—have contributed to the tendency in moral theory to view emotion as irrelevant or, at worst, distorting. Some, including many feminist thinkers, however, have argued that appropriate emotion (eg, empathy) is indispensable to moral reasoning in the ethical conduct of medical care. This position, bolstered further by recent empirical research (13, 14), is consistent with the perspective represented by the ethic of care (see previous section). Third, in calling attention to and attempting to redress the ways that gendered concepts have produced constraints on women, feminism is concerned with oppression as a pervasive and insidious moral wrong (15, 16). The tools of feminist ethics can help to identify and challenge dominance and oppression not only of women, but also of other groups oppressed because of race, class, or other characteristics. These tools also can help to detect more subtle gender and other biases and assist in addressing significant health disparities. Rather than rejecting such principles as respect for autonomy and justice, feminist thinkers may interpret and apply these principles to highlight and redress various kinds of domination, oppression, and bias.

Communitarian Ethics

Communitarian ethics challenges the primacy often attributed to personal autonomy in contemporary biomedical ethics (17). A communitarian ethic emphasizes a community's other shared values, ideals, and goals and suggests that the needs of the larger community may take precedence, in some cases, over the rights and desires of individuals. If proponents of a communitarian ethic accept the four principles of Beauchamp and Childress (1), they will tend to interpret those principles through the lens of community, stressing, for example, benefits and harms to community and communities as well as the need to override autonomy in some cases. Major examples arise in the context of public health. However, in considering the proper framework for communitarian ethics, questions arise in a pluralistic society about which community is relevant. For instance, is the relevant community one embodied in particular traditions (eg, one religion) or is it the broader, pluralistic society? Even though there is a broad consensus that communal values and interests sometimes trump personal autonomy, disputes persist about exactly when it is justifiable to override personal autonomy. To take one example, apart from laws that specify which diseases are reportable, physicians may have to balance a patient's claims of privacy and confidentiality against risks to others. Different judgments about the appropriate balance often hinge on an assessment of risks: How probable and serious must the harm be to justify a breach of privacy and confidentiality?

Case-Based Reasoning

In a final approach, case-based reasoning (sometimes called casuistry), ethical decision making builds on precedents set in specific cases (18, 19). This is analogous to the role of case law in jurisprudence in that an accumulated body of influential cases and their interpretation provide moral guidance. This approach analyzes current cases requiring decisions in light of relevantly similar cases that have already been settled or gained a rough consensus. Case-based reasoning asserts the priority of practice over both ethical theory and moral principles. It recognizes the principles that emerge by a process of generalization from the analysis of cases but views these principles as always open to future revision. In considering a particular case, someone taking this approach would seek to determine whether there are any relevantly similar cases, either positive or negative, that enjoy an ethical consensus. If, for example, a new research protocol is relevantly similar to an earlier and widely condemned one (eg, the Tuskegee Syphilis Study), that similarity is a reason for moral suspicion of the new protocol. A question for this approach is how to identify relevant similarities and differences among cases and whether ethical principles are sometimes useful in this process.

Ethics as Toolbox

An example of how the different ethical frameworks and perspectives might address a particular case is shown in the box. From this analysis of different approaches, it is plausible to derive the following conclusion: enlightened ethical decision making in clinical medicine cannot rely exclusively on any single fundamental approach to biomedical ethics. The metaphor of toolbox or toolkit may provide a useful way to think about these different approaches to ethical decision making (20). Some ethical tools may fit some contexts, situations, and cases better than others, and more than one—or even all of them—usually are valuable.

It is helpful to have access to a variety of ethical tools because clinical problems often are too complex to be resolved by using simple rules or by rigidly applying ethical principles. Indeed, virtues such as prudence, fairness, and trustworthiness enable clinicians to apply ethical principles sensitively and wisely in situations of conflict. The specific virtues that are most important may vary from one circumstance to another, but in women's health care, there must be particular sensitivity to the needs of women. Furthermore, in many, perhaps most, difficult situations requiring ethical insight, tensions exist between the well-being and interests of the individual patient and the interest of the "community," however that is defined. Finally, current ethical decisions can be improved by awareness of and guidance from existing precedents.

In short, even though a principle-based approach may provide a reasonable starting point for ethical decision making, it is not adequate by itself and needs the valuable contributions and insights of other approaches. Principles often serve as initial points of reference in ethical decision making in obstetrics and gynecology, however, and the next section examines several ethical principles in detail.

Ethical Principles

Clinicians and others often make decisions without appealing to principles for guidance or justification. But when they experience unclear situations, uncertainties, or conflicts, principles often can be helpful. The major principles that are commonly invoked as guides to profes-sional action and for resolving conflicting obligations in health care are respect for autonomy, beneficence and nonmaleficence, and justice (1). Other principles or rules, such as fidelity, honesty, privacy, and confidentiality, also are important, whether they are viewed as derived from the four broad principles or as independent.

Respect for Autonomy

Autonomy, which derives from the Greek *autos* ("self") and *nomos* ("rule" or "governance"), literally means self-rule. In medical practice, the principle of respect for autonomy implies personal rule of the self that is free both from controlling interferences by others and from personal limitations that prevent meaningful choice, such as inadequate understanding (1). Respect for a patient's autonomy acknowledges an individual's right to hold views, to make choices, and to take actions based on her own personal values and beliefs. Respect for autonomy provides a strong moral foundation for informed consent, in which a patient, adequately informed about her medical condition and the available therapies, freely chooses specific treatments or nontreatment. Respect for patient autonomy, like all ethical principles, cannot be regarded as absolute. At times it may conflict with other principles or values and sometimes must yield to them.

Beneficence and Nonmaleficence

The principle of beneficence, which literally means doing or producing good, expresses the obligation to promote the well-being of others. It requires a physician to act in a way that is likely to benefit the patient. Nonmaleficence is the obligation not to harm or cause injury, and it is best known in the maxim, *primum non nocere* ("First, do no harm."). Although there are some subtle distinctions between nonmaleficence and beneficence, they often are considered manifestations of a single principle. These two principles taken together are operative in almost every treatment decision because every medical or surgical pro-

---

One Case Study: Five Approaches

Although the several approaches to ethical decision making may all produce the same answer in a situation that requires a decision, they focus on different, though related, aspects of the situation and decision. Consider, for instance, how they might address interventions for fetal well-being if a pregnant woman rejects medical recommendations or engages in actions that put the fetus at risk.*

A *principle-based approach* would seek to identify the principles and rules pertinent to the case. These might include beneficence–nonmaleficence to both the pregnant woman and her fetus, justice to both parties, and respect for the pregnant woman's autonomous choices. These principles cannot be applied mechanically. After all, it may be unclear whether the pregnant woman is making an autonomous decision, and there may be debates about the balance of probable benefits and risks of interventions to all the stakeholders as well as about which principle should take priority in this conflict. Professional codes and commentaries may offer some guidance about how to resolve such conflicts.

A *virtue-based approach* would focus on the courses of action to which different virtues would and should dispose the obstetrician–gynecologist. For instance, which course of action would follow from compassion? From respectfulness? And so forth. In addition, the obstetrician–gynecologist may find it helpful to ask more broadly: Which course of action would best express the character of a good physician?

An *ethic of care* would concentrate on the implications of the virtue of caring in the obstetrician–gynecologist's special relationship with the pregnant women and with the fetus. In the process of deliberation, individuals using this approach generally would resist viewing the relationship between the pregnant woman and her fetus as adversarial, acknowledging that most of the time women are paradigmatically invested in their fetus' well-being and that maternal and fetal interests usually are aligned.* If, however, a real conflict does exist, the obstetrician–gynecologist should resist feeling the need to take one side or the other. Instead, he or she should seek a solution in identifying and balancing his or her duties in these special relationships, situating these duties in the context of a pregnant woman's

values and concerns, instead of specifying and balancing abstract principles or rights.

To take one example, in considering a case of a pregnant woman in preterm labor who refuses admission to the hospital for bed rest or tocolytics, Harris combines a care or relational perspective with a feminist perspective to provide a "much wider gaze" than a principle-based approach might*:

> The clinician would focus attention on important social and family relationships, contexts or constraints that might come to bear on [a] pregnant [woman's] decision making, such as her need to care for other children at home or to continue working to support other family members, or whatever life project occupied her, and attempt to provide relief in those areas….[Often] fetal well-being is achieved when maternal well-being is achieved.

As this example suggests, a *feminist ethics* approach would attend to the social structures and factors that limit and control the pregnant woman's options and decisions in this situation and would seek to alter any that can be changed.* It also would consider the implications any intervention might have for further control of women's choices and actions—for instance, by reducing a pregnant woman, in extreme cases, to the status of "fetal container" or "incubator."

Finally, a *case-based approach* would consider whether there are any relevantly similar cases that constitute precedents for the current one. For instance, an obstetrician–gynecologist may wonder whether to seek a court order for a cesarean delivery that he or she believes would increase the chances of survival for the child-to-be but that the pregnant woman continues to reject. In considering what to do, the physician may ask, as some courts have asked, whether there is a helpful precedent in the settled consensus of not subjecting a nonconsenting person to a surgical procedure to benefit a third party, for instance, by removing an organ for transplantation.†

*Harris LH. Rethinking maternal-fetal conflict: gender and equality in perinatal ethics. Obstet Gynecol 2000;96:786–91.

†In re A.C., 572 A.2d 1235 (D.C. Ct. App. 1990).

---

cedure has both benefits and risks, which must be balanced knowledgeably and wisely. Beneficence, the obligation to promote the patient's well-being, may sometimes conflict with the obligation to respect the patient's autonomy. For example, a patient may desire to deliver a fatally malformed fetus by cesarean because she believes that this procedure will increase the newborn's chance of surviving, if only for a few hours. However, in the physician's best judgment, the theoretical benefit to a "nonviable" infant may not justify the risks of the surgical delivery to the woman. In such a situation, the physician's task is further complicated by the need to consider the patient's psychologic, physical, and spiritual well-being.

Justice

Justice is the principle of rendering to others what is due to them. It is the most complex of the ethical principles to be considered because it deals not only with the physician's obligation to render to a patient what is owed but also with the physician's role in the allocation of limited medical resources in the broader community. In addition, various criteria such as need, effort, contribution, and merit are important in determining what is owed and to whom it is owed. Justice is the obligation to treat equally those who are alike or similar according to whatever criteria are selected. Individuals should receive equal treatment unless scientific and clinical evidence establishes that they differ from others in ways that are relevant to the treatments in question. Determination of the criteria on which these judgments are based is a highly complex moral process, as exemplified by the ethical controversies about providing or withholding renal dialysis and organ transplantation.

The principle of justice applies at many levels. At the societal level, it addresses the criteria for allocating scarce resources, such as organs for transplantation. At a more local level, it is relevant to questions such as which patients (and physicians) receive priority for operating room times. Even at the level of the physician–patient relationship, the principle of justice applies to matters such as the timing of patient discharge. The principle also governs relationships between physicians and third parties, such as payers and regulators. In the context of the physician–patient relationship, the physician should be the patient's advocate when institutional decisions about allocation of resources must be made.

Balancing the Principles

In order to guide actions, each of these broad principles needs to be made more concrete. Sometimes the principles can be addressed in more definite rules—for instance, rules of voluntary, informed consent express requirements of the principle of respect for personal autonomy, and rules of confidentiality rest on several principles (see "Common Ethical Issues and Problems in Obstetrics and Gynecology"). Nevertheless, conflicts may arise among these various principles and rules. In cases of conflict, physicians have to determine which principle(s) should have priority. Some ethical theories view all of these principles as prima facie binding, resist any effort to prioritize them apart from particular situations, and call for balancing in particular situations (1). Some other theories attempt to rank principles in advance of actual conflicts (21).

Obstetrician–gynecologists, like other physicians, often face a conflict between principles of beneficence–nonmaleficence in relation to a patient and respect for that patient's personal autonomy. In such cases, the physician's judgment about what is in the patient's best interests conflicts with the patient's preferences. The physician then has to decide whether to respect the patient's choices or to refuse to act on the patient's preferences in order to achieve what the physician believes to be a better outcome for the patient. Paternalistic models of physician–patient relationships have been sharply challenged and often supplanted by other models. At the other end of the spectrum, however, the model of following patients' choices, whatever they are, as long as they are informed choices, also has been criticized for reducing the physician to a mere technician (22). Other models have been proposed, such as negotiation (23), shared decision making (24), or a deliberative model, in which the physician integrates information about the patient's condition with the patient's values to make a cogent recommendation (22). Whatever model is selected, a physician may still, in a par-

ticular situation, have to decide whether to act on the patient's request that does not appear to accord with the patient's best interests. These dilemmas are considered in greater detail elsewhere (25).

Common Ethical Issues and Problems in Obstetrics and Gynecology

Almost everything obstetrician–gynecologists do in their professional lives involves one or more of the ethical principles and personal virtues to a greater or lesser degree. Nevertheless, several specific areas deserve special attention: the role of the obstetrician–gynecologist in the society at large; the process of voluntary, informed consent; confidentiality; and conflict of interest.

The Obstetrician–Gynecologist's Role in Society at Large

In addition to their ethical responsibilities in direct patient care, obstetrician–gynecologists have ethical responsibilities related to their involvement in the organization, administration, and evaluation of health care. They exercise these broader responsibilities through membership in professional organizations; consultation with and advice to community leaders, government officials, and members of the judiciary; expert witness testimony; and education of the public. Justice is both the operative principle and the defining virtue in decisions about the distribution of scarce health care resources and the provision of health care for the medically indigent and uninsured. Obstetricians and gynecologists should offer their support for institutions, policies, and practices that ensure quality of and more equitable access to health care, particularly, but not exclusively, for women and children. The virtues of truthfulness, fidelity, trustworthiness, and integrity must guide physicians in their roles as expert witnesses, as consultants to public officials, as educators of the lay public, and as health advocates (26).

Informed Consent Process

Often, informed consent is confused with the consent form. In fact, informed consent is "the willing acceptance of a medical intervention by a patient after adequate disclosure by the physician of the nature of the intervention with its risks and benefits and of the alternatives with their risks and benefits" (27). The consent form only documents the process and the patient decision. The primary purpose of the consent process is to protect patient autonomy. By encouraging an ongoing and open communication of relevant information (adequate disclosure), the physician enables the patient to exercise personal choice. This sort of communication is central to a satisfactory physician–patient relationship. Unfortunately, discussions for the purpose of educating and informing patients about their health care options are never completely free of the informant's bias. Practitioners should seek to uncover their own biases and endeavor to maintain objectivity in the face of those biases, while disclosing to the patient any personal biases that could influence the practitioner's recommendations (28, 29). A patient's right to make her own decisions about medical issues extends to the right to refuse recommended medical treatment. The freedom to accept or refuse recommended medical treatment has legal as well as ethical foundations.

As previously noted, one of the most important elements of informed consent is the patient's capacity to understand the nature of her condition and the benefits and risks of the treatment that is recommended as well as those of the alternative treatments (30). A patient's capacity to understand depends on her maturity, state of consciousness, mental acuity, education, cultural background, native language, the opportunity and willingness to ask questions, and the way in which the information is presented. Diminished capacity to understand is not necessarily the same as legal incompetence. Psychiatric consultation may be helpful in establishing a patient's capacity, or ability to comprehend relevant information. Critical to the process of informing the patient is the physician's integrity in choosing the information that is given to the patient and respectfulness in presenting it in a comprehensible way. The point is not merely to disclose information but to ensure patient comprehension of relevant information. Voluntariness—the patient's freedom to choose among alternatives—is also an important element of informed consent, which should be free from coercion, pressure, or undue influence (31).

Confidentiality

Confidentiality applies when an individual to whom information is disclosed is obligated not to divulge this information to a third party. Rules of confidentiality are among the most ancient and widespread components of codes of medical ethics. Confidentiality is based on the principle of respect for patient autonomy, which includes a patient's right to privacy, and on the physician's fidelity-based responsibility to respect a patient's privacy. Rules of confidentiality also are justified by their good effects: Assurance of confidentiality encourages patients to disclose information that may be essential in making an accurate diagnosis and planning appropriate treatment. However, rules of confidentiality are not absolute, either legally or ethically. Legal exceptions to confidentiality include the requirements to report certain sexually transmitted diseases or suspected child abuse. Ethically, breaches of confidentiality also may be justified in rare cases to protect others from serious harm.

The need for storing and transmitting medical information about patients is a serious threat to confidentiality and privacy, a problem made more complex by the use of electronic storage and transmission of patient data. The recent increase in the use of genetic testing and screening also highlights the need for strong protections of confidentiality and patient privacy because genetic information has lifelong implications for patients and their families.

Obstetrician–gynecologists also are confronted with issues of confidentiality in dealing with adolescents, especially regarding the diagnosis and treatment of sexually transmitted diseases, contraceptive counseling, and pregnancy (32). The physician's willingness and ability to protect confidentiality should be discussed with all adolescent patients early in their care. Many state laws protect adolescent confidentiality in certain types of situations, and obstetrician–gynecologists should be aware of the laws in their own states.

Conflict of Interest

It is necessary to distinguish conflicts of interest from conflicts of obligation. A conflict of obligation exists when a physician has two or more obligations that sometimes conflict—for example, an obligation to patients and an obligation to a managed care organization. By contrast, a conflict of interest exists when a primary interest (usually the patient's well-being) is in conflict with a physician's secondary interest (such as his or her financial interest). A conflict of interest is not necessarily wrong, but it creates the occasion and temptation for the physician to breach a primary obligation to the patient.

Many kinds of conflicts of interest arise in obstetrics and gynecology; some are obvious, others more subtle. Following are a few examples: a managed care guideline limits coverage for diagnostic tests that physicians consider necessary for patients and penalizes physicians who order such tests (or rewards physicians who do not order such tests); a physician recommends products to patients that are sold for a profit in his or her office (33); a physician refers patients for tests or procedures at an entity in which the physician has a financial interest; a physician accepts gifts from a pharmaceutical or medical device company (34). It is important for physicians to be attentive to the wide range of actual and perceived conflicts of interest. Even perceived conflicts of interest can threaten patient and societal trust.

There is ever-increasing intrusion into the patient–physician relationship by government and by the marketplace. Care plans, practice guidelines, and treatment protocols may substantially limit physicians' ability to provide what they consider proper care for patients. If the conflict is too great, the physician should withdraw from the organization. In addition to such conflicts of obligation, a conflict of interest exists if the organization's incentive plans create inducements to limit care in the interest of increasing physicians' incomes. At one time, the tension between physicians' financial self-interest and patients' interests often encouraged unnecessary testing and excessive treatment, but the current tension may provide incentives for too little care. Conflicts of interest should be avoided whenever possible, and when they are unavoidable and material to patients' decisions, it is the physician's responsibility to disclose them to patients. Serious ethical problems arise if organizational rules (so-called "gag rules") preclude such disclosures.

Guidelines for Ethical Decision Making

Often, more than one course of action may be morally justifiable. At times, however, no course of action may seem acceptable because each may result in significant harms or compromise important principles or values. Nevertheless, the clinician must select one of the available options, justify that decision by ethical reasons, and apply the same critical thinking faculties that would be applied to issues of medical evidence. An analysis of the various factors involved in ethical decisions can aid attempts to resolve difficult cases. In addition, the involvement of individuals with a variety of backgrounds and perspectives can be useful in addressing ethical questions. Informal or formal consultation with those from related services or with a hospital ethics committee can help ensure that all stakeholders, viewpoints, and options are considered as a decision is made.

It is important for the individual physician to find or develop guidelines for decision making that can be applied consistently in facing ethical dilemmas. Guidelines consisting of several logical steps can aid the practitioner analyzing and resolving an ethical problem. The approach that follows incorporates elements of several proposed schemes (27, 35–38).

1. *Identify the decision makers.* The first step in addressing any problem is to answer the question, "Whose decision is it?" Generally, the patient is presumed to have the authority and capacity to choose among medically acceptable alternatives or to refuse treatment.

   a. Assess the patient's ability to make a decision. At times, this is not clear. An individual's capacity to make a decision depends on that individual's ability to understand information and appreciate the implications of that information when making a personal decision (30). In contrast, competence and incompetence are legal determinations that may or may not truly reflect functional capacity. Assessment of a patient's capacity to make decisions must at times be made by professionals with expertise in making such determinations. Decisions about competence can be made only in a court of law.

   b. Identify a surrogate decision maker for incompetent patients. If a patient is thought to be incapable of making a decision or has been found legally incompetent, a surrogate decision maker must be identified. In the absence of a durable power of attorney, family members have been called on to render proxy decisions. In some situations, the court may be called on to appoint a guardian. A surrogate decision maker should make the decision that the patient would have wanted or, if the patient's wishes are not known, that will promote the best interests of the patient.

   The physician has an obligation to assist the patient's representatives in examining the issues and reaching a resolution.

   c. In the obstetric setting, recognize that a competent pregnant woman is the appropriate decision maker for the fetus that she is carrying.

2. *Collect data, establish facts.*

   a. Be aware that perceptions about what may or may not be relevant or important to a case reflect values—whether personal, professional, institutional, or societal. Hence, one should strive to be as objective as possible when collecting the information on which to base a decision.

   b. Use consultants as needed to ensure that all available information about the diagnosis, treatment, and prognosis has been obtained.

3. *Identify all medically appropriate options.*

   a. Use consultation as necessary.

   b. Identify other options raised by the patient or other concerned parties.

4. *Evaluate options according to the values and principles involved.*

   a. Start by gathering information about the values of the involved parties, the primary stakeholders, and try to get a sense of the perspective each is bringing to the discussion. The values of the patient generally will be the most important consideration as decision making proceeds.

   b. Determine whether any of the options violates ethical principles that all agree are important. Eliminate those options that, after analysis, are found to be morally unacceptable by all parties.

   c. Reexamine the remaining options according to the interests and values of each party. Some alternatives may be combined successfully.

5. *Identify ethical conflicts and set priorities.*

   a. Try to define the problem in terms of the ethical principles involved (eg, beneficence versus respect for autonomy).

   b. Weigh the principles underlying each of the arguments made. Does one of the principles appear more important than others in this conflict? Does one proposed course of action seem to have more merit than the others?

   c. Consider respected opinions about similar cases and decide to what extent they can be useful in addressing the current problem. Look for morally relevant differences and similarities between this and other cases. Usually, physicians find that the basic dilemma at hand is not a new one and that points considered by others in resolving past dilemmas can be useful.

6. *Select the option that can be best justified.* Try to arrive at a rational resolution to the problem, one that can

be justified to others in terms of widely recognized ethical principles.

7. *Reevaluate the decision after it is acted on.* Repeat the evaluation of the major options in light of information gained during the implementation of the decision. Was the best possible decision made? What lessons can be learned from the discussion and resolution of the problem?

Summary

Obstetrician–gynecologists who are familiar with the concepts of medical ethics will be better able to approach complex ethical situations in a clear and structured way. By considering the ethical frameworks involving principles, virtues, care and feminist perspectives, concern for community, and case precedents, they can enhance their ability to make ethically justifiable clinical decisions. They also need to attend to the kinds of ethical issues and problems that arise particularly or with special features in obstetrics and gynecology. Finally, obstetricians and gynecologists can enhance their decision-making process by considering when it would be useful to seek a formal or informal ethics consult as well as which guidelines would be most helpful to them as they move from case to case and decision to decision.

References

1. Beauchamp TL, Childress JF. Principles of biomedical ethics. 5th ed. New York (NY): Oxford University Press; 2001.

2. Childress JF. Methods in bioethics. In: Steinbock B, editor. The Oxford handbook of bioethics. New York (NY): Oxford University Press; 2007. p. 15–45.

3. Pellegrino ED. The metamorphosis of medical ethics. A 30-year retrospective. JAMA 1993;269:1158–62.

4. Steinbock B, Arras JD, London AJ, editors. Ethical issues in modern medicine. 6th ed. Boston (MA): McGraw-Hill; 2003.

5. Beauchamp TL, Walters L, editors. Contemporary issues in bioethics. 6th ed. Belmont (CA): Thomson Wadsworth; 2003.

6. Mappes TA, DeGrazia D, editors. Biomedical ethics. 6th ed. Boston (MA): McGraw-Hill; 2006.

7. McCullough LB, Chervenak FA. Ethics in obstetrics and gynecology. New York (NY): Oxford University Press; 1994.

8. Pellegrino ED, Thomasma DC. The virtues in medical practice. New York (NY): Oxford University Press; 1993.

9. Pellegrino ED. Toward a virtue-based normative ethics for the health professions. Kennedy Inst Ethics J 1995;5: 253–77.

10. Gilligan C. Moral orientation and moral development. In: Kittay EF, Meyers DT, editors. Women and moral theory. Totowa (NJ): Rowman and Littlefield; 1987. p. 19–33.

11. Manning RC. A care approach. In: Kuhse H, Singer P, editors. A companion to bioethics. Malden (MA): Blackwell; 1998. p. 98–105.

12. Little MO. Why a feminist approach to bioethics? Kennedy Inst Ethics J 1996;6:1–18.

13. Koenigs M, Young L, Adolphs R, Tranel D, Cushman F, Hauser M, et al. Damage to the prefrontal cortex increases utilitarian moral judgements [letter]. Nature 2007;446: 908–11.

14. Greene JD, Sommerville RB, Nystrom LE, Darley JM, Cohen JD. An fMRI investigation of emotional engagement in moral judgment. Science 2001;293:2105–8.

15. Tong R. Feminist approaches to bioethics. In: Wolf SM, editor. Feminism and bioethics: beyond reproduction. New York (NY): Oxford University Press; 1996. p. 67–94.

16. Sherwin S. No longer patient: feminist ethics and health care. Philadelphia (PA): Temple University Press; 1992.

17. Callahan D. Principlism and communitarianism. J Med Ethics 2003;29:287–91.

18. Jonsen AR. Casuistry: an alternative or complement to principles? Kennedy Inst Ethics J 1995;5:237–51.

19. Jonsen AR, Toulmin S. The abuse of casuistry: a history of moral reasoning. Berkeley (CA): University of California Press; 1990.

20. Hope T. Medical ethics: a very short introduction. New York (NY): Oxford University Press; 2004.

21. Veatch RM. The basics of bioethics. 2nd ed. Upper Saddle River (NJ): Prentice Hall; 2003.

22. Emanuel EJ, Emanuel LL. Four models of the physician-patient relationship. JAMA 1992;267:2221–6.

23. Childress JF, Siegler M. Metaphors and models of doctor-patient relationships: their implications for autonomy. Theor Med 1984;5:17–30.

24. Katz J. The silent world of doctor and patient. Baltimore (MD): Johns Hopkins University Press; 2002.

25. American College of Obstetricians and Gynecologists. Surgery and patient choice. In: Ethics in obstetrics and gynecology. 2nd ed. Washington, DC: ACOG; 2004. p. 21–5.

26. Expert testimony. ACOG Committee Opinion No. 374. American College of Obstetricians and Gynecologists. Obstet Gynecol 2007;110:445–6.

27. Jonsen AR, Siegler M, Winslade WJ. Clinical ethics: a practical approach to ethical decisions in clinical medicine. 6th ed. New York (NY): McGraw-Hill; 2006.

28. Asch A. Prenatal diagnosis and selective abortion: a challenge to practice and policy. Am J Public Health 1999; 89:1649–57.

29. Parens E, Asch A. The disability rights critique of prenatal genetic testing. Reflections and recommendations. Hastings Cent Rep 1999;29:S1–22.

30. Grisso T, Appelbaum PS. Assessing competence to consent to treatment: a guide for physicians and other health professionals. New York (NY): Oxford University Press; 1998.

31. American College of Obstetricians and Gynecologists. Informed consent. In: Ethics in obstetrics and gynecology. 2nd ed. Washington, DC: ACOG; 2004. p. 9–17.

32. American College of Obstetricians and Gynecologists. Human resources. In: Guidelines for women's health care. 3rd ed. Washington, DC: ACOG; 2007. p. 15–29.

33. Commercial enterprises in medical practice. ACOG Committee Opinion No. 359. American College of Obstetricians and Gynecologists. Obstet Gynecol 2007;109: 243–5.

34. American College of Obstetricians and Gynecologists. Relationships with industry. In: Ethics in obstetrics and gynecology. 2nd ed. Washington, DC: ACOG; 2004. p. 107–10.

35. Pellegrino ED. The anatomy of clinical-ethical judgments in perinatology and neonatology: a substantive and procedural framework. Semin Perinatol 1987;11:202–9.

36. Kanoti GA. Ethics and medical-ethical decisions. Crit Care Clin 1986;2:3–12.

37. Abrams FR. Bioethical considerations for high-risk pregnancy. In: Abrams RS, Wexler P, editors. Medical care of the pregnant patient. Boston (MA): Little, Brown and Co.; 1983. p. 1–12.

38. Fletcher JC, Spencer EM, Lombardo P, editors. Fletcher's introduction to clinical ethics. 3rd ed. Hagerstown (MD): University Publishing Group; 2005.

Ethical decision making in obstetrics and gynecology. ACOG Committee Opinion No. 390. American College of Obstetricians and Gynecologists. Obstet Gynecol 2007;110:1479–87.

ISSN 1074-861X

ACOG COMMITTEE OPINION

Number 395 • January 2008

Surgery and Patient Choice*

Committee on Ethics

ABSTRACT: Acknowledgment of the importance of patient autonomy and increased patient access to information has prompted more patient-generated requests for surgical interventions not necessarily recommended by their physicians. Decision making in obstetrics and gynecology should be guided by the ethical principles of respect for patient autonomy, beneficence, nonmaleficence, justice, and veracity. Each physician should exercise judgment when determining whether information presented to the patient is adequate. When working with a patient to make decisions about surgery, it is important for obstetricians and gynecologists to take a broad view of the consequences of surgical treatment and to acknowledge the lack of firm evidence for the benefit of one approach over another when evidence is limited.

Is it ethical to perform an elective cesarean delivery for a woman with a normal pregnancy, a prophylactic oophorectomy for a 30-year-old patient with no family history of ovarian cancer, or a tubal ligation for an 18-year-old nulligravid woman? How should the physician respond to a patient who requests a specific surgical therapy without having an accepted medical indication? Should health care options be regarded in the same way as choice of cereal in the supermarket: the consumer makes a choice based on appearance, content, and cost, and the grocer takes the money and bags the cornflakes, without providing any direction? Is choosing a medical procedure so radically different and complex that this analogy is inappropriate?

Years ago, patients presented to their physicians with symptoms, and the physicians would establish diagnoses then make recommendations for therapy; usually recommendations were accepted by patients without question. An example of that paternalistic model was the widespread practice of "twilight sleep" for labor and delivery. Physicians administered a narcotic and scopolamine, and decisions during labor and delivery were delegated to the medical team. In contrast, today the first prenatal visit may open with a discussion of the patient's birth plan, including her preferences for anesthesia, episiotomy,

forceps use, cesarean delivery, and breastfeeding. The purpose of this Committee Opinion is to provide the obstetrician–gynecologist with an approach to decision making based on ethics in an environment of increased patient information, recognition of patient autonomy, direct-to-consumer marketing, often incomplete evidence, and a plethora of alternative, investigational, or unproven treatments for many conditions.

Ethical Principles

Decision making in obstetrics and gynecology should be guided by the ethical principles of respect for patient autonomy, beneficence, nonmaleficence, justice, and veracity and as set forth throughout this document and in the "Code of Professional Ethics of the American College of Obstetricians and Gynecologists" (1). Although obligations to the patient are paramount, in addition, the obstetrician–gynecologist must consider resolution of conflicts of interest, acknowledgment of the profession's responsibility to society as a whole, and the maintenance of the dignity and honor of the discipline of obstetrics and gynecology and its standards of care. Issues related to surgery are addressed in this Committee Opinion; however, the ethical principles are the same as for other health care decisions (eg, diagnostic testing or medical therapy).

Patient autonomy and the concept of informed consent or refusal are central to issues regarding patient choice to have or not

The American College of Obstetricians and Gynecologists
Women's Health Care Physicians

---

*Update of "Surgery and Patient Choice," in *Ethics in Obstetrics and Gynecology*, Second Edition, 2004.

have a surgical procedure. It is the obligation of the obstetrician–gynecologist to fully inform the patient regarding treatment options and the potential risks and benefits of those options. In discussing these options, the physician should take into account the context of the patient's decision making, including the potential influences of family and society (2). Once the physician is satisfied that the patient fully comprehends the options, her autonomous decision ordinarily should be respected and supported. Patients should be encouraged to seek second opinions when in doubt or in need of reassurance. However, even though the decision of the patient should be respected, respect might not include supporting the decision, particularly when doing so is in direct conflict with other guiding ethical principles. At times, these other principles may take priority over supporting the patient's decisions.

The principle of beneficence refers to the ethical obligation of the physician to promote the health and welfare of the patient. The complementary principle of nonmaleficence refers to the physician's obligation to not harm the patient. When a patient refuses surgery or another treatment that the obstetrician–gynecologist believes is necessary for her health and welfare, beneficence and nonmaleficence can conflict with respect for patient autonomy. In almost all situations, the patient has a right to refuse unwanted treatment. She does not, however, have a parallel right of access to treatment that the physician believes is unwise or overly risky.

Justice, as an ethical principle, applies to the physician, the hospital, the payer, and society, as well as to the individual patient. Although there are many theories of justice, in the medical context, this principle requires that medical professionals treat individuals fairly. Further, it is important for the physician to consider the impact on not only the individual patient but also society. At the level of the physician–patient relationship, justice implies, for instance, that physicians consider a patient's request for an elective procedure in the context of similar types of requests by other patients. At the societal level, justice directs physicians to consider the impact of their decision to perform a procedure in terms of the allocation of scarce resources.

Veracity, or truth telling, is important in surgical counseling and decision making. When the patient requests a procedure to which the physician is morally opposed (such as abortion or permanent sterilization), the physician may have a limited right to refuse to provide the service; however, the physician must disclose scientifically accurate information, convey to the patient that this refusal is based on moral (not medical) grounds, and refer the patient in a timely manner (3). The obstetrician–gynecologist should not misrepresent his or her experience with the proposed treatment or knowledge regarding potential long-term outcomes.

The Physician–Patient Relationship

Four models of the relationship between the physician and patient have been described: 1) paternalistic, 2) informative,

3) interpretive, and 4) deliberative (4). Depending on which model is used, different ethical principles emerge as relevant to ethical decision making. The ideal model for the physician–patient relationship has been the subject of considerable debate. In fact, physicians probably use all four models, depending on the individual patient, her situation, and the disease process involved (4).

Paternalistic Model

In the paternalistic physician–patient model (4), the physician might present only information on risks and benefits of a procedure that he or she thinks will lead the patient to make the "right" decision (ie, in this model, the physician-supported decision) regarding health care. One example of the paternalistic model would be the ethically and professionally problematic practice of recommending amniocentesis for a 35-year-old pregnant patient but offering no alternatives.

This model is not appropriate when the patient is competent to make informed decisions, but it may be the best choice in situations of last resort, such as unconscious patients in the emergency department when no surrogate decision maker is present. When the patient is ill and unable to engage, either physically or mentally, in a discussion of the risks and benefits of a particular surgical intervention and there is neither an advance directive nor an assigned proxy for health care decisions, a paternalistic physician–patient relationship may be the only way to adhere to the ethical principles of beneficence and nonmaleficence with impaired patient autonomy.

Informative Model

At the opposite end of the spectrum, the informative model describes a physician–patient relationship in which the physician is a provider of objective and technical information regarding the patient's medical problem and its potential therapeutic solutions. The patient has complete control over surgical decision making, and the physician's values are not discussed. An example is a physician offering a patient with an abnormal cervical cytology result the options of watchful waiting, colposcopy, loop electrosurgical excision procedure, laser ablation, cold knife conization, and hysterectomy. The discussion includes a complete description of advantages, disadvantages, risks, and complications of each option. The discussion does not include any statement about the physician's recommendations or prioritization of the options.

A serious drawback of this model is the physician's abandonment of the role of a caring partner and medical expert in the decision-making process. This model also assumes that patients have set values and are able to completely integrate the sometimes complex medical and surgical treatment decisions with those values. However, when the physician–patient relationship is necessarily brief and there are multiple treatment options with comparable risks and benefits, the informative model may be appropriate. One example is the choice of having a genetic amniocentesis for advanced maternal age versus multiple marker testing or no testing.

One of the many unfortunate consequences of the professional liability crisis is the unsubstantiated belief of some physicians that the informative model reduces the physician's risk of liability. Such a belief raises concerns about physicians protecting themselves rather than working in the best interests of their patients.

This model may not be ideal for patient care in most situations because the physician's professional judgment generally is of considerable value to patients. In any case, it probably is impossible for a physician to counsel a patient with complete objectivity and without introducing some implied preference for one of many options (5).

Interpretive Model

Other models for physician–patient relationships strike a middle ground between the extremes of the paternalistic and informative models. In the interpretive model, the physician helps the patient clarify and integrate her values into the decision-making process while acting as an information source regarding the technical aspects of any given medical procedure. In this model, the physician aids the patient in "self-understanding; the patient comes to know more clearly who he or she is and how various medical options bear on his or her identity" (4).

Application of this model to an example of cervical dysplasia might result in the physician noting that the patient had a history of moderate symptoms associated with menses, had completed her childbearing, and was very fearful of cancer. On that basis, the physician recommends hysterectomy over other options, although he or she describes and discusses other options and their potential implications for the patient. When implementing this model, the physician must be careful to help the patient clarify her values while not imposing his or her own values or beliefs on the patient.

Deliberative Model

In the deliberative model, the physician's role is to guide the patient in taking the most admirable or moral (based on her values, needs, and fears) course of treatment or health-related action (4). It is similar to the interpretive model in that it includes a discussion of not only the medical benefits and risks but also the patient's individual priorities, values, and fears. It goes beyond the interpretive model in that the physician must consciously communicate to the patient his or her health values; however, the physician should not use the moral discussion to dictate to the patient the best course of action (4). Because of the potential for an unequal balance of power in the physician–patient relationship, great care should be taken in this model to avoid subjecting the patient to undue pressure.

The case of a patient with a history of tubal ligation considering her fertility options may illustrate the deliberative model. In this case, the patient's understanding of the moral status of the human embryo might influence whether tubal anastomosis or in vitro fertilization is pursued. The physician would provide technical information about the options but might also convey information about how individuals and organizations have formulated the discussion of the moral status of embryos. This deliberation then may assist the patient by providing tools with which the patient might examine her values in support of a treatment decision.

The Process of Decision Making

Each physician should exercise judgment when determining whether information presented to the patient is adequate. The practice of evidence-based medicine involves understanding the scientific basis of treatment and the strength of the evidence and applying the results of the strongest evidence available to medical decision making. Frequently, both surgical and medical decisions need to be made in a context in which the scientific evidence supporting one treatment option over another is incomplete, of poor quality, or totally lacking. There is no ethical imperative to initiate discussion of treatment options that are either unproven or not part of accepted medical practice. The physician may, however, want to discuss investigational options so that the patient understands the unproven nature of these options and can make an informed decision about them. Surgical and medical advice or guidance for many obstetric and gynecologic problems is based in part on science, in part on the experience and values of the physician, and in part on the physician's understanding of the patient's preferences, values, and desired outcome.

When working with a patient to make decisions about surgery, it is important for obstetricians and gynecologists to take a broad view of the consequences of surgical treatment and to acknowledge the lack of firm evidence for the benefit of one approach over another when evidence is limited. For example, a discussion of treatment options for menorrhagia associated with leiomyoma should include the fact that the long-term risks and benefits of some treatment options have not been compared directly (6). Recommendation for a particular option is dictated by many factors, including patient age, leiomyoma size, bleeding severity, and coexisting medical conditions, but in many cases two or more therapeutic options probably would be regarded as equally medically sound. Comparing possible long-term complications of hysterectomy, such as bowel obstruction and loss of vaginal support, with the risks of more conservative surgical approaches, such as the possible need for future treatment of recurrent leiomyomata, is an important part of informed consent. Helping patients understand potential long- and short-term consequences of any given decision as well as giving patients an appreciation of the quality of evidence on which each option is based are critical parts of informed consent. In addition, the physician must be aware of potential personal conflicts of interest that may be present, such as personal financial gain related to the provision or nonprovision of surgical care, and he or she must guard against this as an influence when giving guidance to patients as they make treatment choices.

An Example of the Process

Elective cesarean delivery is offered as an example to illustrate an ethical framework physicians may use in responding to patient requests for treatment for which evidence of benefit is absent or imperfect or which the health care professional would not usually recommend. In using this example, the Committee on Ethics does not mean to comment on the clinical appropriateness of or medical evidence supporting elective cesarean delivery, which would require a review beyond the scope of this document and the Committee on Ethics and have recently been addressed by the Committee on Obstetric Practice (7).

In obstetrics, the ethical issues of informed consent and patient choice are exemplified in the current debate regarding whether elective cesarean delivery should be offered as a birth option in normal pregnancy (8). The wide range of opinion on this issue is reflected in the language that is used, with varying terms reflecting different views of the physician–patient relationship. "Cesarean delivery on demand" reflects the informative model, in which the physician simply describes options and provides the service chosen by the patient. The phrase "elective cesarean delivery" is more suggestive of the deliberative and interpretive models, in which the physician and patient also discuss concerns, needs, and values.

The ethical evaluation is clouded by the limitations of data regarding relative short- and long-term risks and benefits of cesarean delivery versus vaginal delivery (9). For example, limitations that need to be acknowledged on both sides of the debate include evidence for long-term reduction in pelvic floor disorders in women undergoing elective cesarean delivery and lack of extensive morbidity and mortality data comparing routine cesarean delivery with vaginal delivery.

Each of the ethical principles contributes to the decision-making process regarding elective cesarean delivery. However, none alone is sufficient for making the decision.

If taken in a vacuum, the principle of respect for patient autonomy would lend support to the permissibility of elective cesarean delivery in a normal pregnancy (after adequate informed consent). To ensure that the patient's consent is in fact informed, the physician should explore the patient's concerns. For example, a patient may request elective cesarean delivery because she is afraid of discomfort during labor (10). In this case, providing her with information about procedures available for effective pain relief during labor would actually enhance the patient's capacity for autonomous choice and may result in an agreement to proceed without surgery (11).

The ethical principle of justice regarding the allocation of medical resources must be considered in the debate over elective cesarean delivery and informed patient choice. It is not clear whether widespread implementation of elective cesarean delivery would increase or decrease resources required to provide delivery services. Comprehensive analysis of costs and benefits for current and subsequent pregnancies would provide a basis for application of the principle of justice (12).

Application of the principles of beneficence and nonmaleficence (a physician should offer only treatments that promote the health and welfare of the patient) is made problematic by the limitations of the scientific data described previously. Different interpretations of the risks and benefits are the basis for reasonable differences among obstetricians regarding this challenging issue. In addition, different patients may place considerably different values on known risks and benefits. How certain is it that elective cesarean delivery really protects pelvic support 20 years later? How different is the maternal mortality rate of elective or repeat cesarean delivery in healthy women compared with that of women who have had one or two vaginal deliveries? Are there any desirable or undesirable psychosocial effects of elective cesarean delivery? The currently available data do not adequately represent the comparative populations in question. For instance, data regarding outcomes of cesarean delivery usually involve complicated pregnancies or women in whom a trial of labor has failed. These outcomes are compared with those involving probably healthier women who were able to give birth vaginally. As better data accumulate, the principle of beneficence may result in a shift in clinical practice.

Based on these principles, is it ethical to agree to a patient request for elective cesarean delivery in the absence of an accepted medical indication? The response must begin with the physician's assessment of the current data regarding the relative benefits and risks of the two approaches. In the absence of significant data on the risks and benefits of cesarean delivery, the burden of proof should fall on those who are advocates for a change in policy in support of elective cesarean delivery (ie, the replacement of usual care in labor with a major surgical procedure). If the physician believes that cesarean delivery promotes the overall health and welfare of the woman and her fetus more than vaginal delivery, he or she is ethically justified in performing a cesarean delivery. Similarly, if the physician believes that performing a cesarean delivery would be detrimental to the overall health and welfare of the woman and her fetus, he or she is ethically obliged to refrain from performing the surgery. In this case, a referral to another health care provider would be appropriate if the physician and patient cannot agree on a route of delivery.

Given the lack of data, it currently is not ethically necessary to initiate discussion regarding the relative risks and benefits of elective cesarean delivery versus vaginal delivery with every pregnant patient. There is no obligation to initiate discussion about procedures that the physician does not consider medically acceptable or that are unproven.

On the basis of the ethical principles of beneficence and respect for patient autonomy, an algorithm has been proposed for deciding between the performance of a cesarean delivery and making a referral in cases in which the physician's recommendation is vaginal delivery and the informed patient makes the autonomous decision to request a cesarean delivery (13). The Committee on Ethics addresses other special considerations involving patient choice in obstetric decision making elsewhere (14).

Summary

Although informed refusal of care by the patient is a familiar situation for most clinicians in the practice of both obstetrics and gynecology, acknowledgment of the importance of patient autonomy and increased patient access to information, such as information on the Internet, has prompted more patient-generated requests for surgical interventions not necessarily recommended by their physicians. A patient request for elective cesarean delivery, prompted by a perception of lower risk to the woman (of pelvic floor and sexual dysfunction) and her fetus with cesarean delivery, is an obstetric example. Other examples include requests for prophylactic oophorectomy to reduce risk of ovarian cancer in otherwise healthy women at low risk.

The response to such requests must begin with the physician having a good understanding of the scientific evidence for and against the requested procedure. With that information, the physician should counsel the patient within the framework of the ethical principles of respect for autonomy, beneficence, nonmaleficence, veracity, and justice. The ethical models described in this document provide an approach for using these principles. The physician should use the opportunity that this kind of request presents to explore the patient's concerns and values. In most cases, providing information and careful counseling will allow patients and their physicians to reach a mutually acceptable decision. If an acceptable balance cannot be reached by the patient and physician, the patient may choose to continue care with another provider.

References

1. American College of Obstetricians and Gynecologists. Code of professional ethics of the American College of Obstetricians and Gynecologists. Washington, DC: ACOG; 2008. Available at: http://www.acog.org/from_home/acogcode.pdf. Retrieved January 2, 2008.

2. Mackenzie C, Stoljar N. Relational autonomy: feminist perspectives on autonomy, agency, and the social self. New York (NY): Oxford University Press; 2000.

3. The limits of conscientious refusal in reproductive medicine. ACOG Committee Opinion No. 385. American College of Obstetricians and Gynecologists. Obstet Gynecol 2007;110;1203–8.

4. Emanuel EJ, Emanuel LL. Four models of the physician-patient relationship. JAMA 1992;267:2221–6.

5. Mahowald MB. On the treatment of myopia: feminist standpoint theory and bioethics. In: Wolf S, editor. Feminism and bioethics: beyond reproduction. New York (NY): Oxford University Press; 1996. p. 95–115.

6. Myers ER, Barber MD, Gustilo-Ashby T, Couchman G, Matchar DB, McCrory DC. Management of uterine leiomyomata: what do we really know? Obstet Gynecol 2002;100: 8–17.

7. Cesarean delivery on maternal request. ACOG Committee Opinion No. 394. American College of Obstetricians and Gynecologists. Obstet Gynecol 2007;110:1501–4.

8. Minkoff H, Chervenak FA. Elective primary cesarean delivery. N Engl J Med 2003;348:946–50.

9. Cesarean delivery on maternal request March 27–29, 2006. National Institutes of Health state-of-the-science conference statement. Obstet Gynecol 2006;107:1386–97.

10. Bewley S, Cockburn J. Responding to fear of childbirth. Lancet 2002;359:2128–9.

11. Saisto T, Salmela-Aro K, Nurmi JE, Kononen T, Halmesmaki E. A randomized controlled trial of intervention in fear of childbirth. Obstet Gynecol 2001;98:820–6.

12. Morrison J, MacKenzie IZ. Cesarean section on demand. Semin Perinatol 2003;27:20–33.

13. Chervenak FA, McCullough LB. An ethically justified algorithm for offering, recommending, and performing cesarean delivery and its application in managed care practice. Obstet Gynecol 1996;87:302–5.

14. Maternal decision making, ethics, and the law. ACOG Committee Opinion No. 321. American College of Obstetricians and Gynecologists. Obstet Gynecol 2005; 106:1127–37.

Surgery and patient choice. ACOG Committee Opinion No. 395. American College of Obstetricians and Gynecologists. Obstet Gynecol 2008;111:243–7.

ISSN 1074-861X

ACOG COMMITTEE OPINION

Number 397 • February 2008

Surrogate Motherhood*

Committee on Ethics

ABSTRACT: Ethical responsibilities are described for obstetrician–gynecologists who choose to participate in surrogacy arrangements by 1) advising couples who are considering surrogacy, 2) counseling potential surrogate mothers, 3) providing obstetric services for pregnant women participating in surrogacy, or 4) offering assisted reproductive technologies related to surrogacy. Although the obligations of physicians will vary depending on the type and level of their involvement, in all cases physicians should carefully examine all relevant issues related to surrogacy, including medical, ethical, legal, and psychologic aspects.

Although the practice of surrogate motherhood has become more common since the American College of Obstetricians and Gynecologists (ACOG) issued its first statement on this subject in 1983, it continues to be controversial. There are those who believe that surrogacy should be permitted because such arrangements can be beneficial to all parties, and to prohibit them would limit the autonomy of infertile couples and women who wish to help them through surrogate gestation. Others believe that the risks outweigh the benefits or that because of shifting emotions and attitudes toward the fetus during gestation, it is not possible for a pregnant woman to give truly informed consent to relinquish an infant until after birth has occurred (1).

Many issues related to surrogate motherhood have not been resolved, and considerable disagreement persists within the medical profession, the medical ethics community, state legislatures, the courts, and the general public. Similarly, no one position reflects the variety of opinions on surrogacy within ACOG's membership. Although these differences of opinion are recognized, the purpose of this Committee Opinion is to focus on the ethical responsibilities of obstetrician–gynecologists who choose to participate in surrogacy arrangements on a variety of levels, including caring for the pregnant woman and her fetus.

The American College of Obstetricians and Gynecologists

Women's Health Care Physicians

---

*Update of "Surrogate Motherhood" in *Ethics in Obstetrics and Gynecology*, Second Edition, 2004.

The first part of this Committee Opinion provides an overview of public policy issues, descriptions of the types of surrogacy, arguments supporting and opposing surrogacy arrangements, and particular concerns related to payment and commercialization. The second part offers ethical recommendations to physicians and patients who may participate in surrogacy. The ethical obligations of physicians will vary depending on the type and level of their involvement in surrogacy arrangements.

General Issues

Public Policy

In some states, the practice of surrogate motherhood is not clearly covered under existing law. There is a split among the states that have statutes. Some states prohibit surrogacy contracts or make them void and unenforceable, whereas others permit such agreements (2, 3).

When a court is asked to decide a dispute regarding parental rights or custody of a child born as a result of a surrogacy arrangement, existing statutes may not prove adequate given the complexity of the problem. Courts faced with such decisions have given preference to different factors: the best interest of the child, the rights of the birth mother (as in adoption situations), the genetic link between the child and the genetic parents, and the intent of the couple who entered into a surrogacy contract to become parents. Often two or more of these factors conflict with each other, and there is not a consensus in the legal or ethical communities as to which factor should have priority (2, 4–7).

The obstetrician–gynecologist who facilitates surrogacy arrangements should be aware of any statutes or court cases in the state in which he or she practices. In counseling individuals seeking a child through surrogacy or a woman who is considering surrogate gestation, the physician should encourage consideration of the possible consequences of a surrogacy arrangement, including potential legal complications.

Types of Surrogacy

Surrogacy can be classified on the basis of the source of the genetic material. Eggs, sperm, or both may be donated, thereby altering the "intended parents'" biologic relationship to the child.

In one type of surrogacy arrangement, the intended parents are a couple who reach an agreement with a woman (the "surrogate mother") who will be artificially inseminated with sperm provided by the male partner of the couple seeking surrogacy services. Thus, the genetic and gestational mother of any resultant child is the surrogate mother, and the genetic father is the intended father. The intended parents plan to be the "social" or "rearing" parents of the child. Although this Committee Opinion refers to intended parents as a couple, individual men and women also may seek surrogacy services.

In another type of surrogacy, in vitro fertilization and embryo transfer are combined with surrogacy arrangements. In this case, it is possible for both the intended father and the intended mother to be the genetic parents of the child, and the surrogate fulfills only the role of gestational mother. This type of arrangement originally was called surrogate gestational motherhood, and now the carrying woman is called the "gestational carrier" or "gestational surrogate."

The different types of relationships that are possible—genetic (either, both, or neither intended parent), gestational (the surrogate mother), and social or rearing (the intended parents)—give rise to both conceptual challenges regarding the nature of parenthood and legal problems as to who should be considered the parents responsible for the child.

Major Arguments for and Against Surrogacy Arrangements

Surrogacy can allow a couple to have a child when they would otherwise be unable to do so except by adoption because of an inability to achieve pregnancy or medical contraindications to pregnancy for the intended mother. Adoption, however, does not provide a genetic link to the child, an important consideration for some prospective parents. Surrogacy is chosen by some prospective parents because of a desire for genetic linkage or for practical reasons, such as the scarcity of adoptable children.

Arguments based on reproductive liberty also support surrogacy arrangements. In the United States, the freedom to decide whether and when to conceive or bear a child is highly valued and protected. Thus, some have argued that intended parents and surrogate mothers should be free to cooperate in procreating, at least in cases of medical need and where care is taken to avoid harming others, especially the prospective child. Furthermore, women willing to participate in surrogacy may derive satisfaction from helping the intended parents. Many women participate in surrogacy primarily for altruistic reasons and see their services as a gift.

The primary arguments against surrogate motherhood are based on the harms that the practice may be thought to produce—harms to the child that is born, harms to the surrogate mother herself, harms to her existing children if she has children, and harms to society as a whole. It is surely harmful to any child to be the object of a custody dispute. In addition, the rejection of an infant—for example, rejection of an infant with a disability by both intended parents and surrogate mother—is a significant harm. If an existing relationship is used to coerce relatives or close friends to become surrogate mothers, that coercion is a harm resulting from the practice of surrogate motherhood. The existing children of a surrogate mother may be harmed if her pregnancy and relinquishment result in high levels of stress for the surrogate mother or her family. These children and society as a whole may be harmed by the perception that reproduction is trivialized by transactions that translate women's reproductive capacities and the infants that result into commodities to be bought and sold. Depersonalization of a pregnant woman as a "vehicle" for the genetic perpetuation of other individuals may harm not only surrogate mothers but also the status of women as a whole. There also is a concern that redefining concepts of motherhood may threaten traditional understandings of parenting and family.

Children are much more vulnerable than adults. Harms to children who have no choice in a matter are more serious, from an ethical standpoint, than harms to adults who make a choice that they later regret. Further, a distinction should be drawn between harms that inevitably, or almost invariably, are associated with a practice and harms that likely could be avoided through advance planning, appropriate counseling, or oversight mechanisms.

Few studies provide data about harms and benefits resulting from surrogacy arrangements. Absent such data, discussion about possible outcomes does not provide a solid foundation for ethical conclusions and clinical guidelines. It is important to know whether these outcomes actually occur and, if so, how frequently. Studies that will provide more data of this type are needed (8, 9).

In summary, there are strong arguments both for and against the practice of surrogacy. Physicians will be on both sides of this debate. If, after careful consideration of the arguments, a physician chooses to facilitate or recommend surrogacy arrangements, then precautions should be taken to prevent medical, psychologic, and legal harms to the intended parents, the potential surrogate mother, and the prospective child.

Payment to the Surrogate Mother

Perhaps no topic related to surrogate motherhood is more contentious than compensation of the surrogate mother by the intended parents (10). Payment often is substantial because of the duration and complexity of involvement. As noted previously, some states specifically prohibit surrogacy contracts that involve payment. Several questions about payment for surrogacy have been raised:

For what is payment made? Although there is debate on this point, it is clear that payment must not be made contingent on the delivery of an "acceptable product"—a live-born, healthy child. Rather, payment should be construed as compensation for the surrogate mother's time and effort, her initiating and carrying the pregnancy, her participation in labor and delivery, her acceptance of the risks of pregnancy and childbirth, and her possible loss of employment opportunities.

Why is payment offered or requested? In many surrogacy arrangements among close friends or relatives, there is no payment for the services of the surrogate mother. Rather, she may provide her services as an act of altruism, and the intended parents will be asked to reimburse her only for out-of-pocket expenses connected with the pregnancy. However, most women are understandably reluctant to undertake the burdens and risks of pregnancy on behalf of strangers without some kind of compensation for their time, effort, and risk.

Is payment likely to lead to the exploitation of potential surrogate mothers? Surrogacy arrangements often take place between parties with unequal power, education, and economic status (11). Unless independent legal representation and mental health counseling are mandated, women serving as surrogate mothers may be particularly vulnerable to being exploited. If a payment offered to a candidate for surrogacy is too low, it may be said to exploit her by not providing adequate compensation; if the payment is too high, it may be said to exploit her by being irresistible and coercive. Opponents of surrogate motherhood also have argued that if a fee must be paid to the surrogate mother, only affluent couples will be able to seek surrogacy services. This access barrier, however problematic, exists for most services related to infertility, for certain other medical procedures, and for adoption and, thus, is not specific to surrogacy agreements.

Responsibilities of Obstetrician–Gynecologists

In this Committee Opinion, the Committee on Ethics makes ethical recommendations for four categories of physician involvement: 1) advising couples who are considering surrogacy, 2) counseling potential surrogate mothers, 3) providing obstetric services for pregnant surrogates, and 4) offering assisted reproductive technologies related to surrogacy. Although the obligations of physicians will vary depending on the type and level of their involvement, in all cases physicians should carefully examine all relevant issues related to surrogacy, including medical, ethical, legal, and psychologic aspects.

Intended parents and surrogate mothers have both divergent and common interests. Because of these divergent interests, one professional individual (eg, physician, attorney, or psychologist) or agency should not represent the interests of both major parties in surrogacy arrangements. The physician who treats the intended parents should not have the surrogate mother as an obstetric patient because conflicts of interest may arise that would not allow the physician to serve all parties properly.

Responsibilities of Physicians to Couples Considering Surrogacy

When approached by a couple considering surrogacy, the physician should, as in all other aspects of medical care, be certain that there will be a full discussion of ethical and legal issues as well as medical risks, benefits, and alternatives, many of which have been addressed in this statement. An obstetrician–gynecologist who is not familiar with these issues should refer the couple for appropriate counseling. Additional recommendations for advising couples considering surrogacy are as follows:

- Because of the risks inherent in surrogacy arrangements, such arrangements should be considered only in the case of infertility or serious health-related needs, not for convenience alone.

- A physician may justifiably decline to participate in initiating surrogacy arrangements for personal, ethical, or medical reasons.

- If a physician decides to become involved in facilitating surrogate motherhood arrangements, the following guidelines should be used:

    —The physician should be assured that appropriate procedures are used to screen the intended parents and the surrogate mother. Such screening should include appropriate fertility studies, medical screening, and psychologic assessment.

    —Mental health counseling should be provided before initiation of a pregnancy 1) to permit the potential surrogate mother and the intended parents to explore the range of outcomes and possible long-term effects and 2) to consider possible psychologic risks to and vulnerabilities of both parties and the prospective child.

    —It is preferable that surrogacy arrangements be overseen by private nonprofit agencies with credentials similar to those of adoption agencies. However, many existing agencies are entrepreneurial and for-profit (9). A physician making a referral to an agency must have assurance that the agency is medically and ethically reputable and that it is committed to protecting the interests of all parties involved.

— The physician should receive only usual compensation for medical services. Referral fees and other arrangements for financial gain beyond usual fees for medical services are inappropriate.

— The physician should not refer patients to surrogacy programs in which the financial arrangements are likely to exploit any of the parties.

- The obstetrician–gynecologist should urge the intended parents to discuss preconditions and possible contingencies with the surrogate mother or her representative and to agree in advance on the response to them. These issues include, but may not be limited to, the expected health-related behaviors of the surrogate mother; the prenatal diagnosis of a genetic or chromosomal abnormality; the inability or unwillingness of the surrogate mother to carry the pregnancy to term; the death of one of the intended parents or the dissolution of the couple's marriage during the pregnancy; the birth of an infant with a disability; a decision by the surrogate mother to abrogate the contract and to contest custody of an infant conceived with the sperm of the intended father; or, in the case of gestational surrogacy, the option of registering the intended parents as the legal parents.

- The obstetrician–gynecologist should urge the parties involved to record in writing the preconditions and contingency plans on which they have agreed to make explicit the intentions of the parties, to facilitate later recollection of these intentions, and to help promote the interests of the future child. In the preparation of this agreement, both parties should be encouraged to have independent legal representation.

- Whatever compensation is provided to the surrogate mother should be paid solely on the basis of her time and effort, her initiation and continued gestation of the pregnancy, her participation in labor and delivery, her acceptance of the risks of pregnancy and childbirth, and her possible loss of employment opportunities. Compensation must not be contingent on a successful delivery or on the health of the child.

- Where possible, obstetrician–gynecologists should cooperate with and participate in research intended to provide data on outcomes of surrogacy arrangements.

Responsibilities of Physicians to Potential Surrogate Mothers

When approached by a patient considering becoming a surrogate mother, the physician should address ethical and legal concerns fully along with medical risks and ben-

efits as part of the initial consultation. In particular, the physician should be sure that preconditions and contingencies, such as those outlined in the previous section, have been thoroughly considered and that the potential surrogate mother recognizes the importance of having explicit written precondition and contingency agreements. In the preparation of this agreement, both the intended parents and the potential surrogate mother should be encouraged to have independent legal representation. Additional recommendations for counseling and providing other services for potential surrogate mothers are as follows:

- To avoid conflict of interest, the physician should not facilitate a woman's becoming a surrogate mother for a couple whom the physician also is treating.

- The physician should ensure that appropriate procedures are used to screen and counsel both the intended parents and the surrogate mother. Referral for mental health counseling should be provided before initiation of a pregnancy 1) to permit the potential surrogate mother to explore the range of outcomes and possible long-term effects and 2) to evaluate her psychologic risks and vulnerabilities as well as the possible effects of surrogacy on her existing relationships and on any existing children.

- A physician who provides examinations and performs procedures for an agency that arranges surrogacy contracts should be aware of the policies of the agency and should decline involvement with any agency whose policies are not consistent with the ethical recommendations of this Committee Opinion and those of other professional organizations related to reproductive medicine, such as the American Society for Reproductive Medicine (formerly known as the American Fertility Society) (8, 9, 12).

- Whatever compensation is provided to the surrogate mother should be paid solely on the basis of her time and effort, her initiation and continued gestation of the pregnancy, her participation in labor and delivery, her acceptance of the risks of pregnancy and childbirth, and her possible loss of employment opportunities. Compensation must not be contingent on a successful delivery or on the health of the child.

- The physician should avoid participation in medical care arising from surrogacy arrangements in which the financial or other arrangements are likely to exploit any of the parties. The physician, therefore, is obliged to become as informed as possible about the financial and other arrangements between the surrogate mother and intended parents to make ethical decisions about providing medical care. A physician who agrees to provide medical care in what he or she later recognizes as clearly exploitative circumstances has a responsibility to discuss and, if possible, resolve problematic arrangements with all parties and may choose to transfer care when it is possible to do so.

Responsibilities of Physicians to Pregnant Women Participating in Surrogacy

When a woman participating in surrogacy seeks medical care for an established pregnancy, the obstetrician should explore with the woman her understanding of her contract with the intended parents and any provisions of it that may affect her care. If the physician believes that provisions of the contract may conflict with his or her professional judgment, the physician may refuse to accept the patient under those terms. Once accepted as a patient, she should be cared for as any other obstetric patient, regardless of the method of conception, or referred to an obstetrician who will provide that care. Even if she has already undergone screening by an agency, a physician–patient relationship exists between her and the obstetrician. The obstetrician has the attendant obligations of this relationship. Additional recommendations regarding the provision of obstetric services in this setting are as follows:

- The obstetrician's professional obligation is to support the well-being of the pregnant woman and her fetus, to support the pregnant woman's goals for the pregnancy, and to provide appropriate care regardless of the patient's plans to keep or relinquish the future child. If a physician's discomfort with surrogacy arrangements might interfere with that obligation, the patient should be referred to another obstetrician.

- The pregnant woman should be the sole source of consent regarding clinical intervention and management of the pregnancy, labor, and delivery.

- Agreements the surrogate mother has made with the intended parents regarding her care and behavior during pregnancy and delivery should not affect the physician's care of the patient. The obstetrician must make recommendations that are in the best interests of the pregnant woman and her fetus, regardless of prior agreements between her and the intended parents.

- Confidentiality between the physician and the pregnant patient should be maintained. The intended parents may have access to the patient's medical information only with the pregnant woman's explicit consent.

- Obstetrician–gynecologists are encouraged to assist in the development of hospital policies to address labor, delivery, postpartum, and neonatal care in situations in which surrogacy arrangements exist.

Responsibilities of Infertility Specialists and Reproductive Endocrinologists to Intended Parents and Surrogate Mothers

In providing medical services related to surrogate motherhood arrangements, infertility specialists and reproductive endocrinologists should follow the recommendations in the two previous sections. In particular, these specialists should ensure that appropriate procedures are used to screen the intended parents and the surrogate mother and that mental health counseling is provided to all parties before initiation of a pregnancy. Additional recommendations regarding the provision of assisted reproductive technologies are as follows:

- A physician who performs artificial insemination or in vitro fertilization as a part of surrogacy services necessarily will be involved with both the intended parents and the surrogate mother. However, the intended parents and the surrogate mother should have independent counseling and independent legal representation, and the surrogate mother should obtain obstetric care from a physician who is not involved with the intended parents.

- A physician who provides examinations and performs procedures for an agency that arranges surrogacy contracts should be aware of the policies of the agency and should decline involvement with any agency whose policies are not consistent with the ethical recommendations of this Committee Opinion and those of other professional organizations related to reproductive medicine (8, 9, 12).

- Specialists in infertility and reproductive endocrinology are encouraged to participate in research that is intended to provide data on the outcomes of surrogacy arrangements.

Summary

The obstetrician–gynecologist has an ethical responsibility to review the risks and benefits of surrogacy fully and fairly with couples who are considering surrogacy arrangements. The obstetrician who is consulted by a pregnant woman who is participating in a surrogacy arrangement owes her the same care as any pregnant woman and must respect her right to be the sole source of consent for all matters regarding prenatal care and delivery. The gynecologist or specialist in reproductive endocrinology who performs procedures required for surrogacy should be guided by the same ethical principles aimed at safeguarding the well-being of all participants, including the future child.

References

1. Lederman RP. Psychosocial adaptation in pregnancy: assessment of seven dimensions of maternal development. 2nd ed. New York (NY): Springer Publishing Company; 1996.

2. The American Surrogacy Center. Legal: state by state overview. Kennesaw (GA): TASC; 2005. Available at: http://www.surrogacy.com/Articles/cate_list.asp?ID=7&n=Legal%3A++State+by+State+Overview. Retrieved July 10, 2007.

3. National Conference of Commissioners on Uniform State Laws. Gestational agreement. Article 8. In: Uniform parentage act. Chicago (IL): NCCUSL; 2002. p. 68–78.

4. Andrews LB. Alternative modes of reproduction. In: Cohen S, Taub N, editors. Reproductive laws for the 1990s. Clifton (NJ): Humana Press; 1989. p. 361–403.

5. Serratelli A. Surrogate motherhood contracts: should the British or Canadian model fill the U.S. legislative vacuum? George Washington J Int Law Econ 1993;26:633–74.

6. Field M. Reproductive technologies and surrogacy: legal issues. Creighton Law Rev 1992;25:1589–98.

7. New York State Task Force on Life and the Law. Assisted reproductive technologies: analysis and recommendations for public policy. New York (NY): NYSTF; 1998.

8. Surrogate gestational mothers: women who gestate a genetically unrelated embryo. American Fertility Society. Fertil Steril 1994;62(suppl 1):67S–70S.

9. Surrogate mothers. American Fertility Society. Fertil Steril 1994;62(suppl 1):71S–77S.

10. Moody-Adams MM. On surrogacy: morality, markets, and motherhood. Public Aff Q 1991;5:175–90.

11. Harrison M. Financial incentives for surrogacy. Womens Health Issues 1991;1:145–7.

12. Family members as gamete donors and surrogates. Ethics Committee Report. American Society for Reproductive Medicine. Fertil Steril 2003;80:1124–30.

Surrogate motherhood. ACOG Committee Opinion No. 397. American College of Obstetricians and Gynecologists. Obstet Gynecol 2008;111:465–70.

ISSN 1074-861X

ACOG COMMITTEE OPINION

Number 401 • March 2008

Relationships With Industry*

Committee on Ethics

ABSTRACT: Although physicians and their professional organizations have routinely accepted gifts from the health care industry, evidence now indicates that such gifts may misdirect physicians from their primary responsibility to act in the best interests of their patients. The American College of Obstetricians and Gynecologists' Committee on Ethics offers revised recommendations for relationships with industry. Physicians should understand the potential for influence when considering accepting gifts, including those of apparently nominal value. If any gifts are accepted, they should primarily entail benefit to patients or be related to the physician's work and should not be of substantial value. Sample drugs (or vouchers) may be dispensed but preferably as a full course of therapy on the basis of true need. Physicians are obligated to seek the most accurate, up-to-date, evidence-based, and balanced source of information about products. Neither patient referral nor industry support of institutions should be contingent on physician use or advocacy of a product. Physicians should disclose their financial interests to patients and colleagues. Support from industry for continuing medical education and professional meetings may be accepted, but subsidies should be disclosed and should not be accepted directly by physicians. Speakers may receive reasonable honoraria. Reimbursement for research should not exceed reasonable direct and indirect costs, and reasonable compensation for subsequent consulting and lecturing is permissible. Investigators who are or may become involved in a company's research may not buy or sell its stock until their involvement ends and the research is published or disseminated.

**The American College
of Obstetricians
and Gynecologists**

*Women's Health Care
Physicians*

Industrial development of products is important to continuing improvement in health care. Manufacturers of pharmaceutical agents and medical devices assist physicians in the pursuit of their educational goals and objectives through financial support of various medical, research, and educational programs. The goals of corporations, however, may conflict with physicians' duties to their patients. Corporations are primarily responsible to their stockholders, whereas physicians are primarily responsible to their patients.

In the past, physicians and their professional organizations often have uncritically accepted gifts from the health care industry in the belief that such gifts did not necessarily create undue influence on medical practice. Evidence has accumulated, however, about the extent to which gifts from industry may misdirect physicians from their primary

*Update of "Relationships With Industry" in *Ethics in Obstetrics and Gynecology*, Second Edition, 2004

responsibility, which is to act consistently in the best interests of their patients. Studies demonstrate that the prescribing practices of physicians are commonly influenced by both subtle and obvious marketing messages and gifts, even when delivered in an educational context, and even when the physicians studied did not recognize or admit to any changes in their practice of medicine (1, 2).

When members of industry interact with professional societies and their members, corporate activities may generate biases or obligations unrelated to product merit, creating the actuality or the appearance of inappropriate and undue interest on the part of physicians or organizations. In addition to selling drugs, medical devices, and tests, corporations are significantly involved in support of medical practice at all levels, leading to a considerable risk of conflict of interest. In 2002, pharmaceutical companies spent $11.5 billion to provide physicians with free samples (3). Sixty percent of biomedical research is privately funded, of which 70% is directly supported by the pharmaceutical industry. Fifty percent of continuing medical education (CME) is funded primarily through educational grants by the pharmaceutical industry (4, 5). Biomedical research expenditures by industry exceed those of the federal government. In a survey of more than 3,000 physicians, 78% reported receiving pharmaceutical samples, 83% received meals, 35% received reimbursement for CME expenses, and 28% received payment for consulting or serving on an advisory board or speakers bureau (6). This widespread industry support, funding, and involvement has the strong potential to affect treatment practices and may lead to decisions based on factors other than the merit of the product alone.

The public expects physicians to avoid conflicts of interest in decisions about patient care, which usually involve the direct treatment of patients. Conflicts also may involve physician participation in purchasing decisions by medical organizations, such as hospitals and group practices. When any product promotion or research project leads to inappropriate or unbalanced medical advice to patients, an ethical problem exists. Sponsorship of medical activities by industrial companies and by other agencies seeking to influence medical care patterns must not distort the accuracy, completeness, or balanced presentation of medical advice to patients. Disclosure of conflict may not be sufficient to nullify its effect.

Evidence of the subtle and often unrecognized influence over prescribing behavior is part of an important ethical argument. Physicians have long been held to a high moral standard in the patient–physician relationship. This relationship is not egalitarian. Instead, the physician has control over knowledge of and, often, access to treatment, creating an obligation of fidelity, the ethical obligation not to abandon the patient. In this relationship the patient is given priority, and there is a responsibility to serve as personal advocate for the patient and to eliminate impediments to the promotion of patient welfare. The physician is obligated to ensure that the best medical advice is transmitted to the patient and is not prejudiced in any manner by industry incitements of gifts, support, or advertisement.

Recommendations of Other Organizations

Several professional and regulatory organizations have put forth positions related to industry's relationship to individual physician practices and educational activities (7–16). There has been movement within the profession to further restrict relationships with industry, particularly in the setting of academic medical centers. The American Medical Student Association launched the "PharmFree Campaign" initiative in 2002 to encourage medical students toward evidence-based prescribing and to avoid all

pharmaceutical advertisements and sponsorships (17). A growing number of professional leaders have called for similar restrictions for those in settings other than training programs. They are proposing that, despite the restrictions put in place by industry, professional societies, and government agencies, conflict of interest is inherent in all educational ventures promoted by the health care industry (18). For example, several prominent teaching institutions have taken the step of banning gifts, lunches, and educational events sponsored by industry (19).

In addition, and at least in part in response to this move toward regulation, the Pharmaceutical Research and Manufacturers of America (PhRMA) has developed guidelines for the pharmaceutical industry's relationship with clinicians (13) and for the conduct of clinical trials and the communication of clinical trial results (14). These voluntary guidelines took effect in 2002. Similarly, in 2004 the Advanced Medical Technology Association (AdvaMed) adopted a code of ethics to guide its members (medical technology companies) in interacting with health care professionals. This code of ethics generally addresses the same issues as the PhRMA guidelines (15).

Finally, guidance has been issued by the federal government. In 2003, the Office of Inspector General (OIG) at the U.S. Department of Health and Human Services issued a notice regarding voluntary compliance programs for pharmaceutical manufacturers. Among the written policies and procedures that the OIG suggests be addressed are 1) a code of conduct and 2) potential risks, including relationships with purchasers, physicians, and sales agents (ie, gifts, entertainment, personal compensation, education grants, and research funding). The OIG guidance references and endorses the voluntary PhRMA guidelines (16).

Recommendations of the American College of Obstetricians and Gynecologists' Committee on Ethics

The American College of Obstetricians and Gynecologists is committed to work toward ensuring that its educational mission is evidence based and free from undue bias from all outside influence. The following are recommended to address the College's and Fellows' relationships with industry.

Industry–physician interactions can be divided into five major types, as characterized in the following sections. Ethical implications specific to each type of interaction are discussed. In providing recommendations, the Committee on Ethics is mindful both of the effort Fellows have made to meet past recommendations and the challenges in meeting the ideal behaviors outlined. In presenting these paradigms, the Committee wishes to set goals that will not only eliminate undue influence on Fellows' practice and behavior but also promote continued confidence in the provider and specialty.

Product Promotion to Individual Physicians by Advertising, Personal Communication, and Provision of Samples

Physicians have an obligation to go beyond the information provided through advertising or other marketing strategies in selecting the best product for care of the patient. Substantial evidence exists that even small gifts influence prescribing practices and thereby have an impact on patient care (18). The provision of samples similarly influences prescribing practice (20). To preclude inappropriate influence, the Committee on Ethics recommends the following:

- Physicians have an obligation to seek the most accurate, up-to-date, evidence-based, and balanced sources of information about new products that they contemplate using. They should not base decisions solely or primarily on information provided by the products' marketers. Physicians must recognize that promotional items provided by vendors have been carefully produced or promoted to advocate use of their products.

- Although the provision of pharmaceutical samples offers potential benefits to patients, particularly for those who are uninsured or for whom purchase of medications otherwise represents a burden, such samples also may influence prescribing behavior inappropriately. Until a means is found to ensure that all patients have access to medications, physicians may choose to provide samples or vouchers but should be aware of these influences. In particular, physicians should be mindful of providing samples to cover just a portion of a course of needed treatment, a practice that may promote patients' ongoing use of a particular medication, when other potential alternatives exist. When vouchers or samples are dispensed, consideration should be given to providing them preferentially to those patients with a true need and dispensing a supply sufficient for a full course of therapy.

- Providers should understand that gifts tied to promotional information, even small gifts and meals, are designed to influence provider behavior. Fellows should be mindful of such intents and influences when deciding whether to accept gifts, including gifts of apparently nominal value. Cash gifts should not be accepted.

- Any gifts accepted by an individual physician should primarily entail a benefit to patients or be related to the physician's work and should not be of substantial value. Accordingly, textbooks, study aids, and similar gifts may be acceptable only if they serve a genuine educational function.

Donations, Parties, Trips, Services, and Opportunities for Investment

The health care industry also has promoted its products to individual physicians and groups of physicians, such as medical specialty societies, by provision of donations, parties, trips, services, and opportunities for investment. Such promotional practices, whether directed toward professional groups or individual physicians, must be assumed to have as their purpose the creation of attitudes or practices favorable to the donor. This may result in a real or perceived conflict of interest for the individual recipient or organization. Such ethical conflicts can interfere with patient care and may not be in keeping with the standards of professional conduct to which physicians are expected to adhere. In this regard, the Committee on Ethics recommends the following:

- Any individual or group should weigh carefully the risks of ethical conflicts and adverse public opinion before accepting donations, parties, trips, and services directly from industry.

- When the obstetrician–gynecologist has a significant financial interest in or receives anything of substantial material value, including royalties, from companies in the health care industry, such as a manufacturer of pharmaceuticals and medical devices, this information should be disclosed to patients and colleagues (21). Physicians should not engage in agreements in which referral of patients to them is contingent on their use or advocacy of a product.

- Physicians should not engage in agreements in which companies make substantial donations to a third party (eg, a hospital or charitable organization) that is contingent on their use or advocacy of a product.

Support of Educational Activities, Awards, and Development Contracts

The health care industry has promoted its products to individual physicians and groups, including specialty societies, hospitals, and medical schools, through the support of educational activities, awards, and development contracts. Support of educational programs and the provision of awards, grants, and contracts should follow, in principle, the guidelines of the American Medical Association (7, 8) and the Accreditation Council for Continuing Medical Education (12), which are adapted by the Committee on Ethics as follows:

- Subsidies to underwrite the costs of CME conferences or professional meetings can contribute to the improvement of patient care and, therefore, are permissible. Payments to defray the costs of a conference should not be accepted directly from the company by the physicians who are attending the conference. Funds from a commercial source should be in the form of an educational grant made payable to the accredited provider for the support of programs. The ultimate decision about funding arrangements for CME activities must be the responsibility of the accredited provider. It is most desirable if these funds are allocated from a central repository.

- Subsidies from industry should not be accepted directly to pay for the costs of travel, lodging, or other personal expenses of the physicians who are attending the conferences or meetings; subsidies should not be accepted to compensate physicians for their time.

- The gift of special funds to permit medical students, residents, and fellows to attend carefully selected educational conferences may be permissible as long as the selection of the students, residents, or fellows who will receive the funds is made by the academic or training institution or by the accredited CME provider with the full concurrence of the academic or training institution. These funds should be deposited at a central office within the training institution that could dispense these funds directly to the designated trainee.

- When companies underwrite medical conferences or lectures other than under their own labels, the physicians responsible for organizing these activities should be responsible for and control the selection of content, faculty, educational methods, and materials.

- Subsidies of educational activities, including activities linked to meals, should not include direct promotion or requisite contact with company representatives.

- Accredited CME providers are responsible for the content, quality, and scientific integrity of all CME activities and materials certified for credit. Commercially supported social events should be separated clearly from CME programs, and social activities should not compete with, or take precedence over, the educational events.

- Presentations should give a balanced view of therapeutic options. Use of generic names will contribute to this impartiality. If trade names are used, those of several companies should be used rather than only those of a single company.

- When commercial exhibits are part of the overall program, arrangements for these should not influence the planning or interfere with the presentation of CME activities. Exhibit placement should not be a condition of support for a CME activity.

- Subsidized professional presentations related to pharmaceutical products should avoid commercial advertisements or biased exposure at the same setting.

- All financial support for meetings and educational activities should be clearly disclosed, but physicians should be mindful that disclosure in itself may not eliminate the potential for influence or bias.

Industrial Sponsorship of Research

Companies must conduct clinical testing to obtain approval for the marketing of new products. This involves collaboration with physicians and clinical institutions when conducting such work. The Committee on Ethics recommends the following guidelines for engaging in industry-sponsored research:

- Research trials should be conducted in accordance with the federal guidelines for the protection of human participants (22). Approval by the institutional review board of a medical school or hospital provides adequate ethical and scientific review. If the project is to be conducted in a private medical office, investigators must ascertain the nature of the ethical and scientific review process by the sponsoring corporation. Submission of the project to the researcher's institution usually is required and helpful. If there is any question about the adequacy or efficacy of this review, investigators should seek independent consultation for research oversight.

- Reimbursement to investigators and their institutions for involvement in research, including recruitment of participants, should not exceed reasonable direct and indirect costs. Investigators may accept reasonable compensation for consultation or lecturing that follows participation in research.

- Once a clinical investigator becomes involved in a research project for a company or knows that he or she might become involved, the investigator, as an individual, cannot ethically buy or sell the company's stock until the involvement ends and the results of the research are published or otherwise disseminated to the public (23).

- The following guidelines should govern control over information gained from research (24):

  — All obligations of investigators and sponsors should be contractually defined.

  — Scientific freedom of independent investigators (those not employed by the funding organization) should be preserved.

  — Principal investigators should be involved in decisions regarding the publication of data from their trials. Short delays in the dissemination of data generated by industry-sponsored research are acceptable to protect a patent or related proprietary interests. Prolonged delays, or suppression of information harmful to the sponsor's interests, are unethical.

  — Investigators should control the use of their names in promotions.

  — Project funding should not be contingent on results.

  — Investigators should disclose their relationships with industry funders in publications or lectures based on the research.

Speakers Bureaus, Consulting Services, and Ghostwriting

Speakers bureaus are a common marketing strategy to promote a particular product through the use of recognized professional leaders as paid spokespersons. Speakers bureaus are an efficient way to communicate information about a specific product but are subject to a high potential for bias and unbalanced information and conflict of interest. Audiences may not be able to identify bias when it occurs (18). Physicians who participate in industry-sponsored speaking should adhere to the following specific ethical guidelines to reduce the risk of undue influence:

- Speakers should fully disclose the extent of their relationship with the sponsoring entity.

- Speakers should ensure that the information in their presentation is accurate, balanced, evidence based, and free of undue commercial influence.

- Speakers should take responsibility for the material presented and ensure that the material has not been regulated by the sponsoring corporation.

- Speakers should accept only reasonable honoraria commensurate with the value of their time and reimbursement for travel, lodging, and expenses derived from predetermined policies.

- Speakers should recognize that they may be influenced through their relationship with the sponsoring corporation.

Consulting with industry on the development of new medical devices or pharmaceutical agents can play an important role in the progress of scientific discovery. It also is appropriate for consultants who provide genuine services to receive reasonable reimbursement for travel, lodging, and meal expenses, as well as value of their time. Token consulting or advisory arrangements cannot be used to justify the compensation of physicians for their time or their travel, lodging, and other out-of-pocket expenses. It must be recognized, however, that industry may use consulting arrangements in order to influence the consultant.

The practice of "ghostwriting" or unacknowledged medical writing that may be sponsored by the pharmaceutical or other industry is unacceptable because it is inherently deceptive and may bias the presentation of research results. Authors should write and assume responsibility for the content of all publications for which they receive authorship credit. Ghostwriting, in which a writer produces content attributed to another, should be distinguished from acknowledged authorship and peer editing, which may serve important communication functions.

Summary

Support from the pharmaceutical and device industry continues to provide substantial and potentially valuable support for physician education. Obstetrician–gynecologists' relationships with industry should be structured in a manner that will enhance, rather than detract from, their obligations to their patients. The guidelines set forth in this Committee Opinion will contribute to this goal.

References

1. Wazana A. Physicians and the pharmaceutical industry: is a gift ever just a gift? JAMA 2000;283:373–80.

2. Morgan MA, Dana J, Loewenstein G, Zinberg S, Schulkin J. Interactions of doctors with the pharmaceutical industry. J Med Ethics 2006;32:559–63.

3. Kumar P, Zaugg AM. IMS review: steady but not stellar. MM&M May 2003. p. 50–63. Available at: http://www. imshealth.com/vgn/images/portal/cit_40000873/42912029 Business%20Watch.pdf. Retrieved November 8, 2007.

4. Studdert DM, Mello MM, Brennan TA. Financial conflicts of interest in physicians' relationships with the pharmaceutical industry—self-regulation in the shadow of federal prosecution. N Engl J Med 2004;351:1891–900.

5. Katz D, Caplan AL, Merz JF. All gifts large and small: toward an understanding of the ethics of pharmaceutical industry gift-giving. Am J Bioeth 2003;3:39–46.

6. Campbell EG, Gruen RL, Mountford J, Miller LG, Cleary PD, Blumenthal D. A national survey of physician–industry relationships. N Engl J Med 2007;356:1742–50.

7. American Medical Association. Gifts to physicians from industry. In: Code of medical ethics of the American Medical Association: current opinions with annotations. 2006-2007 ed. Chicago (IL): AMA; 2006. p. 212–6.

8. American Medical Association. Clarification of opinion 8.061 "gifts to physicians from industry." In: Code of medical ethics of the American Medical Association: current opinions with annotations. 2006-2007 ed. Chicago (IL): AMA; 2006. p. 216–24.

9. Coyle SL. Physician-industry relations. Part 1: individual physicians. Ethics and Human Rights Committee, American College of Physicians–American Society of Internal Medicine. Ann Intern Med 2002;136:396–402.

10. Coyle SL. Physician-industry relations. Part 2: organizational issues. Ethics and Human Rights Committee, American College of Physicians–American Society of Internal Medicine. Ann Intern Med 2002;136:403–6.

11. Accreditation Council for Graduate Medical Education. Principles to guide the relationship between graduate medical education and industry. Chicago (IL): ACGME; 2002. Available at: http://www.acgme.org/acWebsite/position Papers/ pp_GMEGuide.pdf. Retrieved November 8, 2007.

12. Accreditation Council for Continuing Medical Education. ACCME standards for commercial support. Standards to ensure the independence of CME activities. Chicago (IL): ACCME; 2004. Available at: http://www.accme.org/dir_docs/doc_upload/68b2902a-fb73-44d1-872580a1504e520c_uploaddocument.pdf. Retrieved November 8, 2007.

13. Pharmaceutical Research and Manufacturers of America. Code on interactions with healthcare professionals. Washington, DC: PhRMA; 2002. Available at: http://www.phrma.org/files/PhRMA%20Code.pdf. Retrieved November 8, 2007.

14. Pharmaceutical Research and Manufacturers of America. Principles on conduct of clinical trials and communication of clinical trial results. Washington, DC: PhRMA; 2002. Available at: http://www.phrma.org/files/Clinical%20Trials. pdf. Retrieved November 8, 2007.

15. Advanced Medical Technology Association. Code of ethics on interactions with health care professionals. Washington, DC: AdvaMed; 2003. Available at: http://www.advamed. org/NR/rdonlyres/FA437A5F-4C75-43B2-A900-C9470BA8DFA7/0/coe_with_faqs_41505.pdf. Retrieved November 8, 2007.

16. OIG compliance program guidance for pharmaceutical manufacturers. Department of Health and Human Services, Office of Inspector General. Fed Regist 2003;68:23731–43.

17. American Medical Student Association. National Pharm Free Day. Reston (VA): AMSA; 2006. Available at: http://www.amsa.org/prof/pharmfree.cfm. Retrieved November 8, 2007.

18. Brennan TA, Rothman DJ, Blank L, Blumenthal D, Chimonas SC, Cohen JJ, et al. Health industry practices that create conflicts of interest: a policy proposal for academic medical centers. JAMA 2006;295:429–33.

19. Stanford University School of Medicine. Policy and guidelines for interactions between the Stanford University School of Medicine, the Stanford Hospital and Clinics, and Lucile Packard Children's Hospital with the pharmaceutical, biotech, medical device, and hospital and research equipment and supplies industries ("industry"). Stanford (CA): SUSM; 2006. Available at: http://med.stanford. edu/coi/siip/documents/siip_policy_aug06.pdf. Retrieved November 8, 2007.

20. Adair RF, Holmgren LR. Do drug samples influence resident prescribing behavior? A randomized trial. Am J Med 2005;118:881–4.

21. American College of Obstetricians and Gynecologists. Code of professional ethics of the American College of Obstetricians and Gynecologists. Washington, DC: ACOG; 2004. Available at: http://www.acog.org/from_home/ acogcode.pdf. Retrieved November 8, 2007.

22. Protection of human subjects, 42 C.F.R. §46 (2006).

23. American Medical Association. Conflicts of interest: biomedical research. In: Code of medical ethics of the American Medical Association: current opinions with annotations. 2006-2007 ed. Chicago (IL): AMA; 2006. p. 185–7.

24. Chren MM. Independent investigators and for-profit companies. Guidelines for biomedical scientists considering funding by industry. Arch Dermatol 1994;130:432–7.

Relationships with industry. ACOG Committee Opinion No. 401. American College of Obstetricians and Gynecologists. Obstet Gynecol 2008;111:799–804.

ISSN 1074-861X

ACOG COMMITTEE OPINION

Number 403 • April 2008

End-of-Life Decision Making*

Committee on Ethics

ABSTRACT: The purpose of this Committee Opinion is to discuss issues related to end-of-life care, including terms and definitions, ethical principles, legal constructs, physician–patient communication, and educational opportunities pertinent for specialists in obstetrics and gynecology. Assumptions about the objectives of care—which may be understood differently by the patient and her caregivers—inevitably shape perceptions about appropriate treatment. Because unarticulated commitments to certain goals may lead to misunderstanding and conflict, the goals of care should be identified through shared communication and decision making and should be reexamined periodically. A good opportunity to initiate the discussion of caregiving goals, including end-of-life care, is during well-patient care. Physicians must be careful not to impose their own conception of benefit or burden on a patient. End-of-life care is particularly challenging for pregnant women, whose autonomy is limited in many states. Many apparent conflicts will be averted by recognizing the shared interests of the woman and her fetus. When interests diverge, however, pregnant women's autonomous decisions should be respected.

Obstetricians and gynecologists, including those in training, care for women throughout their life span and not infrequently need to participate in end-of-life decision making. Tragic accidents occasionally threaten the life of a pregnant woman and her fetus, and terminal outcomes occur for some patients with gynecologic cancer. As a result, physicians are expected to present options and guide patients as they make decisions in the face of such events. Life-threatening situations are never easy to deal with, even for the well trained. The purpose of this Committee Opinion is to discuss issues related to end-of-life care, including terms and definitions, ethical principles, legal constructs, physician–patient communication, and educational opportunities pertinent for specialists in obstetrics and gynecology.

The Ethical Basis of Medical Practice

The moral foundation of medicine includes three values central to the healing relationship. These are patient benefit, patient self-determination, and the moral and ethical integrity of the health care professional (1, 2).

Patient Benefit

The obligation to promote the good of the patient is a basic presumption of medical caregiving and a defining feature of the physician's ethical responsibility. The ethical principle of beneficence upholds the physician's duty to seek to promote the patient's good, providing care in which benefits outweigh burdens or harms. Providing benefit at the end of life when further medical intervention may be deemed futile may at first seem challenging, but further consideration suggests that the principle of beneficence may be manifested in many dimensions. In some situations, it may be manifested by providing treatment to improve health or prolong life. In other situations, it may be exhibited through the elimination of false hope, avoidance of unwarranted tests and therapies, and assistance for patients and their families in reconciling themselves to the limitations of available medical options and achieving peace of mind. Indeed, in considering end-of-life care, benefits are understood only relative to the goals that the patient and physician hope to achieve through medical care. At times, what is beneficent in the patient's eyes may seem to the physician to cause more suffering or involve the inappropriate use of medical

The American College of Obstetricians and Gynecologists
Women's Health Care Physicians

*Update of "End-of-Life Decision Making" in *Ethics in Obstetrics and Gynecology*, Second Edition, 2004

resources. These complicated issues of futility are addressed further elsewhere (3).

Patient Self-Determination

The inherent value of individual autonomy or self-determination is one of the fundamental principles of democracy and represents the basis for many individual rights and protections in the United States. In health care, the value of individual autonomy is affirmed in the ethical and legal doctrine of informed consent (4, 5). Under this doctrine, the patient has a right to control what happens to her body. This means that in nonemergent situations, no treatment may be given to the patient without her consent (or, if she lacks decision-making capacity, the consent of her valid surrogate). Treatment otherwise given to the patient without her consent may be judged in some cases to be assault and battery. A patient's right to informed consent or refusal is not contingent on the presence or absence of terminal illness, on the agreement of family members, or on the approval of physicians or hospital administrators.

In the medical context, physician respect for patient self-determination consists of an active inclusion of the patient in decisions regarding her own care. This involves frank discussion of diagnoses and prognoses (an essential part of an informed consent); the relative risks and benefits of alternatives, including the option of refusing all curative treatments; and, based on these discussions, a mutual identification of the operative goals of care. Studies suggest that most patients want to know the reality of their conditions and benefit from an honest communication with the physician (6, 7). It is unethical for a physician to deny patients important information in order to avoid physician–patient interactions that are difficult or uncomfortable. Moreover, appropriate regard for patient autonomy involves respecting the patient's considered choice to change therapeutic modalities to better meet her current goals of care. The patient's choice may be conveyed through an instructional directive or a surrogate with power of attorney (see box). Advance directives will be discussed in later sections.

Ethical Integrity of the Health Care Professional

Because physicians, like patients, are autonomous agents, they usually cannot be compelled to violate personal ethical or religious commitments in service to the patient (8). If physicians have moral reservations about providing certain forms of caregiving or about stopping treatment, they should (if appropriate to the circumstances) make that known at the outset. Physicians must not stand in the way of patients' desires to seek other caregivers and should, where possible, help guide the transition.

The profession of medicine is guided by its moral commitment to avoid subjecting a patient to harms that are greater than potential benefits (the principle of nonmaleficence). On this basis, physicians have a presumptive obligation not to provide treatments that are untested, contraindicated, or useless. For this reason, a patient's demand for care that she deems desirable is not sufficient to impose on providers an absolute obligation to provide care that is futile or likely to be harmful without offering corresponding benefit.

Legal Developments That Bear on End-of-Life Decision Making

In addition to the emotional and medical challenges that accompany decisions at the end of life, care in such situations may be shaped by statute and legislation. Laws governing such situations vary from state to state. In the 1990s, there were a number of developments in law that influence end-of-life decision making.

First, in June 1990, in *Cruzan v. Director of the Missouri Dept. of Health*, the United States Supreme Court affirmed that patients have a constitutionally protected right to refuse unwanted medical treatments (9). The ruling also affirms the states' authority to adopt procedural requirements for the withdrawal and withholding of life-prolonging medical interventions.

A second legal development was the passage of the federal Patient Self-Determination Act (PSDA), which went into effect December 1, 1991 (10). The PSDA requires Medicaid- and Medicare-participating health care institutions to inform all adult patients of their rights "to make decisions concerning medical care, including the right to accept or refuse medical or surgical treatment and the right to formulate an advance directive." Under the PSDA, institutions that receive Medicare or Medicaid reimbursement are legally required to provide this information to patients on admission for care or on enrollment in a health maintenance organization. The institution must note in the medical record the existence of an advance directive and must respect these directives to the fullest extent under state law. Put simply, the aim of the PSDA is to empower patients to make decisions regarding their medical care.

Advance Directives

An advance directive is the formal mechanism by which a patient may express her values regarding her future health status. It may take the form of a proxy directive or an instructional directive or both:

- Proxy directives, such as the durable power of attorney for health care, designate a surrogate to make medical decisions on behalf of the patient who is no longer competent to express her choices. The terms *health care proxy*, *health care agent*, and *surrogate* can be used interchangeably. The term *surrogate* is used in this Committee Opinion.

- Instructional directives, such as living wills, focus on the types of life-sustaining treatment that a patient would or would not choose in various clinical circumstances.

A third development is found in legislation and legal rulings concerning the autonomy of the pregnant woman to refuse treatment. Although courts at times have intervened to impose treatment on a pregnant woman, currently there is general agreement that a pregnant woman who has decision-making capacity has the same right to refuse treatment as a nonpregnant woman (11). When a pregnant woman does not have decision-making capacity, however, legislation frequently limits her ability to refuse treatment through an advance directive. As of 2006, 31 states had living will statutes that explicitly forbid the withholding or withdrawal of life support either from all pregnant patients or from pregnant patients whose fetuses could become, or currently are, viable (12). Only four states specifically permit a woman to choose to refuse life-sustaining treatment if she is pregnant. The other states either have no living will statute or make no mention of pregnancy. Similar types of restrictions exist in some states with respect to a surrogate who is appointed to make decisions on behalf of a pregnant woman (11). Statutes that prohibit pregnant women from exercising their right to determine or refuse current or future medical treatment are unethical. (An ethical framework for addressing end-of-life decisions in pregnant women is discussed later in this Committee Opinion.)

A final development pertains to euthanasia and physician-assisted suicide. Euthanasia refers to the administration of drugs with the intention of ending a patient's life at her request (13). Physician-assisted suicide refers to supplying a patient with drugs or a prescription for drugs knowing one is enabling a patient to kill herself. Oregon's 1997 Death With Dignity Act, which permits physicians to write prescriptions for a lethal dosage of medication to people with a terminal illness, was upheld January 2006 by the Supreme Court. No other state in the United States allows such acts, but other countries that authorize physician-assisted suicide or euthanasia include Belgium, The Netherlands, and Australia.

In contrast to the previous decisions and legislation, some have argued that irrespective of the individuals' specific circumstances, support should be offered to maintain life. These arguments were made perhaps most prominently in debate and legislation surrounding the care of Terry Schiavo. As discussed in the following section, more than perhaps anything else, this case illustrated the advantage of all individuals providing advance, written instructions concerning their wishes for end-of-life care.

Physician–Patient Communication and the Goals of Care

The practice of obstetrics and gynecology involves many different types of care. These include but are not limited to preventive care; periodic examinations; family planning; the provision of prenatal and delivery care; medical and surgical intervention for conditions that threaten a patient's fertility, life, or quality of life; long-term care for patients with chronic illness; and palliative care for patients whose illnesses offer no chance of cure or remission. The combination of medical and surgical treatment approaches, as well as the intimate nature of the specialized care offered by obstetrician–gynecologists, allows for a long-term close relationship with many opportunities for communication with patients. Questions about the use of specific therapeutic modalities become meaningful often only in relation to the goals of management for a particular patient (14). Goals of care in obstetrics and gynecology include:

- Relief of symptoms, pain, and suffering
- Achievement of cure or remission
- Achievement or prevention of pregnancy
- Optimization of pregnancy outcomes
- Prevention of illness in a woman or her fetus or both
- Maintenance or restoration of biologic function
- Performance of palliative surgery or chemotherapy
- Maximization of comfort
- Achievement or maintenance of a certain quality of life
- Education of the patient about her medical condition

The ultimate goals of care are properly identified through a process of shared and ongoing communication and decision making between the patient and physician (15–17). Skilled, honest communication is key in this process. Explicit discussion about the goals of care is important for a number of reasons. First, assumptions about the objectives of care inevitably shape perceptions about the appropriate course of treatment. Second, these objectives may be understood differently by the patient and her caregivers. Third, unarticulated commitments to certain goals may lead to misunderstanding and conflict. Finally, the goals of care are fluid and may evolve and change in response to clinical or other factors.

A comprehensive and ongoing process of communication not only advances patient self-determination but also is the basis for "preventive ethics"; that is, the establishment of a moral common ground that may prevent ethical conflict and crisis (18). The benefits of engaging in and becoming skilled at such conversations are many and include optimizing care, diminishing family burden, diminishing stress among members of the health care team, and utilizing resources more effectively. Inadequate communication, whether from inappropriate training, personal provider discomfort with death, or differences in personal or cultural values, has the potential to impair the process of informed consent and may result in overtreatment, pain and suffering, undue burden on the patient and family, misuse of resources, and loss of the peace of mind that can result from including interdisciplinary care such as hospice and palliative care departments.

The well-publicized and discussed case of Terri Schiavo emphasizes the need to discuss these issues with loved ones and also the need to put them in writing. In this case, the diagnosis of a permanent vegetative state and the unwritten wishes of the patient contributed to painful conflicts between the patient's husband and her parents regarding the effort to keep her alive by tube feedings (19). Even if patients do all they can to make their wishes known, conflicts may still occur.

Shared Decision Making Regarding the End of Life

The process of decision making regarding the end of life may take place under two different circumstances. In the first, decisions are made in an acute situation of present health crisis; these are immediate choices that determine actual end-of-life treatment. In the second, decisions are made that proactively provide for possible future end-of-life situations; these decisions are expressed through advance directives. In practice, however, the distinction may not be drawn sharply, and such decision making often is more appropriately thought of as an ongoing process or conversation. Because circumstances may change, goals also may change over time and will need to be readdressed with all involved parties on a regular basis.

Communication Regarding Immediate Health Status

An ongoing process of informed consent requires physicians to communicate information regarding the patient's health status and comparative risks and benefits of treatment (including no treatment) so that she or, if she lacks decision-making capacity, her surrogate may determine goals of her care. If the patient decides that the maximization of comfort is her desired goal of care, the practitioner's responsibilities will focus on palliative strategies, such as pain relief, attentive and responsive communication with the patient about her health status, and the facilitation of communication with the patient's involved family and loved ones. These components of care are essential to the physician's positive therapeutic role and are often the most valuable services that can be offered. The expression "nothing more can be done" is misleading shorthand that improperly equates care with cure and, in so doing, ignores the importance of the physician's role in providing comfort to the dying patient (20–22).

If the patient or surrogate and physician finally disagree on the goals that should guide care, a clearly defined process of discussion and consultation should be followed to resolve the disagreement. Examples of a process are available (3, 23). In many institutions, such disagreements are first addressed by an ethics consultation service or an ethics committee. By using consultative services to clarify the cultural, religious, or personal considerations that shape decision making, the parties may be able to resolve apparent conflict. The specific details of this process may vary by institution and locality.

Results of such a consultation may include the transfer of care to another physician. In other circumstances, the assistance of a palliative care team to bridge the transition to palliative care may be helpful. Some patients who are near the end of life and who anticipate ever-increasing pain and suffering may inquire about the alternative of physician-assisted suicide. It currently is not legal for physicians to participate in physician-assisted suicide in states other than Oregon. When a patient inquires about physician-assisted suicide as a possible option, the physician should explore with her the nature of her fears and her expectations and should be prepared to offer reassurances regarding palliative care plans for relieving distress at the end of life. Physicians should be aware that a request for physician-assisted suicide may be a marker for treatable depression or inadequately treated pain.

Communication Regarding Future Health Status: Advance Directives

In many cases, it is the obstetrician–gynecologist who not only acts as the principal physician for female patients but also has the most contact with them throughout their lives. For these reasons, the obstetrician–gynecologist is in an ideal position to discuss with the patient her values and wishes regarding future care and to encourage her to formulate an advance directive (see box).

A good opportunity to initiate the discussion of caregiving goals, including end-of-life care, is during well-patient care, either at the time of the periodic examination or during pregnancy. Because a patient's wishes regarding care might change over time or under different conditions of illness, these discussions should include occasional reexamination of values and goals and, if necessary, updating of her advance directives and other documentation. Decision making should be treated as a process rather than an event.

To facilitate the initiation of these discussions, the patient history form could contain questions about a patient's execution of an instructional directive and her designation of a surrogate or next of kin as her medical proxy. If the patient has an instructional directive or durable power of attorney or both, they should become part of her medical record. If the patient does not have an advance directive, assistance in executing one might be provided by the social services or nursing staff of a hospital or clinical practice.

Ideally, these discussions serve an educational purpose for both patient and physician. For the physician, these discussions establish a basis for future care and provide an opportunity for the candid expression of personal values regarding care. For the patient, the discussions provide the opportunity to learn about advance directives, to formulate and articulate her values regarding the goals of care, and to understand the compatibility of these goals with the values of the health care provider.

Although it is the physician's responsibility to educate patients about possible future health status and rights regarding medical care, it is the responsibility of the patient to thoughtfully assess her values and goals and to make them clearly known to those involved in her care. Again, the explicit discussion and continued reevaluation of caregiving goals provides an optimal mechanism for shared decision making.

Potential Physician Influence

In the face of end-of-life decision making, physicians trained to prize interventionist strategies must be especially careful not to impose their own conception of benefit or burden on a patient or to use coercive means to establish or achieve goals that are not shared by the patient. The obstetrician–gynecologist should recognize that the harms associated with prolonged attempts at cure may not be acceptable to some patients. However, neither the presence of a "do not resuscitate" order nor specific directives regarding limitation of other treatments remove the responsibility for providing palliative care. Moreover, the physician should not rely on the presence or absence of a do-not-resuscitate order to make assumptions about the appropriateness of other treatment but rather should be guided by the explicitly identified goals of care.

There is considerable evidence that sociocultural and gender differences between patients and their physicians may subtly influence the style and content of physician–patient communication and the care that patients receive (24–31). Physicians who are aware of these potential problems can guard against the influence of bias in judgments concerning patient choices. Differences in gender and in ethnic, social, religious, and economic background between patients and physicians may complicate communication, but they should not compromise care.

An additional area of potential conflict is research. The dual role that physicians often assume as research scientists and clinical practitioners can be challenging because the goals and priorities of science and clinical practice may be different (32). For example, one should not overlook the potential conflict that may arise during a patient's end-of-life transition when the primary physician is also a primary investigator for an oncology trial for which the patient is eligible. Both the researcher and the primary caregiver should guard against inflating the patient's perception of the therapeutic benefit expected from participating in clinical trials. Studies have shown that research participants tend to believe, despite careful explanation of research protocols, that they will likely benefit from participation or that the level of actual benefit will be greater than stated in the consent process (33). A patient's decision to participate in research should be consistent with her end-of-life goals.

Surrogate Decision Making

If the patient who lacks decision-making capacity has not designated a surrogate, state law may dictate the order in which relatives should be asked to serve in this role. The individual selected should be someone who knows the patient's values and wishes and will respect them in his or her role as surrogate decision maker. If there is conflict regarding the designation of a surrogate, it may be appropriate to seek the advice of an ethics committee or consultant or, possibly, the courts. The benefit of choosing a surrogate is immeasurable because this individual has the same authority the patient would if she were able to make decisions. The surrogate has the legal right to all confidential medical information and ideally would be someone trusted and chosen by the patient herself. Proactively choosing a surrogate allows the opportunity to discuss pertinent religious or moral beliefs with that individual. One additional precaution a patient can take to be sure her wishes are respected is the execution of a living will.

The surrogate decision maker is ethically obligated to base decisions on the wishes and values of the patient. If these wishes and values have been explicitly stated, either in writing or in oral discussion, the surrogate has to interpret and apply them in the current situation. If wishes and values have not been explicitly stated beforehand, the surrogate has to attempt to extrapolate them from what is known about the patient. In some cases (for example, a never-competent patient), the surrogate will have to decide entirely on the basis of what is in the best interests of this particular patient.

Pregnant Patients and End-of-Life Decisions: Preventing Conflict

For the overwhelming majority of pregnant women, the welfare of the fetus is of the utmost concern. This concern motivates women to modify their behaviors for months at a time and to undergo the discomforts and risks of pregnancy and delivery. This maternal interest in fetal welfare traditionally has been the basis of the fundamental ethical commitment of obstetrician–gynecologists: that they are responsible for both the pregnant woman and her fetus and that they must optimize the benefits to both while minimizing the risks to each.

In recent years, some have advanced the view of the "fetus as patient"—an ethics framework that highlights questions about what should be done in cases in which the pregnant woman's decisions about her own health seem unlikely to optimize fetal well-being. Many of these apparent conflicts will be averted by recognizing the interconnectedness of the pregnant woman and fetus with an approach that emphasizes their shared interests. For cases in which their interests do diverge, however, candid discussion of these matters in advance of a situation, conflict, or crisis is important. Pregnant women's autonomous decisions should be respected, and concerns about the impact of those decisions on fetal well-being should be discussed in the context of medical evidence and understood within the context of the women's values and social context (11).

Within the context of obstetric care, situations rarely arise when a dying pregnant woman must decide between caregiving goals that emphasize palliative management for her own illness or an interventionist strategy, such as cesarean delivery, for the sake of her fetus. Likewise, she might be forced to decide between a curative strategy, such as chemotherapy, for her metastatic breast cancer and a course that poses less risk to her fetus but offers her less anticipated benefit. In either case, it is safe to assume that having been provided with all of the clinical information necessary to make her decision, she regards the choice as a difficult, possibly excruciating one and one that she wishes she did not have to make. The patient with a life-threatening condition identifies treatment goals by considering her beliefs and values in the context of obligations and concerns for her family, her fetus, and her own health and life prospects.

The obstetrician–gynecologist, as the woman's advocate, should attempt to ensure that the wishes of the pregnant patient are followed. Even if the patient is no longer able to make her own decisions, her previously expressed wishes and values (whether expressed as an instructional directive or through the appointment of a surrogate decision maker) should guide the course of treatment, whenever legally possible. When this is not possible, clinicians should advocate changes in the law (34, 35).

Clinician Education

The need for effective end-of-life education for physicians in training is obvious, not only for the benefit of patients but also for physicians, to avoid burnout and to help them manage anxiety with issues of mortality. In a survey of six medical schools, only 22–53% of fourth-year medical students felt prepared by the end-of-life education they received (36). A study of 157 first-year internal medicine residents (interns) identified very little classroom teaching, clinical observation, or clinical experience with end-of-life communication and, perhaps as a consequence, reported low self-perceived comfort and skill in this area (37). Finally, in a study of general surgeons, 84% reported receiving no education in palliative care in residency, and 44% indicated that they had not had sufficient continuing medical education on the topic (38).

One particularly beneficial educational example is that of the Giving Bad News script (39), but also helpful are courses such as the Healer's Art, designed by Rachael Naomi Remen (40), and techniques such as Narrative Medicine (41), designed for physicians to remain self-reflective about issues of humane caring and differences in their own concerns about life and death.

Conclusion

Effective proactive communication between the patient and the physician is the cornerstone of the therapeutic relationship. Explicit identification of the operative goals of care is important for four reasons:

1. Assumptions about the objectives of care inevitably shape perceptions about the appropriate course of treatment.

2. These objectives may be understood differently by the patient and her caregivers.

3. Unarticulated commitments to certain goals may lead to misunderstanding and conflict.

4. The goals of care may evolve and change in response to clinical or other factors.

In the course of providing comprehensive care, obstetrician–gynecologists are in an excellent position to encourage women to formulate advance directives. The discussion of the advance directive should be regarded as integral to the ongoing process of communication to be initiated by the health care provider. Special attention should be given to the discussion of treatment wishes with pregnant women facing end-of-life decisions, especially in view of current state restrictions on the application of advance directives during pregnancy.

Sometimes the maximization of comfort is the chosen therapeutic goal. In this case, the care offered by the physician can continue to benefit the patient in a number of important ways by providing humane and supportive care at the end of life.

References

1. Pellegrino ED, Thomasma DC. For the patient's good: the restoration of beneficence in health care. New York (NY): Oxford University Press; 1988.

2. Beauchamp TL, Childress JF. Principles of biomedical ethics. 5th ed. New York (NY): Oxford University Press; 2001.

3. Medical futility. ACOG Committee Opinion No. 362. American College of Obstetricians and Gynecologists. Obstet Gynecol 2007;109:791–4.

4. American College of Obstetricians and Gynecologists. Informed consent. In: Ethics in obstetrics and gynecology. 2nd ed. Washington (DC): ACOG; 2004. p. 9–17.

5. Faden RR, Beauchamp TL. A history and theory of informed consent. New York (NY): Oxford University Press; 1986.

6. Edinger W, Smucker DR. Outpatients' attitudes regarding advance directives. J Fam Pract 1992;35:650–3.

7. Guidelines on foregoing life-sustaining medical treatment. American Academy of Pediatrics Committee on Bioethics. Pediatrics 1994;93:532–6.

8. The limits of conscientious refusal in reproductive medicine. ACOG Committee Opinion No. 385. American College of Obstetricians and Gynecologists. Obstet Gynecol 2007;110:1203–8.

9. Cruzan v Director of the Missouri Dept. of Health et al, 497 US 261, 262 (1990).

10. Cate FH, Gill BA. The Patient Self-Determination Act: implementation issues and opportunities. Washington, DC: The Annenberg Washington Program; 1991.

11. Maternal decision making, ethics, and the law. ACOG Committee Opinion No. 321. American College of Obstetricians and Gynecologists. Obstet Gynecol 2005;106: 1127–37.

12. FindLaw for the Public. State laws: living wills. Eagan (MN): FindLaw; 2007. Available at: http://print.estate.findlaw.com/estate-planning/living-wills/estate-planning-law-state-living-wills.html. Retrieved July 18, 2007.

13. van der Maas PJ, van der Wal G, Haverkate I, de Graaff CL, Kester JG, Onwuteaka-Philipsen BD, et al. Euthanasia, physician-assisted suicide, and other medical practices involving the end of life in the Netherlands, 1990–1995. N Engl J Med 1996;335:1699–705.

14. American Medical Association, The Robert Wood Johnson Foundation. EPEC: education for physicians on end-of-life care: participant's handbook. Chicago (IL): AMA; Princeton (NJ): RWJF; 1999.

15. Larson DG, Tobin DR. End-of-life conversations: evolving practice and theory. JAMA 2000;284:1573–8.

16. Tulsky JA, Chesney MA, Lo B. How do medical residents discuss resuscitation with patients? J Gen Intern Med 1995; 10:436–42.

17. Tulsky JA, Chesney MA, Lo B. See one, do one, teach one? House staff experience discussing do-not-resuscitate orders. Arch Intern Med 1996;156:1285–9.

18. McCullough LB, Chervenak FA. Ethics in obstetrics and gynecology. New York (NY): Oxford University Press; 1994.

19. Caplan AL, McCartney JJ, Sisti DA, editors. The case of Terri Schiavo: ethics at the end of life. Amherst (NY): Prometheus Books; 2006.

20. Brody H, Campbell ML, Faber-Langendoen K, Ogle KS. Withdrawing intensive life-sustaining treatment—recommendations for compassionate clinical management. N Engl J Med 1997;336:652–7.

21. Faber-Langendoen K, Lanken PN. Dying patients in the intensive care unit: forgoing treatment, maintaining care. Ann Intern Med 2000;133:886–93.

22. Institute of Medicine (US). Approaching death: improving care at the end of life. Washington, DC: National Academy Press; 1997.

23. Medical futility in end-of-life care: report of the Council on Ethical and Judicial Affairs. JAMA 1999;281:937–41.

24. Foss C, Hofoss D. Patients' voices on satisfaction: unheeded women and maltreated men? Scand J Caring Sci 2004; 18:273–80.

25. Gordon HS, Street RL Jr, Sharf BF, Souchek J. Racial differences in doctors' information-giving and patients' participation. Cancer 2006;107:1313–20.

26. Kaplan KJ, Schneiderhan M, Harrow M, Omens R. Autonomy, gender, and preference for paternalistic or informative physicians: a study of the doctor-patient relation. Ethics Med 2002;18:49–60.

27. Liang W, Kasman D, Wang JH, Yuan EH, Mandelblatt JS. Communication between older women and physicians: preliminary implications for satisfaction and intention to have mammography. Patient Educ Couns 2006;64: 387–92.

28. Santoso JT, Engle DB, Schaffer L, Wan JY. Cancer diagnosis and treatment: communication accuracy between patients and their physicians. Cancer J 2006;12:73–6.

29. Schouten BC, Meeuwesen L. Cultural differences in medical communication: a review of the literature. Patient Educ Couns 2006;64:21–34.

30. Teutsch C. Patient-doctor communication. Med Clin North Am 2003;87:1115–45.

31. Uskul AK, Ahmad F. Physician-patient interaction: a gynecology clinic in Turkey. Soc Sci Med 2003;57:205–15.

32. Research involving women. ACOG Committee Opinion No. 377. American College of Obstetricians and Gynecologists. Obstet Gynecol 2007;110:731–6.

33. Appelbaum PS, Roth LH, Lidz CW, Benson P, Winslade W. False hopes and best data: consent to research and the therapeutic misconception. Hastings Cent Rep 1987;17:20–4.

34. American Medical Association. Principles of medical ethics. In: Code of medical ethics of the American Medical Association: current opinions with annotations. 2006–2007 ed. Chicago (IL): AMA; 2006. p. xv.

35. American College of Obstetricians and Gynecologists. Code of professional ethics of the American College of Obstetricians and Gynecologists. Washington, DC: ACOG; 2004. Available at: http://www.acog.org/from_home/acogcode.pdf. Retrieved July 10, 2007.

36. Fraser HC, Kutner JS, Pfeifer MP. Senior medical students' perceptions of the adequacy of education on end-of-life issues. J Palliat Med 2001;4:337–43.

37. Ury WA, Berkman CS, Weber CM, Pignotti MG, Leipzig RM. Assessing medical students' training in end-of-life communication: a survey of interns at one urban teaching hospital. Acad Med 2003;78:530–7.

38. Galante JM, Bowles TL, Khatri VP, Schneider PD, Goodnight JE Jr, Bold RJ. Experience and attitudes of surgeons toward palliation in cancer. Arch Surg 2005;140: 873–8; discussion 878–80.

39. Arnold RL, Egan K. Breaking the "bad" news to patients and families: preparing to have the conversation about end-of-life and hospice care. Am J Geriatr Cardiol 2004;13:307–12.

40. Remen RN, Rabow MW. The Healer's Art: professionalism, service and mission. Med Educ 2005;39:1167–8.

41. DasGupta S, Charon R. Personal illness narratives: using reflective writing to teach empathy. Acad Med 2004;79: 351–6.

End-of-life decision making. ACOG Committee Opinion No. 403. American College of Obstetricians and Gynecologists. Obstet Gynecol 2008;111:1021–7.

ISSN 1074-861X

ACOG COMMITTEE OPINION

Number 409 • June 2008

Direct-to-Consumer Marketing of Genetic Testing

Committee on Genetics

Committee on Ethics

This document reflects emerging clinical and scientific advances as of the date issued and is subject to change. The information should not be construed as dictating an exclusive course of treatment or procedure to be followed.

ABSTRACT: Marketing of genetic testing, although similar to direct-to-consumer advertising of prescription drugs, raises additional concerns and considerations. These include issues of limited knowledge among patients and health care providers of available genetic tests, difficulty in interpretation of genetic testing results, lack of federal oversight of companies offering genetic testing, and issues of privacy and confidentiality. Until all of these considerations are addressed, direct or home genetic testing should be discouraged because of the potential harm of a misinterpreted or inaccurate result.

With the increase in the number of clinical genetic tests requested by health care providers, there has been an increase in direct-to-consumer advertising and offering of genetic tests, including at-home tests and those provided by private companies. Although similar to direct-to-consumer advertising of prescription drugs, marketing of genetic testing raises additional concerns and considerations. These include issues of limited knowledge among patients and health care providers of available genetic tests, difficulty in interpretation of genetic testing results, lack of federal oversight of companies offering genetic testing, and issues of privacy and confidentiality.

All genetic testing, including at-home tests, should be considered medical testing because results might have an impact on future medical care and clinical decision making. Although some tests have been marketed as nonmedical, such as paternity testing and early fetal sex prediction from maternal blood, these also should be considered medical tests. Decisions based on these results regarding a pregnancy may cause a patient to seek further medical treatment or intervention.

Despite the clear limitations of direct-to-consumer genetic testing, women still use the service. Physicians should acknowledge that one factor that might contribute to this trend is the belief among some patients that adequate privacy safeguards do not exist when genetic testing is performed in the office.

Physicians should use mechanisms in their practice environment that would provide the reassurance that women seek when being tested for gene mutations associated with disease.

Some companies offering direct-to-consumer testing promote the increased privacy of a direct test in their marketing efforts. However, patients are not made aware that failure to indicate results of genetic testing in life insurance or disability applications could be considered fraud. In addition, many laboratories have not indicated their policies on what is done with the DNA sample after analysis. To ensure privacy, DNA samples should be destroyed after the requested test is performed. Those overseeing procedures for testing should continue to work to address patient privacy concerns.

The U.S. Federal Trade Commission, U.S. Food and Drug Administration, and the Centers for Disease Control and Prevention have issued a public message about at-home genetic tests. They advise consumers to be skeptical of the claims of the tests that are offered. Many tests may be of questionable value. The agencies also advise talking to a health care practitioner or genetic counselor before and after testing to help ensure understanding of what the test offers and what the results of testing reveal. In addition, they point out that unlike other home-use medical tests, the U.S. Food and Drug Administration has not reviewed any of the at-home genetic tests. Because of this, the validity and accuracy of many of these tests are unknown.

The American College of Obstetricians and Gynecologists
Women's Health Care Physicians

All genetic testing should be provided only after consultation with a qualified health care professional. For complex testing, this may involve referral to a genetic counselor or a medical geneticist. Appropriate pretest and posttest counseling should be provided, including a discussion of the risks, benefits, and limitations of the testing. It must be recognized that direct-to-consumer genetic testing will create downstream needs for counseling, support, and care for those identified as carriers of genes associated with undesired medical conditions. In many locales, the current health care system is not sufficient to meet those needs. Although some companies offer genetic counseling, concerns have been raised regarding a potential conflict of interest when the company providing the testing employs the genetic counselor because a company advertising directly to consumers may receive no compensation for counseling alone and is compensated only if the test is ordered by the consumer.

Until all of these considerations are addressed, direct and home genetic testing should be discouraged because of the potential harm of a misinterpreted or inaccurate result.

Resources

Bianchi DW. At-home fetal DNA gender testing: caveat emptor. Obstet Gynecol 2006;107:216–8.

Federal Trade Commission (US). At-home genetic tests: a healthy dose of skepticism may be the best prescription. Washington, DC: FTC; 2006. Available at: http://www.ftc.gov/bcp/edu/pubs/consumer/health/hea02.shtm. Retrieved March 10, 2008.

Gollust SE, Wilfond BS, Hull SC. Direct-to-consumer sales of genetic services on the Internet. Genet Med 2003;5:332–7.

Gollust SE, Hull SC, Wilfond BS. Limitations of direct-to-consumer advertising for clinical genetic testing. JAMA 2002;288:1762–7.

Roche PA, Annas GJ. DNA testing, banking, and genetic privacy. N Engl J Med 2006;355:545–6.

Wolfberg AJ. Genes on the Web—direct-to-consumer marketing of genetic testing. N Engl J Med 2006;355:543–5.

Direct-to-consumer marketing of genetic testing. ACOG Committee Opinion No. 409. American College of Obstetricians and Gynecologists. Obstet Gynecol 2008;111:1493–4.

ACOG COMMITTEE OPINION

Number 410 • June 2008

Ethical Issues in Genetic Testing

Committee on Ethics

Committee on Genetics

This document reflects emerging clinical and scientific advances as of the date issued and is subject to change. The information should not be construed as dictating an exclusive course of treatment or procedure to be followed.

ABSTRACT: Genetic testing is poised to play an increasing role in the practice of obstetrics and gynecology. To assure patients of the highest quality of care, physicians should become familiar with the currently available array of genetic tests and the tests' limitations. Clinicians should be able to identify patients within their practices who are candidates for genetic testing. Candidates will include patients who are pregnant or considering pregnancy and are at risk for giving birth to affected children as well as gynecology patients who, for example, may have or be predisposed to certain types of cancer. The purpose of this Committee Opinion is to review some of the ethical issues related to genetic testing and provide guidelines for the appropriate use of genetic tests by obstetrician–gynecologists. Expert consultation and referral are likely to be needed when obstetrician–gynecologists are confronted with these issues.

The American College of Obstetricians and Gynecologists
Women's Health Care Physicians

Although ethical questions related to genetic testing have been recognized for some time, they have gained a greater urgency because of the rapid advances in the field as a result of the success of the Human Genome Project. That project—a 13-year multibillion-dollar program—was initiated in 1990 to identify all the estimated 20,000–25,000 genes and to make them accessible for further study. The project harnessed America's scientists in a quest for rapid completion of a high-priority mission but left a series of ethical challenges in its wake. When developing the authorizing legislation for the federally funded Human Genome Project, Congress recognized that ethical conundrums would result from the project's technical successes and included the need for the development of federally funded programs to address ethical, legal, and social issues. Accordingly, the U.S. Department of Energy and the National Institutes of Health earmarked portions of their budgets to examine the ethical, legal, and social issues surrounding the availability of genetic information.

The purpose of this Committee Opinion is to review some of the ethical issues related to genetic testing and provide guidelines for the appropriate use of genetic tests by obstetrician–gynecologists. It is important to note at the outset, given the increasing complexity of this field and the quickness with which it

advances, that expert consultation and referral are likely to be needed when obstetrician–gynecologists are confronted with many of the issues detailed in this Committee Opinion.

The pace at which new information about genetic diseases is being developed and disseminated is astounding. Thus, the ethical obligations of clinicians start with the need to maintain competence in the face of this evolving science. Clinicians should be able to identify patients within their practices who are candidates for genetic testing. Candidates will include patients who are pregnant or considering pregnancy and are at risk for giving birth to affected children as well as gynecology patients who, for example, may have or be predisposed to certain types of cancer.

If a patient is being evaluated because of a diagnosis of cancer in a biologic relative and is found to have genetic susceptibility to cancer, she should be offered counseling and follow-up, with referral as appropriate, to ensure delivery of care consistent with current standards. In fact, genetic screening for any clinical purpose should be tied to the availability of intervention, including prenatal diagnosis, counseling, reproductive decision making, lifestyle changes, and enhanced phenotype screening.

One of the pillars of professionalism is social justice, which would oblige physicians to "promote justice in the health care system, including the fair distribution of health care resources" (1). In the context of genetic testing, justice would require clinicians to press for resources, independent of an individual's ability to pay, when they encounter barriers to health care for their patients who require care as a consequence of genetic testing and diagnosis (1).

Obstetrician–gynecologists also are ideally positioned to educate women. When they, or experts in genetics to whom they refer, counsel on genetics, they should provide accurate information and, if needed, emotional support for patients burdened by the results or consequences of genetic diagnoses, be they related to preconception or prenatal care, cancer risks, or other implications for health. Finally, clinicians should familiarize their patients with steps that can be taken to mitigate health risks associated with their genetic circumstance (eg, having a colonoscopy if there is a predisposition to colon cancer) (2).

It recently has been suggested that each person's entire genome may be available for use by physicians for diagnostic and therapeutic purposes in the not-too-distant future (3). Although that might seem like a medical panacea, the potential risks associated with wide-scale genetic testing are substantial. Many incidental findings will come to light, and yet, although those tested may be tempted to believe otherwise, genetic findings do not equate directly with either disease or health: "one hundred percent accurate identification of such incidental pathologies will lead to iatrogenic pathology… the belief that genetics completely determines phenotypic outcome must be informed by an understanding that most genetic measurements only shift the probability of an outcome, which often depends on other environmental triggers and chance" (4).

Informed Consent

Genetic Exceptionalism

Before the appropriate process for obtaining consent for genetic tests is considered, it is necessary to confront the broader question of whether the consequences of the results of those tests are substantively different from the consequences of other "medical" tests, for which specific consent is not always obtained. Some ethicists argue against what has been called the "exceptionalism" of genetic tests (5). They maintain that many medical tests have consequences for patients that are similar to those of genetic tests. For example, there can be discrimination by insurance companies against individuals either with a genetic disease or with a disease that is not linked to any particular gene. Results of nongenetic tests, as well as genetic tests, can divulge information about family members (eg, tests for sexually transmitted diseases). Additionally, both genetic and nongenetic tests can provide information about a person's medical future. As such, some authors have concluded that many genetic test results "may cause stigmatization, family discord and psy-

chological distress. Regardless of whether a test is genetic, when this combination of characteristics is present…testing should be performed with particular caution and the highest standards of informed consent and privacy protection should be applied" (6).

However, others argue that genetics should be treated as a unique class and be subject to a more rigorous process for consent. They base their belief on several factors. Genes, they argue, do not merely inform patients and their health care providers about the diagnosis of an extant illness. They also foretell the possibility (or in some cases the certainty) of a future disease, thus allowing "perfectly healthy" individuals to be subject to discrimination based on a predisposing gene. The DNA sample—which can be viewed as "a coded probabilistic medical record"— "makes genetic privacy unique and differentiates it from the privacy of medical records" (7). Some believe that this information is even more sensitive given the uncertainties attached to genetic results (ie, the reliability of tests, the penetrance of genes, and the unavailability of efficacious interventions to reduce the consequences of genetic diseases). Additionally, the consequence of being found to carry a particular gene has resonance not only for the individual who is tested but also for family members.

Patients should be informed that genetic testing could reveal that they have, are at risk for, or are a carrier of a specific disease. The results of testing might have important consequences or require difficult choices regarding their current or future health, insurance coverage, career, marriage, or reproductive options.

Role of the Obstetrician–Gynecologist

In addition to needing to ensure proper consent, the obstetrician–gynecologist who orders genetic tests should be aware of when it is appropriate to test, which particular test to order, and "what information the test can provide, the limitations of the test, how to interpret positive and negative results in light of the patient's medical or family history, and the medical management options available" (8). The health care provider ordering tests has a responsibility to use and interpret those tests correctly or to refer to someone with relevant expertise. Because completing all these tasks is particularly difficult when direct-to-consumer marketing of genetic tests is used, that marketing approach has significant limitations (9). These enterprises receive compensation only if an individual, after counseling, chooses to undergo a test, bringing the standard of neutral counseling into question and further rendering the use of a market-driven approach to testing ethically problematic (10). In the end, the physician plays an important role in providing adequate, neutral counseling; ensuring informed consent; and providing follow-up for genetic tests. Neutral counseling also may be compromised through the use of patient educational materials or counselors that are provided by a company that might profit from a patient's decision to undergo testing.

Particular caution should be exercised when obtaining consent for collecting genetic material that may be stored and, therefore, can have future clinical or research applications. The American College of Medical Genetics (ACMG) recommends that when samples are obtained for clinical tests, counseling should address the anticipated use of samples, including whether their use will be restricted for the purpose for which they were collected and if and when they will be destroyed (11). When samples will be used for research or the development of diagnostic tests, the ACMG recommends that consent should include a description of the work (eg, its purposes, limitations, possible outcomes, and methods for communicating and maintaining confidentiality of results). There should be a discussion with the research participant about whether she wishes to give permission to use her samples without identifiers for other types of research, and she should be informed of the institution's policy regarding recontacting participants in the future. Current and future use of samples for research should follow state and federal regulations governing protection of human participants in research (12). Two authors recently suggested that the "best consumer advice, given current law, is that one should not send a DNA sample to anyone who does not guarantee to destroy it on completion of the specified test" (7). Others argue for the creation of a repository of samples donated by genetic altruists to be used for many different types of research (4).

Genetic Testing in Children and Adolescents

Testing of children presents unique issues in counseling and consent. Although it is most commonly pediatricians or geneticists who are called on to test children for genetic diseases, obstetricians may be asked to test already born children of parents who, through the process of prenatal testing, have been found to be carriers of genetic diseases. In such cases, the physician should balance the rights of the parents to have information that can optimize the ongoing health care of their children against the rights of the children to have their best interests protected. There will be circumstances in which it can be determined that a child is at risk for an untoward clinical event in the future, but there may be no information about interventions that have the potential to reduce the likelihood of that event or the magnitude of its effect. In that circumstance, the benefits of testing a child are not always clear (eg, *BRCA* testing in a young child).

The American Society of Human Genetics (ASHG) and ACMG together have suggested, "Counseling and communication with the child and family about genetic testing should include the following components: 1) assessment of the significance of the potential benefits and harms of the test, 2) determination of the decision-making capacity of the child, and 3) advocacy on behalf of the interests of the child" (13). These societies highlighted additional points about benefits and burdens

that should be included in counseling, some of which follow:

- Timely medical benefit to the child should be the primary justification for genetic testing in children and adolescents. If the medical benefits are uncertain or will be deferred to a later time, this justification for testing is less compelling.
- If the medical or psychosocial benefits of a genetic test will not accrue until adulthood, as in the case of carrier status or adult-onset diseases, genetic testing generally should be deferred. Further consultation with other genetic services providers, pediatricians, psychologists, and ethics committees may be appropriate to evaluate these conditions.
- Testing should be discouraged when the health care provider determines that potential harms of genetic testing in children and adolescents outweigh the potential benefits. A health care provider has no obligation to provide a medical service for a child or adolescent that is not in the best interest of the child or adolescent.

The ASHG and ACMG concluded, "Providers who receive requests for genetic testing in children must weigh the interests of children and those of their parents and families. The provider and the family both should consider the medical, psychosocial, and reproductive issues that bear on providing the best care for children" (8).

Physicians (obstetricians and pediatricians) also have a responsibility to provide information to patients regarding newborn screening. The primacy of the child's welfare should animate these discussions as well. More detail about this issue can be found elsewhere (14).

Prenatal Genetic Testing

Genetic testing of the fetus offers both opportunities and ethical challenges. Preconception and prenatal genetic screening and testing are recommended for a limited number of severe child-onset diseases because such screening and testing provides individuals with the chance to pursue assisted reproductive technology in order to avoid conception of an affected child, to consider termination of a pregnancy, or to prepare for the birth of a chronically ill child. With advancing genetic technology, however, physicians may increasingly face requests for testing of fetuses for less severe child-onset conditions, adult-onset conditions, or genetically linked traits.

Principles regarding testing of children provide some guidance for when prenatal testing might be appropriate but this decision is significantly complicated by the various purposes that prenatal testing can have: to detect a fetal condition for pregnancy termination, to allow patients to prepare for the birth and care of a potentially affected child, or, more rarely, to detect and treat a fetal condition in utero. Furthermore, many times, a woman's intentions regarding pregnancy termination evolve as genetic information becomes available to her. Therefore, testing the fetus for adult-onset disorders with no known therapeutic or preventive treatment (save prevention by pregnancy termination) should raise caution in a way similar to the manner in which testing of children can. In pregnancies likely to be carried to term, consideration should be given to whether, as in the case of testing children, the decision to test should be reserved for the child to make upon reaching adulthood. However, consideration also should be given to personal preference, that is, the interests individuals may have in terminating a pregnancy that may result in a life (such as life that will be affected by Huntington chorea) that they feel morally obliged or prefer not to bring into the world. Because these often are wrenching decisions for parents, referral to parent support networks (eg, National Down Syndrome Society, if that is the diagnosis of concern), counselors, social workers, or clergy may provide additional information and support (15).

Genetic Data and the Family

In a large number of instances, when patients receive the results of genetic tests, they are party to information that directly concerns their biologic relatives as well. This familial quality of genetic information raises ethical quandaries for physicians, particularly related to their duty of confidentiality. In these circumstances, some have posited an ethical tension between obligations the clinician has to protect the confidentiality of the individual who has consented to a test on the one hand and a physician's duty to protect the health of a different individual on the other hand. For example, a woman who discovers that she is a carrier of an X-linked recessive disease during the workup of an affected son might choose not to tell her pregnant sister about her carrier status because she does not believe in abortion and fears that her sister might consider an abortion (16). In another example, a woman identified as a carrier of a gene predisposing individuals to cancer might not wish to share the information with relatives, some of whom might even be patients of the same physician who tested her, because such sharing would disclose her own status as a carrier.

In both the previously cited cases, information obtained with the consent of one individual could assist in the management of another. However, medical ethics as reflected in American Medical Association (AMA) policies recognizes a physician's duty to safeguard patient confidences in such cases (with a few notable exceptions, often mandated by law—for example, communicable diseases and gunshot and knife wounds should be reported as required by applicable statutes or ordinances) (17). How assiduously that confidentiality needs to be guarded is the subject of some debate. Some have argued that genetic information should be subject to stringent safeguards because, even though there may be uncertainty about the ultimate biologic consequence of a given gene, the social consequences (discrimination and stigmatiza-

tion) can be substantial (18). The AMA's Council on Ethical and Judicial Affairs has argued that physicians do indeed have an obligation to pay almost unlimited obeisance to a patient's confidentiality save only for "certain circumstances which are ethically and legally justified because of overriding social considerations" (19).

Conversely, there are those who argue against the withholding of important information from potentially affected family members (20). Those who subscribe to this belief feel that when information applies to family as much as to the proband, an obligation arises that extends from the physician to those potentially affected family members but no further. This view is consistent with court rulings in three states, which have held that a physician owes a duty to the patient's potentially affected family members (21–24). Two of these rulings addressed the question of how physicians must fulfill this duty and reached different conclusions. In one case, the court held that the physician can discharge the duty by informing the patient of the risk and is not required to inform the patient's child (22). In another case, the court did not decide how the physician could satisfy the duty to warn, other than requiring that "reasonable steps be taken to assure that the information reaches those likely to be affected or is made available for their benefit" (23). As these alternate decisions illustrate, the legal limits of privacy are evolving, emphasizing the need for patient communication and case-by-case evaluation.

Recommendations of Other Organizations

Organizations that promulgate guidelines for genetic care and counseling also have proposed different approaches to the disclosure of genetic information. The ASHG tailors its recommendations to the magnitude and immediacy of risk faced by kindred (25), encouraging voluntary disclosure by the proband but also articulating circumstances in which the proband's refusal to do so should not preclude disclosure by the health care provider. According to the ASHG, disclosure is acceptable if "the harm is likely to occur, and is serious, immediate and foreseeable." It adds that the at-risk relative must be identifiable and that there must be some extant intervention that can have a salutary effect on the course of the genetic disease. In summary, "the harm from failing to disclose should outweigh the risk from disclosure." Although this suggestion to disclose seems unequivocal, it also posits circumstances for its exercise that are highly unlikely at the current time (ie, very few genetic diagnoses pose an immediate risk, let alone ones that can be substantively modified with an intervention [25]).

The President's Commission for the Study of Ethical Problems in Medicine and Biomedical and Behavioral Research also suggested circumstances in which a health care provider should disclose information in the absence of the proband's permission to do so (26). The commission indicated that disclosure is required when four conditions are present: 1) efforts to elicit voluntary disclosure by the proband have failed, 2) there is a high probability that harm will occur if disclosure is not made, and intervention can avert that harm, 3) the harm would be serious, and 4) efforts are made to limit disclosed information to genetic information needed for diagnosis and treatment. Although the commission did not cite a requirement for an *immediate* risk, the requirements for a high probability of harm and for the availability of an efficacious intervention make it likely that adherence to these guidelines rarely will result in cases in which a patient's rights of confidentiality are overridden in order to inform relatives at risk.

Role of the Obstetrician–Gynecologist

The best way for the obstetrician–gynecologist to avoid the challenging choice between involuntary disclosure and being passive in the face of risks to kindred is to anticipate the issue and raise it at the first genetic counseling session. At that session, the patient needs to be educated about the implications of findings for relatives and why voluntary disclosure would in many circumstances be encouraged (as well as the possibility that relatives might prefer not to know the results). Some bioethicists have even suggested that these sessions should be used as an opportunity for clinicians to articulate the circumstances under which they would consider disclosure obligatory, thus allowing patients to seek care elsewhere if they found the conditions for testing unacceptable (Macklin has referred to this as the "genetic Miranda warning") (27). Similarly, even if the health care provider would not disclose without consent under any circumstance, the initial counseling session could allow the health care provider to refer the patient elsewhere if they find they have an irreconcilable difference or have an objection of conscience in expectations about disclosure. Physicians also should make themselves available to assist patients at the time of disclosure if that will help assuage their patients' concerns.

A particularly thorny issue related to the ownership of genetic information might be results that bear on paternity. It is possible that prenatal assessments and family testing might reveal that the husband, partner, or other putative father is not the biologic father. In 1994, the Committee on Assessing Genetic Risks of the Institute of Medicine recommended that in such situations the health care provider should inform a woman but should not disclose this information to her partner (28). The Institute of Medicine's reason for withholding such information was that "genetic testing should not be used in ways that disrupt families." Another reason may be that the physician–patient relationship exists solely with the woman. Others have disagreed with the Institute of Medicine's recommendation (29). In some cases, it is not merely a matter of acting to protect families. For example, suppose a child is born with a disease that is caused by an autosomal recessive gene, and the husband does not carry the deleterious gene because he is not actually the father. If the physician were to maintain the charade of paternity,

then the counseling given to both parents (ie, there is one chance in four that each subsequent child will have the same disease) would be false and might lead the husband to argue against more children or for unnecessary amniocenteses in all future pregnancies, or inappropriately lead to concern for others in his family.

Other circumstances exist in which the interests of a pregnant woman and family members might diverge. For example, if the husband's father has Huntington chorea (an autosomal dominant trait), the pregnant woman might wish to test the fetus for the gene. If the father did not want to know his own status, a conflict would arise, pitting her right to know about her fetus against his right not to know about himself. Another example of conflict would be if problems arose during diagnostic linkage studies for prenatal or preclinical diagnosis in a family and some family members did not want to participate in the testing (eg, testing for thalassemia). It might then be impossible to make a diagnosis in the index case. Both ethical and legal precedents, however, argue that individuals cannot be forced to have such testing.

Genetic Data and Insurers and Employers

Concerns about access to health and life insurance in the face of the discovery of a deleterious or predisposing gene is one of the most nettlesome issues facing health care providers who wish to use genetic testing to improve the health of their patients. In some ways, the importance of this issue is more pronounced in the United States because of the manner in which health care coverage is obtained. In countries with universal health care, individuals with the diagnosis of a predisposing gene need not fear the loss of access to health insurance.

In recognition of concerns related to genetic testing, in 1995, the Equal Employment Opportunity Commission issued guidelines stating that individuals who thought they had been discriminated against by an employer because of predictive genetic testing had the right to sue that employer. Additionally, the Health Insurance Portability and Accountability Act (HIPAA), enacted in 1996, prevented insurance companies from denying health care based on predictive testing for individuals transferring from one plan to another (30). Physicians should advocate for patients' ability to obtain health or life insurance uncompromised by the results of any genetic tests they might undergo.

Although there is scant evidence of widespread genetic discrimination, there is clear evidence that fear of that discrimination can drive patients away from needed testing or from participation in research and also may influence physicians' uses of genetic tests (31). In commenting on insurance and discrimination and considering needed protections and legislation, ACMG makes the following points: legislation must not impede the ability of individuals to maximize use of genetic information in their health care and employment decision making, and it must not limit the access of health care providers to genetic information needed to ensure that the care provided is beneficial and specific to the needs of the individual. Furthermore, the privacy of genetic information must be adequately protected. Protection against unfair discrimination on the basis of genetic risk for disease is achieved only by strategies that restrict use of genetic information in enrollment and rate-setting. Protected genetic information must include information based on evaluation, testing, and family histories of individuals and their family members (32). Finally, as discussed before, it must be recognized that the confidentiality of these data has become difficult to guarantee in this era of electronic medical records.

Genetics and Assisted Reproductive Technology

There are at least two issues that relate to the intersection of genetics and assisted reproductive technology (ART). In the first instance, there is the need to consider whether all individuals, regardless of genotype, should have access to ART using their own gametes. In the past, individuals who were infected with deleterious viruses that have the potential to be passed to their children (eg, human immunodeficiency virus) were denied access to ART, in part because, before the advent of a variety of interventions, as many as one in four of their offspring would acquire an ultimately fatal infection, a risk similar to that if both parents are carriers for a serious autosomal recessive disease. Others have argued, however, that "procreative liberty should enjoy presumptive primacy when conflicts about its exercise arise because . . . [it] is central to personal identity, to dignity and to the meaning of one's life" (33). Such principles would support allowing prospective parents to be arbiters of the level of risk to which a child could be exposed.

Second is the question of the extent to which preimplantation genetics should be used in pursuit of the "genetically ideal" child. The American College of Obstetricians and Gynecologists (ACOG) already opposes all forms of sex selection not related to the diagnosis of sex-linked genetic conditions (34). In the near future, other potentially controversial genetic manipulations may be available. Complex genetic systems such as cognition and aging soon may be determinable and may be constituents of potentially desirable characteristics, such as intelligence or longevity. They could, therefore, be used or misused as parameters for prenatal diagnosis (35). Some have argued for a permissive approach, allowing parents to choose from a menu of possible children the one with the chance for the "best life." That approach would allow selection for both disease-related genes (eg, eliminating carriers of BRCA genes) and nondisease genes "even if this maintains or increases social inequality" (36). One author has referred to this as "procreative beneficence," defining it as couples selecting, from the possible children they could have, the child who is expect-

ed to have the best life, or at least as good a life as the others, based on the relevant, available information (36). Conversely, in the United Kingdom, strict limits are set on the use of prenatal genetic diagnosis, and clinics must apply for a license for every new disease they want to include in screening. However, even in that country, the list of allowable preimplantation genetic diagnosis tests has been expanded recently to include susceptibilities for certain cancers (37, 38).

Parents' requests to select a certain genetic trait may pose even greater challenges for reproductive endocrinologists and embryologists when parents' choices seem to be antithetical to the best interests of the future child. For example, deaf parents may prefer to select for an embryo that will yield a child who will also be deaf. Couples who have short stature due to skeletal dysplasia might feel they would prefer to have a child of similar stature. The technical ability to provide these choices is not far from reality, but the ethical roadmap that will offer direction to physicians is not as clearly laid out.

Conclusions

Genetic testing is poised to play a greater and greater role in the practice of obstetrics and gynecology. To assure patients of the highest quality of care, physicians should be familiar with the currently available array of genetic tests, as well as with their limitations. They also should be aware of the untoward consequences their patients might sustain because of a genetic diagnosis. The physician should work to minimize those consequences. Genetic information is unique in being shared by a family. Physicians should inform their patients of that fact and help them to prepare for dealing with their results, including considering disclosure to their biologic family. If the genetic information could potentially benefit family members (eg, allow them to improve their own prognosis), physicians should guide their patients toward voluntary disclosure while assiduously guarding their right to confidentiality.

Recommendations

The ACOG Committees on Ethics and Genetics recommend the following guidelines:

1. Clinicians should be able to identify patients within their practices who are candidates for genetic testing and should maintain competence in the face of increasing genetic knowledge.

2. Obstetrician–gynecologists should recognize that geneticists and genetic counselors are an important part of the health care team and should consult with them and refer as needed.

3. Discussions with patients about the importance of genetic information for their kindred, as well as a recommendation that information be shared with potentially affected family members as appropriate, should be a standard part of genetic counseling.

4. Obstetrician–gynecologists should be aware that genetic information has the potential to lead to discrimination in the workplace and to affect an individual's insurability adversely. In addition to including this information in counseling materials, physicians should recognize that their obligation to professionalism includes a mandate to prevent discrimination. Steps that physicians can take to fulfill this obligation could include, among others, advocacy for legislation to ban genetic discrimination.

References

1. Medical professionalism in the new millennium: a physician charter. ABIM Foundation; American Board of Internal Medicine; ACP-ASIM Foundation. American College of Physicians–American Society of Internal Medicine; European Federation of Internal Medicine. Ann Intern Med 2002;136:243–6.

2. Burke W, Press N. Ethical obligations and counseling challenges in cancer genetics. J Natl Compr Canc Netw 2006; 4:185–91.

3. Wade N. The quest for the $1,000 human genome. New York Times, July 18, 2006. Available at: http://www.nytimes.com/2006/07/18/science/18dna.html. Retrieved January 9, 2008.

4. Kohane IS, Masys DR, Altman RB. The incidentalome: a threat to genomic medicine [published erratum appears in JAMA 2006;296:1466]. JAMA 2006;296:212–5.

5. Gostin LO, Hodge JG. Genetic privacy and the law: an end to genetics exceptionalism. Jurimetrics 1999;40:21–58.

6. Green MJ, Botkin JR. "Genetic exceptionalism" in medicine: clarifying the differences between genetic and nongenetic tests. Ann Intern Med 2003;138:571–5.

7. Roche PA, Annas GJ. DNA testing, banking, and genetic privacy. N Engl J Med 2006;355:545–6.

8. Genetics and Public Policy Center. Genetic testing practice guidelines: translating genetic discoveries into clinical care. Washington, DC: GPPC; 2006. Available at: http://www.dnapolicy.org/images/issuebriefpdfs/Professional_Guidelines_Issue_Brief.pdf. Retrieved January 9, 2008.

9. Direct-to-consumer genetic testing. ACOG Committee Opinion No. 409. American College of Obstetricians and Gynecologists. Obstet Gynecol 2008;111:1493–4.

10. Wolfberg AJ. Genes on the Web—direct-to-consumer marketing of genetic testing. N Engl J Med 2006;355:543–5.

11. Statement on storage and use of genetic materials. ACMG statement. American College of Medical Genetics Storage of Genetics Materials Committee. Am J Hum Genet 1995;57: 1499–500.

12. Protection of human subjects. 46 C.F.R. § 46 (2007).

13. Points to consider: ethical, legal, and psychosocial implications of genetic testing in children and adolescents. American Society of Human Genetics Board of Directors, American College of Medical Genetics Board of Directors. Am J Hum Genet 1995;57:1233–41.

14. Newborn screening. ACOG Committee Opinion No. 393. American College of Obstetricians and Gynecologists. Obstet Gynecol 2007;110:1497–500.

15. Invasive prenatal testing for aneuploidy. ACOG Practice Bulletin No. 88. American College of Obstetricians and Gynecologists. Obstet Gynecol 2007;110:1459–67.

16. Minkoff H, Ecker J. Genetic testing and breach of patient confidentiality: law, ethics, and pragmatics. Am J Obstet Gynecol 2008;198:498.e1–498.e4.

17. American Medical Association. Principles of medical ethics. In: Code of medical ethics of the American Medical Association: current opinions with annotations. 2006-2007 ed. Chicago (IL): AMA; 2006. p. xv–lvii.

18. Annas GJ, Glantz LH, Roche PA. Drafting the Genetic Privacy Act: science, policy, and practical considerations. J Law Med Ethics 1995;23:360–6.

19. American Medical Association. Confidentiality. In: Code of medical ethics of the American Medical Association: current opinions with annotations. 2006-2007 ed. Chicago (IL): AMA; 2006. p. 136–50.

20. Wachbroit R. Rethinking medical confidentiality: the impact of genetics. Suffolk Univ Law Rev 1993;27:1391–410.

21. Offit K, Groeger E, Turner S, Wadsworth EA, Weiser MA. The "duty to warn" a patient's family members about hereditary disease risks. JAMA 2004;292:1469–73.

22. Pate v. Threlkel, 661 So.2d 278 (Fla. 1995).

23. Safer v. Estate of Pack, 291 N.J. Super. 619, 677 A.2d 1188 (1996).

24. Molloy v. Meier, 679 N.W.2d 711, 718 (Minn. 2004).

25. Professional disclosure of familial genetic information. ASHG statement. The American Society of Human Genetics Social Issues Subcommittee on Familial Disclosure. Am J Hum Genet 1998;62:474–83.

26. President's Commission for the Study of Ethical Problems in Medicine and Biomedical and Behavioral Research. Screening and counseling for genetic conditions: a report on the ethical, social, and legal implications of genetic screening, counseling, and education programs. Washington, DC: U.S. Government Printing Office; 1983.

27. Macklin R. Privacy and control of genetic information. In: Annas GJ, Elias S, editors. Gene mapping: using law and ethics as guides. New York (NY): Oxford University Press; 1992. p. 157–72.

28. Institute of Medicine (US). Assessing genetic risks: implications for health and social policy. Washington, DC: National Academy Press; 1994.

29. Ross LF. Disclosing misattributed paternity. Bioethics 1996;10:114–30.

30. Fulda KG, Lykens K. Ethical issues in predictive genetic testing: a public health perspective. J Med Ethics 2006;32:143–7.

31. Hudson KL. Prohibiting genetic discrimination. N Engl J Med 2007;356:2021–3.

32. Watson MS, Greene CL. Points to consider in preventing unfair discrimination based on genetic disease risk: a position statement of the American College of Medical Genetics. Genet Med 2001;3:436–7.

33. Robertson JA. Children of choice: freedom and the new reproductive technology. Princeton (NJ): Princeton University Press; 1994.

34. Sex selection. ACOG Committee Opinion No. 360. American College of Obstetricians and Gynecologists. Obstet Gynecol 2007;109:475–8.

35. Henn W. Consumerism in prenatal diagnosis: a challenge for ethical guidelines. J Med Ethics 2000;26:444–6.

36. Savulescu J. Procreative beneficence: why we should select the best children. Bioethics 2001;15:413–26.

37. Braude P. Preimplantation diagnosis for genetic susceptibility. N Engl J Med 2006;355:541–3.

38. Human Fertilisation and Embryology Authority. Authority decision on the use of PGD for lower penetrance, later onset inherited conditions. London (UK): HFEA; 2006. Available at: http://www.hfea.gov.uk/docs/The_Authority_decision_-_Choices_and_boundaries.pdf. Retrieved January 9, 2008.

Ethical issues in genetic testing. ACOG Committee Opinion No. 410. American College of Obstetricians and Gynecologists. Obstet Gynecol 2008;111:1495–502.

ACOG COMMITTEE OPINION

Number 422 • December 2008   *(Replaces No. 294, May 2004)*

At-Risk Drinking and Illicit Drug Use: Ethical Issues in Obstetric and Gynecologic Practice

Committee on Ethics

ABSTRACT: Drug and alcohol abuse is a major health problem for American women regardless of their socioeconomic status, race, ethnicity, and age. It is costly to individuals and to society. Obstetrician–gynecologists have an ethical obligation to learn and use a protocol for universal screening questions, brief intervention, and referral to treatment in order to provide patients and their families with medical care that is state-of-the-art, comprehensive, and effective. In this Committee Opinion, the American College of Obstetricians and Gynecologists' Committee on Ethics proposes an ethical rationale for this protocol in both obstetric and gynecologic practice, offers a practical aid for incorporating such care, and provides guidelines for resolving common ethical dilemmas related to drug and alcohol use that arise in the clinical setting.

The American College of Obstetricians and Gynecologists
Women's Health Care Physicians

Drug and alcohol abuse is a major health problem for American women regardless of their socioeconomic status, race, ethnicity, and age. It is costly to individuals and to society. Among 18–25-year-old women, 34% binge drink and 10% are heavy drinkers. These rates are lower among women aged 26 years or older (12.8% binge drink and 2.4% are heavy drinkers), but 6.3% of females aged 12 years or older have been classified as dependent on alcohol or illegal drugs (1). Heavy drinking (five or more drinks on one occasion on five or more days in the last 30 days) carries a higher risk of cardiac and hepatic complications for women than men. The alcohol-associated mortality rate is 50–100 times higher, and there is an increased burden of mental and physical disability (2). Among pregnant women aged 15–44 years, 11.8% admit to drinking some alcohol during the previous month (1), which may put the fetus at risk for fetal alcohol syndrome (FAS), the leading cause of mental retardation in the United States (3), and 0.7% reported heavy drinking (1). Maternal alcoholism is one of the leading preventable causes of fetal neurodevelopmental disorders (4). The economic costs of FAS for 2003 are estimated at $5.4 billion.

Each case prevented is predicted to save $860,000 in lifetime direct and indirect costs (5). Illicit drug use has major physical and mental health consequences and is associated with increased rates of sexually transmitted infections in women, including hepatitis and human immunodeficiency virus (HIV), as well as depression, domestic violence, poverty, and significant prenatal and neonatal complications (6, 7). Overall, 10% of nonpregnant women and 4% of pregnant women report illicit drug use, but among pregnant women aged 15–17 years, the rate of use is 15.5% (8). Drug abuse costs are estimated at more than $180 billion yearly, including $605 million associated with health care costs for drug-exposed newborns (9).

As a result of intensive research in addiction over the past decade, evidence-based recommendations have been consolidated into a protocol for universal screening questions, brief intervention, and referral to treatment (10). The abstinence rate after drug abuse treatment (the treatment success rate) is now comparable to the level of medication compliance achieved in diabetes, hypertension, or other chronic illnesses (11). Brief physician advice has been shown unequivocally to be both powerful and feasible in a clinical office setting (10, 12, 13). The American Medical Association has endorsed universal screening (14), and health services researchers have determined that treatment saves $7 for every dollar spent (15). For these reasons, the American College of Obstetricians and Gynecologists (ACOG) collaborated with the Physician Leadership on National Drug Policy at Brown University to produce a slide–lecture presentation that addresses the identification and treatment of drug abuse (16). The presentation was distributed to obstetric–gynecologic clerkship and residency program directors and is available at www.acog.org.

Physicians have been slow to implement universal screening, and rates of detection and referral to treatment among nonpregnant women remain very low (17). Studies using simulated patients have demonstrated that women are less likely than men to be screened or referred (18, 19). Physicians lack accurate knowledge about physiology (ie, the equivalency of 1.5 oz of distilled spirits, 12 oz of beer or wine cooler, and 5 oz of wine), risk factors, and sex differences in problem presentation and treatment response (20). These knowledge gaps are compounded by state laws designed to criminalize drug use during pregnancy, by women's fears that they might lose custody of their children, and by the social stigma experienced by women who abuse alcohol or use illicit drugs (21, 22). In one study, for example, the physicians surveyed defined "light drinking" as an average of 1.2 drinks per day, an amount that exceeds the National Institute on Alcohol Abuse and Alcoholism's (NIAAA) guidelines for at-risk drinking for women (23). Furthermore, communicating about difficult issues takes time, requires skills, and is poorly reimbursed by procedure-oriented insurance coverage. Physicians are concerned about the consequences of legally mandated reporting, they lack familiarity with treatment resources, and they do not have the extensive time required to make an appropriate referral (11). These are all problems that must be solved in order to provide medically appropriate and ethically necessary care to women who engage in at-risk drinking or use illicit drugs.

Many physicians are understandably reluctant to take on a new responsibility in the context of time constraints and the already intense demands of practice (24), but there are practical measures that can be taken to make screening and brief intervention feasible for many, if not all, patients. Universal screening can be accomplished by adding a few questions to a standard intake form (see box "Substance Abuse Screening"). In an office practice, 1 in 20 patients will require further intervention (25, 26). Intervention for these patients can be started effectively in 5 minutes, as demonstrated in a busy academic emergency department setting (27). Referrals can be provided as a handout, with a nurse or office assistant available to help the patient make contact with treatment if desired. Because more women than men are hidden drinkers, and many see the obstetrician or gynecologist as their principle source of care, the opportunity to screen and inter-

vene, with benefits to women, their children, and society, are too great to be missed. In recognition of the importance of this activity, *Current Procedural Terminology* and Healthcare Common Procedure Coding System (Medicare) codes have been established for screening, brief intervention, and referral performed by a physician or by an educator under the physician's direction. Further, the Centers for Medicare & Medicaid Services and many non-Medicare payers provide coverage for these services.

Substance abuse presents complex ethical issues and challenges. This Committee Opinion proposes an ethical rationale for universal screening questions, brief intervention, and referral to treatment in both obstetric and gynecologic practice, offers a practical aid for incorporating such care (see box "BNI-ART Institute Intervention Algorithm"), and provides guidelines for resolving common ethical dilemmas that arise in the clinical setting.

The Ethical Rationale for Universal Screening Questions, Brief Intervention, and Referral to Treatment

Support for universal screening questions, brief intervention, and referral to treatment is derived from four basic principles of ethics. These principles are 1) beneficence, 2) nonmaleficence, 3) justice, and 4) respect for autonomy.

Beneficence

Therapeutic intent, or beneficence, is the foundation of medical knowledge, training, and practice. Experts at the NIAAA and the National Institute on Drug Abuse confirm that addiction is not primarily a moral weakness, as it has been viewed in the past, but a "brain disease" that should be included in a review of systems just like any other biologic disease process (28). A medical diagnosis of addiction requires medical intervention in the same manner that a diagnosis of diabetes requires nutritional counseling or therapeutic agents or both. Positive behavior change arises from the trust implicit in the physician–patient relationship, the respect that patients have for physicians' knowledge, and the ability of physicians to help patients see the links between substance use behaviors and real physical consequences. Brief physician advice has been shown to be as effective as conventional treatment for substance abuse and can produce dramatic reductions in drinking and drug use, improved health status, and decreased costs to society (10, 13, 15, 17, 29–31). The Center for Substance Abuse Prevention has now implemented more than 147 projects for pregnant and postpartum women and their children (32), and there are several different successful models for prevention and treatment for women and their families: AR-Cares (34), Choices (35), SafePort (36), Early Start (37), and the Mom/Kid Trial (38).

Given this capacity for dramatic improvement in health status, physicians have an obligation to be therapeutic—in this case to learn the techniques of screening

---

Substance Abuse Screening

T-ACE

T Tolerance: How many drinks does it take to make you feel high? *More than 2 drinks is a positive response—score 2 points.*

A Have people **A**nnoyed you by criticizing your drinking? *If "Yes"—score 1 point.*

C Have you ever felt you ought to **C**ut down on your drinking? *If "Yes"—score 1 point.*

E **E**ye opener: Have you ever had a drink first thing in the morning to steady your nerves or get rid of a hangover? *If "Yes"—score 1 point.*

A total score of 2 or more points indicates a positive screen for pregnancy risk drinking.

Reprinted from the American Journal of Obstetrics & Gynecology, Vol 160, Sokol RJ, Martier SS, Ager JW, The T-ACE questions: practical prenatal detection of risk drinking, 863–8; discussion 868–70, Copyright 1989, with permission from Elsevier.

TWEAK

T Tolerance: How many drinks can you hold? *If 6 or more drinks, score 2 points.*

W Have close friends or relatives **W**orried or complained about your drinking in the past year? *If "Yes" 2 points.*

E **E**ye opener: Do you sometimes take a drink in the morning when you get up? *If "Yes" 1 point.*

A **A**mnesia: Has a friend or family member ever told you about things you said or did while you were drinking that you could not remember? *If "Yes" 1 point.*

K(C) Do you sometimes feel the need to **C**ut down on your drinking? *If "Yes" 1 point.*

The TWEAK is used to screen for pregnant at-risk drinking, defined here as the consumption of 1 oz or more of alcohol per day while pregnant. A total score of 2 points or more indicates a positive screen for pregnancy risk drinking.

Adapted from Russell M. New assessment tools for risk drinking during pregnancy: T-ACE, TWEAK, and others. Alcohol Health Res World 1994;18:55–61.

NIAAA Questionnaire

Do you drink?

Do you use drugs?

On average, how many days per week do you drink alcohol (beer, wine, liquor)?

On a typical day when you drink, how many drinks do you have?

Positive score: >14 drinks per week for men and >7 drinks per week for women

What is the maximum number of drinks you had on any given occasion during the past month?

Positive score: >4 for men and >3 for women

National Institute on Alcohol Abuse and Alcoholism. Helping patients who drink too much: a clinician's guide. Updated 2005 ed. NIH Publication No. 07-3769. Bethesda (MD): NIAAA; 2007. Available at: http://pubs.niaaa.nih.gov/publications/Practitioner/CliniciansGuide 2005/guide.pdf. Retrieved January 23, 2008.

---

and brief intervention—and to inform themselves as they would if a new test or therapy were developed for any other recognized disease entity. The practice of universal screening questions, brief intervention, and referral to treatment falls well within the purview of the obstetrician–gynecologist's role as a provider of primary care to women and has potential for major impact on recognized obstetric and gynecologic outcomes. Furthermore, if the topic is raised respectfully, the physician–patient relationship may be substantially enhanced, even if no substantive changes in lifestyle are achieved immediately. Therapy is called "patient care" because both physicians and patients recognize and value the commitment of the medical profession to engage in a nurturing relationship in the course of providing carefully selected therapeutic modalities. Nurturance of healthy behaviors through universal screening questions, brief intervention, and referral to treatment is, thus, part of the traditional healing role and an appropriate focus for the obstetrician–gynecologist's role as a primary care provider.

Nonmaleficence

The obligation to do no harm, or nonmaleficence, also applies to universal screening questions, brief intervention, and referral to treatment. Medical care can be compromised if physicians are unaware of a patient's alcohol or drug abuse and, thus, miss related diagnoses or medication interactions with alcohol or illegal substances. If the problem is not identified, major health risks, such as HIV exposure and depression, also may be missed. These are examples of harms that may occur as a result of omission (nondetection of a serious problem). Furthermore, patients may be harmed when substance abuse is treated by a physician as a moral rather than medical issue (38). Women who abuse alcohol or use illicit drugs are more likely than men to be stigmatized and labeled as hopeless (39). In particular, physicians should avoid using humiliation as a tool to force change because such behavior is ethically inappropriate, engenders resistance, and may act as a barrier to successful treatment and recovery.

BNI-ART Institute Intervention Algorithm

The BNI-ART Institute (Brief Negotiated Interview and Active Referral to Treatment) is a program of Boston University School of Public Health and the Youth Alcohol Prevention Center in collaboration with Boston Medical Center. Among its tools is a two-sided card that summarizes the process of a brief intervention and referral for treatment.

Front of Card

BNI STEPS	DIALOGUE/PROCEDURES
1. Raise subject and ask permission	• Would you mind taking a few minutes to talk with me confidentially about your use of [X]? <<PAUSE and LISTEN>>
	• Before we start, could you tell me a little about your goals for yourself…What's important to you?
2. Provide feedback • Review screen	• From what I understand, you are using [insert screening data]… We know that drinking above certain levels, smoking and/or use of illicit drugs can cause problems, such as [insert medical info].
• For alcohol… Show NIAAA guidelines & norms	• These are the upper limits of low risk drinking for your age and sex. By low risk we mean you would be less likely to experience illness or injury if you stay within the guidelines.
• Make connection (no arguing)	• If there is a possible connection between use of [X] and today's medical problem, ask, "What connection (if any) do you see between your use of [X] and this visit today?" If patient does not see connection: make one using specific medical information
3. Enhance motivation • Explore Pros and Cons	Ask pros and cons • Help me to understand what you enjoy about [X]? <<PAUSE AND LISTEN>>
• Use reflective listening	• Now tell me what you enjoy less about [X] or regret about your use of [X] <<PAUSE AND LISTEN>> On the one hand you said… <<RESTATE PROS>> On the other hand you said… <<RESTATE CONS>>
• Readiness to change	• So tell me, where does this leave you? [show readiness ruler] On a scale from 1-10, how ready are you to change any aspect of your use of [X]?
• Reinforce positives	• Ask: Why did you choose that number and not a lower one like a 1 or a 2? Other reasons for change?
• Develop discrepancy between ideal and present self	• Ask: How does this fit with where you see yourself in the future?
4. Negotiate & advise • Negotiate goal	What's the next step? • What do you think you can do to stay healthy and safe?
• Benefits of change	• If you make these changes what do you think might happen?
• Reinforce resilience/resources	• What have you succeeded in changing in the past? How? Could you use these methods to help you with the challenges of changing?
• Summarize	• This is what I've heard you say…Here's an action plan I would like you to fill out, reinforcing your new goals. This is really an agreement between you and yourself.
• Provide handouts	• Provide agreement and information sheet
	• Thank patient for his/her time.

Boston University School of Public Health. BNI-ART Institute intervention algorithm. Available at: http://www.ed.bmc.org/sbirt/docs/aligo_adult.pdf. Retrieved January 23, 2008.

(continued)

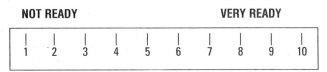

Justice

The ethical principle of justice governs access to care and fair distribution of resources. Elimination of health disparities and promotion of quality care for all are at the top of the list of goals for *Healthy People 2010*, the nation's health agenda. Injustice may result from a variety of sources.

Physicians may fail to apply principles of universal screening. When women are less likely to be screened or referred for treatment, their burden of disability is increased and health status decreased. The principle of justice requires that screening questions related to alcohol and drug use should be asked equally of men and women, regardless of race or economic status. It also requires that women be screened with tests such as TWEAK, T-ACE, or the NIAAA quantity and frequency questions that are more accurate in detecting women's patterns of substance abuse, which differ from those of men (40) (see box "Substance Abuse Screening"). Women, for example, are more likely to be hidden drinkers and frequently underreport alcohol use, especially during pregnancy. Tests to detect the problem in women must include questions about tolerance, which are not included in the most commonly used screen, CAGE, which has a sensitivity of only 75% compared with 87% for TWEAK (41).

Pregnant women are more likely to be screened than nonpregnant women. Although the vulnerability of the fetus is an important concern, the lives of nonpregnant women also have compelling value, and there is much evidence to suggest that women who abuse alcohol or use illicit drugs have coexisting or preexisting conditions (ie, mental health disorders, domestic violence, stress, childhood sexual abuse, poverty, and lack of resources) that put them in a vulnerable status (6, 42, 43). Universal application of screening questions, brief intervention, and referral to treatment eliminates these disparities related to justice.

Additionally, failure to diagnose and treat substance abuse with the same evidence-based approach applied to other chronic illnesses reduces patients' access to health services and resources. Justice requires that physicians counsel patients who have drug or alcohol problems and refer them to an appropriate treatment resource when available. No physician would withhold hypertension therapy because the medication adherence rate is only 60%. Physicians who detect the serious medical condition of addiction are equally obligated to intervene.

Respect for Autonomy

No person has a right to use illegal drugs, and a pregnant woman has a moral obligation to avoid the use of both illicit drugs and alcohol in order to safeguard the welfare of her fetus. At the same time, effective intervention with respect to substance abuse by a pregnant or a nonpregnant woman requires that a climate of respect and trust exist within the physician–patient relationship. Patients who begin to disclose behaviors that are stigmatized by society may be harmed if they feel that their trust is met with disrespect. Criticism and shaming statements actually increase resistance and impede change. Effective interventions, as summarized in the NIAAA Treatment Improvement Protocol number 35, are designed to increase motivation to change by respecting autonomy, supporting self-efficacy, and offering hope and resources (10).

Effective intervention also requires that universal screening questions, brief intervention, and referral to treatment be conducted with full protection of confidentiality. Patients who fear that acknowledging substance abuse may lead to disclosure to others will be inhibited from honest reporting to their physicians (44). A difficult dilemma is created by state laws that require physicians to report the nonmedical use of controlled substances by a pregnant woman or that require toxicology tests after delivery when there is evidence of possible use of a controlled substance (eg, Minnesota statutes 626.5561 and 626.5562). Although such laws have the goals of referring the pregnant woman for assessment and chemical dependency treatment if indicated and of protecting fetuses and newborns from harm, these laws may unwittingly result in pregnant women not seeking prenatal care or concealing drug use from their obstetricians. Although it is always appropriate for a physician to negotiate with a patient about her willingness to accept a medical recommendation, respect for autonomy includes respect for refusal to be screened.

Special Responsibilities to Pregnant Patients

Federal warnings about the need to abstain from alcohol use in pregnancy were first issued in 1984. The American College of Obstetricians and Gynecologists recommended screening early in pregnancy in its 1977 *Standards for Ambulatory Obstetric Care*, and a pamphlet was issued in 1982 entitled "Alcohol and Your Unborn Baby." Screening during pregnancy was subsequently supported in a variety of documents and is recommended in a joint publication issued by ACOG and the American Academy of Pediatrics (AAP) (45). Although obstetricians report screening 97% of pregnant women for alcohol use, only 25% used any of the standard screening tools, and only 20% of those surveyed knew that abstinence is the only known way to avoid all four adverse pregnancy outcomes (spontaneous abortion, nervous system impairment, birth defects, and FAS). This is a particularly significant gap in knowledge because there is no level of alcohol use, even minimal drinking, that has been determined to be absolutely safe. More than one half of the respondents (63%) reported that they lacked adequate information about referral resources (46). Screening rates for illicit drugs are lower than for alcohol (89%, according to unpublished ACOG survey data).

Ethical issues related to beneficence and nonmaleficence and the ethics of care (47) are similar for pregnant and nonpregnant women and for women who do and do not have children. In each of these cases, universal screening questions, brief intervention, and referral to treatment enables physicians to collaborate with patients to improve their own health, reduce the likelihood of preterm birth and neonatal complications in both current and future pregnancies, and improve the parenting capacity of the family unit.

As noted previously, autonomy issues are particularly challenging in pregnancy. In a survey of obstetricians, pediatricians, and family practice physicians, more than one half of the respondents believed that pregnant women have a legal as well as moral responsibility to ensure that they have healthy newborns (48). Although 61% were concerned that fear of criminal charges would be a barrier to receiving prenatal care, more than one half supported a statute that would permit removal of children from any woman who abused alcohol or drugs (48). This position is particularly troubling because these physicians did not state that there needed to be evidence of physical or emotional neglect (adverse effects on basic needs and safety) for children to be so removed. Both ethical and legal perspectives require that the best interests of the child be served, which requires both protecting children and assisting their mothers to be healthy so as to provide an optimal situation for growth and development.

Physicians' concerns about mothers who abuse alcohol or drugs undoubtedly reflect a desire to protect children. However, recommended screening and referral protocols may be perceived as punitive measures when they are connected with legally mandated testing, or reporting, or both. Such measures endanger the relationship of trust between physician and patient, place the obstetrician in an adversarial relationship with the patient, and possibly conflict with the therapeutic obligation. If pregnant women become reluctant to seek medical care because they fear being reported for alcohol or illegal drug use, these strategies will actually increase the risks for the woman and the fetus rather than reduce the consequences of substance abuse. Furthermore, threats and incarceration have proved to be ineffective in reducing the incidence of alcohol or drug abuse, and removing children from the home may only subject them to worse risks in the foster care system (49). Treatment is both more effective and less expensive than restrictive policies (50), and it results in a mean net saving of $4,644 in medical expenses per mother–infant pair (51). Moreover, women who have custody of their children complete treatment at a higher rate than those who do not. Putting women in jail, where drugs may be available but treatment is not, jeopardizes the health of pregnant women and that of their existing and future children (52).

Referral to treatment, especially if combined with training in parenting skills, is the clinically appropriate recommendation, both medically and ethically (37). Criminal charges against pregnant women on grounds of child abuse have been struck down in almost all cases because courts have upheld the right to privacy, which includes the right to decide whether to have a child, the right to bodily integrity, and the right to "be let alone" (53), and have found that states could better protect fetal health through "education and making available medical care and drug treatment centers for women" (54). The United States Supreme Court recognized the importance of privacy to the physician–patient relationship when it ruled in 2001 to prohibit a public hospital from performing nonconsensual drug tests on pregnant women without a warrant and providing police with positive results (55). Despite more than a decade of efforts and the 1992 passage of a federal Alcohol Drug Abuse and Mental Health Administration Reorganization Act explicitly prohibiting pregnancy discrimination, few treatment programs focus on the needs of pregnant women. In the absence of appropriate and adequate drug treatment services for pregnant women, criminal charges on grounds of child abuse are unjust in that they indict women for failing to seek treatment that actually may not be available to them.

Justice issues also are problematic in that punitive measures are not applied evenly across sex, race, and socioeconomic status. Although several types of legal sanctions against pregnant women who abuse alcohol or drugs are being tested in the courts, there has been no attempt to impose similar sanctions for paternal drug use (56), despite the significant involvement of male partners in pregnant women's substance abuse (57). In a landmark study among pregnant women anonymously tested for drug use, drug prevalence was similar between African-American women and white women, but African-American women were 10 times more likely than white women to be reported as a result of positive screen results (58). Similar patterns of injustice have been noted for the types of drugs for which sanctions exist in the legal system. For example, mandatory incarceration and more severe penalties are applied to crack cocaine, which is primarily used by African Americans, than to powder cocaine or heroin, which is primarily used by whites. In the case of *Ferguson v. City of Charleston*, an overwhelming majority of the pregnant women arrested in the immediate postpartum period because of cocaine-positive drug screen results were African American. When the results of similarly drawn drug screens were positive for methamphetamine or heroin, which were more commonly used by white patients, physicians were more likely to refer to social services rather than to the courts (55).

Some physicians are reluctant to record information related to alcohol or drug abuse in medical records because of competing obligations. On the one hand, the physician may be concerned about nonmaleficence. Because medical records may not be safe from inappropriate disclosure despite federal and state privacy protections, the patient may experience real harms—such as job loss unrelated to workplace performance issues, eviction from public housing, or termination of insurance—if a diagnosis of dependency is recorded in the medical record. Although legal redress for harms that result from inappropriate transfer of information may be possible, it may not be feasible for a woman in straitened circumstances. On the other hand, the principle of beneficence often requires disclosure of information needed by the medical team to provide appropriate medical care. Without this disclosure, a physician treating the patient for a problem unrelated to pregnancy or an emergency department physician seeing the patient for the first time may miss a major complication related to substance abuse. Concerns about protection of confidentiality and nonmaleficence can be addressed most appropriately by including only medically necessary, accurate information in the medical record and informing the patient about the purpose of any disclosure.

Responsibilities to Neonates

The use of illicit drugs and alcohol during pregnancy has demonstrated adverse effects on the neonate, and these newborns are subsequently at risk for altered neurodevelopmental outcome and poor health status (59). Detection and treatment are essential precursors of appropriate therapeutic intervention in the immediate setting. Early recognition of parental substance abuse also may lead to interventions designed to decrease associated risks to a child's physical and psychologic health and safety (32–37). Doing so may obviate the necessity for placement in an already overburdened foster care system (60). Underrecognition of prenatal alcohol and drug effects is common, however (61). A toxicology screen and scoring for craniofacial features suggestive of FAS should be performed by the neonate's physician whenever clinically indicated. According to the AAP's statement on neonatal drug withdrawal (62), maternal characteristics that suggest a need for biochemical screening of the neonate include no prenatal care, previous unexplained fetal demise, precipitous labor, abruptio placentae, hypertensive episodes, severe mood swings, cerebrovascular accidents, myocardial infarction, and repeated spontaneous abortions. Infant characteristics that may be associated with maternal drug use include preterm birth, unexplained intrauterine growth restriction, neurobehavioral abnormalities, congenital abnormalities, atypical vascular incidents, myocardial infarction, and necrotizing enterocolitis in otherwise healthy term infants. The legal implications of testing and the need for maternal consent vary from state to state; therefore, physicians should be aware of local laws that may influence regional practice.

Biophysical testing, however, has major limitations (63–65). Both urine and meconium screens have a high rate of false-negative results because of factors related to the timing and amount of the last maternal drug use (for urine) and the failure to detect drug metabolites (for meconium). Hair is associated with a substantial false-positive rate because of passive exposure to minute quantities of illicit substances in the environment. Physicians and nurses often fail to recognize the physical manifestations of FAS (66). Maternal self-report of use or consent to testing, elicited using nonjudgmental, supportive interview techniques within a physician–patient relationship of trust, can thus provide the best information for guiding neonatal treatment and the best prognosis for family intervention. Maternal substance abuse does not by itself guarantee child neglect or prove inadequate parenting capacity (67, 68). Parenting skills programs, assistance with employment and housing issues, and access to substance abuse treatment have been shown to be successful support mechanisms for families of affected neonates, and these elements should be part of a comprehensive approach to substance abuse problems. If there is evidence to suggest the likelihood of neglect or abuse, referral to children's protective services may be indicated (69). A children's protective services referral should never be undertaken as a punitive measure, but with the aim of evaluating circumstances, protecting the child, and providing services to maintain or reunify the family unit if at all possible.

Special Issues for Girls and Young Women

Use of alcohol and illicit drugs among youth is prevalent, and studies that included both male and female youth indicate that age of first use is decreasing. Youth who begin drinking at age 14 years are at least three times more likely to experience dependence (using criteria from the *Diagnostic and Statistical Manual of Mental Disorders*, 4th Edition) than those who delay drinking to age 21 years (70). Early onset of drinking increases the likelihood of alcohol-related unintentional injuries (71), motor vehicle crash involvement after drinking (72), unprotected intercourse (73), and getting into fights after drinking, even after controlling for frequency of heavy drinking, alcohol dependence, and other factors related to age of onset (74). A study among a large community sample of lifetime drinkers showed that those who reported first drinking at the ages of 11–14 years experienced a rapid progression to alcohol-related harm, and 16% developed dependence by age 24 years (75). Among youth aged 21–25 years surveyed in 2006, 27.3% drove under the influence of alcohol (1). The use of alcohol and illicit substances by youth and the impact of parental alcohol and substance use on children have adverse health outcomes (76, 77). Prevention (universal screening questions, brief intervention, and referral to treatment) has thus been described by leaders in obstetrics and gynecology and by pediatricians as a moral obligation (78). In 1993, the AAP developed substance abuse guidelines for clinical practice. These guidelines have now been refined and developed into competencies that provide practical direction for clinicians engaged in educating, supporting, and treating patients and families affected by substance abuse (79).

Confidentiality is as essential to the physician–patient relationship with children as it is with adults. Many state laws protect the confidentiality of minors with regard to substance abuse detection and treatment (79). Autonomy issues are of particular importance in the detection and treatment of substance abuse for adolescents, who are at a developmental stage in which it is a normative task to test new identities and engage in risk-taking in the process (80). The ACOG Committee on Adolescent Health Care lists the following key points concerning informed consent, parental permission, and assent (81):

- Concern about confidentiality is a major obstacle in the delivery of health care to adolescents. Physicians should address confidentiality issues with the adolescent patient to build a trusting relationship with her and to facilitate a candid discussion regarding her health and health-related behaviors.

- Physicians also should discuss confidentiality issues with the parent(s) or guardian(s) of the adolescent patient. Physicians should encourage their involve-ment in the patient's health and health care decisions and, when appropriate, facilitate communication between the two.

- The right of a "mature minor" to obtain selected medical care has been established in most states.

In a document about testing for drugs of abuse in children and adolescents, AAP states that the goal of care is a therapeutic, rather than adversarial, relationship with the child and, therefore, makes the following recommendations (82):

- Screening or testing under any circumstances is improper if clinicians cannot be reasonably certain that the laboratory results are valid and that patient confidentiality is ensured.

- Diagnostic testing for the purpose of drug abuse treatment is within the ethical tradition of health care, and in the competent patient, it should be conducted noncovertly, confidentially, and with informed consent in the same context as for other medical conditions.

- Parental permission is not sufficient for involuntary testing of the adolescent with decisional capacity.

- Suspicion that an adolescent is using a psychoactive drug does not justify involuntary testing, and testing adolescents requires their consent unless 1) the patient lacks decision-making capacity or 2) there are strong medical indications or legal requirements to do so.

- Minors should not be immune from the criminal justice system, but physicians should not initiate or participate in a criminal investigation, except when required by law, as in the case of court-ordered drug testing or child abuse reporting.

Guidance for Physicians

The health care system as it is currently constituted creates barriers to the practice of universal screening questions, brief intervention, and referral to treatment for alcohol and drug abuse. Because of a lack of medical school curricular content about addiction, physicians often are unfamiliar with screening procedures. Many institutions do not have appropriate protocols in place for intervention and referral. Time constraints, mandatory reporting laws, and lack of treatment resources may impede both screening and referral, and some of these problems may be beyond the ability of the individual physician to modify. Nevertheless, in fulfillment of the therapeutic obligation, physicians must make a substantial effort to:

- Learn established techniques for rapid, effective screening, intervention, and referral, and practice universal screening questions, brief intervention, and referral to treatment in order to provide benefit and do no harm. Where possible, create a team approach to deal with barriers of time limitations, using the skills of social workers, nurses, and peer educators for universal screening questions, brief intervention, and referral to treatment. Use external resources (eg, hospital social worker, health department, addiction specialist) to develop a list of treatment resources.

- Treat the patient with a substance abuse problem with dignity and respect in order to form a therapeutic alliance.

- Protect confidentiality and the integrity of the physician–patient relationship wherever possible within the requirements of legal obligations, and communicate honestly and directly with patients about what information can and cannot be protected. In states where there are laws requiring disclosure, inform patients in advance about specific items for which disclosure is mandated.

- Recognize that the most effective safeguard for children is treatment for family members who have a substance abuse problem.

- Balance competing obligations carefully, consulting with other physicians or an ethicist if troubling situations arise.

- Participate, whenever possible, in the policy process at institutional, state, and national levels as an advocate for the health care needs of patients.

- Consider whether elements of personal beliefs and values may be resulting in biases in medical practice. Be aware that some physicians minimize the universality and impact of alcohol or prescription drug abuse to protect against evaluating their own alcohol or substance abuse problems. A physician who has questions about his or her own use should seek help.

Conclusion

Substance abuse is a common medical condition that can have devastating physical and emotional consequences for women and their children. The traditional role of healer, the contemporary role of medical expert, and the newer role of primary care physician all require obstetrician–gynecologists to develop an evidence-supported knowledge base about methods for detection and treatment of substance abuse. The close working relationship between the physician and the patient that is both a goal of care and a means to improved health outcomes offers tremendous potential to influence patients' lifestyles positively. Despite this relationship, physicians seldom practice universal screening because of a lack of appreciation of prevalence, misunderstandings about treatment success rates, unfamiliarity with treatment resources, and inadequate knowledge about sex differences in presentation and the course of the disease. However, common barriers to universal screening questions, brief intervention, and referral to treatment can and should be addressed. Physicians have an ethical obligation to learn and use techniques for universal screening questions, brief intervention, and referral to treatment in order to provide patients and their families with medical care that is state-of-the-art, comprehensive, and effective.

References

1. Substance Abuse and Mental Health Services Administration. Results from the 2006 National Survey on Drug Use and Health: national findings. Office of Applied Studies, NSDUH Series H-32, DHHS Publication No. SMA 07-4293. Rockville (MD): SAMHSA; 2007. Available at: http://www.oas.samhsa.gov/nsduh/2k6nsduh/2k6Results.pdf. Retrieved January 23, 2008.

2. Smith WB, Weisner C. Women and alcohol problems: a critical analysis of the literature and unanswered questions. Alcohol Clin Exp Res 2000;24:1320–1.

3. Fetal alcohol exposure and the brain. National Institute on Alcohol Abuse and Alcoholism. Alcohol Alert 2000;50:1–6.

4. Fetal alcohol syndrome and alcohol-related neurodevelopmental disorders. American Academy of Pediatrics. Committee on Substance Abuse and Committee on Children with Disabilities. Pediatrics 2000;106:358–61.

5. Substance Abuse and Mental Health Services Administration. The financial impact of fetal alcohol syndrome. Rockville (MD): SAMHSA; 2003. Available at: http://www.fascenter.samhsa.gov/publications/cost.cfm. Retrieved May 28, 2008.

6. Amaro H, Fried LE, Cabral H, Zuckerman B. Violence during pregnancy and substance use. Am J Public Health 1990; 80:575–9.

7. Hutchins E, DiPietro J. Psychosocial risk factors associated with cocaine use during pregnancy: a case-control study. Obstet Gynecol 1997;90:142–7.

8. Substance Abuse and Mental Health Services Administration. 2006 National Survey on Drug Use and Health: detailed tables. Rockville (MD): SAMHSA; 2007. Available at: http://www.oas.samhsa.gov/NSDUH/2k6NSDUH/tabs/Sect7peTabs48to93.htm. Retrieved May 28, 2008.

9. Office of National Drug Control Policy. The economic costs of drug abuse in the United States, 1992-2002. Publication No. 207303. Washington, DC: Executive Office of the President; 2004. Available at: http://www.whitehousedrugpolicy.gov/publications/economic_costs/economic_costs.pdf. Retrieved January 23, 2008.

10. Substance Abuse and Mental Health Services Administration. Enhancing motivation for change in substance abuse. Treatment Improvement Protocol (TIP) series; 35. Rockville (MD): SAMHSA; 1999.

11. McLellan AT, Lewis DC, O'Brien CP, Kleber HD. Drug dependence, a chronic medical illness: implications for treatment, insurance, and outcomes evaluation. JAMA 2000;284:1689–95.

12. Bien TH, Miller WR, Tonigan JS. Brief interventions for alcohol problems: a review. Addiction 1993;88:315–35.

13. Fleming MF, Mundt MP, French MT, Manwell LB, Stauffacher EA, Barry KL. Benefit-cost analysis of brief physician advice with problem drinkers in primary care settings. Med Care 2000;38:7–18.

14. Blum LN, Nielsen NH, Riggs JA. Alcoholism and alcohol abuse among women: report of the Council on Scientific Affairs. American Medical Association. J Womens Health 1998;7:861–71.

15. Hubbard RL, French MT. New perspectives on the benefit-cost and cost-effectiveness of drug abuse treatment. NIDA Res Monogr 1991;113:94–113.

16. Chez RA, Andres RL, Chazotte C, Ling FW. Illicit drug use and dependence in women: a slide lecture presentation. Washington, DC: American College of Obstetricians and Gynecologists; 2002. Available at: http://www.acog.org/from_home/departments/underserved/Dependencein Women.ppt. Retrieved January 23, 2008.

17. Fleming MF, Barry KL. The effectiveness of alcoholism screening in an ambulatory care setting. J Stud Alcohol 1991;52:33–6.

18. Wilson L, Kahan M, Liu E, Brewster JM, Sobell MB, Sobell LC. Physician behavior towards male and female problem drinkers: a controlled study using simulated patients. J Addict Dis 2002;21:87–99.

19. Volk RJ, Steinbauer JR, Cantor SB. Patient factors influencing variation in the use of preventive interventions for alcohol abuse by primary care physicians. J Stud Alcohol 1996;57:203–9.

20. Gearhart JG, Beebe DK, Milhorn HT, Meeks GR. Alcoholism in women. Am Fam Physician 1991;44:907–13.

21. Gomberg ES. Women and alcohol: use and abuse. J Nerv Ment Dis 1993;181:211–9.

22. Marcenko MO, Spense M. Social and psychological correlates of substance abuse among pregnant women. Soc Work Res 1995;19:103–9.

23. Abel EL, Kruger ML, Friedl J. How do physicians define "light," "moderate," and "heavy" drinking? Alcohol Clin Exp Res 1998;22:979–84.

24. Yarnall KS, Pollak KI, Ostbye T, Krause KM, Michener JL. Primary care: is there enough time for prevention? Am J Public Health 2003;93:635–41.

25. Bernstein J, Bernstein E, Tassiopoulos K, Heeren T, Levenson S, Hingson R. Brief motivational intervention at a clinic visit reduces cocaine and heroin use. Drug Alcohol Depend 2005;77:49–59.

26. Fleming M, Manwell LB. Brief intervention in primary care settings. A primary treatment method for at-risk, problem, and dependent drinkers. Alcohol Res Health 1999;23:128–37.

27. The impact of screening, brief intervention, and referral for treatment on emergency department patients' alcohol use. Academic ED SBIRT Research Collaborative. Ann Emerg Med 2007;50:699–710, 710.e1–6.

28. National Institute on Drug Abuse. NIDA for teens: the science behind drug abuse: mind over matter. Bethesda (MD): NIDA; 2005. Available at: http://teens.drugabuse.gov/mom/index.asp. Retrieved January 23, 2008.

29. Chang G, Goetz MA, Wilkins-Haug L, Berman S. A brief intervention for prenatal alcohol use: an in-depth look. J Subst Abuse Treat 2000;18:365–9.

30. Bernstein E, Bernstein J, Levenson S. Project ASSERT: an ED-based intervention to increase access to primary care, preventive services, and the substance abuse treatment system. Ann Emerg Med 1997;30:181–9.

31. Manwell LB, Fleming MF, Mundt MP, Stauffacher EA, Barry KL. Treatment of problem alcohol use in women of childbearing age: results of a brief intervention trial. Alcohol Clin Exp Res 2000;24:1517–24.

32. Rosensweig MA. Reflections on the Center for Substance Abuse Prevention's pregnant and postpartum women and their infants program. Womens Health Issues 1998;8:206–7.

33. Whiteside-Mansell L, Crone CC, Conners NA. The development and evaluation of an alcohol and drug prevention and treatment program for women and children. The AR-CARES program. J Subst Abuse Treat 1999;16:265–75.

34. Ingersoll K, Floyd L, Sobell M, Velasquez MM. Reducing the risk of alcohol-exposed pregnancies: a study of a motivational intervention in community settings. Project CHOICES Intervention Research Group. Pediatrics 2003; 111: 1131–5.

35. Metsch LR, Wolfe HP, Fewell R, McCoy CB, Elwood WN, Wohler-Torres B, et al. Treating substance-using women and their children in public housing: preliminary evaluation findings. Child Welfare 2001;80:199–220.

36. Armstrong MA, Gonzales Osejo V, Lieberman L, Carpenter DM, Pantoja PM, Escobar GJ. Perinatal substance abuse intervention in obstetric clinics decreases adverse neonatal outcomes. J Perinatol 2003;23:3–9.

37. Peterson L, Gable S, Saldana L. Treatment of maternal addiction to prevent child abuse and neglect. Addict Behav 1996;21:789–801.

38. Boyd CJ, Guthrie B. Women, their significant others, and crack cocaine. Am J Addict 1996;5:156–66.

39. Ehrmin JT. Unresolved feelings of guilt and shame in the maternal role with substance-dependent African American women. J Nurs Scholarsh 2001;33:47–52.

40. Chang G, Wilkins-Haug L, Berman S, Goetz MA, Behr H, Hiley A. Alcohol use and pregnancy: improving identification. Obstet Gynecol 1998;91:892–8.

41. Cherpitel CJ. Screening for alcohol problems in the emergency department. Ann Emerg Med 1995;26:158–66.

42. Berenson AB, Wiemann CM, Wilkinson GS, Jones WA, Anderson GD. Perinatal morbidity associated with violence experienced by pregnant women. Am J Obstet Gynecol 1994;170:1760–6; discussion 1766–9.

43. Sheehan TJ. Stress and low birth weight: a structural modeling approach using real life stressors. Soc Sci Med 1998;47:1503–12.

44. Poland ML, Dombrowski MP, Ager JW, Sokol RJ. Punishing pregnant drug users: enhancing the flight from care. Drug Alcohol Depend 1993;31:199–203.

45. American Academy of Pediatrics, American College of Obstetricians and Gynecologists. Guidelines for perinatal care. 6th ed. Elk Grove Village (IL): AAP; Washington, DC: ACOG; 2007.

46. Diekman ST, Floyd RL, Decoufle P, Schulkin J, Ebrahim SH, Sokol RJ. A survey of obstetrician-gynecologists on their

patients' alcohol use during pregnancy. Obstet Gynecol 2000;95:756–63.

47. Ethical decision making in obstetrics and gynecology. ACOG Committee Opinion No. 390. American College of Obstetricians and Gynecologists. Obstet Gynecol 2007; 110:1479–87.

48. Abel EL, Kruger M. Physician attitudes concerning legal coercion of pregnant alcohol and drug abusers. Am J Obstet Gynecol 2002;186:768–72.

49. Drug exposed infants: recommendations. Center for the Future of Children. Future Child 1991;1:8–9.

50. Rydell CP, Everingham SS. Controlling cocaine: supply versus demand programs. Santa Monica (CA): RAND; 1994.

51. Svikis DS, Golden AS, Huggins GR, Pickens RW, McCaul ME, Velez ML, et al. Cost-effectiveness of treatment for drug-abusing pregnant women. Drug Alcohol Depend 1997;45:105–13.

52. Paltrow LM. Punishing women for their behavior during pregnancy: an approach that undermines the health of women and children. In: Wetherington CL, Roman AB, editors. Drug addiction research and the health of women. Rockville (MD): National Institute on Drug Abuse; 1998. p. 467–501. Available at: http://www.nida.nih.gov/PDF/ DARHW/467-502_Paltrow.pdf. Retrieved January 23, 2008.

53. Olmstead v. U.S., 277 U.S. 438 (1928).

54. Gostin LO. The rights of pregnant women: the Supreme Court and drug testing. Hastings Cent Rep 2001;31:8–9.

55. Ferguson v. City of Charleston, 532 U.S. 67 (2001).

56. Nelson LJ, Marshall MF. Ethical and legal analyses of three coercive policies aimed at substance abuse by pregnant women. Charleston (SC): Medical University of South Carolina, Program in Bioethics; 1998.

57. Frank DA, Brown J, Johnson S, Cabral H. Forgotten fathers: an exploratory study of mothers' report of drug and alcohol problems among fathers of urban newborns. Neurotoxicol Teratol 2002;24:339–47.

58. Chasnoff IJ, Landress HJ, Barrett ME. The prevalence of illicit-drug or alcohol use during pregnancy and discrepancies in mandatory reporting in Pinellas County, Florida. N Engl J Med 1990;322:1202–6.

59. Wagner CL, Katikaneni LD, Cox TH, Ryan RM. The impact of prenatal drug exposure on the neonate. Obstet Gynecol Clin North Am 1998;25:169–94.

60. United States General Accounting Office. Foster care: health needs of many young children are unknown and unmet. GAO/HEHS-95-114. Washington, DC: GAO; 1995. Available at: http://www.gao.gov/archive/1995/he95114.pdf. Retrieved January 23, 2008.

61. Stoler JM, Holmes LB. Under-recognition of prenatal alcohol effects in infants of known alcohol abusing women. J Pediatr 1999;135:430–6.

62. Neonatal drug withdrawal. American Academy of Pediatrics Committee on Drugs [published erratum appears in Pediatrics 1998;102:660]. Pediatrics 1998;101: 1079–88.

63. Lester BM, ElSohly M, Wright LL, Smeriglio VL, Verter J, Bauer CR, et al. The Maternal Lifestyle Study: drug use by meconium toxicology and maternal self-report. Pediatrics 2001;107:309–17.

64. Millard DD. Toxicology testing in neonates. Is it ethical, and what does it mean? Clin Perinatol 1996;23:491–507.

65. Ostrea EM Jr, Knapp DK, Tannenbaum L, Ostrea AR, Romero A, Salari V, et al. Estimates of illicit drug use during pregnancy by maternal interview, hair analysis, and meconium analysis. J Pediatr 2001;138:344–8.

66. Lyons Jones K. Early recognition of prenatal alcohol effects: A pediatrician's responsibility. J Pediatr 1999;135:405–6.

67. Davis SK. Comprehensive interventions for affecting the parenting effectiveness of chemically dependent women. J Obstet Gynecol Neonatal Nurs 1997;26:604–10.

68. Smith BD, Test MF. The risk of subsequent maltreatment allegations in families with substance-exposed infants. Child Abuse Negl 2002;26:97–114.

69. MacMahon JR. Perinatal substance abuse: the impact of reporting infants to child protective services. Pediatrics 1997;100(5):E1.

70. Grant BF. The impact of a family history of alcoholism on the relationship between age at onset of alcohol use and DSM-IV alcohol dependence: results from the National Longitudinal Alcohol Epidemiologic Survey. Alcohol Health Res World 1998;22:144–7.

71. Hingson RW, Heeren T, Jamanka A, Howland J. Age of drinking onset and unintentional injury involvement after drinking. JAMA 2000;284:1527–33.

72. Hingson R, Heeren T, Zakocs R, Winter M, Wechsler H. Age of first intoxication, heavy drinking, driving after drinking and risk of unintentional injury among U.S. college students. J Stud Alcohol 2003;64:23–31.

73. Hingson R, Heeren T, Winter MR, Wechsler H. Early age of first drunkenness as a factor in college students' unplanned and unprotected sex attributable to drinking. Pediatrics 2003;111:34–41.

74. Substance Abuse and Mental Health Services Administration. The relationship between mental health and substance abuse among adolescents. National Household Survey on Drug Abuse Series: A-9. Rockville (MD): SAMHSA; 1999. Available at: http://www.oas.samhsa.gov/ NHSDA/A-9/ comorb3c.htm. Retrieved January 23, 2008.

75. DeWit DJ, Adlaf EM, Offord DR, Ogborne AC. Age at first alcohol use: a risk factor for the development of alcohol disorders. Am J Psychiatry 2000;157:745–50.

76. Alcohol use and abuse: a pediatric concern. American Academy of Pediatrics: Committee on Substance Abuse. Pediatrics 2001;108:185–9.

77. Fishman M, Bruner A, Adger H Jr. Substance abuse among children and adolescents. Pediatr Rev 1997;18:394–403.

78. Chasnoff IJ. Silent violence: is prevention a moral obligation? Pediatrics 1998;102:145–8.

79. Adger H Jr, Macdonald DI, Wenger S. Core competencies for involvement of health care providers in the care of children and adolescents in families affected by substance abuse. Pediatrics 1999;103:1083–4.

80. Donovan JE, Jessor R, Costa FM. Adolescent problem drinking: stability of psychosocial and behavioral correlates across a generation. J Stud Alcohol 1999;60:352–61.

81. American College of Obstetricians and Gynecologists. Health care for adolescents. Washington, DC: ACOG; 2003.

82. Testing for drugs of abuse in children and adolescents. American Academy of Pediatrics Committee on Substance Abuse. Pediatrics 1996;98:305–7.

At-risk drinking and illicit drug use: ethical issues in obstetric and gynecologic practice. ACOG Committee Opinion No. 422. American College of Obstetricians and Gynecologists. Obstet Gynecol 2008; 112:1449–60.

ISSN 1074-861X

COMMITTEE ON GENETICS

COMMITTEE ON GENETICS

ACOG COMMITTEE OPINION

Number 383 • October 2007

(Replaces No. 257, May 2001)

Evaluation of Stillbirths and Neonatal Deaths

Committee on Genetics

This document reflects emerging clinical and scientific advances as of the date issued and is subject to change. The information should not be construed as dictating an exclusive course of treatment or procedure to be followed.

ASTRACT: A complete evaluation of a stillbirth or neonatal death may explain the cause of death, direct further investigation of the family, and be particularly valuable in counseling parents about recurrence risks in future pregnancies. The results of the autopsy, placental examination, laboratory tests, and cytogenetic studies should be communicated to the involved clinicians and to the family of the deceased infant in a timely manner.

A stillbirth or fetal death is a death before the complete expulsion or extraction of a product of human conception from its mother, regardless of the duration of pregnancy, that is not an induced termination of pregnancy. Such losses are reported according to varying state guidelines, although many states use a fetal weight of 350 g or more or, if weight is unknown, a gestational age of 20 completed weeks or more, calculated from the date of the last menstrual period, as requirements for reporting (1). As of 2003, the fetal mortality rate overall in the United States was 6.2 per 1,000 live births and fetal deaths (2). Neonatal death is the death of a liveborn neonate before the neonate becomes 28 days old. Perinatal death includes the deaths of neonates that are less than 28 days old and deaths of fetuses at 20 weeks or more of gestation. In 2003, the perinatal mortality rate was 10.83 per 1,000 live births and fetal deaths (2). A complete evaluation of a stillbirth or neonatal death may explain the cause of death, direct further investigation of the family, and be particularly valuable in counseling parents about recurrence risks in future pregnancies. Each institution may use these guidelines to establish an appropriate referral team and protocol for management and evaluation of a fetal death.

Initial Parental Discussion

Sensitivity is needed when discussing evaluation with the family. In discussing options, clinicians should refer to the fetus by name, if one was given. Grief-stricken parents may be reluctant to consent to evaluation or autopsy examination, and some may have religious or cultural objections. Parents should be informed about the reasons for autopsy, procedures (eg, the face is usually not touched), and potential costs. Even though the bereaved parents may not want the information initially, health care providers should strongly emphasize that results of the evaluation may be useful to the patient and her family in planning future pregnancies. The family should be informed of the value of less invasive methods of evaluation, including the use of photographs, X-ray imaging, ultrasonography, magnetic resonance imaging, and sampling of tissues, such as blood or skin. These methods may help to identify a syndrome or chromosomal abnormality even without full autopsy data. Congenital anomalies are a significant cause of fetal death; 15–20% of stillborn fetuses have a major malformation (3). Approximately 8% of stillborn fetuses have chromosomal abnormalities and approximately 20% have dysmorphic features or skeletal abnormalities (3, 4). Malformations often are present in patterns that permit classification into a particular syndrome. Syndrome identification may delineate etiologic and pathogenetic factors that could have predictive significance for recurrence risk and the risk of other associated anomalies (5).

Management

After a stillbirth or neonatal death, proper management includes obtaining a complete perinatal and family history, performing a physical examination of the fetus or neonate

The American College of Obstetricians and Gynecologists
Women's Health Care Physicians

139

(with documentation by description and photography, if possible), and obtaining laboratory studies (see Fig. 1 and the box). To ascertain the etiology and provide appropriate counseling to the family, clinical–pathologic correlation is best accomplished by a team comprising obstetricians, pediatricians, neonatologists, pathologists, and geneticists. Initial evaluation by a geneticist, neonatologist, or pathologist may help the team coordinate the evaluation and the needed follow-up.

History

When stillbirth or neonatal death occurs, the obstetric history, including exposures (eg, medications and viral infections) and family history with a three-generation pedigree, if possible, should be reviewed. Any pertinent

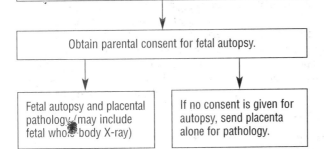

Fig. 1. Flow chart for fetal and placental evaluation

Maternal Evaluation Checklist

Family history
- Recurrent spontaneous abortions
- Venous thromboembolism or pulmonary embolism
- Congenital anomaly or abnormal karyotype
- Hereditary condition or syndrome
- Developmental delay
- Consanguinity

Maternal history
- Personal history of venous thromboembolism or pulmonary embolism
- Diabetes mellitus
- Chronic hypertension
- Thrombophilia
- Systemic lupus erythematosus
- Autoimmune disease
- Epilepsy
- Severe anemia
- Heart disease
- Tobacco, alcohol, drug or medication use

Obstetric history
- Recurrent miscarriages
- Previous child with anomaly, hereditary condition, or growth restriction
- Previous gestational hypertension or preeclampsia
- Previous gestational diabetes mellitus
- Previous abruptio placentae
- Previous fetal demise

Current pregnancy
- Maternal age
- Gestational age at fetal death
- Medical conditions complicating pregnancy
  —Hypertension
  —Gestational diabetes mellitus
  —Systemic lupus erythematosus
  —Cholestasis
- Pregnancy weight gain and body mass index
- Complications of multi-fetal gestation, such as twin–twin transfusion syndrome, twin reversed arterial perfusion syndrome, and discordant growth
- Abruptio placentae
- Abdominal trauma
- Preterm labor or rupture of membranes
- Gestational age at onset of prenatal care
- Abnormalities seen on an ultrasound image
- Infections or chorioamnionitis
- Alloimmunization

(continued)

Maternal Evaluation Checklist *(continued)*

Maternal laboratory evaluation at time of identification of demise
- Complete blood count
- Kleihauer–Betke test (or comparable test for fetal cells in maternal circulation)
- Parvovirus B-19 immunoglobulin G and immunoglobulin M
- Syphilis
- Lupus anticoagulant
- MTHFR gene mutation
- Anticardiolipin antibodies
- Thrombophilia
  —Factor V Leiden
  —Prothrombin gene mutation
  —Protein C activity
  —Antithrombin III
- Thyroid-stimulating hormones and free thyroxine

Maternal laboratory evaluation at follow-up
- Parental karyotypes if desired
- Protein S activity

information in the maternal or paternal pedigree should be documented and investigated further. Relevant original medical records and documentation should be obtained whenever possible. The gestational age by last menstrual period, maternal examinations, laboratory data, and ultrasonograms should be recorded for correlation with the physical examination of the neonate. Possible nongenetic causes, such as infection, abruptio placentae, and umbilical cord abnormality also should be considered.

Examination of the Stillborn Fetus

The general examination of the stillborn fetus should be done promptly, noting any dysmorphic features and obtaining measurements of weight, length, and head circumference (6–9). Foot length may be especially useful before 23 weeks of gestation to ascertain gestational age. Photographs of the whole body (unclothed); frontal and profile views of the face, extremities, and palms; and close-up photographs of specific abnormalities are vital for subsequent review and consultation with a specialist, particularly if no geneticist is available at the institution. Even if parents have declined an autopsy, a description of any obvious abnormalities of the stillborn fetus should be included in the medical record. Measurements may be accomplished by the obstetrician, pathologist, or other specialist, such as a neonatologist, depending on the institutional protocol.

Autopsy as well as examination of the placenta should be offered. This is especially true when dysmor-

phic features, inconsistent growth measurements, anomalies, hydrops, or growth restriction are present. Parents should be given the opportunity to hold the baby and perform cultural activities, such as baptism, before the autopsy. If no previous anatomic ultrasound image was obtained during pregnancy, whole-body X-ray with anterior–posterior and lateral views may reveal an unrecognized skeletal abnormality or further define a grossly apparent deformity.

When a full autopsy is performed, it should follow the guidelines for perinatal autopsy published by the College of American Pathologists (www.cap.org) or other standard references (9, 10). The pathologist should be aware of the clinical history and suspected genetic diagnoses; any need to obtain samples for cytogenetic studies should be explained.

Examination of the Placenta

Gross and microscopic examination of the placenta, including membranes for amniotic bands and other anomalies, and umbilical cord specimen and blood vessels for knots or constrictions may corroborate autopsy findings or explain apparent fetal deformity. Even if the family declines fetal autopsy, histologic study of the placenta usually is not problematic and is extremely valuable in identifying underlying etiologies (11, 12).

Fetal Laboratory Studies

Chromosomal information is particularly valuable if the fetus displays dysmorphic features, inconsistent growth measurements, anomalies, hydrops, or growth restriction or if a parent carries a balanced chromosomal rearrangement (eg, translocation or inversion) or has a mosaic karyotype. Samples of amniotic fluid, umbilical cord, fetal tissue, or placenta may be obtained for chromosomal and any other relevant tests. Generally, the most viable tissue is placental, followed by fetal cartilage obtained from the costochondral junction or patella (see Fig. 1) (13–15). Appropriate history and physical findings should be sent to the laboratory for the laboratory to choose any appropriate cytogenetic tests. These additional tests may be needed, depending on the results of the first study.

Maternal Evaluation

Numerous other maternal conditions, such as systemic lupus erythematosus, renal disease, uncontrolled thyroid disease, obesity, infection, maternal diabetes mellitus, hypertension, and thrombophilias have been associated with increased risk for stillbirth compared with the absence of these conditions (16). Immediate investigation for fetal–maternal hemorrhage should be conducted shortly after the diagnosis of the demise because this also may be a cause for fetal death (17). Maternal testing for lupus anticoagulant, anticardiolipin antibodies, Parvovirus B19 immunoglobulin G and immunoglobulin M, thyroid stimulating hormone, free thyroxine, factor V Leiden and prothrombin mutations, antithrombin III,

MTHFR gene mutation, and protein C and protein S activity may provide information that could affect future pregnancy management (18–20).

Counseling

The results of the autopsy, placental examination, laboratory tests, and cytogenetic studies should be communicated to the involved clinicians and to the family of the deceased infant in a timely manner. Feelings of guilt or anger in parents who have experienced a perinatal death are common and may be magnified when there is an abnormal child or a genetic defect. However, some parents may welcome discussion and find relief in autopsy results. The results of the tests are important even when no specific diagnosis is identified (21). If there was no growth of the fetal chromosomes (or these were not obtained), further consultation with a genetics professional or high-risk pregnancy (maternal–fetal medicine) specialist is advised to discuss the need for parental chromosomal testing. A copy of the results of the tests and a list of diagnoses excluded should be provided to the patients for counseling. Referral to a bereavement counselor, religious leader, peer support group, or mental health professional may be advisable for management of grief and depression.

References

1. National Center for Health Statistics. State definitions and reporting requirements for live births, fetal deaths, and induced terminations of pregnancy. 1997 revision. Hyattsville (MD): NCHS; 1997. Available at: http://www.cdc.gov/nchs/data/misc/itop97.pdf. Retrieved March 21, 2007.

2. MacDorman MF, Hoyert DL, Martin JA, Munson ML, Hamilton BE. Fetal and perinatal mortality, United States, 2003. Natl Vital Stat Rep 2007;55(6):1–17.

3. Pauli RM, Reiser CA. Wisconsin Stillbirth Service Program: II. Analysis of diagnoses and diagnostic categories in the first 1,000 referrals. Am J Med Genet 1994;50:135–53.

4. Pauli RM, Reiser CA, Lebovitz RM, Kirkpatrick SJ. Wisconsin Stillbirth Service Program: I. Establishment and assessment of a community-based program for etiologic investigation of intrauterine deaths. Am J Med Genet 1994; 50:116–34.

5. Leppig KA, Werler MM, Cann CI, Cook CA, Holmes LB. Predictive value of minor anomalies. I. Association with major malformations. J Pediatr 1987;110:531–7.

6. Reed GB, Claireaux AE, Cockburn F, editors. Diseases of the fetus and newborn: pathology, imaging, genetics and management. 2nd ed. London (UK): Chapman & Hall Medical; 1995.

7. Stocker JT, Dehner LP, editors. Pediatric pathology. 2nd ed. Philadelphia (PA): Lippincott Williams & Wilkins; 2001.

8. Naeye RL. Disorders of the placenta, fetus, and neonate: diagnosis and clinical significance. St. Louis (MO): Mosby Year Book; 1992.

9. Valdes-Dapena MA, Huff DS. Perinatal autopsy Manual. Washington (DC): Armed Forces Institute of Pathology; 1983.

10. Bove KE. Practice guidelines for autopsy pathology: the perinatal and pediatric autopsy. Autopsy Committee of the College of American Pathologists. Arch Pathol Lab Med 1997;121:368–76.

11. Benirschke K, Kaufman P. Pathology of the human placenta. 4th ed. New York (NY): Springer; 2000.

12. Genest DR. Estimating the time of death in stillborn fetuses: II. Histologic evaluation of the placenta; a study of 71 stillborns. Obstet Gynecol 1992;80:585–92.

13. Smith A, Bannatyne P, Russell P, Ellwood D, den Dulk G. Cytogenetic studies in perinatal death. Aust N Z J Obstet Gynaecol 1990;30:206–10.

14. Baena N, Guitart M, Ferreres JC, Gabau E, Corona M, Mellado F, et al. Fetal and placenta chromosome constitution in 237 pregnancy losses. Ann Genet 2001;44:83–8.

15. Gelman-Kohan Z, Rosensaft J, Ben-Hur H, Haber A, Chemke J. Cytogenetic analysis of fetal chondrocytes: a comparative study. Prenat Diagn 1996;16:165–8.

16. Fretts RC. Etiology and prevention of stillbirth. Am J Obstet Gynecol 2005;193:1923–35.

17. Biankin SA, Arbuckle SM, Graf NS. Autopsy findings in a series of five cases of fetomaternal haemorrhages. Pathology 2003;35:319–24.

18. Fretts RC. Etiology and prevention of stillbirth. Am J Obstet Gynecol 2005;193:1923–35.

19. Leduc L, Farine D, Armson BA, Brunner M, Crane J, Delisle MF, et al. Stillbirth and bereavement: guidelines for stillbirth investigation. Maternal-Fetal Medicine Committee; Clinical Practice Obstetrics Committee. J Obstet Gynaecol Can 2006;28:540–52.

20. Alonso A, Soto I, Urgelles MF, Corte JR, Rodriguez MJ, Pinto CR. Acquired and inherited thrombophilia in women with unexplained fetal losses. Am J Obstet Gynecol 2002;187:1337–42.

21. Rushton DI. Prognostic role of the perinatal postmortem. Br J Hosp Med 1994;52:450–4.

Evaluation of stillbirths and neonatal deaths. ACOG Committee Opinion No. 383. American College of Obstetricians and Gynecologists. Obstet Gynecol 2007;110:963–6.

ISSN 1074-861X

ACOG COMMITTEE OPINION

Number 393 • December 2007   *(Replaces No. 287, October 2003)*

Newborn Screening

Committee on Genetics

This document reflects emerging clinical and scientific advances as of the date issued and is subject to change. The information should not be construed as dictating an exclusive course of treatment or procedure to be followed.

ABSTRACT: Newborn screening tests are designed to detect infants with specific conditions whose families also would benefit from early diagnosis and treatment. These conditions include disorders of metabolism, endocrinopathies, hemoglobinopathies, hearing loss, and cystic fibrosis. Each state program must have a system in place for notification, timely follow-up, and evaluation of any infant with a positive screening result. Newborn screening programs have enormous public health benefits and have been effective in identifying newborns that can benefit from early treatment.

The American College of Obstetricians and Gynecologists
Women's Health Care Physicians

Obstetricians need to be aware of the status of newborn screening in their states and should be prepared to address questions or refer their patients to appropriate sources for additional information. Newborn screening tests are designed to detect infants with specific conditions whose families also would benefit from early diagnosis and treatment. These conditions include disorders of metabolism, endocrinopathies, hemoglobinopathies, hearing loss, and cystic fibrosis. These screening tests secondarily may identify couples who are carriers of inherited conditions. Currently, state public health agencies fund and implement newborn screening programs for their own residents, leading to variations in practice nationwide.

Technologic advances in combination with new genetic information have led to a re-examination of the implementation and standardization of newborn screening practices across the United States. These efforts are lead by the Health and Human Resources Services Administration Maternal Child and Health Bureau. As providers of obstetric services, obstetrician–gynecologists are advocates for women and play an expanded role in newborn screening (1–4). A recent report by the American Academy of Pediatrics "highlights the need for a more uniform national policy for the selection of newborn screening tests." In response, the American College of Medical Genetics was commissioned by the Health and Human Resources Services Administration Maternal Child and Health Bureau to determine a uniform panel of core conditions appropriate for newborn

screening. Each of the 29 conditions in the core panel (Table 1) has a screening test that can be performed within 24–48 hours after birth, can be treated, and has a known natural history. It is intended that this core panel remain flexible and criteria yet to be established will be used to expand this panel in the future. Secondary targets (supplemental conditions) are conditions that can be detected using the same technology as in the detection of core conditions (Table 1). Although secondary targets are clinically important, they may lack known treatments or their natural histories may not be well understood.

Most states require newborn screening for the core panel, and a number of states require newborn screening for some conditions on the secondary panel. However, the list of conditions screened for in each state can be expected to change over time; a listing of the most current panel of conditions screened for by states can be viewed at the web site of the National Newborn Screening and Genetics Resource Center (http://genes-r-us.uthscsa. edu).

Collection of newborn heel stick-derived blood onto filter paper specimens remains the method of sample collection. Technologic advances have enabled newborn screening to rely less on single platform tests and more on multiplex technology, such as tandem mass spectrometry (MS/MS), immunoassay, and spectrophotometry. Newborn screening may now include 1) screening for genetic conditions that relies on polymerase chain reaction and immunoassay (eg, cystic fibrosis), 2) screening for hemo-

Table 1. Newborn Screening Panel: Core Panel and Secondary Targets

Tandem Mass Spectrometry				
Acylcarnitines		Amino Acids		
Conditions of Organic Acid Metabolism	Conditions of Fatty Acid Metabolism	Conditions of Amino Acid Metabolism	Hemoglobinopathies	Others
CORE PANEL				
Isovaleric acidemia	Medium-chain acyl-CoA dehydrogenase deficiency	Phenylketonuria	Hb SS disease (sickle cell anemia)	Congenital hypo-thyroidism
Glutaric acidemia type 1	Very long-chain acyl-CoA dehydrogenase deficiency	Maple syrup (urine) disease	Hb S/β-thalassemia	Biotinidase deficiency
3-hydroxy 3-methyl glutaric aciduria	Long-chain 3-OH acyl-CoA dehydrogenase deficiency	Homocystinuria	Hb S/C disease	Congenital adrenal hyperplasia
Multiple carboxylase deficiency	Trifunctional protein deficiency	Citrullinemia		Classic galactosemia
Methylmalonic acidemia (mutase)	Carnitine uptake defect	Argininosuccinic acidemia		Hearing loss
3-Methylcrotonyl-CoA carboxylase deficiency		Tyrosinemia type I		Cystic fibrosis
Methylmalonic acidemia (Cbl A, B)				
Propionic acidemia				
β-Ketothiolase deficiency				
SECONDARY TARGETS				
Methylmalonic acidemia (Cbl C, D)	Short-chain acyl-CoA dehydrogenase deficiency	Benign hyperpheny-lalaninemia	Other variant hemo-globinopathies (including Hb E)	Galactokinase deficiency
Malonic aciduria Isobutyryl-CoA dehydrogenase deficiency	Glutaric acidemia type II	Tyrosinemia type II		Galactose epimerase deficiency
2-Methyl 3-hydroxy butyric aciduria	Medium/short-chain 3-OH acyl-CoA DH deficiency	Defects of biopterin cofactor biosynthesis		
2-Methylbutyryl-CoA carboxylase deficiency	Medium chain ketoacyl-CoA thiolase deficiency	Argininemia		
3-Methylglutaconic aciduria	Carnitine palmitoyltrans-ferase II deficiency	Tyrosinemia type III		
	Carnitine/acylcarnitine translocase deficiency	Defects of biopterin cofactor regeneration		
	Carnitine palmitoyltrans-ferase la deficiency (L)	Hypermethioninemia		
	Dienoyl-CoA reductase deficiency	Citrullinemia type II		

Abbreviations: Cbl indicates cobalamin; Hb, hemoglobin.

Maternal and Child Health Bureau. Newborn screening: toward a uniform screening panel and system. Executive summary. Rockville (MD): MCHB; 2005. Available at: http://mchb.hrsa.gov/screening/summary.htm. Retrieved September 10, 2007.

globinopathies that uses isoelectric focusing, high-performance liquid chromatography, or electrophoresis, 3) screening for hearing loss that incorporates either otoacoustic emissions or auditory brainstem response, and 4) screening for infectious diseases (eg, human immunodeficiency virus [HIV] and toxoplasmosis) using immuno-assays for disease specific immunoglobulin G and immunoglobulin M antibodies.

Newborn screening programs are expected to operate with maximal sensitivity and specificity within a public health model that must account for population-based challenges that are distinct from the more familiar challenges of a single-patient diagnosis. There are at least eight different testing platforms used in screening for the 29 conditions listed in Table 1 (eg, MS/MS screens for 22 of the listed conditions). Although patients may inquire regarding the detection rate (sensitivity) and the positive predictive value, these data are not readily available for the aggregate of tests. Performance data for specific screening tests or platforms require discussions with the state screening laboratory. State-specific contact information for newborn screening programs can be found at the web site of the National Newborn Screening and Genetics Resource Center (http://genes-r-us.uthscsa.edu).

Statistical uncertainty is driven in large part by the addition of MS/MS technology used to screen for rare metabolic conditions (Table 1). With any technology, the rate of false-positive results are reduced as experience grows (5). Defining detection rates using MS/MS is complicated by incomplete data reporting, variation in testing procedures, variation in definition of false-positive results, variation in case definition, and nonuniform screening thresholds. Calculating detection rates is made difficult by the nature of the disorders being screened for and the inability to determine prevalence with confidence. For example, it is not uncommon for children with rare metabolic disorders to succumb before a diagnosis can be made. These aspects are compounded by the problems commonly encountered in clinical laboratory settings, including inadequate clinical information and mislabeled samples. Performance goals for newborn screening using MS/MS have been suggested (6). On average, the number of neonates that must be tested to detect one affected patient should be approximately 3,000. A performance goal is used to ensure that at least one fifth of patients (20%) with a positive screening result will, after follow-up testing, be determined to be affected (positive predictive value). Finally, by addressing causes of false-positive rates, these may be reduced to approximately 3 per 1,000 results. These screening test performance goals compare with first-trimester screening for aneuploidy as follows: 1) at least 6–7 individuals per 3,000 screened individuals are affected, 2) the positive predictive value for patients aged 35 years is approximately 4–5%, 3) the false-positive rate for first trimester screening is approximately 5% for women younger than 35 years at the time of delivery (7–9).

Each state program must have a system in place for notification, timely follow-up, and evaluation of any infant with a positive screening result. Furthermore, the system should incorporate protocols for more evaluation, treatment, and long-term follow-up for any infant whose positive screening result suggests a likely risk of the condition. Positive newborn screening results typically are reported to the newborn's primary care provider and, subsequently, the custodial parent(s).

Patients typically are not billed for their participation in newborn screening programs. Newborn screening is mandated by state statute or regulation, and, in most states,

parents are informed that testing will be done as part of standard care unless they specifically decline ("opt out" consent process); Maryland, the District of Columbia, and Wyoming currently require written consent ("opt in"). Many states allow parents to refuse testing based on religious or personal grounds. Hospitals and newborn nurseries usually provide written materials to parents immediately postpartum to inform them of the newborn screening their children will undergo. Survey data suggest that patients are underinformed regarding newborn screening (10) and desire information during the prenatal period. Prenatal education about newborn screening not only provides parents with the reasons for obtaining their newborn's blood specimen, but also informs them that an initial positive test result does not necessarily mean that their child has the condition for which the screening result was positive. Materials are available on the web site of the American College of Obstetricians and Gynecologists (http://www.acog.org/from_home/misc/dept_pubs.cfm).

Newborn screening programs have enormous public health benefits and have been effective in identifying newborns that can benefit from early treatment. In addition, many couples have been made aware of their carrier status because of diagnoses in their newborns. There are many important issues surrounding the debate on universal screening, including financial resources, level of screening, continuity of care, and informed consent. To date, policy on newborn screening has been fragmented, but efforts are underway to ensure uniformity and equity for all newborns. Obstetrician–gynecologists are encouraged to make written or video materials or electronic information available to parents regarding the availability of newborn screening tests.

References

1. Newborn screening: toward a uniform screening panel and system—executive summary. American College of Medical Genetics Newborn Screening Expert Group. Pediatrics 2006;117:S296–307.

2. Lloyd-Puryear MA, Tonniges T, van Dyck PC, Mann MY, Brin A, Johnson K, et al. American Academy of Pediatrics Newborn Screening Task Force recommendations: how far have we come? Pediatrics 2006;117(suppl):S194–211.

3. Larsson A, Therrell BL. Newborn screening: the role of the obstetrician. Clin Obstet Gynecol 2002;45:697–710; discussion 730–2.

4. Campbell ED, Ross LF. Incorporating newborn screening into prenatal care. Am J Obstet Gynecol 2004;190:876–7.

5. Feuchtbaum L, Faulkner L, Verghese S. Tandem mass spectrometry program implementation challenges for state newborn screening programs: national survey of barriers and issues. Pediatrics 2006;117(suppl):S253–60.

6. Rinaldo P, Zafari S, Tortorelli S, Matern D. Making the case for objective performance metrics in newborn screening by tandem mass spectrometry. Ment Retard Dev Disabil Res Rev 2006;12:255–61.

7. Screening for fetal chromosomal abnormalities. ACOG Practice Bulletin No. 77. American College of Obstetricians and Gynecologists. Obstet Gynecol 2007;109:217–27.

8. Malone FD, Canick JA, Ball RH, Nyberg DA, Comstock CH, Bukowski R, et al. First-trimester or second-trimester screening, or both, for Down's syndrome. First- and Second-Trimester Evaluation of Risk (FASTER) Research Consortium. N Engl J Med 2005;353:2001–11.

9. Gardner RJ, Sutherland GR. Parental age counseling and screening for fetal trisomy. In: Chromosome abnormalities and genetic counseling. 3rd ed. New York (NY): Oxford University Press; 2004. p. 363–72.

10. Davis TC, Humiston SG, Arnold CL, Bocchini JA Jr, Bass PF 3rd, Kennen EM, et al. Recommendations for effective newborn screening communication: results of focus groups with parents, providers, and experts. Pediatrics 2006;117 (suppl): S326–40.

Newborn screening. ACOG Committee Opinion No. 393. American College of Obstetricians and Gynecologists. Obstet Gynecol 2007;110:1497–500.

ISSN 1074-861X

ACOG COMMITTEE OPINION

Number 399 • February 2008   *(Replaces No. 183, April 1997)*

Umbilical Cord Blood Banking

Committee on Obstetric Practice

Committee on Genetics

This document reflects emerging clinical and scientific advances as of the date issued and is subject to change. The information should not be construed as dictating an exclusive course of treatment or procedure to be followed.

ABSTRACT: Two types of banks have emerged for the collection and storage of umbilical cord blood—public banks and private banks. Public banks promote allogenic (related or unrelated) donation, analogous to the current collection of whole blood units in the United States. Private banks were initially developed to store stem cells from umbilical cord blood for autologous use (taken from an individual for subsequent use by the same individual) by a child if the child develops disease later in life. If a patient requests information on umbilical cord blood banking, balanced and accurate information regarding the advantages and disadvantages of public versus private banking should be provided. The remote chance of an autologous unit of umbilical cord blood being used for a child or a family member (approximately 1 in 2,700 individuals) should be disclosed. The collection should not alter routine practice for the timing of umbilical cord clamping. Physicians or other professionals who recruit pregnant women and their families for for-profit umbilical cord blood banking should disclose any financial interests or other potential conflicts of interest.

The American College of Obstetricians and Gynecologists
Women's Health Care Physicians

Introduction

Once considered a waste product that was discarded with the placenta, umbilical cord blood is now known to contain potentially life-saving hematopoietic stem cells. When used in hematopoietic stem cell transplantation, umbilical cord blood offers several distinct advantages over bone marrow or peripheral stem cells. Biologically, a greater degree of human leukocyte antigen mismatch is tolerated by the recipient and the incidence of acute graft-versus-host reaction is decreased when umbilical cord blood is used (1, 2). The predominant disadvantage of umbilical cord blood use is related to the low number of stem cells acquired per unit. However, the use of combined units of umbilical cord blood allows for the expansion of umbilical cord blood volume (and increased number of stem cells) to be used for adult hematopoietic transplants. Studies are currently underway evaluating the feasibility of ex vivo expansion of the units (3, 4). Since the first successful umbilical cord blood transplant in 1988, it has been estimated that more than 7,000 transplants have been performed in children and adults for the correction of inborn errors of metabolism, hematopoietic malignancies, and genetic disorders of the blood and immune system (5).

Two types of banks have emerged for the collection and storage of umbilical cord blood—public banks and private banks. The first public bank was established at the New York Blood Center in 1991 and other public banks have since been established in various regions of the country. In 1999, the National Bone Marrow Donor Program established a network of these banks listing their units on the National Bone Marrow Donor Program Registry and established the Center for Cord Blood in 2005 (6). As part of this effort, specific subcommittees have been established to address issues related to umbilical cord blood banking, such as standards, quality improvement, donor recruitment, collection, testing, and processing methodology. In December 2005, federal legislation was enacted that provides funding for continued growth of a national umbilical cord blood registry in the United States through the C.W. Bill Young Cell Transplantation Act. Some states have passed legislation requiring physicians to inform their patients about umbilical cord blood banking options. Clinicians should consult their state medical associations for more information regarding state laws.

Public banks promote allogenic (related or unrelated) donation, analogous to the current collection of whole blood units in the United States. These banks typically are associated with a local network of obstetric hospitals that send their units of blood to a central processing facility. A minority of public banks will accept units from any provider through shipment by an overnight express courier (7). Units of umbilical cord blood collected for public banks must meet rigorous standards of donor screening and infectious disease testing as outlined by the U.S. Food and Drug Administration. Initial human leukocyte antigen typing of these units allows them to be entered into computerized registries so that when the need arises, a specific unit can be rapidly located for a patient.

Private banks were initially developed to store stem cells from umbilical cord blood for autologous use (taken from an individual for subsequent use by the same individual) by a child if the child develops disease later in life. There is a cost associated with the initial specimen processing and an annual storage fee for for-profit umbilical cord blood banks (8).

The utility of long-term storage of autologous umbilical cord blood has been questioned. There is no accurate estimate of an individual's likelihood of using an autologous unit of umbilical cord blood. One estimate is approximately 1 in 2,700 individuals, whereas others argue that the rate would be even lower (9). Stem cells obtained from banked umbilical cord blood cannot currently be used to treat inborn errors of metabolism or other genetic diseases in the same individual from whom they were collected because the genetic mutation would already be present in the stem cells. Autologous umbilical cord blood is not used as a source of stem cells to treat childhood leukemia because chromosomal translocations in fetal blood have been detected in some children who ultimately develop leukemia (10, 11). In addition, the use of autologous stem cells would negate the beneficial graft-versus-leukemic effect that occurs with allogenic stem cell transplants (9).

Recommendations and Conclusions

- If a patient requests information on umbilical cord banking, balanced and accurate information regarding the advantages and disadvantages of public versus private umbilical cord blood banking should be provided. The remote chance of an autologous unit being used for a child or a family member (approximately 1 in 2,700 individuals) should be disclosed.

- Discussion may include information regarding maternal infectious disease and genetic testing, the ultimate outcome of use of poor quality units of umbilical cord blood, and a disclosure that demographic data will be maintained on the patient.

- Some states have passed legislation requiring physicians to inform their patients about umbilical cord blood banking options. Clinicians should consult their state medical associations for more information regarding state laws.

- Directed donation of umbilical cord blood should be considered when there is a specific diagnosis of a disease known to be treatable by hematopoietic transplant for an immediate family member.

- Obstetric providers are not obligated to obtain consent for private umbilical cord blood banking.

- The collection should not alter routine practice for the timing of umbilical cord clamping.

- Physicians or other professionals who recruit pregnant women and their families for for-profit umbilical cord blood banking should disclose any financial interests or other potential conflicts of interest.

References

1. Laughlin MJ, Eapen M, Rubinstein P, Wagner JE, Zhang MJ, Champlin RE, et al. Outcomes after transplantation of cord blood or bone marrow from unrelated donors in adults with leukemia. N Engl J Med 2004;351:2265–75.

2. Rocha V, Labopin M, Sanz G, Arcese W, Schwerdtfeger R, Bosi A, et al. Transplants of umbilical-cord blood or bone marrow from unrelated donors in adults with acute leukemia. Acute Leukemia Working Party of European Blood and Marrow Transplant Group; Eurocord-Netcord Registry. N Engl J Med 2004;351:2276–85.

3. Barker JN, Weisdorf DJ, DeFor TE, Blazar BR, McGlave PB, Miller JS, et al. Transplantation of 2 partially HLA-matched umbilical cord blood units to enhance engraftment in adults with hematologic malignancy. Blood 2005;105: 1343–7.

4. Jaroscak J, Goltry K, Smith A, Waters-Pick B, Martin PL, Driscoll TA, et al. Augmentation of umbilical cord blood (UCB) transplantation with ex vivo-expanded UCB cells: results of a phase 1 trial using the AastromReplicell System. Blood 2003;101:5061–7.

5. Moise KJ Jr. Umbilical cord stem cells. Obstet Gynecol 2005;106:1393–407.

6. National Marrow Donor Program. Where to donate cord blood. Minneapolis (MN): NMDP; 2007. Available at: http://www.marrow.org/HELP/Donate_Cord_Blood_Share _Life/How_to_Donate_Cord_Blood/CB_Participating_Hos pitals/nmdp_cord_blood_hospitals.pl. Retrieved August 22, 2007.

7. Parent's Guide to Cord Blood. Public cord blood banks in the USA. Available at: http://parentsguidecordblood.org/ content/usa/banklists/publicbanks_new.shtml?navid=9. Retrieved August 22, 2007.

8. Parent's Guide to Cord Blood. Family cord blood banks in the USA. Available at: http://parentsguidecordblood.org/ content/usa/banklists/listusa.shtml?navid=11. Retrieved August 22, 2007.

9. Johnson FL. Placental blood transplantation and autologous banking—caveat emptor. J Pediatr Hematol Oncol 1997;19:183–6.

10. Rowley JD. Backtracking leukemia to birth. Nat Med 1998;4:150–1.

11. Greaves MF, Wiemels J. Origins of chromosome transloca-tions in childhood leukaemia. Nat Rev Cancer 2003;3: 639–49.

Additional Resources

National Marrow Donor Program
3001 Broadway Street, NE
Minneapolis, MN 55413
612-627-5000 or 1-800-627-7692
http://www.marrow.org

Parent's Guide to Cord Blood Banks
http://parentsguidecordblood.org

American Academy of Pediatrics
141 Northwest Point Boulevard.
Elk Grove Village, IL 60007
847-434-4000
http://www.aap.org

American Association of Blood Banks
8101 Glenbrook Road
Bethesda, MD 20814
301-907-6977
http://www.aabb.org

Umbilical cord blood banking. ACOG Committee Opinion No. 399. American College of Obstetricians and Gynecologists. Obstet Gynecol 2008;111:475–7.

ISSN 1074-861X

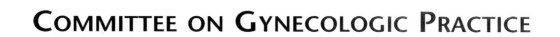

COMMITTEE ON GYNECOLOGIC PRACTICE

COMMITTEE ON GYNECOLOGIC PRACTICE

ACOG COMMITTEE OPINION

Number 372 • July 2007

The Role of Cystourethroscopy in the Generalist Obstetrician–Gynecologist Practice

Committee on Gynecologic Practice

This document reflects emerging clinical and scientific advances as of the date issued and is subject to change. The information should not be construed as dictating an exclusive course of treatment or procedure to be followed.

ABSTRACT: Cystourethroscopy can be performed for diagnostic and a few operative indications by obstetrician–gynecologists to help improve patient care. Perhaps the most important indications for cystourethroscopy are to rule out cystotomy and intravesical or intraurethral suture or mesh placement and to verify bilateral ureteral patency during or after certain gynecologic surgical procedures. The granting of privileges for cystourethroscopy and other urogynecologic procedures should be based on training, experience, and demonstrated competence. Postgraduate education, including residency training programs in obstetrics and gynecology and continuing medical education, should include education in the instrumentation, technique, and evaluation of findings of cystourethroscopy, and in the pathophysiology of diseases of the lower urinary tract.

The American College of Obstetricians and Gynecologists
Women's Health Care Physicians

Although many of the pioneers of cystourethroscopy, most notably Howard Kelly, were gynecologists, for decades the procedure has been performed mainly by urologists. However, cystourethroscopy can be performed for diagnostic and a few operative indications by obstetrician–gynecologists to help improve patient care. This document reviews the definition and indications for cystourethroscopy and discusses the evidence and recommendations for its use in the generalist obstetrician–gynecologist practice.

Cystoscopy

Cystoscopy is a surgical procedure in which a rigid or flexible fiberoptic endoscope is used to examine the lumen of the bladder. Urethroscopy, in which the urethral lumen is examined for urethral diseases or abnormalities, is a related procedure. For cystoscopy, the endoscope is introduced through the urethra, allowing the surgeon to visualize both the bladder and urethra, thus the term *cystourethroscopy*.

Operative Technique

When performing cystourethroscopy for diagnostic indications, the surgeon should follow a technical routine in which the entire lumen of the urethra and bladder are examined systematically. The instrumentation, surgical technique, and typical findings (normal and abnormal) have been reviewed in most textbooks on urogynecology and female urology. Briefly, diagnostic cystourethroscopy is performed using sterile techniques, usually with local anesthesia, while the patient is awake and in the supine lithotomy position. It also can be performed during or after gynecologic surgery with the patient under general or regional anesthesia. The urine should be free of infection before the procedure. After sterile preparation of the urethral meatus and surrounding vulvar vestibule, 2% lidocaine jelly can be introduced into the urethra and then used as lubrication for the endoscope. Sterile water or saline is used to fill the bladder by gravity during the procedure. If electrocautery is to be performed, a nonconducting solution, such as glycine, should be used.

Depending on the indication for the cystourethroscopy, the surgeon generally starts with a 30-degree endoscope and, with the solution running, introduces it through the urethra under direct vision with or without video assistance. After partial distention of the bladder, the trigone is examined for mucosal abnormalities, lesions, or foreign bodies, as indicated. The interureteric ridge is noted above the trigone, and both ureteral orifices are visualized. If the goal is to examine for ureteral patency, 5 mL of indigo carmine can be given intravenously 10–15 minutes before the cystoscopy, followed by observation of blue-stained urine from the ureteral orifices. An in–out technique is used to circumferentially examine sections of the bladder surface, usually starting at the trigone at the 6-o'clock position, progressing clockwise around the right bladder surface to the dome at the 12-o'clock position, and then back to the trigone on the left side of the bladder (1). After the entire bladder examination is accomplished, the urethra is reexamined with removal of the endoscope. If the specific goal is to examine for lesions or for suture or mesh material in the lateral edges of the bladder, a 70-degree rigid or flexible endoscope can be reintroduced to reexamine the bladder. If the specific goal is to examine the urethra, a 0-degree or 25-degree endoscope can be used. The findings should be documented carefully, noting the systematic nature of the procedure.

Shortly before the procedure, a single dose of prophylactic antibiotics is recommended to prevent urinary tract infection or septicemia for patients at moderate or high risk of endocarditis, those who are neutropenic, and those with preoperative bacteriuria or an indwelling catheter (2, 3).

Indications and Complications

The indications for cystourethroscopy, like hysteroscopy, are both diagnostic and operative and are for symptoms and diseases related to the lower urinary tract. Diagnostic cystourethroscopy can be performed as part of an evaluation of abnormal symptoms, signs, or laboratory findings; intraoperatively during gynecologic or urogynecologic surgery to rule out bladder, urethral, or ureteral trauma; and as part of staging or surgery for gynecologic malignancy. A list of possible indications for diagnostic cystourethroscopy during gynecologic surgery is shown in the box. Operative cystoscopy usually involves the introduction of additional instruments, such as biopsy forceps or scissors, through an operating channel in the

---

Possible Indications for Diagnostic Cystourethroscopy During Gynecologic Surgery

- During or after surgery for pelvic organ prolapse or stress urinary incontinence to rule out cystotomy and intravesical or intraurethral suture or mesh placement
- Verification of bilateral ureteral flow during or after obstetric, gynecologic, urogynecologic, or gynecologic oncologic surgery
- Evaluation of suspected urine leak during or after laparotomy, laparoscopy, or vaginal surgery
- Verification of suprapubic catheter placement, if desired

---

cystoscope to perform procedures or interventions. It also can be done as part of a reparative procedure to the bladder or urethra, such as vesicovaginal fistula or urethral diverticulum repair. Operative procedures generally are performed by urologists and selectively by urogynecologists and gynecologic oncologists. However, generalist obstetrician–gynecologists with special expertise and experience may perform minor operative procedures such as passage of ureteral stents and injection of urethral bulking agents.

Complications after cystourethroscopy are few. These generally involve minor pain related to the procedure and the small risk of postoperative urinary tract infection. These risks usually are negligible with use of local anesthesia and single-dose prophylactic antibiotics in patients at moderate or high risk for endocarditis. Other rare complications include perforation of the urethra or bladder or ureteral perforation if instruments or stents are placed into the ureter.

There is a small risk that the surgeon will not recognize abnormalities that are present, such as bladder lesions or mesh or sutures in the bladder. For example, in one study, urologists had less than perfect agreement between cystoscopic and histologic diagnoses when biopsies were performed for suspicious bladder lesions (4). Because routine intraoperative cystourethroscopy examines only the bladder and urethral mucosal surfaces and ureteral orifices, it does not guarantee recognition of all lower urinary tract injuries (5). Nonobstructive, partially obstructive, or late ureteral injuries may not be recognized or prevented (6–8). When cystourethroscopy is performed, there are minimal additional costs and time spent in the operating room.

Recommendations for the Generalist Obstetrician–Gynecologist

Few studies have been conducted that provide evidence-based recommendations for the use of cystourethroscopy in a general obstetric and gynecologic practice. Typically, recommendations for the use of cystourethroscopy in general obstetric and gynecologic practice imply that the physician has knowledge and competency in the instrumentation and surgical technique; can recognize normal and abnormal bladder and urethral findings; and has knowledge of pathology, diagnosis, and treatment of specific diseases of the female lower urinary tract. Specialists in female pelvic medicine and reconstructive surgery and gynecologic oncology have an expanded use of cystourethroscopy based on their additional training and resulting greater level of expertise and experience.

The granting of privileges for cystourethroscopy and other urogynecologic procedures should be based on training, experience, and demonstrated competence. Obstetrician–gynecologists who are appropriately trained in a technique, have sufficient experience performing it, and have demonstrated current clinical competence should be granted privileges accordingly.

In 1996, the Agency for Healthcare Research and Quality (then known as the Agency for Healthcare Policy and Research) provided recommendations for cystoscopy (regardless of specialty), but none of the recommendations were supported by scientific evidence from properly designed and implemented controlled trials and are no longer considered current (9). In that document, cystoscopy was recommended for the evaluation of patients who have sterile hematuria or pyuria; new-onset irritative voiding symptoms such as frequency, urgency, and urge incontinence in the absence of any reversible causes; bladder pain; recurrent cystitis; suspected presence of a foreign body; or when urodynamic testing failed to duplicate symptoms of urinary incontinence. Cystoscopy was not recommended in the basic evaluation of urinary incontinence. Likewise, routine cystoscopy in women with urinary incontinence to exclude neoplasia was not indicated because the risk of bladder lesions is less than 2% (9, 10).

Cystourethroscopy is indicated during or after some surgical procedures performed 1) to treat stress urinary incontinence and anterior vaginal prolapse, such as Burch colposuspension, paravaginal defect repair, pubovaginal sling procedure, and tension-free vaginal tape procedure; 2) to rule out intravesical placement of sutures or mesh; and 3) to verify ureteral patency. Tension-free vaginal tape and related mid-urethral sling procedures that pass through the retropubic space especially require routine cystourethroscopy to detect intraoperative bladder perforation, which occurs in 3–9% of cases (11, 12). As noted earlier, certain other surgical procedures usually performed by specialists, such as repair of vesicovaginal fistula or urethral diverticulum, routinely require cystourethroscopy to aid the surgical repair.

The issue of whether cystourethroscopy should be performed during and after gynecologic surgery to evaluate for bladder integrity and for ureteral patency remains unresolved. Intraoperative cystotomies usually are noted at the time of the injury, especially if retrograde bladder filling is used to aid recognition. However, sutures or mesh placed in the bladder or urethral lumen during surgical procedures usually are not recognized unless cystourethroscopy is performed.

Ureteral injuries are of particular concern to practicing obstetrician–gynecologists. Although the incidence of bladder and ureteral injury during common gynecologic procedures is low, wide ranges have been reported in the literature making estimation of risk difficult for individual surgical procedures. A recent systematic review of urinary tract injuries during gynecologic surgery with routine intraoperative cystourethroscopy for benign disease reported crude ureteral injury rates for laparoscopic hysterectomy with bilateral salpingo-oophorectomy of 17.3 per 1,000 procedures (95% confidence interval [CI], 0.3–66.3); for other gynecologic and urogynecologic surgical procedures, including other types of hysterectomy, the overall ureteral injury rate was 8.8 per 1,000 proce-

dures (95% CI, 2.3–12.6) (13). The overall bladder injury rate per 1,000 laparoscopic hysterectomies with bilateral salpingo-oophorectomy was 29.2 (95% CI, 7.5–148.0); after other gynecologic and urogynecologic surgical procedures, the rate was 16.3 (95% CI, 4.3–26.6) (13).

Factors that should be considered when deciding when to perform diagnostic cystourethroscopy include complication rates associated with the procedure and the difficulty of the individual surgical case. Cystourethroscopy is indicated during or after tension-free vaginal tape procedure, Burch colposuspension, and high uterosacral ligament vaginal vault suspension. Surgical procedures such as McCall culdoplasty, colpocleisis, and perhaps certain advanced and difficult vaginal and laparoscopic procedures and hysterectomies may be indications for intraoperative diagnostic cystourethroscopy.

Conclusions

Cystourethroscopy is a low-risk operative procedure used to examine the lumen of the bladder and urethra. Perhaps the most important indications for cystourethroscopy are to rule out cystotomy and intravesical or intraurethral suture or mesh placement and to verify bilateral ureteral patency during or after certain gynecologic surgical procedures. The procedures that have a relatively high risk for these complications (at least 1–2%) may benefit from cystourethroscopy to help avoid additional surgery, permanent loss of renal function, fistulas, and other abnormalities. Because intraoperative cystourethroscopy examines only the bladder and urethral mucosal surfaces and ureteral orifices, it does not guarantee recognition of all lower urinary tract injuries. Nonobstructive, partially obstructive, or late ureteral or bladder injuries may not be recognized or prevented. Whether the routine use of intraoperative cystourethroscopy during hysterectomy and other gynecologic surgical procedures with a lower risk of urinary tract injury is advisable requires further study.

Postgraduate education, including residency training programs in obstetrics and gynecology and continuing medical education, should include education in the instrumentation, technique, and evaluation of findings of cystourethroscopy, and in the pathophysiology of diseases of the lower urinary tract.

References

1. Cundiff GW, Bent AE. Endoscopic evaluation of the lower urinary tract. In: Walters MD, Karram MM, editors. Urogynecology and reconstructive pelvic surgery. 3rd ed. Philadelphia (PA): Mosby Elsevier; 2007. p. 114–23.

2. Dajani AS, Taubert KA, Wilson W, Bolger AF, Bayer A, Ferrieri P, et al. Prevention of bacterial endocarditis. Recommendations by the American Heart Association. JAMA 1997;277:1794–801.

3. Olson ES, Cookson BD. Do antimicrobials have a role in preventing septicemia following instrumentation of the urinary tract? J Hosp Infect 2000;45:85–97.

4. Mitropoulos D, Kiroudi-Voulgari A, Nikolopoulos P, Manousakas T, Zervas A. Accuracy of cystoscopy in predicting histologic features of bladder lesions. J Endourol 2005;19:861–4.

5. Dwyer PL, Carey MP, Rosamilia A. Suture injury to the urinary tract in urethral suspension procedures for stress incontinence. Int Urogynecol J Pelvic Floor Dysfunct 1999;10:15–21.

6. Councell RB, Thorp JM Jr, Sandridge DA, Hill ST. Assessments of laparoscopic-assisted vaginal hysterectomy. J Am Assoc Gynecol Laparosc 1994;2:49–56.

7. Dandolu V, Mathai E, Chatwani A, Harmanli O, Pontari M, Hernandez E. Accuracy of cystoscopy in the diagnosis of ureteral injury in benign gynecologic surgery. Int Urogynecol J Pelvic Floor Dysfunct 2003;14:427–31.

8. Gustilo-Ashby AM, Jelovsek JE, Barber MD, Yoo EH, Paraiso MF, Walters MD. The incidence of ureteral obstruction and the value of intraoperative cystoscopy during vaginal surgery for pelvic organ prolapse. Am J Obstet Gynecol 2006;194:1478–85.

9. Agency for Health Care Policy and Research. Urinary incontinence in adults: acute and chronic management. Clinical Practice Guideline, No. 2, 1996 update. AHCPR Publication No. 96-0682. Rockville (MD): AHCPR; 1996.

10. Ouslander J, Leach G, Staskin D, Abelson S, Blaustein J, Morishita L, et al. Prospective evaluation of an assessment strategy for geriatric urinary incontinence. J Am Geriatr Soc 1989;37:715–24.

11. Ward K, Hilton P. Prospective multicentre randomised trial of tension-free vaginal tape and colposuspension as primary treatment for stress incontinence. United Kingdom and Ireland Tension-Free Vaginal Tape Trial Group. BMJ 2002;325:67–70.

12. Tamussino KF, Hanzal E, Kolle D, Ralph G, Riss PA. Tension-free vaginal tape operation: results of the Austrian registry. Austrian Urogynecology Working Group. Obstet Gynecol 2001;98:732–6.

13. Gilmour DT, Das S, Flowerdew G. Rates of urinary tract injury from gynecologic surgery and the role of intraoperative cystoscopy. Obstet Gynecol 2006;107:1366–72.

The role of cystourethroscopy in the generalist obstetrician–gynecologist practice. ACOG Committee Opinion No. 372. American College of Obstetricians and Gynecologists. Obstet Gynecol 2007;110:221–4.

ISSN 1074-861X

ACOG COMMITTEE OPINION

Number 375 • August 2007

Brand Versus Generic Oral Contraceptives

**Committee on
Gynecologic
Practice**

This document reflects emerging clinical and scientific advances as of the date issued and is subject to change. The information should not be construed as dictating an exclusive course of treatment or procedure to be followed.

ABSTRACT: The U.S. Food and Drug Administration considers generic and brand name oral contraceptive (OC) products clinically equivalent and interchangeable. The American College of Obstetricians and Gynecologists supports patient or clinician requests for branded OCs or continuation of the same generic or branded OCs if the request is based on clinical experience or concerns regarding packaging or compliance, or if the branded product is considered a better choice for that individual patient.

To control pharmaceutical costs and standardize national practice, the U.S. Food and Drug Administration (FDA) was given the authority to approve generic versions of branded pharmaceutical products by the Drug Price Competition and Patent Term Restoration Act. Before 1984, manufacturers of generic products had to submit clinical safety and efficacy data for their products just as the innovator drug manufacturer had to do for initial approval. Since 1984, generic products, including generic oral contraceptive (OC) products, must demonstrate pharmaceutical equivalence, meaning that this new generic product contains the same active ingredients, identical in strength and dosage, as the branded product. This generic product also must be bioequivalent, meaning that blood levels obtained in clinical trials demonstrate a rate and extent of absorption not substantially different from the branded product (1).

Studies demonstrating bioequivalence of generic OC products are submitted by the generic pharmaceutical company after a crossover study of adequate power (usually of 20–24 women) with pharmacokinetic calculations of serial blood levels of the progestin or its active metabolite and ethinyl estradiol, plasma concentration time curves (AUC), peak concentration, and the time to peak concentration. The average blood level deviation from the brand must be in the range of 80–125%. If these criteria are met, the FDA Office of Generic Drugs does not request or recommend clinical efficacy or safety studies for the generic product before granting marketing approval, and it considers the generic product to be interchangeable

with the branded product. No clinical trial is needed given that the safety and efficacy of the generic product is expected to be that of the clinically tested and FDA-approved branded product. Brand name and generic drug facilities are required to meet the same standards of good manufacturing practices.

Patients and clinicians have questioned whether generic and brand name OC products are clinically equivalent and interchangeable, as effective in preventing pregnancy, and have similar occurrences of side effects, such as breakthrough bleeding. The FDA considers generic and brand name OC products clinically equivalent and interchangeable; however, others imply that this may not be true (2). The statistical methods used by the FDA to determine bioequivalence have been challenged. The FDA Center for Drug Evaluation and Research has taken a firm stand upholding the therapeutic equivalence and interchangeability of generic and branded products (3).

Oral contraceptive pills are the most commonly used form of reversible contraception in the United States. Overall, the FDA lists more than 90 combination hormonal contraceptives containing ethinyl estradiol. Most OCs are no longer patent protected and are available for the development of generic pharmaceutical copies. The 2007 27th edition of *Approved Drug Products With Therapeutic Equivalence Evaluations,* the so-called "Orange Book," lists only seven combination OCs that do not have a generic alternative (4). Although new OC formulations are protected by patent for 20 years from initial patent filing, in practice there is a much shorter inter-

**The American College
of Obstetricians
and Gynecologists**

*Women's Health Care
Physicians*

val from final approval and marketing to loss of patent protection.

Although considered clinically equivalent by the FDA, branded and generic OCs may differ in shape, packaging, color, flavor, and shelf life. In addition, nonactive ingredients such as preservatives and labeling and storage requirements also may differ. Products are considered bioequivalent if they fall within the required parameters; the mean bioequivalence cannot be more than 20% lower or 25% higher, with 95% certainty. In practice, the reported ranges of generics are much narrower. Given the range of acceptable generic bioequivalence, switching between generic OCs or from branded to generic OCs might be associated with increased side effects or other problems, but similar problems theoretically might occur when switching between two batches made by the same manufacturer. Additionally, some firms package their own branded drugs and sell them under a generic or other brand label.

When taken correctly and consistently, combination OCs and other hormonal contraceptives have failure rates of less than one pregnancy per 100 couples over 1 year. Published studies report different failure rates for various brands, but few head-to-head studies have been performed, and there is no evidence that with perfect use different combination products have different failure rates (5).

Although there are no clinical data on any difference in compliance between different branded OCs or between generic and branded OCs, patients and clinicians anecdotally report problems when switching occurs. It is possible that side effects or pregnancy occur as a result of poor compliance because patients are confused by new packaging, they fear that they received the wrong pill, or they lack confidence in generics. Although this likely affects compliance and effectiveness, there are no evidence-based data addressing these issues. Even though some patients may perceive generic products to be less effective, there are no clinical data on how this perception affects continuation rates.

Given an individual's variations in metabolism, it is probably impossible to improve our knowledge of OCs by completing larger studies; effectiveness and side effects will tend to be overwhelmed by other nonpharmaceutical effects. Breakthrough bleeding, which is a common cause of OC discontinuation, is related to missed pills, smoking, infection, and possibly drug interactions, which will tend to overwhelm subtle variations between already confirmed bioequivalent and pharmaceutically equivalent products. As the FDA has pointed out, patients may be more likely to be aware of symptoms when substitutions occur or if they have been told they are taking a generic brand.

Oral contraceptive pills are obtained by patients in a variety of settings and with different reimbursement plans, and cost clearly influences access and use. For a patient whose insurance will pay only for a generic product on formulary or in cases where a patient is paying out of pocket, the difference in price can be as much as 70% less for a generic, especially when multiple generic choices for a specific branded product are available. Often, the difference is much less. Cost has been shown to be among the most important factors in OC continuation, and less expensive generic OCs may have better continuation rates than more expensive alternatives (6).

Generic OCs approved by the FDA have been shown to be bioequivalent and pharmaceutically equivalent to the branded product and are interchangeable. There are no evidence-based data to challenge this conclusion. However, because of possible effects on patient compliance, the American College of Obstetricians and Gynecologists supports patient or clinician requests for branded OCs or continuation of the same generic or branded OC if the request is based on clinical experience or concerns regarding packaging or compliance, or if the branded product is considered a better choice for that individual patient. Women should be informed when a different OC is substituted for a previously prescribed OC.

References

1. Welage LS, Kirking DM, Ascione FJ, Gaither CA. Understanding the scientific issues embedded in the generic drug approval process. J Am Pharm Assoc 2001;41: 856–67.

2. Bioequivalence between brand-name and generic OCs. Contracept Rep 2002;13(2):6–9.

3. U.S. Food and Drug Administration. Therapeutic equivalence of generic drugs. Letter to health practitioners. Rockville (MD): FDA; 1998. Available at: http://www.fda.gov/cder/news/nightgenlett.htm. Retrieved April 3, 2007.

4. U.S. Food and Drug Administration. Approved drug products with therapeutic equivalence evaluations. 27th ed. Rockville (MD): FDA; 2007. Available at: http://www.fda.gov/cder/ob. Retrieved April 3, 2007.

5. Rosenberg MJ, Waugh MS. Oral contraceptive discontinuation: a prospective evaluation of frequency and reasons. Am J Obstet Gynecol 1998;179:577–82.

6. Shrank WH, Hoang T, Ettner SL, Glassman PA, Nair K, DeLapp D, et al. The implications of choice: prescribing generic or preferred pharmaceuticals improves medication adherence for chronic conditions. Arch Intern Med 2006; 166:332–7.

Brand versus generic oral contraceptives. ACOG Committee Opinion No. 375. American College of Obstetricians and Gynecologists. Obstet Gynecol 2007;110:447–8.

ISSN 1074-861X

ACOG COMMITTEE OPINION

Number 378 • September 2007

Vaginal "Rejuvenation" and Cosmetic Vaginal Procedures

Committee on Gynecologic Practice

This document reflects emerging clinical and scientific advances as of the date issued and is subject to change. The information should not be construed as dictating an exclusive course of treatment or procedure to be followed.

ABSTRACT: So-called "vaginal rejuvenation," "designer vaginoplasty," "revirgination," and "G-spot amplification" are vaginal surgical procedures being offered by some practitioners. These procedures are not medically indicated, and the safety and effectiveness of these procedures have not been documented. Clinicians who receive requests from patients for such procedures should discuss with the patient the reason for her request and perform an evaluation for any physical signs or symptoms that may indicate the need for surgical intervention. Women should be informed about the lack of data supporting the efficacy of these procedures and their potential complications, including infection, altered sensation, dyspareunia, adhesions, and scarring.

There have been an increasing number of practitioners offering various types of vaginal surgeries marketed as ways to enhance appearance or sexual gratification. Among the types of procedures being promoted are so-called "vaginal rejuvenation," "designer vaginoplasty," "revirgination," and "G-spot amplification." Often the exact procedure performed is not clear because standard medical nomenclature is not used. Some procedures, such as vaginal rejuvenation, appear to be modifications of traditional vaginal surgical procedures. Other procedures are performed to alter the size or shape of the labia majora or labia minora. Revirgination involves hymenal repair in an attempt to approximate the virginal state. G-spot amplification involves the injection of collagen into the anterior wall of the vagina.

Medically indicated surgical procedures may include reversal or repair of female genital cutting and treatment for labial hypertrophy or asymmetrical labial growth secondary to congenital conditions, chronic irritation, or excessive androgenic hormones. Other procedures, including vaginal rejuvenation, designer vaginoplasty, revirgination, and G-spot amplification, are not medically indicated, and the safety and effectiveness of these procedures have not been documented. No adequate studies have been published assessing the long-term satisfaction, safety, and complication rates for these procedures.

Also of concern are ethical issues associated with the marketing of these procedures and the national franchising in this field. Such a business model that controls the dissemination of scientific knowledge is troubling.

Clinicians who receive requests from patients for such procedures should discuss with the patient the reason for her request and perform an evaluation for any physical signs or symptoms that may indicate the need for surgical intervention. A patient's concern regarding the appearance of her genitalia may be alleviated by a frank discussion of the wide range of normal genitalia and reassurance that the appearance of the external genitalia varies significantly from woman to woman (1). Concerns regarding sexual gratification may be addressed by careful evaluation for any sexual dysfunction and an exploration of nonsurgical interventions, including counseling.

It is deceptive to give the impression that vaginal rejuvenation, designer vaginoplasty, revirgination, G-spot amplification, or any such procedures are accepted and routine surgical practices. Absence of data supporting the safety and efficacy of these procedures makes their recommendation untenable. Patients who are anxious or insecure about their genital appearance or sexual function may be further traumatized by undergoing an unproven surgical procedure with obvi-

The American College of Obstetricians and Gynecologists
Women's Health Care Physicians

ous risks. Women should be informed about the lack of data supporting the efficacy of these procedures and their potential complications, including infection, altered sensation, dyspareunia, adhesions, and scarring.

Reference

1. Lloyd J, Crouch NS, Minto CL, Liao LM, Creighton SM. Female genital appearance: "normality" unfolds. BJOG 2005;112:643–6.

Vaginal "rejuvenation" and cosmetic vaginal procedures. ACOG Committee Opinion No. 378. American College of Obstetricians and Gynecologists. Obstet Gynecol 2007;110:737–8.

ISSN 1074-861X

ACOG COMMITTEE OPINION

Number 384 • November 2007

Colonoscopy and Colorectal Cancer Screening and Prevention

Committee on Gynecologic Practice

This document reflects emerging clinical and scientific advances as of the date issued and is subject to change. The information should not be construed as dictating an exclusive course of treatment or procedure to be followed.

ABSTRACT: Most colorectal cancer can be detected by screening modalities and treated at a preinvasive or early invasive stage, before it has developed to a fully invasive and potentially fatal disease. Obstetrician–gynecologists should counsel all patients aged 50 years and older about the benefits of colorectal cancer screening and should encourage colonoscopy as the preferred method of screening for women at either average risk or high risk. The advantages and limitations of other appropriate colorectal cancer screening methods also should be discussed so that women may choose to be tested by whichever method they are most likely to accept and complete.

More than 74,000 women develop colorectal cancer in the United States each year, almost as many as the number of women who receive diagnoses of gynecologic cancers. Each year more than 26,000 women die from colorectal cancer, making it the third leading cause of cancer death in women, after lung cancer and breast cancer (1). Most colorectal cancer can be detected by screening modalities and treated at a preinvasive or early invasive stage, before it has developed to a fully invasive and potentially fatal disease. The purpose of this document is to review colonoscopy and the other available screening methods to enable the obstetrician–gynecologist to appropriately and adequately counsel patients about the indications for and benefits of colorectal cancer screening.

Screening for colorectal cancer, using one of the methods listed in the box, is indicated for all women aged 50 years or older who are at average risk. It is important to note that digital rectal examination and in-office stool sample collection for fecal occult blood testing are not recommended screening methods for the detection of colorectal cancer. For women at increased risk, screening and surveillance guidelines also have been published (Table 1). Although the guidelines for women at increased risk primarily will be used by physicians who perform colonoscopy, it may be useful for the obstetrician–gynecologist to be aware that there are specific guidelines for women who are not considered to be at average risk.

The American College of Obstetricians and Gynecologists
Women's Health Care Physicians

Colorectal Cancer Screening for Women at Average Risk Starting at Age 50 Years*

Preferred method

- Colonoscopy every 10 years

Other appropriate methods

- Fecal occult blood testing or fecal immunochemical testing[†] every year
- Flexible sigmoidoscopy every 5 years
- Fecal occult blood testing or fecal immunochemical testing[†] every year plus flexible sigmoidoscopy every 5 years
- Double contrast barium enema every 5 years

*American College of Gastroenterology recommends that African Americans begin screening at age 45 years with colonoscopy because of increased incidence and earlier age of onset of colorectal cancer. (Agrawal S, Bhupinderjit A, Bhutani MS, Boardman L, Nguyen C, Romero Y, et al. Colorectal cancer in African Americans. Committee of Minority Affairs and Cultural Diversity, American College of Gastroenterology [published erratum appears in Am J Gastroenterol 2005;100:1432]. Am J Gastroenterol 2005; 100:515–23; discussion 514.)

†Both fecal occult blood testing and fecal immunochemical testing require two or three samples of stool collected by the patient at home and returned for analysis. A single stool sample for fecal occult blood testing or fecal immunochemical testing obtained by digital rectal examination is not adequate for the detection of colorectal cancer.

Table 1. American Cancer Society Guidelines for Colorectal Cancer Screening and Surveillance for Women at Increased Risk or High Risk

Risk Category	Age to Begin	Recommendation	Comment
Increased Risk			
Women with a single, small (less than 1 cm) adenoma	At 3–6 years after the initial polypectomy	Colonoscopy*	If the examination result is normal, the patient can thereafter be screened as per average risk guidelines.
Women with a large (1 cm or larger) adenoma, multiple adenomas, or adenomas with high-grade dysplasia or villous change	Within 3 years after the initial polypectomy	Colonoscopy*	If normal, repeat examination in 3 years; if normal then, the patient can thereafter be screened as per average risk guidelines.
Personal history of curative-intent resection of colorectal cancer	Within 1 year after cancer resection	Colonoscopy*	If normal, repeat examination in 3 years; if normal then, repeat examination every 5 years.
Either colorectal cancer or adenomatous polyps in any first-degree relative before age 60 years or in two or more first-degree relatives at any age (if not a hereditary syndrome)	Age 40 years or 10 years before the youngest case in the immediate family	Colonoscopy*	Every 5–10 years. Colorectal cancer in relatives more distant than first degree does not increase risk substantially above the average risk group.
High Risk			
Family history of familial adenomatous polyposis	Puberty	Early surveillance with endoscopy and counseling to consider genetic testing	If the genetic test result is positive, colectomy is indicated. These patients are best referred to a center with experience in the management of familial adenomatous polyposis.
Family history of hereditary nonpolyposis colon cancer	Age 21 years	Colonoscopy and counseling to consider genetic testing	If the genetic test result is positive or if the patient has not had genetic testing, colonoscopy every 1–2 years until age 40 and then annually. These patients are best referred to a center with experience in the management of hereditary nonpolyposis colon cancer.
Inflammatory bowel disease, chronic ulcerative colitis, or Crohn's disease	Cancer risk begins to be significant 8 years after the onset of pancolitis or 12–15 years after the onset of left-sided colitis	Colonoscopy with biopsies for dysplasia	Every 1–2 years. These patients are best referred to a center with experience in the surveillance and management of inflammatory bowel disease.

*If colonoscopy is unavailable, not feasible, or not desired by the patient, double contrast barium enema alone or the combination of flexible sigmoidoscopy and double contrast barium enema are acceptable alternatives. Adding flexible sigmoidoscopy to double contrast barium enema may provide a more comprehensive diagnostic evaluation than double contrast barium enema alone in finding considerable lesions. A supplementary double contrast barium enema may be needed if a colonoscopic examination fails to reach the cecum, and a supplementary colonoscopy may be needed if a double contrast barium enema identifies a possible lesion or does not adequately visualize the entire colorectum.

Smith R, von Eschenbach A, Wender R, Levin B, Byers T, Rothenberger D, et al. American Cancer Society guidelines for the early detection of cancer: update of early detection guidelines for prostate, colorectal, and endometrial cancers. CA Cancer J Clin 2001;51:38–75.

Understanding the advantages and limitations of each screening method is necessary to adequately counsel women. Because superiority of any one method with regard to risks, benefits, or cost-effectiveness has not been clearly documented (2), all methods are acceptable options for screening. However, many experts prefer colonoscopy.

For women at either average risk or high risk, colonoscopy is the preferred method for colorectal cancer screening. Colonoscopy offers direct visualization of all colonic surfaces and the ability to remove any precancerous lesions that are detected (3). Colonoscopy gives access to right-sided lesions, which comprise a considerable proportion (65%) of advanced colorectal neoplasia in women that would be missed by other screening methods (4). In one study, it was shown that the incidence of colorectal cancer was reduced by 76–90% among individuals undergoing colonoscopy with polypectomy compared with individuals in a general population registry (5). Abnormalities found with any of the other screening methods necessitate referral for diagnostic colonoscopy. Limitations of colonoscopy include cost, inconvenience of the preparation required of the patient, and the risk of complications. In the United States, the capacity for colonoscopy is limited by an inadequate number of trained endoscopists to perform the estimated 41 million colonoscopies required to reach the currently unscreened population at average risk (6).

Flexible sigmoidoscopy is technically easier, requires less preparation, and has a lower risk of complications than colonoscopy but is limited to examining the most distal portion of the colon and will miss a significant number of right-sided colonic lesions, particularly in women (4). Because of these limitations, the combination of yearly fecal occult blood testing or fecal immunochemical testing with flexible sigmoidoscopy every 5 years may be preferable to either method alone (7).

Fecal occult blood testing and fecal immunochemical testing detect occult blood in the stool from a polyp or cancer disrupting the mucosal barrier. Fecal immunochemical testing specifically detects lower-tract bleeding; thus, fecal immunochemical testing does not require changes in diet or medications before testing (8). Although fecal occult blood testing and fecal immunochemical testing are the least invasive colorectal cancer screening methods, both of these methods require samples obtained by the patient at home using a kit that must be returned for analysis.

Both fecal occult blood testing and fecal immunochemical testing require two to three samples of stool. In a recent study, the sensitivity of a single stool sample for fecal occult blood testing obtained during an office visit by digital rectal examination was 4.9%, compared with 23.9% for the recommended at-home fecal occult blood testing series (9). Therefore, fecal occult blood testing of a single stool sample from a rectal examination performed during an office visit is not adequate for the detection of colorectal cancer and is not recommended.

Noninvasive methods of colorectal cancer screening currently being evaluated include computed tomography colonography or "virtual colonoscopy" and fecal DNA testing. Virtual colonoscopy requires bowel preparation similar to colonoscopy. In randomized trials, virtual colonoscopy has shown 39% sensitivity and 90.5% specificity in detecting lesions of at least 6 mm, significantly lower than the 99% sensitivity and 100% specificity of colonoscopy (10). Fecal DNA testing for genetic mutations associated with colorectal cancer requires only a single stool sample. In a recent prospective randomized trial, the DNA test was found to be more sensitive than fecal occult blood testing in detecting both precancerous and cancerous colonic lesions in persons at average risk for developing colorectal cancer (11). However, neither computed tomography colonography nor fecal DNA testing have been recommended for use in routine screening for colorectal cancer. Pending further data supporting their effectiveness, neither should be recommended as a screening modality for women at average risk outside of a research setting.

Colorectal cancer accounts for a considerable number of preventable cancer deaths of women in the United States each year. Despite consensus among health care organizations about the value of screening for colorectal cancer, less than 50% of U.S. women older than 50 years are screened by any of the recommended methods (12). As providers of longitudinal care, obstetrician–gynecologists have a unique opportunity to increase colorectal cancer screening rates among their patients and thus decrease the rate of colorectal cancer mortality in women. Obstetrician–gynecologists should counsel all patients aged 50 years and older about the benefits of colorectal cancer screening and should encourage the use of colonoscopy as the preferred method of screening for women at either average risk or high risk. The advantages and limitations of other appropriate colorectal cancer screening methods also should be discussed so that women may choose to be tested by whichever method they are most likely to accept and complete.

References

1. Jemal A, Siegel R, Ward E, Murray T, Xu J, Thun MJ. Cancer statistics, 2007. CA Cancer J Clin 2007;57:43–66.

2. Screening for colorectal cancer: recommendation and rationale. U.S. Preventive Services Task Force. Ann Intern Med 2002;137:129–31.

3. Smith RA, von Eschenbach AC, Wender R, Levin B, Byers T, Rothenberger D, et al. American Cancer Society guidelines for the early detection of cancer: update of early detection guidelines for prostate, colorectal, and endometrial cancers. Also: update 2001—testing for early lung cancer detection. ACS Prostate Cancer Advisory Committee, ACS Colorectal Cancer Advisory Committee, ACS Endometrial Cancer Advisory Committee [published erratum appears in CA Cancer J Clin 2001;51:150]. CA Cancer J Clin 2001;51: 38–75; quiz 77–80.

4. Schoenfeld P, Cash B, Flood A, Dobhan R, Eastone J, Coyle W, et al. Colonoscopic screening of average-risk women for colorectal neoplasia. CONCeRN Study Investigators. N Engl J Med 2005;352:2061–8.

5. Winawer SJ, Zauber AG, Ho MN, O'Brien MJ, Gottlieb LS, Sternberg SS, et al. Prevention of colorectal cancer by colonoscopic polypectomy. The National Polyp Study Workgroup. N Engl J Med 1993;329:1977–81.

6. Seeff LC, Manninen DL, Dong FB, Chattopadhyay SK, Nadel MR, Tangka FK, et al. Is there endoscopic capacity to provide colorectal cancer screening to the unscreened population in the United States? Gastroenterology 2004;127: 1661–9.

7. Smith RA, Cokkinides V, Eyre HJ. American Cancer Society guidelines for the early detection of cancer, 2006. CA Cancer J Clin 2006;56:11–25; quiz 49–50.

8. Allison JE. Colon Cancer Screening Guidelines 2005: the fecal occult blood test option has become a better FIT. Gastroenterology 2005;129:745–8.

9. Collins JF, Lieberman DA, Durbin TE, Weiss DG. Accuracy of screening for fecal occult blood on a single stool sample obtained by digital rectal examination: a comparison with recommended sampling practice. Veterans Affairs Cooperative Study #380 Group. Ann Intern Med 2005;142: 81–5.

10. Cotton PB, Durkalski VL, Pineau BC, Palesch YY, Mauldin PD, Hoffman B, et al. Computed tomographic colonography (virtual colonoscopy): a multicenter comparison with standard colonoscopy for detection of colorectal neoplasia. JAMA 2004;291:1713–9.

11. Imperiale TF, Ransohoff DF, Itzkowitz SH, Turnbull BA, Ross ME. Fecal DNA versus fecal occult blood for colorectal-cancer screening in an average-risk population. Colorectal Cancer Study Group. N Engl J Med 2004;351: 2704–14.

12. Meissner HI, Breen N, Klabunde CN, Vernon SW. Patterns of colorectal cancer screening uptake among men and women in the United States. Cancer Epidemiol Biomarkers Prev 2006;15:389–94.

Colonoscopy and colorectal cancer screening and prevention. ACOG Committee Opinion No. 384. American College of Obstetricians and Gynecologists. Obstet Gynecol 2007;110:1199–1202.

ISSN 1074-861X

ACOG COMMITTEE OPINION

Number 387 • November 2007

Pharmaceutical Compounding

Committee on Gynecologic Practice

This document reflects emerging clinical and scientific advances as of the date issued and is subject to change. The information should not be construed as dictating an exclusive course of treatment or procedure to be followed.

ABSTRACT: Compounding is the preparation of an individualized drug product in response to a physician's prescription to create a medication tailored to the specialized needs of an individual patient. There are currently no specific prohibitions by the U.S. Food and Drug Administration on what constitutes a legitimate claim for compounded drug products, even if there is no efficacy, risk, or safety evidence to support an advertised claim. Physicians and patients should exercise caution in prescribing and using products that are largely untested for safety and efficacy.

The American College of Obstetricians and Gynecologists
Women's Health Care Physicians

An increase in the marketing and media coverage of compounded pharmaceutical products has resulted in questions from many Fellows of the American College of Obstetricians and Gynecologists and their patients regarding the preparation, regulation, efficacy, and safety of compounded drug products. Compounding is the preparation of an individualized drug product in response to a physician's prescription to create a medication tailored to the specialized needs of an individual patient. Compounded drug products may fill gaps in the commercially available armamentarium. For example, a compounded drug may be prepared for the pediatric patient who is not able to swallow solid oral dosage forms, yet for whom no liquid preparation is commercially available or for the patient who may be allergic to an inactive ingredient in a commercially available product. The use of 17α-hydroxyprogesterone to reduce preterm birth is another example where compounding may be necessary. Despite evidence that 17α-hydroxyprogesterone may be useful in preventing preterm birth in a select high-risk population, the formulation of this drug used in research currently is not commercially available (1). Far removed from these traditional uses of compounding are products that simply blend commercially available drug products in proportions tailored to individual patient information. Many compounded bioidentical hormone products fall into this category (2).

Although technically all compounded prescription drug products could be considered unapproved new drugs, the U.S. Food

and Drug Administration has adopted a policy of "enforcement discretion," allowing legitimate preparation of compounded formulations as regulated by state boards of pharmacy, with a provision of stepping in when dangerous practices must be addressed and when drug manufacturing occurs under the guise of compounding. In general, states regard compounding to be part of the practice of pharmacy. In addition, there normally is a provision in individual states' pharmacy acts to permit other licensed practitioners (eg, physicians, nurse practitioners, and others with prescriptive authority) to engage in the practice of pharmacy compounding for their own patients. According to the American Pharmacists Association, the essence of pharmaceutical compounding is the "triangular" relationship between the individual health practitioner, his or her patient, and the compounding pharmacy. It is this individual prescriber–individual patient–compounder triad that distinguishes compounding from manufacturing, which involves the mass production of medication "with no connection between the producer of the medication and the ultimate user" (3). Thus, the key in distinguishing compounding from manufacturing is whether the product is created in response to an individual patient's need.

There are currently no specific prohibitions by the U.S. Food and Drug Administration on what constitutes a legitimate claim for compounded drug products, even if there is no efficacy, risk, or safety evidence to support an advertised claim. Significant quality concerns may exist for compounded agents, particularly when sterility is important (eg, injectable or inhalational agents), and questions about the safety of certain compounded drug products have been raised (4). Although it is required that manufactured drugs be consistent from batch to batch, there are no similar quality control measures for compounded drugs to ensure that the bioavailability of active ingredients is consistent. Therefore, although interest in and requests for compounded pharmaceutical products appear to be increasing, physicians and patients should exercise caution in prescribing and using products that are largely untested for safety and efficacy.

References

1. Use of progesterone to reduce preterm birth. ACOG Committee Opinion No. 291. American College of Obstetricians and Gynecologists. Obstet Gynecol 2003;102:1115–6.

2. Compounded bioidentical hormones. ACOG Committee Opinion No. 322. American College of Obstetricians and Gynecologists. Obstet Gynecol 2005;106:1139–40.

3. American Pharmacists Association. Testimony of the American Pharmacists Association on federal and state role in pharmacy compounding and reconstitution: exploring the right mix to protect patients. Before the Committee on Health, Education, Labor and Pensions, United States Senate, October 23, 2003. Washington (DC): APA; 2003. Available at: http://www.aphanet.org/AM/Template.cfm?Section=Federal_Government_Affairs&CONTENTID=2932&TEMPLATE=/CM/ContentDisplay.cfm. Retrieved July 20, 2007.

4. Food and Drug Administration (US). Report: limited FDA survey of compounded drug products. Rockville (MD): FDA; 2003. Available at: http://www.fda.gov/cder/pharmcomp/survey.htm. Retrieved July 20, 2007.

Resources

Compounded bioidentical hormones. ACOG Committee Opinion No. 322. American College of Obstetricians and Gynecologists. Obstet Gynecol 2005;106:1139–40.

Food and Drug Administration (US). The practice of pharmacy compounding. Rockville (MD): FDA; 2005. Available at: http://www.fda.gov/cder/pharmcomp. Retrieved July 20, 2007.

Pharmaceutical compounding. ACOG Committee Opinion No. 387. American College of Obstetricians and Gynecologists. Obstet Gynecol 2007;110:1213–4.

ISSN 1074-861X

ACOG COMMITTEE OPINION

Number 388 • November 2007

Supracervical Hysterectomy

**Committee on
Gynecologic
Practice**

This document reflects
emerging clinical and scientific advances as of the
date issued and is subject
to change. The informa-
tion should not be con-
strued as dictating an
exclusive course of treatment or procedure to be
followed.

ABSTRACT: Women with known or suspected gynecologic cancer, current or recent cervical dysplasia, or endometrial hyperplasia are not candidates for a supracervical proce-dure. Patients electing supracervical hysterectomy should be carefully screened preopera-tively to exclude cervical or uterine neoplasm and should be counseled about the need for long-term follow-up, the possibility of future trachelectomy, and the lack of data demon-strating clear benefits over total hysterectomy. The supracervical approach should not be recommended by the surgeon as a superior technique for hysterectomy for benign disease.

Hysterectomy remains one of the most com-monly performed surgical procedures in the United States, with the most frequent indica-tions being abnormal uterine bleeding and symptomatic uterine leiomyomata. Variations in surgical technique have been described in an attempt to reduce operative morbidity and reduce the effects of hysterectomy on urinary and sexual function. Supracervical hysterectomy is one such technique in which there has been renewed interest among patients and some gynecologic surgeons. Historically, the supracervical hysterectomy was abandoned in favor of total hysterectomy because of problems related to the retained cervix. The purpose of this document is to review the scientific data for elective supra-cervical hysterectomy in which it is the pref-erence of the patient or physician to preserve the cervix at the time of hysterectomy unre-lated to the indications for surgery.

Techniques for supracervical hysterec-tomy, defined as removal of the uterine cor-pus with preservation of the cervix, are well described for both the abdominal and laparoscopic approaches (1, 2). Features common to both the laparoscopic and open techniques of supracervical hysterectomy are removal of the corpus at or below the level of the internal os and attempted ablation of the endocervical canal after removal of the cor-pus (1). In laparoscopic supracervical hys-terectomy, morcellation of the uterine fun-dus is performed to facilitate its removal through the port site incisions (1).

Women with known or suspected gyne-cologic cancer, current or recent cervical dys-

plasia, or endometrial hyperplasia are not candidates for a supracervical procedure (3–5). Candidates for elective supracervical hysterectomy must have normal results from a recent cytologic cervical examination and normal gross appearance of the cervix docu-mented before surgery (3–5). Clinicians also should consider testing for high-risk human papillomavirus to identify patients who could be at risk for future cervical neoplasia. Amputation of the uterine corpus in the abdominal approach and morcellation of the corpus in the laparoscopic approach require adequate preoperative assessment of the endometrial cavity to exclude neoplasm (3–5).

Possible benefits of supracervical hys-terectomy with regard to perioperative mor-bidity are not supported by recent evidence. In three prospective randomized controlled trials that did not include laparoscopic pro-cedures, no difference in complications, including infection; blood loss requiring transfusion; or urinary tract, bowel, or vascu-lar injury, was seen between women random-ized to total abdominal hysterectomy (TAH) and supracervical abdominal hysterectomy (3–5). Length of hospital stay (5.2 versus 6 days, $P = .04$) and duration of surgical proce-dure (59.5 versus 71.1 minutes $P < .001$) were significantly shorter for women randomized to supracervical hysterectomy in European studies, but no significant difference was seen in any outcome measured in the only prospective randomized trial of TAH versus supracervical hysterectomy conducted in the United States (3–5). Reported rates of post-

**The American College
of Obstetricians
and Gynecologists**
*Women's Health Care
Physicians*

operative cyclical vaginal bleeding in women randomized to supracervical hysterectomy were 5–20% in these three prospective trials. Of the two trials that reported reoperation rates, 1.5% of the participants had a second operation to remove the cervix less than 3 months from the time of hysterectomy.

Choosing to preserve the cervix to reduce adverse effects of hysterectomy on sexual and urinary function also is not supported by data from prospective randomized trials. Differences in preoperative and postoperative stress or urge incontinence, urinary frequency, and incomplete bladder emptying were not statistically significant between women randomized to supracervical hysterectomy or TAH in either the U.S. or British trials (3, 4). The Danish Hysterectomy Group found a higher incidence of urinary incontinence in women randomized to supracervical hysterectomy ($P = .043$) (5). Sexual satisfaction was reported with similar frequency preoperatively and 1 year postoperatively by women in the Danish study, irrespective of type of hysterectomy performed (5). Frequency of intercourse, frequency of orgasm, and rating of sexual relationship with a partner measured preoperatively and postoperatively were similar for the supracervical hysterectomy and TAH groups in the British study (4). In the U.S. study, there were no differences between the supracervical hysterectomy and the TAH groups in sexual functioning and measure of health-related quality of life, including sexual desire, orgasm frequency and quality, and body image, measured 2 years after surgery (6).

Because there have been no randomized, controlled trials of laparoscopic supracervical hysterectomy compared with either TAH or laparoscopically assisted vaginal hysterectomy (LAVH), evidence regarding the potential benefits of this technique is limited to retrospective series. In a retrospective comparison of laparoscopic supracervical hysterectomy with LAVH, less blood loss, shorter operating time, and fewer complications were found in the patients who had supracervical hysterectomy (7). In contrast, the recent experience of a large managed care organization was documented, indicating longer operating time for laparoscopic supracervical hysterectomy compared with TAH but less blood loss, shorter hospital stay, and fewer major complications for laparoscopic supracervical hysterectomy compared with TAH (8). Although only reported in series with small numbers of patients, the long-term complications of laparoscopic supracervical hysterectomy include cyclical vaginal bleeding in 11–17% of cases and the need for trachelectomy because of symptoms in 23% of cases at a mean of 14 months from the time of hysterectomy (9, 10). The potential risks as well as benefits of laparoscopic supracervical hysterectomy should be carefully considered by the individual surgeon and patient until data from prospective randomized controlled trials comparing this technique with LAVH or TAH are available.

An additional risk of supracervical hysterectomy relates to the development of benign or neoplastic conditions that require future removal of the cervical stump. Complications of trachelectomy reported in the largest published series (310 cases) include a 9% incidence of infection and perioperative bleeding and a 2% incidence of intraoperative bowel injury. Fewer complications were seen with vaginal trachelectomy than with abdominal trachelectomy (11).

Although data from uncontrolled series may suggest a benefit from preserving the cervix, review of recently published Level I evidence reveals no advantage to the supracervical abdominal technique with regard to surgical complications, urinary symptoms, or sexual function in women undergoing hysterectomy for symptomatic uterine leiomyomata or abnormal uterine bleeding (3–5). Despite the potential advantages of shorter hospital stay and less blood loss afforded by the laparoscopic supracervical approach, there are no prospective data comparing laparoscopic supracervical hysterectomy with either LAVH or TAH.

Patients electing supracervical hysterectomy should be carefully screened preoperatively to exclude cervical or uterine neoplasm and should be counseled about the need for long-term follow-up, the possibility of future trachelectomy, and the lack of data demonstrating clear benefits over total hysterectomy. The supracervical approach should not be recommended by the surgeon as a superior technique for hysterectomy for benign disease.

References

1. Jenkins TR. Laparoscopic supracervical hysterectomy. Am J Obstet Gynecol 2004;191:1875–84.

2. Parker WH. Total laparoscopic hysterectomy and laparoscopic supracervical hysterectomy. Obstet Gynecol Clin North Am 2004;31:523–37, viii.

3. Learman LA, Summitt RL Jr, Varner RE, McNeeley SG, Goodman-Gruen D, Richter HE, et al. A randomized comparison of total or supracervical hysterectomy: surgical complications and clinical outcomes. Total or Supracervical Hysterectomy (TOSH) Research Group. Obstet Gynecol 2003;102:453–62.

4. Thakar R, Ayers S, Clarkson P, Stanton S, Manyonda I. Outcomes after total versus subtotal abdominal hysterectomy. N Engl J Med 2002;347:1318–25.

5. Gimbel H, Zobbe V, Andersen BM, Filtenborg T, Gluud C, Tabor A. Randomised controlled trial of total compared with subtotal hysterectomy with one-year follow up results. BJOG 2003;110:1088–98.

6. Kuppermann M, Summitt RL Jr, Varner RE, McNeeley SG, Goodman-Gruen D, Learman LA, et al. Sexual functioning after total compared with supracervical hysterectomy: a randomized trial. Total or Supracervical Hysterectomy Research Group. Obstet Gynecol 2005;105:1309–18.

7. El-Mowafi D, Madkour W, Lall C, Wenger JM. Laparoscopic supracervical hysterectomy versus laparoscopic-assisted vaginal hysterectomy. J Am Assoc Gynecol Laparosc 2004; 11:175–80.

8. Hoffman CP, Kennedy J, Borschel L, Burchette R, Kidd A. Laparoscopic hysterectomy: the Kaiser Permanente San Diego experience. J Minim Invasive Gynecol 2005;12:16–24.

9. Okaro EO, Jones KD, Sutton C. Long term outcome following laparoscopic supracervical hysterectomy. BJOG 2001; 108:1017–20.

10. Ghomi A, Hantes J, Lotze EC. Incidence of cyclical bleeding after laparoscopic supracervical hysterectomy. J Minim Invasive Gynecol 2005;12:201–5.

11. Hilger WS, Pizarro AR, Magrina JF. Removal of the retained cervical stump. Am J Obstet Gynecol 2005;193:2117–21.

Supracervical hysterectomy. ACOG Committee Opinion No. 388. American College of Obstetricians and Gynecologists. Obstet Gynecol 2007;110:1215–7.

ISSN 1074-861X

ACOG COMMITTEE OPINION

Number 396 • January 2008

Intraperitoneal Chemotherapy for Ovarian Cancer

Committee on Gynecologic Practice

This document reflects emerging clinical and scientific advances as of the date issued and is subject to change. The information should not be construed as dictating an exclusive course of treatment or procedure to be followed.

ABSTRACT: Postoperative intravenous (IV) chemotherapy for advanced stage ovarian cancer has been the standard treatment. Recent studies have found significant survival advantages with the use of adjuvant intraperitoneal (IP) chemotherapy. Combination IV/IP chemotherapy may be an option for well counseled, carefully selected patients with optimally debulked stage III ovarian cancer. However, IV/IP treatment also has increased rates of pain, fatigue, and hematologic, gastrointestinal, metabolic, and neurologic toxicities. Given the balance of efficacy, quality of life, and toxicity, the decision to use IP chemotherapy must be individualized.

The American College of Obstetricians and Gynecologists

Women's Health Care Physicians

Epithelial ovarian cancer is the second most common gynecologic malignancy, but is the leading cause of death from gynecologic cancer in the United States. In 2007, an estimated 22,430 new cases of ovarian cancer and 15,280 deaths from ovarian cancer will occur in the United States (1). Most patients with ovarian cancer present with either stage III or stage IV disease.

Patients with early stage disease need to have comprehensive surgical staging to assess risks and to direct adjuvant chemotherapy. In addition, for advanced ovarian cancer, primary surgical cytoreduction plays an important role. The goal of cytoreductive surgery is to achieve optimal tumor reduction, ideally with individual aggregates of residual disease less than 1 cm. Postoperative intravenous (IV) chemotherapy in advanced stage ovarian cancer has been the standard treatment. Recent trials have suggested that patients with optimally debulked stage III ovarian cancer may be candidates to receive part of their chemotherapy intraperitoneally. Patients with newly diagnosed ovarian cancer may solicit input from their generalist obstetrician–gynecologist regarding treatment options. The purpose of this Committee Opinion is to provide the generalist obstetrician–gynecologist with information regarding the use of intraperitoneal (IP) chemotherapy in the treatment of ovarian cancer and a summary of recent trial results.

Intraperitoneal chemotherapy as a therapeutic strategy for patients with ovarian cancer was based on pharmacologic modeling studies performed in the late 1970s (2). The rationale was based on the findings of high intraperitoneal concentration of drugs and longer half-life of the drug in the peritoneal cavity, which resulted in a prolonged exposure of the chemotherapy agents. One of the concerns of the use of IP chemotherapy has been uniform distribution of the drug, which may not occur because of adhesions that result from surgery.

To study these concerns, randomized clinical trials of IV chemotherapy versus IP chemotherapy began approximately 20 years ago. The results of Gynecologic Oncology Group (GOG) Protocol 172 were published in early 2006 (3). This trial compared IV chemotherapy with an experimental regimen containing both IV and IP chemotherapy in women with optimally debulked stage III ovarian cancer. The treatment regimen was administered every 3 weeks for six cycles (see box). The results of this trial are summarized in Table 1.

The survival advantage of approximately 16 months in GOG Protocol 172 was considered to be a significant advance. The results of this trial and six other randomized trials prompted the National Cancer Institute (NCI) to issue a Clinical Announcement pertaining to IP chemotherapy for epithelial ovarian cancer (4). Seven randomized trials

---

Gynecologic Oncology Group Protocol 172 Treatment Schedules

Standard Therapy	**Experimental Arm**
IV administration of paclitaxel, 135 mg/m^2 over 24 h	IV administration of paclitaxel, 135 mg/m^2 over 24 h
plus	**plus**
IV administration of cisplatin, 75 mg mg/m^2 every 3 wk × 6	IP administration of cisplatin, 100 mg/m^2
	plus
	IP administration of paclitaxel, 60 mg/m^2 on d 8 every 3 wk × 6

Table 1. Gynecologic Oncology Group Protocol 172 Results

	Therapy		
	Standard	**Experimental**	**P Value**
Progression-free survival	18.3 mos	23.8 mo	.05
Survival	49.7 mos	65.8 mo	.03

found that women who received adjuvant IP chemotherapy had greater overall survival rates than women who did not receive such treatment.

However, in GOG Protocol 172, the complication rate of the experimental IV/IP regimen was significantly greater than the complication rate of IV therapy alone. The IV/IP chemotherapy group had more severe toxicities, which included pain and fatigue and hematologic, gastrointestinal, metabolic, and neurologic toxicities. Quality of life was lower in the IV/IP chemotherapy group during the first year after initial treatment. In addition, only 42% of the patients randomized to IV/IP chemotherapy completed the recommended six cycles. The most common reason for discontinuation of IP therapy was catheter-related problems (34%) (5). Nine percent of patients refused additional IP treatment.

There has not been widespread acceptance of IV/IP therapy because of toxicities, catheter problems, and a complicated treatment regimen. Acceptance of the IV/IP regimen is further complicated because the IV-only regimen used in GOG Protocol 172 was not the current preferred treatment of IV administration of paclitaxel, 175 mg/m^2 over 3 hours, and IV administration of carboplatin (area under the curve, 7.5). Intravenous administration of paclitaxel, 175 mg/m^2 over 3 hours, and IV administration of carboplatin (area under the curve, 7.5) was one of the treatments compared with 24-hour IV administration of paclitaxel and cisplatin in GOG Protocol 158. The paclitaxel (given over 3 hours) and car-

boplatin treatment arm of GOG Protocol 158 demonstrated improved survival compared with 24-hour IV administration of paclitaxel and cisplatin, which was the IV-only regimen used in GOG Protocol 172 (6). Women in GOG Protocol 172 and GOG Protocol 158 had optimally debulked stage III ovarian cancer. Robust exploratory cross-trial comparisons of IV administration of carboplatin and IV administration of paclitaxel compared with IV/IP regimens suggest similar efficacy (7). A recent international consensus conference recommended IV administration of carboplatin and paclitaxel as the standard regimen against which new treatments should be compared (8).

Patients with optimally debulked stage III epithelial ovarian cancer who would be potential candidates for IP chemotherapy should be well counseled regarding the risks and benefits of IV plus IP chemotherapy versus IV chemotherapy alone. Clinically, many patients are being treated with IP chemotherapy, but probably are not using the GOG Protocol 172 dosing regimen. Consequently, women may be treated with IV/IP chemotherapy regimens that have no scientific evidence of better outcomes. The NCI Clinical Announcement summary stated that despite the positive findings of the trials, the ideal combination of drugs for IV/IP therapy had not been identified. The NCI Clinical Announcement suggested consideration of IP cisplatin therapy, 100 mg/m^2, and IV-only taxane administration or by IV plus IP administration. The Gynecology Oncology Group is currently evaluating other IV/IP chemotherapy regimens to identify a less toxic, more tolerable, and less complicated treatment regimen.

In summary, combination IV/IP chemotherapy may be an option for well counseled, carefully selected patients with optimally debulked stage III ovarian cancer when provided by a physician with the requisite training and experience in administering this treatment. However, given the balance of efficacy, quality of life, and toxicity, the decision to use IP chemotherapy must be individualized.

References

1. American Cancer Society. Cancer facts and figures 2007. Atlanta (GA): ACS; 2007. Available at: http://www.cancer.org/downloads/STT/CAFF2007PWSecured.pdf. Retrieved August 22, 2007.

2. Dedrick RL, Myers CE, Bungay PM, DeVita VT Jr. Pharmacokinetic rationale for peritoneal drug administration in the treatment of ovarian cancer. Cancer Treat Rep 1978;62:1–11.

3. Armstrong DK, Bundy B, Wenzel L, Huang HQ, Baergen R, Lele S, et al. Intraperitoneal cisplatin and paclitaxel in ovarian cancer. Gynecologic Oncology Group. N Engl J Med 2006;354:34–43.

4. National Cancer Institute. Clinical announcement on intraperitoneal chemotherapy in ovarian cancer. Cancer Therapy Evaluation Program. Bethesda (MD): NCI; 2006. Available at: http://ctep.cancer.gov/highlights/clin_annc_010506.pdf. Retrieved September 28, 2007.

5. Walker JL, Armstrong DK, Huang HQ, Fowler J, Webster K, Burger RA, et al. Intraperitoneal catheter outcomes in a phase III trial of intravenous versus intraperitoneal chemotherapy in optimal stage III ovarian and primary peritoneal cancer: a Gynecologic Oncology Group Study. Gynecol Oncol 2006;100:27–32.

6. Ozols RF, Bundy BN, Greer BE, Fowler JM, Clarke-Pearson D, Burger RA, et al. Phase III trial of carboplatin and paclitaxel compared with cisplatin and paclitaxel in patients with optimally resected stage III ovarian cancer: a Gynecologic Oncology Group study. Gynecologic Oncology Group. J Clin Oncol 2003;21:3194–200.

7. Ozols RF, Bookman MA, du Bois A, Pfisterer J, Reuss A, Young RC. Intraperitoneal cisplatin therapy in ovarian cancer: comparison with standard intravenous carboplatin and paclitaxel. Gynecol Oncol 2006;103:1–6.

8. du Bois A, Quinn M, Thigpen T, Vermorken J, Avall-Lundqvist E, Bookman M, et al. 2004 consensus statements on the management of ovarian cancer: final document of the 3rd International Gynecologic Cancer Intergroup Ovarian Cancer Consensus Conference (GCIG OCCC 2004). Gynecologic Cancer Intergroup; AGO-OVAR; ANZGOG; EORTC; GEICO; GINECO; GOG; JGOG; MRC/NCRI; NCIC-CTG; NCI-US; NSGO; RTOG; SGCTG; IGCS; Organizational team of the two prior International OCCC. Ann Oncol 2005;16(suppl 8):viii7–viii12.

Intraperitoneal chemotherapy for ovarian cancer. ACOG Committee Opinion No. 396. American College of Obstetricians and Gynecologists. Obstet Gynecol 2008;111:249–51.

ISSN 1074-861X

ACOG COMMITTEE OPINION

Number 405 • May 2008

Ovarian Tissue and Oocyte Cryopreservation

Committee on Gynecologic Practice

This document reflects emerging clinical and scientific advances as of the date issued and is subject to change. The information should not be construed as dictating an exclusive course of treatment or procedure to be followed.

ABSTRACT: As more young women are cured of cancer with chemotherapy and radiotherapy, which can be gonadotoxic, interest is growing in treatments that may preserve fertility. In vitro fertilization with cryopreservation of embryos is currently the best option for fertility preservation when treatment for cancer is anticipated. Ovarian tissue cryopreservation and oocyte cryopreservation are two options with the potential to preserve fertility. Although these methods are developing rapidly, their use as a means to have a child after cancer treatment must be considered investigational and offered only with appropriate informed consent in a research setting and under the auspices of an institutional review board.

The American College of Obstetricians and Gynecologists

Women's Health Care Physicians

The number of oocytes in the ovaries declines naturally and progressively through the process of atresia. Chemotherapy and radiotherapy have the potential to accelerate this process, placing women who require these treatments at risk of premature ovarian failure.

A number of techniques have been used to protect the ovaries and preserve fertility in women at risk of losing ovarian function prematurely as a consequence of cancer therapy. For women who would otherwise lose function from radiation treatment, ovarian transposition (moving the ovary as far as possible outside the field of radiation while maintaining the blood supply) may be useful (1). Treatment with oral contraceptives and gonadotropin-releasing hormone agonists to preserve ovarian function has been advocated but does not have proven efficacy.

In vitro fertilization (IVF) with cryopreservation of embryos is a proven method and is the most successful approach. In all reported procedures (not just those for women with cancer), this technique affords a live-birth rate of 15.9–31.7% with the transfer of two or three cryopreserved embryos (2) and may offer the opportunity to carry out several attempts at embryo transfer from a single oocyte retrieval. Oocyte retrieval and IVF require several weeks of preparation and the availability of sperm. Elevated estrogen levels have the potential to be detrimental to women with some cancers, and consultation with a repro-

ductive medicine specialist and the oncologist is recommended.

Two investigational methods, oocyte cryopreservation for future IVF and ovarian tissue cryopreservation, have garnered increased interest for preserving fertility in the patient with cancer (3). Clinical pregnancy rates with oocyte cryopreservation and subsequent IVF are significantly lower than rates with embryo cryopreservation. In oocytes, the rate of survival and subsequent fertilization depends on the maturational stage and method of cryopreservation. The mature metaphase-II oocyte is extremely fragile because of its large size, water content, and chromosomal arrangement along the meiotic spindle. This spindle apparatus is damaged easily by intracellular ice formation during the freezing and thawing process. Oocytes frozen at an early germinal vesicle stage have a lower rate of cryopreservation-induced abnormalities of the spindle apparatus, but they must undergo the relatively new process of in vitro maturation. Vitrification, a cryopreservation method that limits the formation of ice crystals, has been shown to improve survival and fertilization rates after thawing. To date, the number of live births reported from oocyte cryopreservation is limited, with one report calculating a live-birth rate per thawed oocyte of only 4% (4). Current data are insufficient to allow any valid estimate of the likelihood of success for an individual woman. Similar to the cryopreservation of embryos, in order to cryopreserve oocytes, the ovaries must be stimulated, and this process will lead to increased estrogen levels and may delay the initiation of treatment.

Orthotopic transplantation (autograft placed near the infundibulopelvic ligament or residual ovarian tissue) and heterotopic transplantation (autograft placed above the fascia in the forearm) of previously cryopreserved ovarian tissue are other investigational options that have been shown to restore ovarian function at least temporarily. Human live births have been reported after orthotopic transplantation of cryopreserved ovarian tissue (5) and the transplantation of ovarian cortical tissue between monozygotic twins (6). Potential risks of the transplantation of cryopreserved tissue in the patient with cancer include reseeding of tumor cells in cancer types such as leukemia, malignant transformation of the transplanted tissue, and recurrence of the malignancy during pregnancy (7). Further research defining patient suitability, methods of tissue collection, cryopreservation protocols, and methods of processing human ovarian tissue after thawing will determine whether fertility can be restored reliably with ovarian tissue transplantation.

In conclusion, ovarian tissue and oocyte cryopreservation hold promise for fertility preservation. However, cryopreservation of ovarian tissue and oocytes is investigational. At this time, these procedures may be offered only with appropriate informed consent in a research setting and under the auspices of an institutional review board. Further research is necessary to determine patient selection, methods of tissue collection, and optimal cryopreservation protocols.

References

1. Morice P, Castaigne D, Haie-Meder C, Pautier P, El Hassan J, Duvillard P, et al. Laparoscopic ovarian transposition for pelvic malignancies: indications and functional outcomes. Fertil Steril 1998;70:956–60.

2. Centers for Disease Control and Prevention. Assisted reproductive technology (ART) report: 2005 preliminary national summary. Atlanta (GA): CDC; 2007. Available at: http://apps.nccd.cdc.gov/ART2005/nation05.asp. Retrieved November 20, 2007.

3. Borini A, Bonu MA, Coticchio G, Bianchi V, Cattoli M, Flamigni C. Pregnancies and births after oocyte cryopreservation. Fertil Steril 2004;82:601–5.

4. Porcu E, Venturoli S. Progress with oocyte cryopreservation. Curr Opin Obstet Gynecol 2006;18:273–9.

5. Donnez J, Dolmans MM, Demylle D, Jadoul P, Pirard C, Squifflet J, et al. Livebirth after orthotopic transplantation of cryopreserved ovarian tissue [published erratum appears in Lancet 2004;364:2020]. Lancet 2004;364:1405–10.

6. Silber SJ, Lenahan KM, Levine DJ, Pineda JA, Gorman KS, Friez MJ, et al. Ovarian transplantation between monozygotic twins discordant for premature ovarian failure. N Engl J Med 2005;353:58–63.

7. Ovarian tissue and oocyte cryopreservation. Practice Committee of the American Society for Reproductive Medicine; Practice Committee of the Society for Assisted Reproductive Technology. Fertil Steril 2006;86(suppl): S142–7.

Ovarian tissue and oocyte cryopreservation. ACOG Committee Opinion No. 405. American College of Obstetricians and Gynecologists. Obstet Gynecol 2008;111:1255–6.

ACOG COMMITTEE OPINION

Number 407 • May 2008

Low Bone Mass (Osteopenia) and Fracture Risk

Committee on Gynecologic Practice

This document reflects emerging clinical and scientific advances as of the date issued and is subject to change. The information should not be construed as dictating an exclusive course of treatment or procedure to be followed.

ABSTRACT: Diagnosis of low bone mass or osteopenia, defined by measures of bone mineral density (BMD), has generated much confusion. Because BMD alone is not sufficient to describe risk of fracture, clinicians face challenges in interpreting BMD and clinical risk factors, counseling patients on absolute risk of fracture, and determining the need for pharmacologic intervention. For fracture risk assessment, the most valuable risk factors appear to be BMD, age, prior fracture history, and risk of falling. Until better models of fracture risk exist, postmenopausal women in their 50s with T scores in the osteopenia range and without risk factors may well benefit from counseling on calcium and vitamin D intake and risk factor reduction to delay the initiation of pharmacologic intervention.

Diagnosis of low bone mass or osteopenia has generated much confusion related to counseling, follow-up, and the need for pharmacologic intervention. An estimated 26 million American women have osteopenia, defined as bone mineral density (BMD) T scores between −1 and −2.5 (Table 1). Although the risk of fracture is higher in women with osteoporosis, the total number of fractures is greater in postmenopausal women with osteopenia because of the

Table 1. World Health Organization Definition of Osteoporosis Based on Bone Mineral Density of Total Hip*

Bone Classification	T Score[†]
Normal	Greater than or equal to −1
Osteopenia (low bone mass)	−1 to −2.5
Osteoporosis	Less than or equal to −2.5

*These definitions were used to describe a Caucasian cohort of women to define risk. This classification was not intended to be applicable to non-Caucasians and men or to peripheral bone density screening devices. The use of the World Health Organization guidelines and definitions nonetheless has become generalized.

[†]Standard deviations from the average value of the mean peak bone mineral density of a normal, young adult population

Data from Assessment of fracture risk and its application to screening for postmenopausal osteoporosis. Report of a WHO Study Group. World Health Organ Tech Rep Ser 1994;843:1–129.

greater numbers of these women (1). Given that women with T scores between −1 and −2.5 account for the majority of fractures, women with low bone mass represent the greatest opportunity to reduce fractures.

After menopause, bone density values decline and the incidence of most fractures increases. Large prospective studies have demonstrated that bone density is an important predictor of fracture risk in untreated populations (2, 3). However, treatment currently is not recommended uniformly for women with osteopenia. Mechanisms to stratify fracture risk within this group are needed to determine appropriate intervention. Reliance on BMD measurements alone to determine fracture risk has been described as analogous to the relationship between blood pressure and cardiovascular disease risk. For example, although cardiovascular disease risk is increased with hypertension, many patients with hypertension will never experience a heart attack or stroke, and some with normal blood pressure will (4). Osteopenia may be considered similar to prehypertension, defining an intermediate risk group that should be offered preventive therapy. Clearly, there are risk factors other than hypertension in the development of cardiovascular disease. Similarly, many factors other than BMD affect fracture risk.

The American College of Obstetricians and Gynecologists
Women's Health Care Physicians

Bone mineral density is only one component of bone integrity, and it is a reflection of bone quantity but not quality. Bone quality is determined by trabecular architecture, bone turnover, degree of matrix mineralization, and other physiologic, molecular, and material processes. This partly explains the loose correlation between fracture risk reduction (significant) and BMD increases (often minimal) after pharmacologic intervention. Not observing an increase in BMD after pharmacologic intervention is not evidence of treatment failure. Loss of bone mass is a continuum, and cutoffs used to define normal versus low bone mass are arbitrary.

The diagnostic category of osteopenia is problematic. The range for normally distributed measures usually is defined as the values within two standard deviations of the mean (T scores −2 and +2). Approximately 16% of young healthy adults have T score values lower than −1 and are most commonly smaller women (5). In interpreting T scores in younger women, it is important to realize that original World Health Organization (WHO) definitions of osteoporosis and osteopenia were based on T scores in postmenopausal Caucasian women. Although relative risk of fracture may increase with decreasing BMD in younger women, absolute risk of fracture may still remain minimal. Relative risk describes risk in a comparative way between two populations, usually expressed as a ratio (eg, "twice as likely" = relative risk of 2), whereas absolute risk describes the probability of a given event occurring over a specific interval of time and usually is expressed as a percentage or a ratio (eg, 5% per year). Differentiating between relative risk and absolute risk is critical when contemplating pharmacologic intervention for osteopenia. For example, given the same BMD T score of −2, the 10-year risk of hip fracture has been estimated to vary from 3% (at age 50 years) to 9% (at age 75 years) (6). Put another way, a 50-year-old patient with a T score of −3 has the same absolute fracture risk as an 80-year-old patient with a T score of −1. Age is clearly a factor that must be considered when interpreting BMD. Overestimating fracture risk in younger, osteopenic women is likely when BMD is used alone because age increases absolute fracture risk.

Various models that incorporate BMD and other clinical factors have been suggested to help the clinician predict both short-term and long-term fracture risks (7). For fracture risk assessment, the most valuable risk factors appear to be BMD, age, prior fracture, and risk of falling (5). The World Health Organization and other organizations are developing tools that incorporate BMD and clinical risk factors to calculate 5- or 10-year absolute risks of fracture. The WHO fracture model may well become the standard because it is reportedly applicable to both sexes, uses a broad age range, includes those exposed to glucocorticoids, and provides absolute fracture risks that have been developed and tested (8, 9). If absolute risk could be calculated easily in an office setting, clinicians

and patients could better understand the cost versus the benefit of pharmacologic intervention.

Listed as follows are recommendations of the American College of Obstetricians and Gynecologists (ACOG) for BMD testing (10):

- Bone mineral density testing should be recommended to all postmenopausal women aged 65 years or older regardless of risk factors.
- Bone mineral density testing may be recommended for postmenopausal women younger than 65 years who have one or more risk factors for osteoporosis (see box). According to these risk factors, all Caucasian postmenopausal women younger than 65 years would be candidates for BMD testing.
- Bone mineral density testing should be performed on all postmenopausal women with fractures to confirm the diagnosis of osteoporosis and determine disease severity.

However, because BMD alone is not sufficient to describe risk of fracture, clinicians face challenges in interpreting BMD, incorporating clinical risk factors, and counseling patients on absolute risk of fracture. This is particularly challenging in the large category of low bone mass or osteopenia, in which patients with various levels

---

Risk Factors for Osteoporotic Fracture in Postmenopausal Women

History of prior fracture

Family history of osteoporosis

Caucasian race

Dementia

Poor nutrition

Smoking

Low weight and body mass index

Estrogen deficiency*

—Early menopause (age younger than 45 years) or bilateral oophorectomy

—Prolonged premenopausal amenorrhea (>1 year)

Long-term low calcium intake

Alcoholism

Impaired eyesight despite adequate correction

History of falls

Inadequate physical activity

*A patient's current use of hormone therapy does not preclude estrogen deficiency.

Data from Osteoporosis prevention, diagnosis, and therapy. NIH Consens Statement 2000;17(1):1–45. Available at: http://consensus.nih.gov/2000/2000Osteoporosis111PDF.pdf. Retrieved November 28, 2007.

of risk can be found. Current recommendations advise all individuals to obtain an adequate intake of dietary calcium and vitamin D and encourage lifestyle practices that reduce the risk of bone loss and osteoporotic fractures, including regular weight-bearing and muscle-strengthening exercise, smoking cessation, moderation of alcohol intake, and fall prevention strategies.

Pharmacotherapy is recommended by ACOG (10) for the following women:

- Postmenopausal women who have experienced a fragility or low-impact fracture
- Postmenopausal women with no risk factors who have a BMD T score determined by central dual energy X-ray absorptiometry of less than −2
- Postmenopausal women with risk factors for fracture (see box) who have a BMD T score by central dual energy X-ray absorptiometry of less than −1.5

For now, the recommendation to treat postmenopausal women with T scores lower than −2 appears to be reasonable, assuming age is strongly considered. T scores between −1.5 and −2.0 require interpretation with existing risk factors, understanding that absolute risk may still be low. Clinicians must be careful because the diagnosis of osteopenia often is interpreted as indicating a pathologic skeletal condition or significant bone loss, neither of which is necessarily true. Until better models of absolute fracture risk exist, postmenopausal women in their 50s with T scores in the osteopenia range and without risk factors may well benefit from counseling on calcium and vitamin D intake and risk factor reduction to delay initiation of pharmacologic intervention.

References

1. Siris ES, Miller PD, Barrett-Connor E, Faulkner KG, Wehren LE, Abbott TA, et al. Identification and fracture outcomes of undiagnosed low bone mineral density in postmenopausal women: results from the National Osteoporosis Risk Assessment. JAMA 2001;286:2815–22.

2. Johnell O, Gullberg B, Kanis JA, Allander E, Elffors L, Dequeker J, et al. Risk factors for hip fracture in European women: the MEDOS Study. Mediterranean Osteoporosis Study. J Bone Miner Res 1995;10:1802–15.

3. Cummings SR, Black DM, Nevitt MC, Browner W, Cauley J, Ensrud K, et al. Bone density at various sites for prediction of hip fractures. The Study of Osteoporotic Fractures Research Group. Lancet 1993;341:72–5.

4. Goldstein SR. Osteopenia: sorting out the confusion. Menopause Manage 2006;15(1):10–7.

5. McClung MR. The relationship between bone mineral density and fracture risk. Curr Osteoporos Rep 2005;3:57–63.

6. Kanis JA, Johnell O, Oden A, Dawson A, De Laet C, Jonsson B. Ten year probabilities of osteoporotic fractures according to BMD and diagnostic thresholds. Osteoporos Int 2001; 12:989–95.

7. Ettinger B, Hillier TA, Pressman A, Che M, Hanley DA. Simple computer model for calculating and reporting 5-year osteoporotic fracture risk in postmenopausal women. J Womens Health 2005;14:159–71.

8. Ettinger B. Making the most of managed care dollars spent for postmenopausal osteoporosis. Manag Care Interface 2005;18(12):55–9.

9. FRAX WHO fracture risk assessment tool. Sheffield (UK): World Health Organization Collaborating Centre for Metabolic Bone Diseases. University of Sheffield; 2008. Available at: http://www.shef.ac.uk/FRAX/index.htm. Retrieved March 6, 2008.

10. Osteoporosis. ACOG Practice Bulletin No. 50. American College of Obstetricians and Gynecologists. Obstet Gynecol 2004;103:203–16.

Low bone mass (osteopenia) and fracture risk. ACOG Committee Opinion No. 407. American College of Obstetricians and Gynecologists. Obstet Gynecol 2008;111:1259–61.

ACOG COMMITTEE OPINION

Number 408 • June 2008

(Replaces No. 288, October 2003)

Professional Liability and Gynecology-Only Practice

**Committee on
Gynecologic
Practice**

**Committee on
Obstetric Practice**

**Committee on
Professional Liability**

ABSTRACT: Fellows of the American College of Obstetricians and Gynecologists may choose to limit the scope of their practices to gynecology. The College considers early pregnancy care (often up to 12–14 weeks of gestation) to be within the scope of gynecology and gynecologic practice. Liability insurers who provide coverage for "gynecology-only" practices should provide coverage for clinical practice activities that involve the management of early pregnancy and its complications.

Fellows of the American College of Obstetricians and Gynecologists may choose to limit the scope of their practices to gynecology and, accordingly, may choose not to request professional liability coverage for obstetrics. However, the College considers early pregnancy care (often up to 12–14 weeks of gestation) to be within the scope of gynecology and gynecologic practice. Management of conditions such as ectopic pregnancy as well as spontaneous and elective abortion, including early midtrimester abortion, may be properly undertaken in such practices. Liability insurers who provide coverage for "gynecology-only" practices should provide coverage for clinical practice activities that involve the management of early pregnancy and its complications.

Professional liability and gynecology-only practice. ACOG Committee Opinion No. 408. American College of Obstetricians and Gynecologists. Obstet Gynecol 2008;111:1491.

**The American College
of Obstetricians
and Gynecologists**
*Women's Health Care
Physicians*

ACOG COMMITTEE OPINION

Number 411 • August 2008

Routine Human Immunodeficiency Virus Screening

**Committee on
Gynecologic
Practice**

This document reflects emerging clinical and scientific advances as of the date issued and is subject to change. The information should not be construed as dictating an exclusive course of treatment or procedure to be followed.

ABSTRACT: The American College of Obstetricians and Gynecologists recommends routine human immunodeficiency virus (HIV) screening for women aged 19–64 years and targeted screening for women with risk factors outside of that age range. Ideally, opt-out HIV screening should be performed, in which the patient is notified that HIV testing will be performed as a routine part of gynecologic and obstetric care, unless the patient declines testing (1). The American College of Obstetricians and Gynecologists recommends that obstetrician–gynecologists annually review patients' risk factors for HIV and assess the need for retesting.

**The American College
of Obstetricians
and Gynecologists**

*Women's Health Care
Physicians*

An estimated one quarter of all individuals infected with the human immunodeficiency virus (HIV) in the United States are unaware of their HIV status. In order to identify individuals with undiagnosed HIV infection, the U.S. Centers for Disease Control and Prevention (CDC) recommends HIV screening for all patients aged 13–64 years in health care settings (1). Because obstetrician–gynecologists provide primary and preventive care for women, they are ideally suited to play an important role in promoting HIV screening for their patients. Although most obstetrician–gynecologists are familiar with routine HIV testing of their pregnant patients, physicians should incorporate routine HIV testing into their gynecologic practices as well.

There are a number of reasons why it is critical that women, who represent an increasing proportion of overall HIV and acquired immunodeficiency syndrome (AIDS) cases, know their HIV status. Early diagnosis and treatment of HIV can improve survival and reduce morbidity (2). In addition, women who are infected with HIV can take steps to avoid unintended pregnancy, protect their sexual partners, and reduce the likelihood of mother-to-child transmission should pregnancy occur (3). Therefore, the American College of Obstetricians and Gynecologists (ACOG) recommends routine HIV screening for women aged 19–64 years

and targeted screening for women with risk factors outside of that age range, for example, sexually active adolescents younger than 19 years.

Ideally, opt-out HIV screening should be performed, in which the patient is notified that HIV testing will be performed as a routine part of gynecologic and obstetric care, unless the patient declines testing (1). In opt-out screening, neither specific signed consent nor prevention counseling is required. However, women should be provided with oral or written information about HIV and the meaning of positive and negative test results and given the opportunity to ask questions and decline testing. If a patient declines HIV testing, this should be documented in the medical record and should not affect access to care (4). Although ACOG recommends opt-out screening where legally possible, state and local laws may have specific requirements for HIV testing that are not consistent with such an approach. Therefore, obstetrician–gynecologists should be aware of and comply with legal requirements regarding HIV testing in their jurisdictions. Legal requirements for HIV testing may be verified by contacting state or local health departments. The National HIV/AIDS Clinicians' Consultation Center at the University of California San Francisco maintains an online compendium of state HIV testing laws that can be a useful resource (www.nccc.ucsf.edu).

The use of rapid HIV tests may provide test results to women in a more timely manner and may reduce the resources necessary to follow-up with patients regarding their test results. Although a positive rapid test result is preliminary and must be confirmed with additional testing, a negative rapid test result does not require any additional testing. Therefore, rapid testing may be a feasible and acceptable approach for an HIV screening program in an obstetric–gynecologic practice (5). To code for rapid testing, the modifier 92 is added to the basic HIV testing *Current Procedural Terminology** (CPT®) codes (86701–86703).

Although CDC and ACOG both recommend that reproductive-aged women be tested at least once in their lifetime, there is no consensus regarding how often women should be retested. The American College of Obstetricians and Gynecologist recommends that obstetrician–gynecologists annually review patients' risk factors for HIV and assess the need for retesting. Repeat HIV testing should be offered at least annually to women who:

- Are injection drug users
- Have sex partners who are injection drug users or are infected with HIV
- Exchange sex for drugs or money
- Have received a diagnosis of another sexually transmitted disease in the past year
- Have had more than one sex partner since their most recent HIV test

Obstetrician–gynecologists also should encourage women and their prospective sex partners to be tested before initiating a new sexual relationship. In addition, periodic retesting could be considered even in the absence of risk factors depending on clinical judgment and the patient's wishes because patients may be concerned about their status but not know about or want to disclose risk-taking behavior to their physicians.

Although HIV-negative test results may be conveyed without direct personal contact, HIV-positive test results should be communicated confidentially and in person by a physician, nurse, or other skilled staff member. Women who are infected with HIV should receive or be referred for appropriate clinical and supportive care.

Rapid test results usually will be available during the same clinical visit that the specimen (eg, blood or oral swab sample) is collected. Obstetrician–gynecologists who use these tests must be prepared to provide counseling to women who receive positive rapid test results the same day that the specimen is collected (ie, women with posi-

tive rapid test results should be counseled regarding the meaning of these preliminarily positive test results and the need for confirmatory testing) (4). Obstetrician–gynecologists should develop links with individuals who can provide these counseling services on an emergent basis or train their own staff to handle the initial encounter and, thereafter, transition infected individuals to professionals who can serve as ongoing resources to them. Women whose confirmatory testing yields positive results and, therefore, are infected with HIV should receive or be referred to appropriate clinical and supportive care.

Resources

American College of Obstetricians and Gynecologists
409 12th Street SW, PO Box 96920
Washington, DC 20090-6920
202-638-5577
ACOG HIV resources: www.acog.org/goto/HIV

National HIV/AIDS Clinicians' Consultation Center
UCSF Department of Family and Community Medicine at San Francisco General Hospital
1001 Potrero Ave., Bldg. 20, Ward 22
San Francisco, CA 94110
415-206-8700

National HIV Telephone Consultation Service:
1-800-933-3413 (M–F, 8 AM–8 PM [EST])
www.nccc.ucsf.edu

American Academy of HIV Medicine, American Medical Association. Coding guidelines for routine HIV testing in health care settings. Washington, DC: AAHIVM; Chicago (IL): AMA; 2008. Available at: http://aahivm.org/images/stories/pdfs/brochure_reimburse_guide_routinehivtest.pdf. Retrieved May 6, 2008.

References

1. Branson BM, Handsfield HH, Lampe MA, Janssen RS, Taylor AW, Lyss SB, et al. Revised recommendations for HIV testing of adults, adolescents, and pregnant women in health-care settings. Centers for Disease Control and Prevention (CDC). MMWR Recomm Rep 2006;55(RR-14):1–17; quiz CE1–4.

2. Palella FJ Jr, Deloria-Knoll M, Chmiel JS, Moorman AC, Wood KC, Greenberg AE, et al. Survival benefit of initiating antiretroviral therapy in HIV-infected persons in different CD4+ cell strata. HIV Outpatient Study Investigators. Ann Intern Med 2003;138:620–6.

3. U.S. Public Health Service Task Force. Recommendations for use of antiretroviral drugs in pregnant HIV-infected women for maternal health and interventions to reduce perinatal HIV transmission in the United States. Rockville (MD): USPHSTF; 2007. Available at: http://www.aidsinfo.nih.gov/contentfiles/PerinatalGL.pdf. Retrieved March 7, 2008.

4. Human immunodeficiency virus. ACOG Committee Opinion No. 389. American College of Obstetricians and Gynecologists. Obstet Gynecol 2007;110:1473–8.

---

5. Jamieson DJ, Cohen MH, Maupin R, Nesheim S, Danner SP, Lampe MA, et al. Rapid human immunodeficiency virus-1 testing on labor and delivery in 17 US hospitals: the MIRIAD experience. Am J Obstet Gynecol 2007;197(suppl 1):S72–S82.

Routine human immunodeficiency virus screening. ACOG Committee Opinion No. 411. American College of Obstetricians and Gynecologists. Obstet Gynecol 2008;112:401–3.

ISSN 1074-861X

ACOG COMMITTEE OPINION

Number 412 • August 2008

Aromatase Inhibitors in Gynecologic Practice

Committee on Gynecologic Practice

This document reflects emerging clinical and scientific advances as of the date issued and is subject to change. The information should not be construed as dictating an exclusive course of treatment or procedure to be followed.

ABSTRACT: Aromatase inhibitors appear to be effective as an adjuvant treatment for early-stage and late-stage breast cancer. Their role in chemoprevention of breast cancer in high-risk patients remains to be defined. Side effects of aromatase inhibitors in postmenopausal women are due to estrogen-lowering action at the target tissues and include hot flushes, vaginal dryness, arthralgias, and decreased bone mineral density. In reproductive-aged women, aromatase inhibitors stimulate gonadotropin secretion and increase ovarian follicular activity. The role of aromatase inhibitors in the treatment of endometriosis and in ovulation induction is still being investigated.

The American College of Obstetricians and Gynecologists

Women's Health Care Physicians

The pharmacologic manipulation of hormone levels has been very successful in the treatment of estrogen-dependent disease processes such as breast cancer, endometriosis, and uterine leiomyomas. As part of this approach, aromatase inhibitors have been introduced for the treatment of breast cancer and, more recently, endometriosis. Aromatase inhibitors also have been used as ovulation induction agents.

The aromatase enzyme is a cytochrome P-450 complex encoded by a single gene, and it is widely expressed in tissues, such as brain, breast, placenta, ovary, testes, endometrium, skin, bone, and fat. Within these tissues, aromatase mediates the conversion of androstenedione to estrone and testosterone to estradiol in situ. Thus, for tissues that express this enzyme, conversion of circulating androgens from an adrenal or ovarian source will significantly increase the in situ estrogen concentrations and provide these tissues with a proliferative advantage.

Three aromatase inhibitors are currently available in the United States. Exemestane is a steroid-derived aromatase inhibitor that binds irreversibly to aromatase and permanently inactivates the available enzyme. Letrozole and anastrozole are reversible inhibitors of aromatase that compete with androgens for aromatase binding sites. All three aromatase inhibitors appear to have similar clinical efficacy despite these differences in pharmacologic properties.

In postmenopausal women, aromatase inhibitors were first introduced for the treatment of advanced breast cancer. Although these compounds did not increase overall survival, they appeared to be similar or better than megestrol when objective responses were the endpoint (1). The early success of these studies led to clinical trials of aromatase inhibitors in breast cancer patients with resectable, estrogen receptor-positive tumors. The largest of these trials compared anastrozole with tamoxifen, alone or in combination, as adjuvant treatment in women with early breast cancer following surgical resection. The study results demonstrated a small but significantly improved 3-year disease-free survival in postmenopausal women with invasive, operable breast cancer who received anastrozole alone compared with tamoxifen (89.4% versus 87.4%, hazard ratio 0.83 [95% confidence interval, 0.71–0.96]) (2). Subsequent trials have been initiated to examine the effectiveness of aromatase inhibitors in other breast cancer clinical scenarios, including the use of aromatase inhibitors as a sequential therapy following tamoxifen, aromatase inhibitors for the treatment of ductal carcinoma in situ, and aromatase inhibitors for the prevention of breast cancer in high-risk patients (3). Although data from these trials are not complete, it appears that aromatase inhibitors will play a significant role in therapy for estrogen receptor-positive breast cancer.

The short-term and long-term adverse effects of aromatase inhibitors in postmenopausal women are related to lack of estrogen action at aromatase-targeted tissue sites. These side effects include hot flushes, vaginal dryness, arthralgias, decreased bone mineral density, and an increased fracture rate (4). The American Society of Clinical Oncologists recommends that bone mineral density screening be repeated annually in all patients receiving aromatase inhibitor adjuvant therapy, and bisphosphonate therapy should be initiated when T scores are –2.5 or lower (5). To reduce the risk of osteoporosis in high-risk patients, bisphosphonates may be co-administered to patients during long-term treatment with aromatase inhibitors.

In contrast to tamoxifen, aromatase inhibitors are associated with a reduced incidence of thrombosis (6) and endometrial cancer (7), and a reduction in vaginal bleeding. Although the results of early studies suggest that aromatase inhibitors have adverse effects on the cardiovascular system and lipid profiles compared with tamoxifen, these effects are milder or have not been seen when comparing aromatase inhibitors with placebo. This suggests that aromatase inhibitors lack the protective effects found with tamoxifen rather than exhibit true toxicity (8). Increased cardiovascular morbidity or mortality through poor lipid profiles or other mechanisms has not been clearly established in patients treated with aromatase inhibitors compared with tamoxifen or placebo (9). More rigorous study is required in this area because most of the trials were not designed to address cardiac disease.

Aromatase inhibitors also have been used as treatment for premenopausal women with early breast cancer who have chemotherapy-induced amenorrhea. This off-label use should be prescribed with caution because case series have described the resumption of ovarian function following initiation of an aromatase inhibitor regimen (10, 11). Serial monitoring of estradiol and gonadotropin levels to identify women who experience a return of ovarian function may be indicated (10).

In premenopausal women, aromatase inhibitors reduce hypothalamic–pituitary estrogen feedback that leads to increased gonadotropin-releasing hormone (GnRH) secretion, concomitant elevations in luteinizing hormone and follicle-stimulating hormone, and increased ovarian follicular development. The gonadotropin-stimulating action of letrozole has been used off-label in the treatment of patients with ovulatory dysfunction, such as polycystic ovary syndrome, and for increasing the number of ovarian follicles recruited for ovulation in women who are already ovulatory (12, 13). In a meta-analysis of four published trials, including 662 women with polycystic ovary syndrome, pregnancy rates were similar between women treated with clomiphene and women treated with letrozole (relative risk, 1.02; 95% confidence interval, 0.83–1.26) (14). Some have raised concerns about this off-label use because letrozole may disrupt the normal aromatase activity in tissues during early fetal development and can be potentially teratogenic if administered inadvertently during early pregnancy. However, a large study of 911 newborns conceived using letrozole for ovulation induction showed no difference in rates of congenital malformations (15). In addition, the half-life of letrozole (approximately 30–60 hours) is shorter than that of clomiphene citrate (5–7 days) and, thus, should be effectively cleared from the body by the time of embryo implantation, likely preventing a teratogenic effect when used in ovulation induction (14). Possible advantages of letrozole over clomiphene citrate include reduced multiple pregnancies, lower estradiol levels, and an absence of antiestrogenic adverse effects on the endometrium. However, there is no evidence that letrozole is more effective than clomiphene for ovulation induction. Letrozole may have a role in the treatment of clomiphene-resistant patients (16).

The recent demonstration that aromatase is expressed at higher levels in endometriosis implants than in normal endometrium has led to pilot studies using anastrozole co-administered with progestins in patients with endometriosis resistant to conventional medical and surgical therapies (17). These small studies suggest that aromatase inhibitors could reduce endometriosis-associated pelvic pain, whereas the progestin could effectively suppress gonadotropins and reduce ovarian activity. Results of subsequent trials have shown similar efficacy for relief of pelvic pain when aromatase inhibitors were combined with combination oral contraceptives (18), or when aromatase inhibitors were given concomitantly with a GnRH agonist (19). There are no randomized controlled trials comparing aromatase inhibitors with traditional medical treatment for endometriosis. Side effect profiles of aromatase inhibitor regimens (including a progestin or oral contraceptive as add-back therapy) are favorable compared with regimens containing GnRH agonists or danazol. These aromatase inhibitor regimens with add-back progestin or oral contraceptives do not appear to be associated with significant bone loss after 6 months of treatment and may be suitable for long-term use (20). Randomized controlled trials are needed to establish the efficacy and side effects of these regimens.

Aromatase inhibitors appear to be effective as an adjuvant treatment for early-stage and late-stage breast cancer. Their role in chemoprevention of breast cancer in high-risk patients remains to be defined. Side effects of aromatase inhibitors in postmenopausal women are due to estrogen-lowering action at the target tissues and include hot flushes, vaginal dryness, arthralgias, and decreased bone mineral density. Although there are no long-term data with regard to side effects and complications associated with the use of aromatase inhibitors in breast cancer patients, the overall safety profile of aromatase inhibitors is good, with less endometrial and thromboembolic toxicity than tamoxifen. In reproductive-aged women, aromatase inhibitors stimulate gonadotropin secretion and increase ovarian follicular activity. The role of aromatase inhibitors in the treatment of endometriosis and in ovulation induction is still being investigated.

References

1. Buzdar AU, Jonat W, Howell A, Jones SE, Blomqvist CP, Vogel CL, et al. Anastrozole versus megestrol acetate in the treatment of postmenopausal women with advanced breast carcinoma: results of a survival update based on a combined analysis of data from two mature phase III trials. Arimidex Study Group. Cancer 1998;83:1142–52.

2. Baum M, Budzar AU, Cuzick J, Forbes J, Houghton JH, Klijn JG, et al. Anastrozole alone or in combination with tamoxifen versus tamoxifen alone for adjuvant treatment of postmenopausal women with early breast cancer: first results of the ATAC randomised trial. Lancet 2002;359: 2131–9.

3. Bickenbach KA, Jaskowiak N. Aromatase inhibitors: an overview for surgeons. J Am Coll Surg 2006;203:376–89.

4. Howell A, Cuzick J, Baum M, Buzdar A, Dowsett M, Forbes JF, et al. Results of the ATAC (Arimidex, Tamoxifen, Alone or in Combination) trial after completion of 5 years' adjuvant treatment for breast cancer. Lancet 2005;365:60–2.

5. Hillner BE, Ingle JN, Chlebowski RT, Gralow J, Yee GC, Janjan NA, et al. American Society of Clinical Oncology 2003 update on the role of bisphosphonates and bone health issues in women with breast cancer. J Clin Oncol 2003;21: 4042–57.

6. Coombes RC, Hall E, Gibson LJ, Paridaens R, Jassem J, Delozier T, et al. A randomized trial of exemestane after two to three years of tamoxifen therapy in postmenopausal women with primary breast cancer. N Engl J Med 2004; 350:1081–92.

7. Jakesz R, Jonat W, Gnant M, Mittlboeck M, Greil R, Tausch C, et al. Switching of postmenopausal women with endocrine-responsive early breast cancer to anastrozole after 2 years' adjuvant tamoxifen: combined results of ABCSG trial 8 and ARNO 95 trial. Lancet 2005;366:455–62.

8. Conte P, Frassoldati A. Aromatase inhibitors in the adjuvant treatment of postmenopausal women with early breast cancer: Putting safety issues into perspective. Breast J 2007; 13:28–35.

9. Gandhi S, Verma S. Aromatase inhibitors and cardiac toxicity: getting to the heart of the matter. Breast Cancer Res Treat 2007;106:1–9.

10. Smith IE, Dowsett M, Yap YS, Walsh G, Lonning PE, Santen RJ, et al. Adjuvant aromatase inhibitors for early breast cancer after chemotherapy-induced amenorrhoea: caution and suggested guidelines. J Clin Oncol 2006;24:2444–7.

11. Burstein HJ, Mayer E, Patridge AH, O'Kane H, Litsas G, Come SE, et al. Inadvertent use of aromatase inhibitors in patients with breast cancer with residual ovarian function: cases and lessons. Clin Breast Cancer 2006;7:158–61.

12. Fisher SA, Reid RL, Van Vugt DA, Casper RF. A randomized double-blind comparison of the effects of clomiphene citrate and the aromatase inhibitor letrozole on ovulatory function in normal women. Fertil Steril 2002;78:280–5.

13. Bedaiwy MA, Forman R, Mousa NA, Al Inany HG, Casper RF. Cost-effectiveness of aromatase inhibitor co-treatment for controlled ovarian stimulation. Hum Reprod 2006; 21:2838–44.

14. Casper RF. Letrozole versus clomiphene citrate: which is better for ovulation induction? Fertil Steril 2007 June 21. DOI: 10.1016/j.fertnstert.2007.03.094.

15. Tulandi T, Martin J, Al-Fadhli R, Kabli N, Forman R, Hitkari J, et al. Congenital malformations among 911 newborns conceived after infertility treatment with letrozole or clomiphene citrate. Fertil Steril 2006;85:1761–5.

16. Badawy A, Abdel Aal I, Abulatta M. Clomiphene citrate or letrozole for ovulation induction in women with polycystic ovarian syndrome: a prospective randomized trial. Fertil Steril 2007 Jun 18. DOI: 10.1016/j.fertnstert.2007.02.062.

17. Ailawadi RK, Jobanputra S, Kataria M, Gurates B, Bulun SE. Treatment of endometriosis and chronic pelvic pain with letrozole and norethindrone acetate: a pilot study. Fertil Steril 2004;81:290–6.

18. Amsterdam LL, Gentry W, Jobanputra S, Wolf M, Rubin SD, Bulun SE. Anastrazole and oral contraceptives: a novel treatment for endometriosis. Fertil Steril 2005;84:300–4.

19. Soysal S, Soysal ME, Ozer S, Gul N, Gezgin T. The effects of post-surgical administration of goserelin plus anastrozole compared to goserelin alone in patients with severe endometriosis: a prospective randomized trial. Hum Reprod 2004;19:160–7.

20. Attar E, Bulun SE. Aromatase inhibitors: the next generation of therapeutics for endometriosis? Fertil Steril 2006;85: 1307–18.

Aromatase inhibitors in gynecologic practice. ACOG Committee Opinion No. 412. American College of Obstetricians and Gynecologists. Obstet Gynecol 2008;112:405–7.

ISSN 1074-861X

ACOG COMMITTEE OPINION

Number 413 • August 2008

Age-Related Fertility Decline

Committee on Gynecologic Practice

This document reflects emerging clinical and scientific advances as of the date issued and is subject to change. The information should not be construed as dictating an exclusive course of treatment or procedure to be followed.

ABSTRACT: Age is a significant factor influencing a woman's ability to conceive. Social trends have led to deferred childbearing, and an increasing number of women are experiencing age-related infertility and pregnancy loss. Women older than 35 years should receive expedited evaluation and treatment after 6 months of failed attempts to conceive, or earlier if clinically indicated.

American Society for Reproductive Medicine

The American College of Obstetricians and Gynecologists
Women's Health Care Physicians

The number of oocytes in the ovaries declines naturally and progressively through the process of atresia. The maximum complement of oocytes is 6–7 million and exists at 20 weeks of gestation in the female fetus. The number of oocytes decreases to approximately 1–2 million oocytes at birth; 300,000–500,000 at puberty; 25,000 at age 37 years; and 1,000 at age 51 years, the average age of menopause in the United States (1–3). Fecundity declines gradually but significantly beginning approximately at age 32 years, and decreases more rapidly after age 37 years, reflecting primarily a decrease in egg quality in association with a gradual increase in the circulating level of follicle-stimulating hormone (3). The mechanisms involved are poorly understood, but appear to include multiple factors encoded by genes on both the X chromosome and the autosomes (4).

Age alone has an impact on fertility. Historical data suggest that among populations that do not use contraception, fertility rates decrease with increasing age of women (Fig. 1). Because sexual activity also declines with age, it is difficult to separate out the effects of sexual behavior from age. However, a classic French study was able to separate behavioral and age effects by studying normal women with azoospermic husbands undergoing donor insemination. The study found that pregnancy rates decreased progressively with increasing age of the recipient female (5). The cumulative pregnancy rate observed across up to 12 insemination cycles was 74% for women younger than 31 years and decreased to 62% for women aged 31–35 years and to 54% for women older than 35

years (5). A similar trend has been observed in analyses of data derived from in vitro fertilization (IVF) embryo transfer programs in the United States. For the year 2006, the percentage of embryo transfers resulting in live births decreased progressively from 44.9% in women younger than 35 years to 37.3% for women aged 35–37 years, 26.6% for women aged 38–40 years, 15.2% for women aged 41–42 years, and 6.7% for women aged 43–44 years (6). By contrast, in cycles using eggs obtained from healthy, young donors, 54% of transfers resulted in a live birth, regardless of the age of the recipient (6). As age increases, the risks of other disorders that may adversely affect fertility, such as fibroids, tubal disease, and endometriosis, also increase. Women with a history of prior ovarian surgery, chemotherapy, radiation therapy, severe endometriosis, smoking, pelvic infection, or a strong family history of early menopause may be at increased risk for having a premature decline in the size of their follicular pool and their fertility.

The age-related decline in fertility is accompanied by a significant increase in the rates of aneuploidy and spontaneous abortion (7). Autosomal trisomy is the most frequent finding and is related, at least in part, to changes in the meiotic spindle (8) that predispose to nondisjunction (9). Even for morphologically normal embryos selected for transfer in IVF cycles, the prevalence of aneuploidy is high in women of advanced maternal age (10). The fetal loss rate also is significantly higher, even after fetal heart rate motion is detected by transvaginal ultrasonography (11). Whereas 9.9% of women

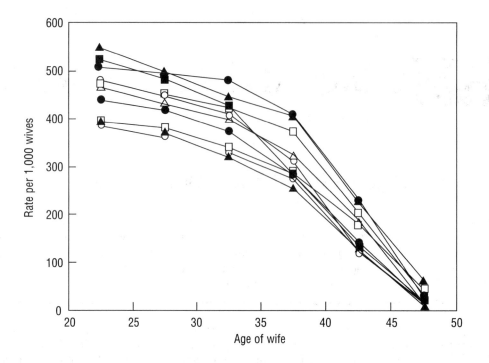

Fig.1. Marital fertility rates by 5-year age groups. The ten populations (in descending order at age 20–24 years) are Hutterites, marriages from 1921–30 (▲); Geneva bourgeoisie, husbands born in 1600–49 (■); Canada, marriages 1700–30 (●); Normandy, marriages 1760–90 (○); Hutterites, marriages before 1921 (□); Tunis, marriages of Europeans 1840–59 (△); Normandy, marriages 1674–1742 (●); Norway, marriages 1874–76 (□); Iran, village marriages, 1940–50 (▲); Geneva bourgeoisie, husbands born before 1600 (○). From Menken J, Trussel J, Larsen U. Age and infertility. Science 1986;233:1389–94. Reprinted with permission from AAAS.

younger than 33 years who conceive during IVF with a fresh embryo transfer experience a pregnancy loss after fetal heart activity is observed, the rate of miscarriage progressively increases to 11.4% for women aged 33–34 years, 13.7% for women aged 35–37 years, 19.8% for women aged 38–40 years, 29.9% for women aged 41–42 years, and 36.6% for women older than age 42 years (11). Therefore, given the anticipated age-related decline in fertility, the increased incidence of disorders that impair fertility, and the higher risk of pregnancy loss, women older than 35 years should receive expedited evaluation and treatment after 6 months of failed attempts to conceive, or earlier if clinically indicated.

In conclusion, fertility in women is closely related to reproductive age and becomes significantly compromised before the onset of perimenopausal menstrual irregularity. Education and enhanced awareness of the impact of age on fertility is essential in counseling the patient who desires pregnancy. Women older than 35 years should receive expedited evaluation and treatment after 6 months of failed attempts to conceive, or earlier if clinically indicated.

References

1. Baker TG. A quantitative and cytological study of germ cells in human ovaries. Proc R Soc Lond B Biol Sci 1963;158: 417–33.

2. Block E. Quantitative morphological investigations of the follicular system in women; variations at different ages. Acta Anat (Basel) 1952;14:108–23.

3. Faddy MJ, Gosden RG, Gougeon A, Richardson SJ, Nelson JF. Accelerated disappearance of ovarian follicles in midlife: implications for forecasting menopause. Hum Reprod 1992;7:1342–6.

4. Simpson JL. Genetic programming in ovarian development and oogenesis. In: Lobo RA, Kelsey J, Marcus R, editors. Menopause: biology and pathobiology. San Diego (CA): Academic Press; 2000. p. 77–94.

5. Schwartz D, Mayaux MJ. Female fecundity as a function of age: results of artificial insemination in 2193 nulliparous women with azoospermic husbands. Federation CECOS. N Engl J Med 1982;306:404–6.

6. Society for Assisted Reproductive Technology. Clinic summary report: all SART member clinics. Birmingham (AL): SART; 2007. Available at: https://www.sartcorsonline.com/rptCSR_PublicMultYear.aspx?ClinicPKID=0. Retrieved March 18, 2008.

7. Newcomb WW, Rodriguez M, Johnson JW. Reproduction in the older gravida. A literature review. J Reprod Med 1991;36:839–45.

8. Battaglia DE, Goodwin P, Klein NA, Soules MR. Influence of maternal age on meiotic spindle assembly in oocytes from naturally cycling women. Hum Reprod 1996;11:2217–22.

9. Pellestor F, Andreo B, Arnal F, Humeau C, Demaille J. Maternal aging and chromosomal abnormalities: new data drawn from in vitro unfertilized human oocytes. Hum Genet 2003;112:195–203.

10. Munne S, Alikani M, Tomkin G, Grifo J, Cohen J. Embryo morphology, developmental rates, and maternal age are correlated with chromosome abnormalities. Fertil Steril 1995;64:382–91.

11. Farr SL, Schieve LA, Jamieson DJ. Pregnancy loss among pregnancies conceived through assisted reproductive technology, United States, 1999-2002. Am J Epidemiol 2007;165:1380–8.

Age-related fertility decline. ACOG Committee Opinion No. 413. American College of Obstetricians and Gynecologists. Obstet Gynecol 2008;112:409–11.

ISSN 1074-861X

ACOG COMMITTEE OPINION

Number 420 • November 2008

Hormone Therapy and Heart Disease

Committee on Gynecologic Practice

This document reflects emerging clinical and scientific advances as of the date issued and is subject to change. The information should not be construed as dictating an exclusive course of treatment or procedure to be followed.

ABSTRACT: The effect of menopausal hormone therapy on coronary heart disease has been the subject of much concern. The Heart and Estrogen/Progestin Replacement Study (HERS) and Women's Health Initiative studies found an increased risk of cardiovascular events with conjugated equine estrogen and medroxyprogesterone acetate use. However, recent evidence suggests that women in early menopause who are in good cardiovascular health are at low risk of adverse cardiovascular outcomes and as such should be considered candidates for the use of conjugated equine estrogen or conjugated equine estrogen and medroxyprogesterone acetate for relief of menopausal vasomotor symptoms. Hormone therapy use should be limited to the treatment of menopausal symptoms at the lowest effective dosage over the shortest duration possible, and continued use should be reevaluated on a periodic basis.

The American College of Obstetricians and Gynecologists
Women's Health Care Physicians

More than two decades of accumulated evidence suggested that women taking estrogen plus progesterone hormone therapy (HT) and estrogen therapy (ET) alone gained protection against coronary heart disease (CHD). Notably criticized, these largely observational studies were confounded by superior cardiovascular health profiles among participants electing to use HT or ET. To assess fully the role of HT and ET for CHD protection among menopausal women, large-scale randomized, controlled clinical trials were begun. Recent evidence suggesting cardioprotective effects of HT and ET has sparked debate regarding the possibility of a "timing hypothesis" (ie, women who recently experienced menopause may be more likely to benefit from HT than women who have been menopausal for a longer period) (1, 2).

Among menopausal women with known CHD, the Heart and Estrogen/Progestin Replacement Study (HERS) examined whether conjugated equine estrogen and medroxyprogesterone acetate altered CHD risk (3). After 4 years of follow-up, the study did not demonstrate an overall reduction in CHD risk. Those receiving conjugated equine estrogen and medroxyprogesterone acetate exhibited a 52% increase in CHD and a 3–4-fold increase in venous thromboem-

bolic events during the first and second years of use.

In 2002, the Women's Health Initiative (WHI), a CHD prevention trial among predominantly healthy menopausal women, published its initial results after 5.2 years of follow-up (4). The study was prematurely terminated because of reports of adverse cardiovascular effects and a worsened global index. Not only did conjugated equine estrogen and medroxyprogesterone acetate not provide protection against CHD, but its use also imparted a 29% increase in CHD-related events (37 versus 30 per 10,000 woman-years) that developed soon after randomization. Notably, most CHD events attributed to conjugated equine estrogen and medroxyprogesterone acetate use were nonfatal myocardial infarctions, and there were no significant differences in overall CHD deaths (hazard ratio (HR): 1.18; 95% CI, 0.70–1.97). Unlike prior randomized studies (5, 6), WHI associated conjugated equine estrogen and medroxyprogesterone acetate use with a 41% increased stroke risk, mostly nonfatal events (29 versus 21 per 10,000 woman-years) that became apparent between the first and second year of use. Consistent with the HERS trial, WHI provided further evidence that conjugated equine estrogen and medroxyprogesterone acetate increased venous thromboembolism and pulmonary embolism risks twofold (venous thromboembolism: 34 versus 16 per 10,000 woman-years; pulmonary embolism: 16 versus 8 per 10,000 woman-years). Time-trend analyses suggested that the risk of CHD and pulmonary embolism began to occur immediately following the initiation of HT. Similar to HERS, the conjugated equine estrogen and medroxyprogesterone acetate arm of the WHI indicated that there was a 26% increase in invasive breast cancer (38 versus 30 per 10,000 woman-years). Benefits associated with conjugated equine estrogen and medroxyprogesterone acetate use in the WHI trial included a 37% reduction in colorectal carcinoma rates (10 versus 16 per 10,000 woman-years) and reduced incidence of hip (10 versus 15 per 10,000 woman-years) and vertebral fractures (9 versus 15 per 10,000 woman-years).

Nearly 2 years later, the conjugated equine estrogen alone study of the WHI was published after a mean of 6.8 years of follow-up, in advance of its designed observation period because of a lack of improvement in CHD risk (the primary outcome) and an increased rate of stroke (7). This conjugated equine estrogen alone trial revealed several notable differences from the initial WHI study publications. No differences in CHD incidence were observed among those receiving conjugated equine estrogen compared with placebo. Although not statistically significant, another notable finding was that invasive breast cancer occurred 23% less frequently in the conjugated equine estrogen alone group compared with the control group (HR=0.77; 95% CI, 0.59–1.01; P=.06). Moreover, no differences were seen in colorectal carcinoma rates. In line with the conjugated equine estrogen and medroxyprogesterone acetate arm of the WHI trial, conjugated equine estrogen alone increased stroke rates by 39% and reduced both hip and vertebral fractures. Although deep vein thrombosis risk was increased (21 versus 15 per 10,000 woman-years), increases in venous thromboembolism and pulmonary embolism risk failed to reach statistical significance. Time-trend analyses demonstrated an increased stroke risk immediately after randomization, but no risk differences could be elucidated for pulmonary embolism or CHD.

Subsequent to the aforementioned studies, the WHI investigators have published several follow-up studies. Consistent with previous reports, analysis directed at extricating the HT effect on CHD risk found superior lipid, insulin, and glucose profiles with conjugated equine estrogen and medroxyprogesterone acetate (8). Subsequent data from the conjugated equine estrogen alone arm suggested an attenuation of venous thromboembolism risk by the exclusion of progestin, yet venous thromboembolism risks were increased with HT use in both the conjugated equine estrogen and conjugated equine estrogen and medroxyprogesterone acetate arms of the study after a longer mean follow-up period (conjugated equine estrogen: 7.1 years; conjugated equine estrogen and medroxyprogesterone acetate: 5.6 years) (9, 10).

Likewise, HT increased the risk of ischemic stroke in both the conjugated equine estrogen and conjugated equine estrogen and medroxyprogesterone acetate arms (11, 12). Overall, the risks associated with long-term primary preventive therapy appeared to outweigh the beneficial effects.

The mean participant age of the WHI trial exceeded 60 years and it has been suggested that the results may not apply to women who recently experienced menopause and for whom treatment would likely be initiated. In an attempt to delineate the impact of age on CHD risk with HT use, WHI data was stratified according to participant age and duration of menopause (13). This study found that the effects of either conjugated equine estrogen or conjugated equine estrogen and medroxyprogesterone acetate on CHD risk might depend, in part, on age at the start of treatment. When analyzed according to treatment type, a trend toward reduced total mortality with conjugated equine estrogen or conjugated equine estrogen and medroxyprogesterone acetate use was noted among those women aged 50–59 years (see Table 1). When individual treatment type data were pooled, total mortality decreased by 30% with conjugated equine estrogen or conjugated equine estrogen and medroxyprogesterone acetate use (95% CI, 0.51–0.96). Whether conjugated equine estrogen or conjugated equine estrogen and medroxyprogesterone acetate administration improves the cardiovascular health of women who recently experienced menopause remains to be determined. Presently, there is insufficient evidence to suggest that long-term conjugated equine estrogen or conjugated equine estrogen and medroxyprogesterone acetate use improves cardiovascular outcomes (1). Nevertheless, recent evidence suggests that women in early menopause who are in good cardiovascular health are at low risk of adverse cardiovascular outcomes and as such should be considered candidates for the use of conjugated equine estrogen or conjugated equine estrogen and medroxyprogesterone acetate for relief of menopausal vasomotor symptoms (2). Ongoing studies, including the Kronos Early Estrogen Prevention Study (KEEPS) are evaluating alterations in surrogate CHD risk markers, including carotid intimal thickness and the accrual of coronary calcium deposition induced by HT, in this case conjugated equine estrogen or transdermal estradiol patches combined with cyclic oral, micronized progesterone.

The WHI Coronary-Artery Calcium Study (WHI-CACS) recently evaluated 1,064 women aged 50–59 years who were previously enrolled in the conjugated equine estrogen arm of WHI (14). Because coronary atherosclerotic plaques have been associated with future CHD risk, the investigators used computed tomography heart imaging to determine the degree of coronary-artery calcium burden. The study results indicated that the overall distribution of coronary-artery calcification scores were lower among those receiving conjugated equine estrogen compared with those receiving placebo (P=.03). Furthermore,

Table 1. Cardiovascular and Global Index Events by Age at Baseline

	Age Group at Randomization									
	50-59 y			**60-69 y**			**70-79 y**			*P* Value for Trend†
	No. of Cases			No. of Cases			No. of Cases			
	Hormone Therapy (n = 4476)	Placebo (n = 4356)	HR (95% CI)*	Hormone Therapy (n = 6240)	Placebo (n = 6122)	HR (95% CI)*	Hormone Therapy (n = 3100)	Placebo (n = 3053)	HR (95% CI)*	
	Combined Trials									
CHD‡	59	61	0.93 (0.65-1.33)	174	178	0.98 (0.79-1.21)	163	131	1.26 (1.00-1.59)	.16
Stroke	44	37	1.13 (0.73-1.76)	156	102	1.50 (1.17-1.92)	127	100	1.21 (0.93-1.58)	.97
Total mortality	69	95	0.70 (0.51-0.96)	240	225	1.05 (0.87-1.26)	237	208	1.14 (0.94-1.37)	.06
Global index§	278	278	0.96 (0.81-1.14)	717	661	1.08 (0.97-1.20)	606	528	1.14 (1.02-1.29)	.09
	CEE Trial									
	CEE (n = 1637)	Placebo (n = 1673)		CEE (n = 2387)	Placebo (n = 2465)		CEE (n = 1286)	Placebo (n = 1291)		
CHD‡	21	34	0.63 (0.36-1.09)	96	106	0.94 (0.71-1.24)	84	77	1.13 (0.82-1.54)	.12
Stroke	18	21	0.89 (0.47-1.69)	84	54	1.62 (1.15-2.27)	66	52	1.21 (0.84-1.75)	.62
Total mortality	34	48	0.71 (0.46-1.11)	129	131	1.02 (0.80-1.30)	134	113	1.20 (0.93-1.55)	.18
Global index§	114	140	0.82 (0.64-1.05)	333	342	1.01 (0.86-1.17)	300	262	1.16 (0.98-1.37)	.01
	CEE + MPA Trial									
	CEE+MPA (n = 2839)	Placebo (n = 2683)		CEE+MPA (n = 3853)	Placebo (n = 3657)		CEE+MPA (n = 1814)	Placebo (n = 1762)		
CHD‡	38	27	1.29 (0.79-2.12)	78	72	1.03 (0.74-1.43)	79	54	1.48 (1.04-2.11)	.70
Stroke	26	16	1.41 (0.75-2.65)	72	48	1.37 (0.95-1.97)	61	48	1.21 (0.82-1.78)	.56
Total mortality	35	47	0.69 (0.44-1.07)	111	94	1.09 (0.83-1.44)	103	95	1.06 (0.80-1.41)	.19
Global index§	164	138	1.10 (0.87-1.38)	384	319	1.15 (0.99-1.34)	306	266	1.13 (0.95-1.33)	.96

Abbreviations: CEE, conjugated equine estrogens; CHD, coronary heart disease; CI, confidence interval; HR, hazard ratio; MPA, medroxyprogesterone acetate.

*Cox regression models stratified according to prior cardiovascular disease and randomization status in the Dietary Modification Trial.

†Test for trend (interaction) using age as continuous (linear) form of categorical coded values. Cox regression models stratified according to active vs placebo and trial, including terms for age and the interaction between trials and age.

‡Defined as CHD death, nonfatal myocardial infarction, or definite silent myocardial infarction (Novacode 5.1 or 5.2).

§Defined as CHD, stroke, pulmonary embolism, breast cancer, colorectal cancer, endometrial cancer for CEE plus MPA trial only, hip fracture, or death from other causes.

Rossouw JE, Prentice RL, Manson JE, Wu L, Barad D, Barnabei VM, et al. Postmenopausal hormone therapy and risk of cardiovascular disease by age and years since menopause. JAMA 2007;297:1465–77. April 4. Copyright © 2007 American Medical Association. All rights reserved.

for those who adhered to the study medication regimen (80% medication adherence for 5 or more years), conjugated equine estrogen use was associated with a significant reduction in the coronary-artery calcification (OR=0.64; 95% CI, 0.46-0.91; *P*=.01). This preliminary evidence, using surrogate outcome markers, needs confirmation of its clinical significance and correlation with clinical outcomes. Nevertheless, it suggests that conjugated equine estrogen therapy may reduce CHD risk factors and may provide cardiovascular protection for select populations of women who experienced menopause recently.

Conclusion

Menopausal HT should not be used for the primary or secondary prevention of CHD at the present. Recent analyses suggest that HT may not increase CHD risk for select populations of women who have experienced menopause recently. Hormone therapy use should be limited to the treatment of menopausal symptoms at the lowest effective dosage over the shortest duration possible and continued use should be reevaluated on a periodic basis. Some women may require extended therapy because of persistent symptoms.

References

1. Barrett-Connor E. Hormones and heart disease in women: the timing hypothesis. Am J Epidemiol 2007;166:506–10.

2. Manson JE, Bassuk SS. Invited commentary: hormone therapy and risk of coronary heart disease why renew the focus on the early years of menopause? Am J Epidemiol 2007;166:511–7.

3. Hulley S, Grady D, Bush T, Furberg C, Herrington D, Riggs B, et al. Randomized trial of estrogen plus progestin for secondary prevention of coronary heart disease in postmenopausal women. Heart and Estrogen/progestin Replacement Study (HERS) Research Group. JAMA 1998; 280(7):605–13.

4. Rossouw JE, Anderson GL, Prentice RL, LaCroix AZ, Kooperberg C, Stefanick ML, et al. Risks and benefits of estrogen plus progestin in healthy postmenopausal women: principal results From the Women's Health Initiative randomized controlled trial. Writing Group for Women's Health Initiative Investigators. JAMA 2002;288(3):321–33.

5. Simon JA, Hsia J, Cauley JA, Richards C, Harris F, Fong J, et al. Postmenopausal hormone therapy and risk of stroke: The Heart and Estrogen-progestin Replacement Study (HERS). Circulation 2001;103:638–42.

6. Grady D, Herrington D, Bittner V, Blumenthal R, Davidson M, Hlatky M, et al. Cardiovascular disease outcomes during 6.8 years of hormone therapy: Heart and Estrogen/progestin Replacement Study follow-up (HERS II). HERS Research Group. JAMA 2002;288:49–57.

7. Anderson GL, Limacher M, Assaf AR, Bassford T, Beresford SA, Black H, et al. Effects of conjugated equine estrogen in postmenopausal women with hysterectomy: the Women's Health Initiative randomized controlled trial. Women's Health Initiative Steering Committee. JAMA 2004;291: 1701–12.

8. Manson JE, Hsia J, Johnson KC, Rossouw JE, Assaf AR, Lasser NL, et al. Estrogen plus progestin and the risk of coronary heart disease. Women's Health Initiative Investigators. N Engl J Med 2003;349:523–34.

9. Curb JD, Prentice RL, Bray PF, Langer RD, Van Horn L, Barnabei VM, et al. Venous thrombosis and conjugated equine estrogen in women without a uterus. Arch Intern Med 2006;166:772–80.

10. Cushman M, Kuller LH, Prentice R, Rodabough RJ, Psaty BM, Stafford RS, et al. Estrogen plus progestin and risk of venous thrombosis. Women's Health Initiative Investigators. JAMA 2004;292:1573–80.

11. Wassertheil-Smoller S, Hendrix SL, Limacher M, Heiss G, Kooperberg C, Baird A, et al. Effect of estrogen plus progestin on stroke in postmenopausal women: the Women's Health Initiative: a randomized trial. WHI Investigators. JAMA 2003 May;289:2673–84.

12. Hendrix SL, Wassertheil-Smoller S, Johnson KC, Howard BV, Kooperberg C, Rossouw JE, et al. Effects of conjugated equine estrogen on stroke in the Women's Health Initiative. WHI Investigators. Circulation 2006;113:2425–34.

13. Rossouw JE, Prentice RL, Manson JE, Wu L, Barad D, Barnabei VM, et al. Postmenopausal hormone therapy and risk of cardiovascular disease by age and years since menopause. JAMA 2007;297:1465–77.

14. Manson JE, Allison MA, Rossouw JE, Carr JJ, Langer RD, Hsia J, et al. Estrogen therapy and coronary-artery calcification. WHI and WHI-CACS Investigators. N Engl J Med 2007;356:2591–602.

Hormone therapy and heart disease. ACOG Committee Opinion No. 420. American College of Obstetricians and Gynecologists. Obstet Gynecol 2008;112:1189–92.

ISSN 1074-861X

ACOG

TECHNOLOGY ASSESSMENT

IN OBSTETRICS AND GYNECOLOGY

NUMBER 5, DECEMBER 2008

(Replaces Technology Assessment No. 3, September 2003)

This Technology Assessment was developed by the ACOG Committee on Gynecologic Practice with the assistance of Daniel Breitkopf, MD, John W. Seeds, MD, and Steven R. Goldstein, MD. This document reflects emerging clinical and scientific advances as of the date issued and is subject to change. The information should not be construed as dictating an exclusive course of treatment or procedure to be followed. Variations in practice may be warranted based on the needs of the individual patient, resources, and limitations unique to the institution or type of practice.

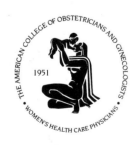

THE AMERICAN COLLEGE
OF OBSTETRICIANS
AND GYNECOLOGISTS
WOMEN'S HEALTH CARE PHYSICIANS

Sonohysterography

ABSTRACT: *The goal of sonohysterography is to visualize the endometrial cavity in more detail than is possible with routine transvaginal ultrasound. The procedure consists of the manual injection of sterile fluid under real-time ultrasonographic imaging. The most common indication for sonohysterography is abnormal uterine bleeding. The procedure should not be performed in a woman who is pregnant or who could be pregnant, or who has a pelvic infection or unexplained pelvic tenderness. Physicians who perform or supervise diagnostic sonohysterography should be skilled in vaginal ultrasonography and transcervical placement of catheters; should have training, experience, and demonstrated competence in gynecologic ultrasonography and sonohysterography; and should keep careful records. Portions of this document were developed jointly with the American College of Radiology and the American Institute of Ultrasound in Medicine.*

Sonohysterography can provide information about the uterus and endometrial cavity. Additional studies may be necessary for a complete diagnosis. Adherence to the following recommendations serves to maximize the diagnostic benefits and safety of sonohysterography.

The clinical aspects of this document include sections addressing indications and contraindications, specifications of the examination, and equipment specifications that were developed collaboratively by the American College of Radiology, the American Institute of Ultrasound in Medicine, and the American College of Obstetricians and Gynecologists and adapted by the American College of Obstetricians and Gynecologists' Committee on Gynecologic Practice. Sections of the document addressing physician qualifications and responsibilities, documentation, quality control, performance improvement, safety, infection control, and patient education are recommendations of the American College of Obstetricians and Gynecologists' Committee on Gynecologic Practice.

Most clinical experience and medical literature to date have focused on the ultrasonographic imaging of the uterus, and specifically the endometrial cavity, using the transcervical injection of sterile fluid. Thus, terms such as saline infusion sonohysterography or simply sonohysterography have been used to describe this technique. The goal of sonohysterography is to visualize the endometrial cavity in more detail than is possible with routine transvaginal ultrasound.

Studies are underway to evaluate fluids other than saline for use in sonohysterography to determine tubal patency, but their use is currently investigational because this application of sonohysterography has not yet been validated.

INDICATIONS AND CONTRAINDICATIONS

The indications for sonohysterography include, but are not limited to, evaluation of

- abnormal uterine bleeding in premenopausal and postmenopausal women
- infertility and habitual abortion
- congenital abnormalities of the uterine cavity
- suspected uterine myomas, polyps, and synechiae
- abnormalities detected on transvaginal ultrasonography, including focal or diffuse endometrial or intracavitary abnormalities
- suboptimally imaged endometrium by transvaginal ultrasonography

The most common indication for sonohysterography is as an adjunct to transvaginal ultrasound in the evaluation of abnormal uterine bleeding in both premenopausal and postmenopausal women.

Sonohysterography should not be performed in a woman who is pregnant or who could be pregnant. This usually is avoided by scheduling the examination in the follicular phase of the menstrual cycle, after the menstrual flow has essentially ceased, but before the patient has ovulated. In a patient with regular menstrual cycles, sonohysterography should, in most cases, be performed by the 10th day of the menstrual cycle. Sonohysterography should not be performed in patients with a pelvic infection or unexplained pelvic tenderness, which could be due to pelvic inflammatory disease. Active vaginal bleeding is not an absolute contraindication to the procedure but may make the interpretation more challenging.

PHYSICIAN QUALIFICATIONS AND RESPONSIBILITIES

Physicians who perform or supervise diagnostic sonohysterography should be skilled in vaginal ultrasonography and transcervical placement of catheters. They should understand the indications, limitations, and possible complications of the procedure. Physicians should have training, experience, and demonstrated competence in gynecologic ultrasonography and sonohysterography. Physicians are responsible for the documentation of the examination, quality control, and patient safety.

SPECIFICATIONS OF THE EXAMINATION

Patient Preparation

The sonohysterography procedure should be fully explained to the patient in advance. Transvaginal ultrasonography is a specialized form of a pelvic examination. Therefore, policies applied locally regarding chaperone or patient privacy issues during a pelvic examination also should be applied during a transvaginal ultrasound examination. Pelvic organ tenderness should be assessed during a preliminary transvaginal ultrasound examination. If adnexal tenderness or pain suspicious for active pelvic infection is found prior to fluid infusion, the examination should be deferred until after an appropriate course of treatment. Although routine use of antibiotic prophylaxis is not recommended, consideration should be given to administering antibiotics based on individual risk factors (eg, in the presence of nontender hydrosalpinges). A pregnancy test is advised when clinically indicated.

Procedure

Preliminary routine transvaginal ultrasonography with measurements of the endometrium and evaluation of the uterus and ovaries should be performed before sonohysterography. A speculum is used to allow visualization of the cervix. The presence of unusual pain, lesions, or purulent vaginal or cervical discharge may require rescheduling the procedure pending further evaluation. After the external os is cleansed, a catheter should be inserted into the cervical canal or uterine cavity or both using aseptic technique. Appropriate sterile fluid should be instilled slowly by means of manual injection under real-time ultrasonographic imaging. Imaging should include real-time scanning of the endometrium and cervical canal.

Images

Appropriate images, in at least two planes, using a high-frequency transvaginal ultrasound probe should be produced and recorded to demonstrate normal and abnormal findings. Precatheterization images should be obtained, including the thickest bilayer endometrial measurement on a sagittal image.

Once the uterine cavity is filled with fluid, representative images with a complete survey of the uterine cavity are obtained as necessary for diagnostic evaluation. If a balloon catheter is used for the examination, images should be obtained at the end of the procedure with the balloon deflated to fully evaluate the endometrial cavity, particularly the cervical canal and lower uterine segment.

Documentation

Appropriate documentation of a sonohysterography examination is essential for clinical care and quality assessment and improvement. An adequate written report should include patient identification, procedural technique, measurements, morphologic descriptions, and interpretation. Images of key findings and written reports from ultrasound examinations are considered part of the medical record and should be documented and stored appropriately. (In *Current Procedural Terminology* [CPT], sonohysterography is referred to as hysterosonography.)

Equipment Specifications

Sonohysterography usually is conducted with a transvaginal transducer. If a patient has an enlarged uterus, additional transabdominal images during infusion may be required to fully evaluate the endometrium. The transducer should be adjusted to operate at the highest clinically appropriate frequency under the ALARA (as low as reasonably achievable) principle.

Quality and Infection Control

Quality control is accomplished through careful record keeping, reliable archiving of reports and images, and clinical correlation with outcomes. Transvaginal transducers always should be covered with a single-use disposable latex or nonlatex cover. However, because no such disposable protective cover is without risk of rupture or defect, transvaginal transducers should undergo appropriate antimicrobial and antiviral reprocessing between patient use.

BIBLIOGRAPHY

Becker E Jr, Lev-Toaff AS, Kaufman EP, Halpern EJ, Edelweiss MI, Kurtz AB. The added value of transvaginal sonohysterography over transvaginal sonography alone in women with known or suspected leiomyoma. J Ultrasound Med 2002; 21:237–47.

Benacerraf BR, Shipp TD, Bromley B. Improving the efficiency of gynecologic sonography with 3-dimensional volumes: a pilot study. J Ultrasound Med 2006;25:165–71.

Bree RL, Bowerman RA, Bohm-Velez M, Benson CB, Doubilet PM, DeDreu S, et al. US evaluation of the uterus in patients with postmenopausal bleeding: a positive effect on diagnostic decision making. Radiology 2000;216:260–4.

Breitkopf DM, Frederickson RA, Snyder RR. Detection of benign endometrial masses by endometrial stripe measurement in premenopausal women. Obstet Gynecol 2004;104:120–5.

Doubilet PM. Society of Radiologists in Ultrasound Consensus Conference statement on postmenopausal bleeding. J Ultrasound Med 2001;20:1037–42.

Dubinsky TJ, Stroehlein K, Abu-Ghazzeh Y, Parvey HR, Maklad N. Prediction of benign and malignant endometrial disease: hysterosonographic-pathologic correlation. Radiology 1999; 210:393–7.

Goldstein RB, Bree RL, Benson CB, Benacerraf BR, Bloss JD, Carlos R, et al. Evaluation of the woman with postmenopausal bleeding: Society of Radiologists in Ultrasound-Sponsored Consensus Conference statement. J Ultrasound Med 2001;20: 1025–36.

Goldstein SR. Use of ultrasonohysterography for triage of perimenopausal patients with unexplained uterine bleeding. Am J Obstet Gynecol 1994;170:565–70.

Hann LE, Gretz EM, Bach AM, Francis SM. Sonohysterography for evaluation of the endometrium in women treated with tamoxifen. AJR Am J Roentgenol 2001;177:337–42.

Laifer-Narin S, Ragavendra N, Parmenter EK, Grant EG. False-normal appearance of the endometrium on conventional transvaginal sonography: comparison with saline hysterosonography. AJR Am J Roentgenol 2002;178:129–33.

Laifer-Narin SL, Ragavendra N, Lu DS, Sayre J, Perrella RR, Grant EG. Transvaginal saline hysterosonography: characteristics distinguishing malignant and various benign conditions. AJR Am J Roentgenol 1999;172:1513–20.

Lev-Toaff AS, Toaff ME, Liu JB, Merton DA, Goldberg BB. Value of sonohysterography in the diagnosis and management of abnormal uterine bleeding. Radiology 1996;201:179–84.

Lindheim SR, Sprague C, Winter TC 3rd. Hysterosalpingography and sonohysterography: lessons in technique. AJR Am J Roentgenol 2006;186:24–9.

Mihm LM, Quick VA, Brumfield JA, Connors AF Jr, Finnerty JJ. The accuracy of endometrial biopsy and saline sonohysterography in the determination of the cause of abnormal uterine bleeding. Am J Obstet Gynecol 2002;186:858–60.

Parsons AK, Lense JJ. Sonohysterography for endometrial abnormalities: preliminary results. J Clin Ultrasound 1993; 21:87–95.

Schwartz LB, Snyder J, Horan C, Porges RF, Nachtigall LE, Goldstein SR. The use of transvaginal ultrasound and saline infusion sonohysterography for the evaluation of asymptomatic postmenopausal breast cancer patients on tamoxifen. Ultrasound Obstet Gynecol 1998;11:48–53.

The American College of Obstetricians and Gynecologists
409 12th Street, SW, PO Box 96920
Washington, DC 20090-6920

Sonohysterography. ACOG Technology Assessment No. 5. American College of Obstetricians and Gynecologists. Obstet Gynecol 2008;112:1467–9.

COMMITTEE ON HEALTH CARE FOR UNDERSERVED WOMEN

COMMITTEE ON HEALTH CARE
FOR UNDERSERVED WOMEN

ACOG COMMITTEE OPINION

Number 361 • February 2007

Breastfeeding: Maternal and Infant Aspects

**Committee on
Health Care for
Underserved
Women**

**Committee on
Obstetric Practice**

*The Committees
would like to thank
Sharon Mass, MD, for
her contributions to
the development of
this document.*

ABSTRACT: Evidence continues to mount regarding the value of breastfeeding for both women and their infants. The American College of Obstetricians and Gynecologists strongly supports breastfeeding and calls on its Fellows, other health care professionals caring for women and their infants, hospitals, and employers to support women in choosing to breastfeed their infants. Obstetrician–gynecologists and other health care professionals caring for pregnant women should provide accurate information about breastfeeding to expectant mothers and be prepared to support them should any problems arise while breastfeeding.

**The American College
of Obstetricians
and Gynecologists**
*Women's Health Care
Physicians*

Research in the United States and throughout the world indicates that breastfeeding and human milk provide benefits to infants, women, families, and society. In 1971, only 24.7% of mothers left the hospital breastfeeding. Since then, breastfeeding initiation rates have been increasing because of a growing awareness of the advantages of breast milk over formula, but they have not yet reached the goal set by the U.S. Public Health Service for Healthy People 2010 (1). In 2005, 72.9% of new U.S. mothers initiated breastfeeding (2). Although this is close to the target rate of 75% in the early postpartum period, there is still a long way to go to achieve target breastfeeding rates of 50% at 6 months and 25% at 12 months (1). Improvement in breastfeeding initiation rates has been uneven as women attempt to overcome practical obstacles. Women and infants who could benefit most from breastfeeding are often within population groups (geographic, racial, economic, and educational) with low rates of breastfeeding. Education and support services can improve rates among these as well as other women. Breastfeeding education and support are an economical investment for health plans and employers because there are lower rates of illness among infants who are breastfed.

Breastfeeding is the preferred method of feeding for newborns and infants. Nearly every woman can breastfeed her child. Exceptions are few and include those women who take street drugs or do not control alcohol use, have an infant with galactosemia, are infected with human immunodeficiency virus (HIV) or human T-cell lymphotropic virus type I or type II, and have active untreated tuberculosis or varicella or active herpes simplex virus with breast lesions (3, 4).

The American College of Obstetricians and Gynecologists strongly supports breastfeeding and calls upon its Fellows, other health care professionals caring for women and their infants, hospitals, and employers to support women in choosing to breastfeed their infants. All should work to facilitate the continuation of breastfeeding in the workplace and public facilities. Health care professionals have a wide range of opportunities to serve as a primary resource to the public and their patients regarding the benefits of breastfeeding and the knowledge, skills, and support needed for successful breastfeeding (5). In addition to providing supportive clinical care for their own patients, obstetrician–gynecologists should be in the forefront of fostering changes in the public environment that will support breastfeeding, whether through change in hospital practices, through community efforts, or through supportive legislation.

The advice and encouragement of the obstetrician–gynecologist during preconception, prenatal, postpartum, and interconception care are critical in making the decision to breastfeed. Good hospital practices surrounding childbirth are significant factors in enabling women to breastfeed. Health care providers should be aware that the giving of gift packs with formula to breastfeeding women is commonly a deterrent to continuation of breastfeeding (4). A professional recommendation of the care and feeding products in the gift pack is implied. For this reason, physicians may conclude that noncommercial educational alternatives or gift packs without health-related items are preferable. After discharge, the obstetrician–gynecologist's office should be a resource for 24-hour assistance, or provide links to other resources in the community. Breastfeeding problems, including breast and nipple pain, should be evaluated and treated promptly. Clinical breast examinations are recommended for breastfeeding women. If any mass or abnormality is detected, it should be fully evaluated.

Contraception is an important topic for early discussion and follow-up for breastfeeding women. Women should be encouraged to consider their future plans for contraception and childbearing during prenatal care and be given information and services that will help them meet their goals. Options that should be explained in detail include nonhormonal methods, hormonal methods, and the lactational amenorrhea method.

Women should be supported in integrating breastfeeding into their daily lives in the community and in the workplace to enable them to continue breastfeeding as long as possible. Maintaining milk supply depends largely on frequency and adequacy of maternal stimulation through breastfeeding and through pumping when mother and baby are separated. The American College of Obstetricians and Gynecologists recommends that exclusive breastfeeding be continued until the infant is approximately 6 months old. A longer breastfeeding experience is, of course, beneficial. The professional objectives are to encourage and enable as many women as possible to breastfeed and to help them continue as long as possible (3, 4). Physicians' offices can set the example in encourag-

ing and welcoming breastfeeding through staff training, office environment, awareness and educational materials, and supportive policies (3, 4).

More detailed information on breastfeeding and practical strategies for support can be found in the *ACOG Clinical Review* "Special Report From ACOG, Breastfeeding: Maternal and Infant Aspects" and in the American Academy of Pediatrics and ACOG resource, *Breastfeeding Handbook for Physicians* (3, 4).

References

1. U.S. Department of Health and Human Services. Increase in the proportion of mothers who breastfeed their babies. In: Healthy people 2010: objectives for improving health. 2nd ed. Washington, DC: U.S. Government Printing Office; 2000. p. 16–46.

2. Centers for Disease Control and Prevention. Breastfeeding: data and statistics: breastfeeding practices—results from the 2005 National Immunization Survey. Atlanta (GA): CDC. Available at: http://www.cdc.gov/breastfeeding/data/NIS_data/data_2005.htm. Retrieved November 14, 2006.

3. American Academy of Pediatrics, American College of Obstetricians and Gynecologists. Breastfeeding handbook for physicians. Elk Grove Village (IL): AAP; Washington, DC: ACOG; 2006.

4. American College of Obstetricians and Gynecologists. Breastfeeding: maternal and infant aspects. Special report from ACOG. ACOG Clin Rev 2007;12(suppl):1S–16S.

5. American College of Obstetricians and Gynecologists. Breastfeeding. ACOG Executive Board Statement. Washington, DC; ACOG: 2003. Available at: http://www.acog.org/departments/underserved/breastfeedingStatement.pdf. Retrieved November 1, 2006.

Breastfeeding: maternal and infant aspects. ACOG Committee Opinion No. 361. American College of Obstetricians and Gynecologists. Obstet Gynecol 2007;109:479–80.

ISSN 1074-861X

ACOG COMMITTEE OPINION

Number 391 • December 2007

Health Literacy

**Committee on
Health Care for
Underserved
Women**

*The Committee would
like to thank Maureen
Phipps, MD and Eve
Espey, MD for their
assistance in the devel-
opment of this docu-
ment.*

This information should
not be construed as dic-
tating an exclusive course
of treatment or procedure
to be followed.

ABSTRACT: According to the U.S. Department of Health and Human Services, health literacy is the degree to which individuals have the capacity to obtain, process, and understand basic health information and services needed to make appropriate health decisions. The American College of Obstetricians and Gynecologists (ACOG) is committed to the promotion of health literacy for all. The purpose of this committee opinion is to outline the complex issues surrounding health literacy and offer strategies for increasing health literacy in clinical practice.

Each day, patients encounter the challenges of interpreting health information presented by health care providers and making decisions based on their understanding of that information. Engaging patients in difficult health care decisions requires that patients listen, understand, read, and analyze information about their health; in essence, we expect patients to be health literate. Health literacy relates to the individual's capacity to obtain, interpret, and understand health information and health care services, and to use such information and services in ways that are health enhancing (1). Because situations regarding an individual's health are often complex and the language used to explain them is often specialized, years of education or reading ability do not necessarily translate into adequate health literacy. Health care professionals often use technical language specific to their areas of expertise with the expectation that people who are not familiar with the professional jargon will understand the meaning of complex ideas and terms. Even individuals highly trained in other fields may have difficulty understanding health information and instructions about their care.

The problem of limited health literacy is widespread. Whereas approximately 10% of Americans have low general literacy (skills necessary to perform simple and everyday literacy activities) (2), 50% of adults are estimated to have marginal to low health literacy skills (3). Multiple studies have demonstrated the seriousness of the problem. Adults with low health literacy are at increased risk for

hospitalization (4), encounter more barriers to receiving necessary health care services (5), and are less likely to understand medical advice that can affect their disease progression (6, 7). Given the scope of the problem, the U.S. Department of Health and Human Services identified several target areas in the *Healthy People 2010* objectives to improve health communication, which incorporated goals related to health literacy and cultural competency (8).

Our current health care delivery system assumes a high level of health literacy. Individuals are expected to understand and apply verbal information, including diagnosis, medical advice, and treatment; have access to and use a computer and the Internet; calculate and interpret numerical data; and interpret graphs and visual information. Patients are expected to be articulate and accurate about their conditions and symptoms, as well as to have sophisticated decision-making skills. Often those individuals with the greatest health care needs have limited skills to synthesize and interpret health information (9).

Patients with specific educational or linguistic challenges also may have limited health literacy. "Nonadherence" to therapeutic and medication recommendations, often pejoratively labeled "noncompliance," can lead to poor outcomes and may be more related to limited health literacy than to patients' indifference toward their health. It may be that nonadherent patients are not following recommendations because they do not understand what is expected of them.

**The American College
of Obstetricians
and Gynecologists**
*Women's Health Care
Physicians*

This is often the case with older patients and those with limited English proficiency or no English proficiency. In the United States, people aged 65 years and older consume 30% of prescriptions and 40% of over-the-counter drugs (10). Senior citizens often have low literacy skills and, therefore, poor comprehension of information on medication labels (2, 11). Low health literacy also may be a problem for immigrant populations for whom English is a second language (12). According to a recent ACOG project focusing on language access solutions in California, 25% of ACOG Fellows reported that one quarter of their patients have limited English proficiency and 38% reported an increase in patients with limited English proficiency during the past 5 years (13).

When the concept of health literacy is taken into consideration, all facets of the medical encounter, including patient education, are important to improving the patient's and the public's health. Patient health literacy includes the ability to understand instructions on prescription drug bottles, appointment slips, patient education brochures, and consent forms, as well as the ability to negotiate complex health care systems.

Multiple factors affect a patient's understanding of health information, including the physician's health knowledge and communication skills, the demands of the situation in which the health information is being conveyed, and time constraints for delivering the information. Other factors include the patient's ability to communicate effectively with the health care team, to manage and commit to his or her own health care, and to comprehend complex concepts such as probability and risk. Understanding the unique capabilities of the individual patient will make the information provided by the health care team more accessible for both the patient and his or her family members. When patients can obtain, process, and understand basic health information, they are more likely to make the most appropriate health decisions.

Responsibility for recognizing and addressing the problem of limited health literacy lies with all entities in the health care profession, from the primary health care team to public health care systems. Making information understandable and accessible to all patients involves a systematic approach toward health literacy in physicians' offices, hospitals, clinics, national organizations, local health organizations, advocacy organizations, medical and allied health professional schools, residency training programs, and continuing medical education programs. Community-based partnerships to help understand and address the needs of the local community and consumer health information organizations to focus on the issue of health literacy are needed in the effort to improve health literacy.

The American College of Obstetricians and Gynecologists supports the following guidelines (adapted from the U.S. Department of Health and Human Services Office of Disease Prevention and Health Promotion Guide to Health Literacy) (14):

1. Tailor speaking and listening skills to individual patients.
   - Ask open-ended questions using the words "what" or "how" to start the sentence. (For example: "What questions do you have for me?" rather than "Do you have any questions?")
   - Use medically trained interpreters.
   - Check for comprehension by asking patients to restate the health information given in their own words. (For example: "Tell me how you are going to take this medication.")
   - Encourage staff and colleagues to obtain training in patient communication and use of plain language along with cultural competency (15). (For more information, please refer to the corresponding chapters in the ACOG publication *Special Issues in Women's Health.*)

2. Tailor health information to the intended user.
   - When developing health information, make sure it reflects the target group's age, social and cultural diversity, language, and literacy skills.
   - When developing information and services, include the target group in the development (pretest) and implementation (posttest) phases to ensure the program is effective.
   - In preparing health information, consider cultural factors and the influence of culture on health, including race, ethnicity, language, nationality, religion, age, gender, sexual orientation, income level, and occupation.

3. Develop written materials.
   - Keep the messages simple.
   - Limit the number of messages (general guideline is four main messages).
   - Focus on action. Give specific recommendations based on behavior rather than the medical principle. (For example, "Take a warm water bath two times a day" instead of "Sitz baths may help healing.")
   - Use the active instead of the passive voice. (For example, "These pills can make you sick to your stomach" instead of "Nausea may be caused by this medication.")
   - Use familiar language and avoid jargon. (For example, "Your may have itching" instead of "You may experience pruritus on your genitalia.")
   - Use visual aids such as drawings or models for key points. Make sure the visual messages are culturally relevant.
   - Use at least 12-point font to make the messages easy to read.
   - Leave plenty of white space around margins and between sections.

Resources

The following online resources may be helpful to physicians in finding resources for patients:

American College of Obstetricians and Gynecologists
www.acog.org/goto/patients

American Academy of Family Physicians
www.familydoctor.org

National Center for Farmworker Health, Inc.
www.ncfh.org/00_nc_rc_pateduc.php

Oregon Health and Science University
www.ohsu.edu/library/patiented/links.shtml#lowlit

U.S. Department of Health and Human Services
www.womenshealth.gov/espanol

University of Washington, Harborview Medical Center
www.ethnomed.org

The resources listed here are for information purposes only. Referral to these web sites does not imply the endorsement of ACOG. Further, ACOG does not endorse any commercial products that may be advertised or available from these organizations or on these web sites. This list is not meant to be comprehensive. The exclusion of a source or web site does not reflect the quality of that source or web site. Please note that web sites and URLs are subject to change without notice.

References

1. Joint Committee on National Health Education Standards. National health education standards: achieving health literacy. Atlanta (GA): American Cancer Society; 1995. Available at: http://eric.ed.gov/ERICDocs/data/ericdocs2sql/content_ storage_01/0000019b/80/14/24/30.pdf. Retrieved September 7, 2007.

2. National Center for Education Statistics. National Assessment of Adult Literacy (NAAL): a first look at the literacy of America's adults in the 21st century. Washington, DC:U.S. Department of Education: 2005. Available at: http://nces.ed.gov/NAAL/PDF/2006470.PDF. Retrieved July 27,2007.

3. Paasche-Orlow MK, Parker RM, Gazmararian JA, Nielsen-Bohlman LT, Rudd RR. The prevalence of limited health literacy. J Gen Intern Med 2005;20:175–84.

4. Baker DW, Parker RM, Williams MV, Clark WS. Health literacy and the risk of hospital admission. J Gen Intern Med 1998;13:791–8.

5. Williams MV, Parker RM, Baker DW, Parikh NS, Pitkin K, Coates WC, et al. Inadequate functional health literacy among patients at two public hospitals. JAMA 1995;274:1677–82.

6. Williams MV, Baker DW, Parker RM, Nurss JR. Relationship of functional health literacy to patients' knowledge of their chronic disease. A study of patients with hypertension and diabetes. Arch Intern Med 1998;158:166–72.

7. Gazmararian JA, Baker DW, Williams MV, Parker RM, Scott TL, Green DC, et al. Health literacy among Medicare enrollees in a managed care organization. JAMA 1999;281:545–51.

8. U.S. Department of Health and Human Services. Health communication. In: Healthy people 2010: objectives for improving health (part A). 2nd ed. Washington, DC: HHS, 2000. p. 11-1–11-25. Available at: http://www.healthypeople.gov/Document/pdf/Volume1/11HealthCom.pdf. Retrieved July 27, 2007.

9. Parker RM, Gazmararian JA, Health literacy: essential for health communication. J Health Commun. 2003;8(suppl 1):116–8.

10. Salom IL, Davis K. Prescribing for older patients: how to avoid toxic drug reactions. Geriatrics 1995;50:37–40, 43; discussion 44–5.

11. Morell RW, Park DC, Poon LW. Effects of labeling techniques on memory and comprehension of prescription information in young and old adults. J Gerontol 1990;45:166–72.

12. Guerra C, Krumholz M, Shea J. Literacy and knowledge, attitudes and behavior about mammography in Latinas. J of Health Care of the Poor and Underserved 2005;16:152–66.

13. American College of Obstetricians and Gynecologists. Strengthening communication capacity: California's OB/GYNs enhance language access for limited English proficient patients. Sacramento (CA): ACOG District IX;2006. Available at: http://www.acog.org/acog_districts/dist9/2006LanguageAccessSolutionsReport.pdf. Retrieved July 27, 2007.

14. U.S. Department of Health and Human Services. Quick guide to health literacy. Washington, DC: HHS; 2006. Available at: http://www.health.gov/communication/literacy/quickguide/Quickguide.pdf. Retrieved July 27, 2007.

15. American College of Obstetricians and Gynecologists. Special issues in women's health. Washington DC: ACOG; 2005.

Health literacy. ACOG Committee Opinion No. 391. American College of Obstetricians and Gynecologists. Obstet Gynecol 2007;110:1489–91.

ISSN 1074-861X

ACOG COMMITTEE OPINION

Number 414 • August 2008

Human Immunodeficiency Virus and Acquired Immunodeficiency Syndrome and Women of Color

Committee on Health Care for Underserved Women

The Committee would like to thank Diana Contreras, MD; Maureen Phipps, MD; and Heather Watts, MD; for their assistance in the development of this document.

This information should not be construed as dictating an exclusive course of treatment or procedure to be followed.

The American College of Obstetricians and Gynecologists
Women's Health Care Physicians

ABSTRACT: In the United States, women of color (primarily African-American and Hispanic women) comprise most new cases of human immunodeficiency virus (HIV) infection and acquired immunodeficiency syndrome (AIDS) among women. Most women of color acquire the disease from heterosexual contact, often from a partner who has undisclosed risk factors for HIV infection. Safe-sex practices, especially consistent condom use, must be emphasized for all women, particularly for women of color. A combination of testing, education, and brief behavioral interventions can help reduce the rate of HIV infection and its complications among women of color.

Impact on Women

Early in the epidemic, human immunodeficiency virus (HIV) and acquired immunodeficiency syndrome (AIDS) were rarely diagnosed in women of all ages, including adolescents. They now account for a growing proportion of new HIV and AIDS diagnoses. In 1985, women represented 8% of HIV/AIDS cases but by 2005 accounted for 27% of the estimated 45,669 new diagnoses of HIV/AIDS (1). (According to this Centers for Disease Control and Prevention report and others cited in this document, HIV/AIDS is defined as infection with or without AIDS.) Heterosexual contact was the source of 80% of these new infections (2). Many women are unaware of their male partners' risk factors for HIV infection (such as unprotected sex with multiple partners, sex with men, or injection drug use).

Of great concern is the number of young women with HIV infection and AIDS. In 2005, 36% of HIV/AIDS cases in the 13–19 year-old age group were in girls, and 28% of HIV/AIDS cases were in women in the 20–24 year-old age group (3). Of women with AIDS, 71% received the diagnosis between the ages of 25 years and 44 years, suggesting that many were infected as adolescents (2).

Older women also represent an increasing proportion of HIV diagnoses. Between 1999 and 2004, the number of women with newly diagnosed HIV infections from heterosexual activity increased by 4.8% per year among women aged 40–49 years, 6.8% per year among women aged 50–59 years, and 4.1% per year among women older than 60 years (4).

There are many reasons why women infected with HIV may have difficulty obtaining health care, including lack of financial resources and health insurance, lack of transportation, and the added responsibility of caring for others, especially children. Lack of access to effective therapy has been associated with an increase in the mortality rate (5).

Women of Color

Women of color comprise most new cases of HIV infection among women in the United States, accounting for more than 80% of new diagnoses in women (2). The rate of AIDS diagnosis for African-American and Hispanic women is disproportionate to the population. Data from the 2005 census show that African-American and Hispanic women represent 24% of all U.S. women; however, both groups accounted for 82% of the estimated total of AIDS diagnoses for women (6). Among African-American women, the rate of AIDS diagnosis is 23 times the rate for white women and four times the rate for Hispanic women (6).

Mortality rates in these groups remain very high. In 2004, HIV infection was the leading cause of death for African-American women aged 25–34 years and the third leading cause of death for African-American women aged 35–44 years (7). HIV was the fourth leading cause of death for Hispanic women aged 35–44 years (7). The death rate from HIV infection among African-American women was higher than for all other groups, both male and female, except for African-American men.

The reasons for the increased risk of HIV infection among women of color are multifactorial. Among African-American and Hispanic women living with HIV/AIDS, the most common exposures were high-risk heterosexual contact and injection drug use (6, 8). The higher prevalence of HIV infection in the African-American community makes women more likely to be exposed to HIV. African-American men who have sex with men have the highest incidence and prevalence of HIV among any ethnic or behavioral risk group in the United States (9). Among men who have sex with men, African-American men are more likely than European-American men to also have sex with women and less likely to disclose their behavior to friends and partners, putting women unknowingly at risk (10). Poverty and economic uncertainty may make it more difficult for women to feel empowered to negotiate condom use and other safe-sex practices (11). In addition, among African-American women, increased rates of other genital infections, including bacterial vaginosis and trichomoniasis vaginalis, may increase susceptibility to HIV infection (12, 13). Racially associated differences in allele frequencies of genes that influence both susceptibility to and progression of HIV infection may increase the risk of HIV infection in African-American women (14).

Many Hispanic women are hesitant to discuss condom use with their partners because they fear emotional or physical abuse or the abandonment of financial support (15). In addition, traditional gender roles hinder open communication of safe-sex practices with male partners (8). Hispanic men and women both are disproportionately likely to face serious socioeconomic barriers, including lack of education, unemployment, inadequate health insurance, and limited access to health care that can increase the risk of HIV infection (8). Language also can be a barrier for this population, thus, culturally and linguistically focused interventions are warranted (8).

Community-Based Interventions for Women of Color

Among women of color, adolescent girls are at high risk of HIV infection. In a recent Centers for Disease Control and Prevention report, among African-American adolescents across 33 states aged 13–24 years in whom HIV/AIDS is diagnosed, approximately 41% are female (16). In a randomized controlled trial that evaluated efficacy of an HIV prevention intervention among sexually experienced African-American adolescent girls, it was found that a gender-tailored and culturally appropriate intervention can enhance HIV-preventive behavior and skills, such as condom use, and psychosocial mediators, such as knowledge, attitudes, and partner communication (17). In another randomized controlled trial it was found that skill-based HIV and sexually transmitted disease (STD) interventions can reduce sexual risk-taking behavior and rates of STDs among African-American and Latino adolescent girls in clinic settings (18). In other studies, similar findings also have been found in which preventive interventions among adolescents that take a cultural approach and take place in groups with ethnic similarity are effective (19, 20). Despite these findings, more intensive interventions and research designed specifically for African-American and Latino adolescents that demonstrate efficacy in reducing behavior associated with HIV risk are necessary (17).

Behavioral interventions targeting adult women of color also are crucial to decrease rates of morbidity and mortality from HIV and AIDS. In a randomized controlled trial testing the efficacy of HIV and STD risk-reduction interventions for African-American women in primary care settings it was found that brief single-session, one-on-one, or group skill-building interventions may reduce behavior associated with HIV and STD risk, such as unprotected sex, and also may reduce rates of STD morbidity (21). In another randomized controlled trial it was found that three small-group sessions decreased rates of chlamydial and gonorrheal infection among Mexican-American and African-American women at high risk of STDs (22). In multiple studies, it has been shown that brief behavioral interventions, including personalized risk assessment, training in negotiation skills, and identification of specific targets for behavioral change, can increase rates of condom use and decrease rates of acquisition of sexually transmitted infections compared with education alone among women of color (21, 23–25). Many interventions range in duration from 1–32 hours, using individual or small-group counseling (26). These findings suggest that targeted and focused programs can be effective among women of color.

Recommendations

Human immunodeficiency virus infection and AIDS can affect all women, but women of color are acquiring the disease at higher rates than other groups. Most of these women are acquiring the disease from heterosexual contact, often from a partner who has undisclosed risk factors for HIV infection. Prevention and early recognition are critical, but women of color are not benefiting maximally from these two interventions. Several approaches can reduce the rate of HIV infection in women and optimize health:

- The American College of Obstetricians and Gynecologists (ACOG) recommends routine HIV screening for women aged 19–64 years and targeted screening for women with risk factors outside of that age range, for example, sexually active adolescents younger than 19 years. Ideally, opt-out HIV screening should be performed, in which the patient is notified that HIV testing will be performed as a routine part of gynecologic and obstetric care, unless the patient declines testing (27). (Please refer to ACOG's Committee Opinion No. 411 "Routine Human Immunodeficiency Virus Screening" for more information.) Obstetrician–gynecologists should be aware of and comply with legal requirements regarding HIV testing in their jurisdictions (28). The National HIV/AIDS Clinicians' Consultation Center at the University of California-San Francisco maintains an online compendium of state HIV testing laws that can be a useful resource (www.nccc.ucsf.edu/).

- Women whose confirmatory testing yields positive results and, therefore, are infected with HIV should receive or be referred for appropriate clinical and supportive care. Early recognition allows initiation of optimal care and medication, when indicated, as well as education to prevent transmission.

- Safe-sex practices, especially consistent condom use, must be emphasized for all women, particularly for women of color. Multiple studies have shown that behavioral interventions can increase rates of condom use, reduce risk-taking behavior, and decrease rates of acquisition of sexually transmitted infections. Most interventions are designed to be provided by nurses or peer educators and often are available through local health departments or community organizations.

- More intensive interventions and research designed specifically for women of color that demonstrate efficacy in reducing behavior associated with HIV risk are necessary.

- Health care providers are urged to identify resources in their community for training of office staff in risk reduction interventions for women of color or for referral of women to these programs.

A combination of testing, education and brief behavioral interventions can help reduce the rate of HIV infection and its complications among women of color.

References

1. Epidemiology of HIV/AIDS—United States, 1981-2005. Centers for Disease Control and Prevention (CDC). MMWR Morb Mortal Wkly Rep 2006;55:589–92.

2. Centers for Disease Control and Prevention. HIV/AIDS surveillance report, 2005. Vol. 17. Rev ed. Atlanta (GA): CDC; 2007. Available at: http://www.cdc.gov/hiv/topics/surveillance/resources/reports/2005report/pdf/2005SurveillanceReport.pdf. Retrieved January 7, 2008.

3. Centers for Disease Control and Prevention. HIV/AIDS surveillance in adolescents and young adults (through 2005). Atlanta (GA): CDC; 2007. Available at: http://www.cdc.gov/hiv/topics/surveillance/resources/slides/adolescents/index.htm. Retrieved January 7, 2008.

4. Espinoza L, Hall HI, Hardnett F, Selik RM, Ling Q, Lee LM. Characteristics of persons with heterosexually acquired HIV infection, United States 1999–2004. Am J Public Health 2007;97:144–9.

5. McFarland W, Chen S, Hsu L, Schwarcz S, Katz M. Low socioeconomic status is associated with a higher rate of death in the era of highly active antiretroviral therapy, San Francisco. J Acquir Immun Defic Syndr 2003;33:96–103.

6. Centers for Disease Control and Prevention. HIV/AIDS among women. CDC HIV/AIDS Fact Sheet. Atlanta (GA): CDC; 2007. Available at: http://www.cdc.gov/hiv/topics/women/resources/factsheets/pdf/women.pdf. Retrieved March 12, 2008.

7. Heron M. Deaths: leading causes for 2004. Natl Vital Stat Rep 2007;56:1–95.

8. Centers for Disease Control and Prevention. HIV/AIDS among Hispanics/Latinos. CDC HIV/AIDS Fact Sheet. Atlanta (GA): CDC; 2007. Available at: http://www.cdc.gov/hiv/resources/factsheets/PDF/hispanic.pdf. Retrieved March 21, 2008.

9. HIV prevalence, unrecognized infection, and HIV testing among men who have sex with men—five U.S. cities, June 2004–April 2005. Centers for Disease Control and Prevention (CDC) MMWR Morb Mortal Wkly Rep 2005; 54:597–601.

10. O'Leary A, Fisher HH, Purcell DW, Spikes PS, Gomez CA. Correlates of risk patterns and race/ethnicity among HIV-positive men who have sex with men. AIDS Behav 2007; 11:706–15.

11. Whyte J 4th. Sexual assertiveness in low-income African American women: unwanted sex, survival, and HIV risk. J Community Health Nurs 2006;23:235–44.

12. Forna FM, Fitzpatrick L, Adimora AA, McLellan-Lemal E, Leone P, Brooks JT, et al. A case–control study of factors associated with HIV infection among black women. J Natl Med Assoc 2006;98:1798–804.

13. Hallfors DD, Iritani BJ, Miller WC, Bauer DJ. Sexual and drug behavior patterns and HIV and STD racial disparities: the need for new directions. Am J Public Health 2007;97: 125–32.

14. Winkler C, An P, O'Brien SJ. Patterns of ethnic diversity among the genes that influence AIDS. Human Mol Genet 2004;13(supp):R9–19.

15. Suarez-Al-Adam M, Raffaelli M, O'Leary A. Influence of abuse and partner hypermasculinity on the sexual behavior of Latinas. AIDS Educ Prev 2000;12:263–74.

16. Racial/ethnic disparities in diagnoses of HIV/AIDS—33 states, 2001-2005. Centers for Disease Control and Prevention (CDC). MMWR Morb Mortal Wkly Rep 2007;56:189–93.

17. DiClemente RJ, Wingood GM, Harrington KF, Lang DL, Davies SL, Hook EW 3rd, et al. Efficacy of an HIV prevention intervention for African American adolescent girls: a randomized controlled trial. JAMA 2004;292:171–9.

18. Jemmott JB 3rd, Jemmott LS, Braverman PK, Fong GT. HIV/STD risk reduction interventions for African American and Latino adolescent girls at an adolescent med-

icine clinic: a randomized controlled trial. Arch Pediatr Adolesc Med 2005;159:440–9.

19. Mullen PD, Ramirez G, Strouse D, Hedges LV, Sogolow E. Meta-analysis of the effects of behavioral HIV prevention interventions on the sexual risk behavior of sexually experienced adolescents in controlled studies in the United States. J Acquir Immune Defic Syndr 2002;30(suppl 1):S94–S105.

20. Salazar LF, DiClemente RJ, Wingood GM, Crosby RA, Harrington K, Davies S, et al. Self-concept and adolescents' refusal of unprotected sex: a test of mediating mechanisms among African American girls. Prev Sci 2004;5:137–49.

21. Jemmott LS, Jemmott JB 3rd, O'Leary A. Effects on sexual risk behavior and STD rate of brief HIV/STD prevention interventions for African American women in primary care settings. Am J Public Health 2007;97:1034–40.

22. Shain RN, Piper JM, Newton ER, Perdue ST, Ramos R, Champion JD, et al. A randomized, controlled trial of a behavioral intervention to prevent sexually transmitted disease among minority women. N Engl J Med 1999;340: 93–100.

23. Kamb ML, Fishbein M, Douglas JM Jr, Rhodes F, Rogers J, Bolan G, et al. Efficacy of risk-reduction counseling to prevent human immunodeficiency virus and sexually transmitted diseases: a randomized controlled trial. Project RESPECT Study Group JAMA 1998;280:1161–7.

24. Ehrhardt AA, Exner TM, Hoffman S, Silberman I, Leu C-S, Miller S, et al. A gender-specific HIV/STD risk reduction intervention for women in a health care setting: short- and long-term results of a randomized clinical trial. AIDS Care 2002;14:147–61.

25. Centers for Disease Control and Prevention. Health disparities in HIV/AIDS, viral hepatitis, sexually transmitted diseases, and tuberculosis in the United States: issues, burden, and response. Atlanta (GA): CDC; 2007. Available at: http://www.cdc.gov/nchhstp/healthdisparities/docs/NCH HSTPHealthDisparitiesReport1107.pdf. Retrieved January 7, 2008.

26. Lyles CM, Kay LS, Crepaz N, et al. Best-evidence interventions: findings from a systematic review of HIV behavioral interventions for the US populations at high risk, 2000–2004. HIV/AIDS Prevention Research Synthesis Team. Am J Public Health 2007;97:133–43.

27. Branson BM, Handsfield HH, Lampe MA, Janssen RS, Taylor AW, Lyss SB, et al. Revised recommendations for HIV testing of adults, adolescents, and pregnant women in health-care settings. Centers for Disease Control and Prevention (CDC) MMWR Recomm Rep 2006;55(RR14): 1–17; quiz CE1–4.

28. Human immunodeficiency virus. ACOG Committee Opinion No. 389. American College of Obstetricians and Gynecologists. Obstet Gynecol 2007;110:1473–8.

Human immunodeficiency virus and acquired immunodeficiency syndrome and women of color. ACOG Committee Opinion No. 414. American College of Obstetricians and Gynecologists. Obstet Gynecol 2008;112:413–6.

ISSN 1074-861X

ACOG COMMITTEE OPINION

Number 416 • September 2008   *(Replaces No. 308, December 2004)*

The Uninsured

Committee on Health Care for Underserved Women

The Committee on Health Care for Underserved Women would like to thank Kerry M. Lewis, MD, and Virginia C. Leslie, MD, for their assistance in the development of this document.

This information should not be construed as dictating an exclusive course of treatment or procedure to be followed.

The American College of Obstetricians and Gynecologists
Women's Health Care Physicians

ABSTRACT: The United States is one of the few industrialized nations in the world that do not guarantee health care for their populations. Access to health care for all women is of paramount concern to obstetrician–gynecologists and the American College of Obstetricians and Gynecologists. Pregnant women and infants are among the most vulnerable populations in the United States and the American College of Obstetricians and Gynecologists believes that providing them with full insurance coverage and access to health care must be a primary step in the process of providing coverage for all individuals within the U.S. borders. Health care professionals can play a pivotal role in improving access to needed health care by helping society and our political representatives understand the importance of broadening health insurance coverage.

The United States is one of the few industrialized nations in the world that do not guarantee health insurance for their populations. Of the 30 countries in the Organization of Economic Cooperation and Development, only Mexico and Turkey have a higher uninsured rate than the United States (1). There are more than 17 million uninsured women (aged 18–64 years) in the United States. This number has increased by 1.2 million since 2004, with one half of this growth occurring among low-income women (2). The number of women in the United States who are uninsured grew three times faster than the number of men without health insurance during the late 1990s and early 2000s (3). In 2006, one in five women of childbearing age—totaling 12.6 million women—was uninsured, showing no improvement from 2005 and accounting for 27% of all uninsured Americans (4). Nearly eight out of ten uninsured women (79%) are in families with at least one part-time or full-time worker (2). Most uninsured women do not qualify for Medicaid, do not have access to employer-sponsored plans, and cannot afford individual policies. Access to health care also is affected by other barriers, including health literacy and cultural differences along with proximity to health care facilities and lack of transportation. Women who are young and low-income are particularly at risk of being uninsured, as are women of color, especially Latina women (2). Most low income uninsured women are not eligible for public programs but cannot afford private coverage (5). This is a problem for both U.S and non-U.S. citizens.

Effect of Lack of Insurance on Women's Reproductive Health and Health Care

Having health insurance does not guarantee good health, but not having insurance is guaranteed to put Americans at higher risk for poor health outcomes and economic hardship. Acquiring health insurance reduces mortality rates for the uninsured by 10–15% (6). The uninsured receive less preventive care, receive diagnoses at more advanced disease stages, and, once diseases are diagnosed, tend to receive less therapeutic care (7). Lack of health insurance may affect women's health in the following ways:

- Uninsured pregnant women receive fewer prenatal care services than their insured counterparts (1) (a total of 18% of uninsured pregnant women reported that they did not receive some needed medical care versus 7.6% of privately insured and 8.1% of Medicaid-enrolled pregnant women [8]).
- Uninsured pregnant women are more likely to experience an adverse maternal outcome (1).

- Uninsured newborns are more likely to experience adverse health outcomes and are more likely to die than insured newborns (1).
- Uninsured women with breast cancer have a 30–50% higher risk of dying than insured women with breast cancer (1).
- Uninsured women's options for contraception are limited (9).
- Uninsured women aged 18–64 years are three times less likely to have had a needed Pap test in the past 3 years (10). This contributes to a 60% greater risk of late-stage diagnosis of cervical cancer among uninsured women compared with insured women (11).

Uninsured Non-U.S. Citizens

As efforts to expand coverage are pursued, assessing the coverage needs of low-income non-citizen adults, who have a high uninsured rate caused by limited access to both private and public coverage, will be an important consideration (12). Following the 1996 welfare reform law, almost all legal immigrants became ineligible for federally matched Medicaid coverage during their first 5 years of residence in the United States. Undocumented immigrants and temporary immigrants generally are ineligible for Medicaid regardless of their length of residence in the country, a restriction that has been in place before welfare reform.

The Capacity of the Health Care System to Serve the Uninsured

The cost of uncompensated care is staggering; in 2004, it was estimated to be $40.7 billion. Most uncompensated care expenses are incurred by hospitals, where services are the most costly. In 2001, hospitals spent 63% of total costs in uncompensated care. Office-based physicians and direct care programs or clinics accounted for 18% and 19% of uncompensated costs, respectively (13). A 2001 Commonwealth Fund study found that the value of care provided by academic health centers to those who were unable to pay for their services increased as a percentage of gross patient revenues by more than 40% in the past decade (14). The number of patients treated at hospitals who are unable to pay is increasing as the number of uninsured individuals grows, threatening the financial viability of some institutions.

The proportion of private physicians providing care to the uninsured is decreasing and those who provide such care are spending less time doing so (15). Specifically, the number of physicians providing any care to individuals unable to pay decreased from 71.5% in 2001 to 68.2% in 2005 (15). A combination of higher office expenses, including professional liability insurance, and stagnant insurance payments reduces the ability of physicians to provide uncompensated care.

Covering the Uninsured

In recent years, there has been bipartisan interest in broadening access to health coverage to the nearly 47 million uninsured Americans. Although there has been relatively little activity at the federal level, a handful of states have recently adopted or are considering adopting proposals to expand coverage. States are using a combination of strategies, such as expanding public programs to cover most children in a state, mandating employers to cover all workers or contribute to a public financing pool, and requiring all individuals to carry health insurance with subsidies for those with lower incomes.

Massachusetts and Vermont passed laws in 2006 to achieve nearly universal coverage as well as address cost and quality. On April 12, 2006, Massachusetts enacted legislation requiring that individuals have health insurance and that the government provide subsidies to ensure affordability (16). Vermont's law, which includes access to subsidized or low-cost insurance, relies on voluntary participation. Approximately 21 states introduced universal coverage bills in 2007 (17).

Conclusion

Access to health care for all women is a paramount concern of the American College of Obstetricians and Gynecologists (see box). Pregnant women and infants are among the most vulnerable populations in the United States and the American College of Obstetricians and Gynecologists believes that providing them with full insurance coverage and access to care must be a priority. Lack of health care coverage creates access issues that affect women, practitioners, and the health care system as a whole. A change in our currently fragmented health care system is warranted to expand coverage to the millions of uninsured individuals within the U.S. borders. Health

---

Principles for Reform of the U.S. Health Care System
January 2007

PREAMBLE: Health care coverage for all is needed to facilitate access to quality health care, which will in turn improve the individual and collective health of society.

1. Health care coverage for all is needed to ensure quality of care and to improve the health status of Americans.

2. The health care system in the U.S. must provide appropriate health care to all people within the U.S. borders, without unreasonable financial barriers to care.

3. Individuals and families must have catastrophic health coverage to provide protection from financial ruin.

4. Improvement of health care quality and safety must be the goal of all health interventions, so that we can assure optimal outcomes for the resources expended.

(continued)

Principles for Reform of the U.S. Health Care System
January 2007 *(continued)*

5. In reforming the health care system, we as a society must respect the ethical imperative of providing health care to individuals, responsible stewardship of community resources, and the importance of personal health responsibility.

6. Access to and financing for appropriate health services must be a shared public/private cooperative effort, with a system which will allow individuals/employers to purchase additional services or insurance.

7. Cost management by all stakeholders, consistent with achieving quality health care, is critical to attaining a workable, affordable and sustainable health care system.

8. Less complicated administrative systems are essential to reduce costs, and increase efficiency.

9. Sufficient funds must be available for research (basic, clinical, translational, and health services), medical education, and comprehensive health information technology infrastructure and implementation.

10. Sufficient funds must be available for public health and other essential medical services to include, but not be limited to, preventive services, trauma care and mental health services.

11. Comprehensive medical liability reform is essential to ensure access to quality health care.

American Academy of Family Physicians, American Academy of Orthopaedic Surgeons, American College of Cardiology, American College of Emergency Physicians, American College of Obstetricians and Gynecologists, American College of Osteopathic Family Physicians, American College of Physicians, American College of Surgeons, American Medical Association, American Osteopathic Association. Principles for reform of the U.S. health care system. Leawood (KS): AAFP; Rosemont (IL): AAOS; Washington, DC: ACC; Irving (TX): ACEP; Washington, DC: ACOG; Arlington Heights (IL): ACOFP; Philadelphia (PA): ACP; Chicago (IL): ACS; Chicago (IL): AMA; Chicago (IL): AOA; 2007. Available at: http://www.acponline.org/pressroom/health_reform.pdf. Retrieved June 10, 2008.

---

professionals can play a pivotal role in improving access to needed health care by helping society understand the importance of universal health care access. For a listing of resources on the topic of the uninsured, go to www.acog.org/goto/underserved.

References

1. Institute of Medicine. Insuring America's health: principles and recommendations. Washington, DC: National Academies Press; 2004.

2. Henry J. Kaiser Family Foundation.Women's health insurance coverage: December 2007. Menlo Park (CA): KFF; 2007. Available at: http://www.kff.org/womenshealth/upload/6000 _06.pdf. Retrieved June 10, 2008.

3. Lambrew JM. Diagnosing disparities in health insurance for women: a prescription for change. New York (NY): The Commonwealth Fund; 2001. Available at: http://www.commonwealthfund.org/usr_doc/lambrew_disparities_493.pdf?section=4039. Retrieved June 10, 2008.

4. March of Dimes. Census data on uninsured women and children. Washington (DC): MOD; 2007. Available at: http://www.marchofdimes.com/Census.pdf. Retrieved June 10, 2008.

5. Henry J. Kaiser Family Foundation. Characteristics of the uninsured: who is eligible for public coverage and who needs help affording coverage? Kaiser Commission on Medicaid and the Uninsured. Washington, DC: KFF; 2007. Available at: http://www.kff.org/uninsured/upload/7613.pdf. Retrieved June 10, 2008.

6. Henry J. Kaiser Family Foundation. Sicker and poorer: the consequences of being uninsured. A review of the research on the relationship between health insurance, health, work, income, and education. Kaiser Commission on Medicaid and the Uninsured. Washington, DC: KFF; 2002. Available at: http://www.kff.org/uninsured/upload/Full-Report.pdf. Retrieved June 10, 2008.

7. American College of Physicians–American Society of Internal Medicine. No health insurance? It's enough to make you sick. Philadelphia (PA): ACP-ASIM; 1999.

8. Bernstein AB. Insurance status and use of health services by pregnant women. Washington, DC: Alpha Center; 1999. Available at: http://www.marchofdimes.com/files/bernstein_paper.pdf. Retrieved June 10, 2008.

9. Sonfield A, Gold RB. New study documents major strides in drive for contraceptive coverage. Guttmacher Rep Public Policy 2004;7(2):4–5, 14.

10. Ayanian JZ, Weissman JS, Schneider EC, Ginsburg JA, Zaslavsky AM. Unmet health needs of uninsured adults in the United States. JAMA 2000;284:2061–9.

11. Ferrante JM, Gonzalez EC, Roetzheim RG, Pal N, Woodard L. Clinical and demographic predictors of late-stage cervical cancer. Arch Fam Med 2000;9:439–45.

12. Henry J. Kaiser Family Foundation. Health insurance coverage and access to care for low-income non-citizen adults. Kaiser Commission on Medicaid and the Uninsured. Washington, DC: KFF; 2007. Available at: http://www.kff.org/uninsured/upload/7651.pdf. Retrieved June 10, 2008.

13. Henry J. Kaiser Family Foundation. The cost of care for the uninsured: what do we spend, who pays, and what would full coverage add to medical spending? Issue update. Kaiser Commission on Medicaid and the Uninsured. Washington, DC: KFF; 2004. Available at: http://www.kff.org/uninsured/upload/The-Cost-of-Care-for-the-Uninsured-What-Do-We-Spend-Who-Pays-and-What-Would-Full-Coverage-Add-to-Medical-Spending.pdf. Retrieved June 10, 2008.

14. The Commonwealth Fund. A shared responsibility: academic health centers and the provision of care to the poor and uninsured. A report of The Commonwealth Fund Task Force on Academic Health Centers. New York (NY): Commonwealth Fund; 2001. Available at: http://www.commonwealthfund.org/usr_doc/AHC_indigentcare_443.pdf?section=4039. Retrieved June 10, 2008.

15. Center for Studying Health System Change. A growing hole in the safety net: physician charity care declines again.

Tracking Report No. 13. Washington, DC: HSC; 2006. Available at: http://www.hschange.com/CONTENT/826/826. pdf. Retrieved June 10, 2008.

16. Henry J. Kaiser Family Foundation. Massachusetts health care reform plan: an update. Kaiser Commission on Medicaid and the Uninsured. Washington, DC: KFF; 2007. Available at: http://www.kff.org/uninsured/upload/7494-02.pdf. Retrieved June 10, 2008.

17. National Conference of State Legislatures. Health reform bills. Denver (CO): NCSL; 2007. Available at: http://www.ncsl.org/programs/health/universalhealth2007.htm. Retrieved June 10, 2008.

The uninsured. ACOG Committee Opinion No. 416. American College of Obstetricians and Gynecologists. Obstet Gynecol 2008;112: 731–4.

ISSN 1074-861X

COMMITTEE ON OBSTETRIC PRACTICE

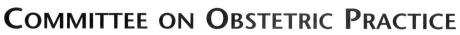

COMMITTEE ON OBSTETRIC PRACTICE

ACOG COMMITTEE OPINION

Number 376 • August 2007

Nalbuphine Hydrochloride Use for Intrapartum Analgesia

Committee on Obstetric Practice

This document reflects emerging clinical and scientific advances as of the date issued and is subject to change. The information should not be construed as dictating an exclusive course of treatment or procedure to be followed.

ABSTRACT: Safety concerns have been raised regarding the use of nalbuphine hydrochloride during labor. The American College of Obstetricians and Gynecologists finds data are insufficient to recommend any changes in nalbuphine hydrochloride administration at this time.

Nalbuphine hydrochloride (formerly marketed as Nubain) is a synthetic opioid agonist–antagonist analgesic commonly used for intrapartum analgesia. Concerns for fetal safety have been raised by one pharmaceutical company that no longer manufactures this agent (www.fda.gov/medwatch/safety/2005/aug_PI/Nubain_PI.pdf). To date there are insufficient data to support these concerns or to recommend any change in the administration of this medication for analgesia in labor.

Nalbuphine hydrochloride use for intrapartum analgesia. ACOG Committee Opinion No. 376. American College of Obstetricians and Gynecologists. Obstet Gynecol 2007;110:449.

ISSN 1074-861X

The American College of Obstetricians and Gynecologists
Women's Health Care Physicians

ACOG COMMITTEE OPINION

Number 379 • September 2007

Management of Delivery of a Newborn With Meconium-Stained Amniotic Fluid

Committee on Obstetric Practice

This document reflects emerging clinical and scientific advances as of the date issued and is subject to change. The information should not be construed as dictating an exclusive course of treatment or procedure to be followed.

ABSTRACT: In accordance with the new guidelines from the American Academy of Pediatrics and the American Heart Association, all infants with meconium-stained amniotic fluid should no longer routinely receive intrapartum suctioning. If meconium is present and the newborn is depressed, the clinician should intubate the trachea and suction meconium and other aspirated material from beneath the glottis.

In 2006, the American Academy of Pediatrics and the American Heart Association published new guidelines on neonatal resuscitation (1). The most significant impact these new guidelines have on obstetricians relates to the management of delivery of a newborn with meconium-stained amniotic fluid. Previously, management of a newborn with meconium-stained amniotic fluid included suctioning of the oropharynx and nasopharynx on the perineum after the delivery of the head but before the delivery of the shoulders (intrapartum suctioning). Current evidence does not support this practice because routine intrapartum suctioning does not prevent or alter the course of meconium aspiration syndrome (1).

The Committee on Obstetric Practice agrees with the recommendation of the American Academy of Pediatrics and the American Heart Association that all infants with meconium-stained amniotic fluid should no longer routinely receive intrapartum suctioning. If meconium is present and the newborn is depressed, the clinician should intubate the trachea and suction meconium or other aspirated material from beneath the glottis. If the newborn is vigorous, defined as having strong respiratory efforts, good muscle tone, and a heart rate greater than 100 beats per minute, there is no evidence that tracheal suctioning is necessary. Injury to the vocal cords is more likely to occur when attempting to intubate a vigorous newborn.

Reference

1. 2005 American Heart Association (AHA) guidelines for cardiopulmonary resuscitation (CPR) and emergency cardiovascular care (ECC) of pediatric and neonatal patients: pediatric basic life support. American Heart Association. Pediatrics 2006;117:e989–1004.

Management of delivery of a newborn with meconium-stained amniotic fluid. ACOG Committee Opinion No. 379. American College of Obstetricians and Gynecologists. Obstet Gynecol 2007;110:739.

ISSN 1074-861X

The American College of Obstetricians and Gynecologists
Women's Health Care Physicians

ACOG **COMMITTEE OPINION**

Number 381 • October 2007

Subclinical Hypothyroidism in Pregnancy

Committee on Obstetric Practice

This document reflects emerging clinical and scientific advances as of the date issued and is subject to change. The information should not be construed as dictating an exclusive course of treatment or procedure to be followed.

ABSTRACT: Subclinical hypothyroidism is diagnosed in asymptomatic women when the thyroid-stimulating hormone level is elevated and the free thyroxine level is within the reference range. Thyroid hormones, specifically thyroxine, are essential for normal fetal brain development. However, data indicating fetal benefit from thyroxine supplementation in pregnant women with subclinical hypothyroidism currently are not available. Based on current literature, thyroid testing in pregnancy should be performed on symptomatic women and those with a personal history of thyroid disease or other medical conditions associated with thyroid disease (eg, diabetes mellitus). Without evidence that identification and treatment of pregnant women with subclinical hypothyroidism improves maternal or infant outcomes, routine screening for subclinical hypothyroidism currently is not recommended.

The American College of Obstetricians and Gynecologists

Women's Health Care Physicians

Subclinical hypothyroidism is diagnosed in asymptomatic women when the thyroid-stimulating hormone (TSH) level is elevated and the free thyroxine (T_4) level is within the reference range. During pregnancy, the diagnosis of thyroid abnormalities is confused by significant but reversible changes in maternal thyroid physiology that lead to alterations in thyroid function tests during gestation. These changes are related to estrogen-mediated increases in maternal thyroid-binding protein, structural homology between TSH and human chorionic gonadotropin, and a relative decrease in availability of iodide during pregnancy (1). There are gestational age-specific normograms and thresholds for evaluating thyroid status during pregnancy (2–4).

Thyroid hormones, specifically T_4, are essential for normal fetal brain development (5). Before 12 weeks of gestation, a time when the fetal thyroid begins to concentrate iodine and synthesize T_4, the fetus is entirely dependent on maternal transfer of thyroid hormones. Brain development begins during this period of fetal dependency in the first trimester and continues throughout pregnancy and on into infancy. In the case of pregnant women who are iodine-deficient, in which thyroxine production in both mother and fetus is insufficient throughout pregnancy, the impact on neurodevelopment of offspring can be dramatic (6). In women with overt hypothyroidism (elevated TSH and low

free T_4 levels), T_4 supplementation during pregnancy also has been associated with improved pregnancy outcomes. However, data indicating fetal benefit from T_4 supplementation in pregnant women with subclinical hypothyroidism are not currently available.

Interest in thyroid disease in pregnancy, especially subclinical hypothyroidism, has escalated in part because of reports suggesting that variously defined thyroid deficiency (including both overt and subclinical disease) during pregnancy results in impaired neurodevelopment in offspring (7, 8). Further, other reports have associated subclinical hypothyroidism with preterm delivery (3, 9). These findings have led some national societies as well as public interest groups to recommend routine thyroid screening during pregnancy (10). The rationale for routine screening of pregnant women is tied both to the prevalence of subclinical hypothyroidism and the potential benefits of treatment during pregnancy. The prevalence of subclinical hypothyroidism could be anticipated to be between 2% and 5% of women screened, depending on the TSH and free T_4 level thresholds applied, and this represents most women who would be identified with thyroid deficiency through routine screening (3). According to criteria established by The U.S. Preventive Services Task Force, before recommending screening of asymptomatic individuals, there must be demonstrated improvement in important health outcomes of those individuals identified through screening (11, 12). As stated previously, benefit of treatment to either mother or fetus has not yet been demonstrated in pregnant women with subclinical hypothyroidism.

Based on current literature, thyroid testing in pregnancy should be performed on symptomatic women and those with a personal history of thyroid disease or other medical conditions associated with thyroid disease (eg, diabetes mellitus). In these women, it is most appropriate to assess TSH levels first and then evaluate other thyroid functions if the TSH level is abnormal. Women with established overt thyroid disease (hyperthyroidism or hypothyroidism) should be appropriately treated to maintain a euthyroid state throughout pregnancy and during the postpartum period. Without evidence that identification and treatment of pregnant women with subclinical hypothyroidism improves maternal or infant outcomes, routine screening for subclinical hypothyroidism is not currently recommended.

References

1. Glinoer D, de Nayer P, Bourdoux P, Lemone M, Robyn C, van Steirteghem A, et al. Regulation of maternal thyroid during pregnancy. J Clin Endocrinol Metab 1990;71: 276–87.

2. Dashe JS, Casey BM, Wells CE, McIntire DD, Byrd EW, Leveno KJ, et al. Thyroid-stimulating hormone in singleton and twin pregnancy: importance of gestational age-specific reference ranges. Obstet Gynecol 2005;106:753–7.

3. Casey BM, Dashe JS, Wells CE, McIntire DD, Byrd W, Leveno KJ, et al. Subclinical hypothyroidism and pregnancy outcomes. Obstet Gynecol 2005;105:239–45.

4. Casey BM, Dashe JS, Spong CY, McIntire DD, Leveno KJ, Cunningham GF. Perinatal significance of isolated maternal hypothyroxinemia identified in the first half of pregnancy. Obstet Gynecol 2007;109:1129–35.

5. Morreale de Escobar G, Obregon MJ, Escobar del Rey F. Is neuropsychological development related to maternal hypothyroidism or to maternal hypothyroxinemia? J Clin Endocrinol Metab 2000;85:3975–87.

6. Glinoer D. Pregnancy and iodine. Thyroid 2001;11:471–81.

7. Haddow JE, Palomaki GE, Allan WC, Williams JR, Knight GJ, Gagnon J, et al. Maternal thyroid deficiency during pregnancy and subsequent neuropsychological development of the child. N Engl J Med 1999;341:549–55.

8. Pop VJ, Kuijpens JL, van Baar AL, Verkerk G, van Son MM, de Vijlder JJ, et al. Low maternal free thyroxine concentrations during early pregnancy are associated with impaired psychomotor development in infancy. Clin Endocrinol 1999;50:149–55.

9. Stagnaro-Green A, Chen X, Bogden JD, Davies TF, Scholl TO. The thyroid and pregnancy: a novel risk factor for very preterm delivery. Thyroid 2005;15:351–7.

10. Gharib H, Tuttle RM, Baskin HJ, Fish LH, Singer PA, McDermott MT. Subclinical thyroid dysfunction: a joint statement on management from the American Association of Clinical Endocrinologists, the American Thyroid Association, and The Endocrine Society. Consensus Statement #1. American Association of Clinical Endocrinologists; American Thyroid Association; The Endocrine Society. Thyroid 2005;15:24–8; response 32–3.

11. Harris RP, Helfand M, Woolf SH, Lohr KN, Mulrow CD, Teutsch SM, et al. Current methods of the US Preventive Services Task Force: a review of the process. Methods Work Group, Third US Preventive Services Task Force. Am J Prev Med 2001;20(suppl):21–35.

12. Surks MI, Ortiz E, Daniels GH, Sawin CT, Col NF, Cobin RH, et al. Subclinical thyroid disease: scientific review and guidelines for diagnosis and management. JAMA 2004; 291:228–38.

Subclinical hypothyroidism in pregnancy. ACOG Committee Opinion No. 381. American College of Obstetricians and Gynecologists. Obstet Gynecol 2007;110:959–60.

ISSN 1074-861X

ACOG COMMITTEE OPINION

Number 382 • October 2007

Fetal Monitoring Prior to Scheduled Cesarean Delivery

Committee on Obstetric Practice

This document reflects emerging clinical and scientific advances as of the date issued and is subject to change. The information should not be construed as dictating an exclusive course of treatment or procedure to be followed.

ABSTRACT: There are insufficient data to determine the value of fetal monitoring prior to scheduled cesarean delivery in patients without risk factors.

With the increasing rate of scheduled cesarean deliveries in the United States, clinicians and hospitals must decide whether there is need to determine fetal status prior to scheduled cesarean delivery. At the present time there are insufficient data to determine the value of fetal monitoring, either by electronic fetal heart rate monitoring or by ultrasound, prior to scheduled cesarean delivery in patients without risk factors. The decision to monitor the fetus prior to scheduled cesarean delivery should be individualized. Presence of fetal heart tones prior to surgery should be documented.

Fetal monitoring prior to scheduled cesarean delivery. ACOG Committee Opinion No. 382. American College of Obstetricians and Gynecologists. Obstet Gynecol 2007;110:961.

ISSN 1074-861X

The American College of Obstetricians and Gynecologists
Women's Health Care Physicians

ACOG COMMITTEE OPINION

Number 394 • December 2007   *(Replaces No. 386, November 2007)*

Cesarean Delivery on Maternal Request

Committee on Obstetric Practice

This document reflects emerging clinical and scientific advances as of the date issued and is subject to change. The information should not be construed as dictating an exclusive course of treatment or procedure to be followed.

ABSTRACT: Cesarean delivery on maternal request is defined as a primary cesarean delivery at maternal request in the absence of any medical or obstetric indication. A potential benefit of cesarean delivery on maternal request is a decreased risk of hemorrhage for the mother. Potential risks of cesarean delivery on maternal request include a longer maternal hospital stay, an increased risk of respiratory problems for the baby, and greater complications in subsequent pregnancies, including uterine rupture and placental implantation problems. Cesarean delivery on maternal request should not be performed before gestational age of 39 weeks has been accurately determined unless there is documentation of lung maturity. Cesarean delivery on maternal request should not be motivated by the unavailability of effective pain management. Cesarean delivery on maternal request is not recommended for women desiring several children, given that the risks of placenta previa, placenta accreta, and the need for gravid hysterectomy increase with each cesarean delivery.

The American College of Obstetricians and Gynecologists
Women's Health Care Physicians

Cesarean delivery on maternal request is defined as a primary cesarean delivery at maternal request in the absence of any medical or obstetric indication. Cesarean delivery rates in the United States are at the highest levels ever, with more than 1.2 million cesarean deliveries (30.2% of live births) performed in 2005 (1). The incidence of cesarean delivery on maternal request and its contribution to the overall increase in the cesarean delivery rate are not known, but it is estimated that 2.5% of all births in the United States are cesarean delivery on maternal request (2).

Cesarean delivery on maternal request is not a well-recognized clinical entity, and there are no accurate means of reporting it for research studies, coding, or reimbursement. There are few studies that directly compare the intended mode of delivery (ie, cesarean delivery on maternal request or planned vaginal delivery). Most of the current knowledge is based on indirect analyses that compare elective cesarean deliveries without labor (instead of cesarean delivery on maternal request) with the combination of vaginal deliveries and unplanned and emergency cesarean deliveries (instead of planned vaginal deliveries) or outcomes of actual modes of delivery.

At the National Institutes of Health State-of-the-Science Conference on Cesarean

Delivery on Maternal Request in 2006, a panel of experts was charged with reviewing the available literature and expert opinions on the subject (2). A systematic literature review of 1,406 recent articles was conducted to evaluate the relevance of existing studies on cesarean delivery on maternal request and the quality of evidence. The panel concluded that the available information comparing the risks and benefits of cesarean delivery on maternal request and planned vaginal delivery does not provide the basis for a recommendation for either mode of delivery. The panel identified the best information available on the short-term and long-term risks and benefits of cesarean delivery on maternal request and planned vaginal delivery for both the mother and her baby.

Benefits and Risks of Cesarean Delivery on Maternal Request Compared With Planned Vaginal Delivery

Maternal Outcomes

Potential short-term maternal benefits of planned vaginal delivery included a shorter maternal length of hospital stay, lower infection rates, fewer anesthetic complications, and higher breastfeeding initiation rates. However, at 3 months and 24 months after delivery, breastfeeding rates did not differ by mode of delivery (3, 4).

Potential short-term maternal benefits of planned cesarean delivery include a decreased risk of postpartum hemorrhage and transfusion, fewer surgical complications, and a decrease in urinary incontinence during the first year after delivery. Analysis of stress urinary incontinence at 2 years (3) and 5 years after delivery (5) showed no difference by mode of delivery. The benefit of a planned cesarean delivery may be eliminated by advanced maternal age and increased body mass index (5).

Maternal outcomes that favored neither delivery route include postpartum pain, pelvic pain, postpartum depression, fistula, anorectal function, sexual function, pelvic organ prolapse, subsequent stillbirth, and maternal mortality. Evidence for thromboembolism was conflicting. Potential risks of cesarean delivery on maternal request include greater complications in subsequent pregnancies, such as uterine rupture, placenta previa, placenta accreta, bladder and bowel injuries, uterine rupture, and the need for hysterectomy. A recent Canadian study of primiparous women with singleton pregnancies showed an increased risk of postpartum cardiac arrest, wound hematoma, hysterectomy, major puerperal infection, anesthetic complications, venous thromboembolism, and hemorrhage requiring hysterectomy in patients who had a planned primary cesarean delivery (6). These are also factors that may be influenced by parity and planned family size. Uterine scars put women at increased risk for uterine rupture in subsequent pregnancies. Although there is no difference between planned cesarean delivery or planned vaginal delivery in risk of peripartum hysterectomy in a woman's first delivery, there is a significant increased risk of placenta previa, placenta accreta, placenta previa with accreta, and the need for gravid hysterectomy after a woman's second cesarean delivery (Table 1). This emphasizes the need to consider the mother's total number of planned or expected pregnancies if cesarean delivery on maternal request is discussed during her first pregnancy, realizing that many pregnancies are unplanned.

Neonatal Outcomes

Potential neonatal benefits of planned vaginal delivery include a lower risk of respiratory problems, fewer problems with iatrogenic prematurity, and shorter length of hospital stay. There are limited studies on cesarean delivery on maternal request and neonatal outcomes, so literature on elective cesarean delivery without labor has been evaluated. The risk of respiratory morbidity, including transient tachypnea of the newborn, respiratory distress syndrome, and persistent pulmonary hypertension, is higher for elective cesarean delivery compared with vaginal delivery when delivery is earlier than 39–40 weeks of gestation (7, 8). The literature on elective cesarean delivery without labor also shows an increased rate of complications related to prematurity, including respiratory symptoms, other neonatal adaptation problems such as hypothermia and hypoglycemia, and neonatal intensive care unit admissions, for infants delivered by cesarean delivery before 39 weeks of gestation (2). Because of these potential complications, cesarean delivery on maternal request should not be performed before gestational age of 39 weeks has been accurately determined unless there is documentation of lung maturity.

Potential neonatal benefits of planned cesarean delivery include lower fetal mortality; lower newborn infection rate; reduced risk of intracranial hemorrhage diagnosis, neonatal asphyxia, and encephalopathy; and fewer birth injuries. In epidemiologic models, cesarean delivery on maternal request by 40 weeks of gestation would reduce fetal mortality because planned vaginal delivery could occur at up to 42 weeks of gestation, and there is a finite risk of stillbirth between 40 and 42 weeks of gestation. Rates of intracranial hemorrhage are similar for spontaneous vaginal deliveries and cesarean deliveries without labor but are higher in operative vaginal deliveries and cesarean deliveries with labor (2).

Table 1. Risk of Placenta Accreta and Hysterectomy by Number of Cesarean Deliveries Compared With the First Cesarean Delivery

Cesarean Delivery	Accreta [n (%)]	Odds Ratio (95% CI)	Hysterectomy [n (%)]	Odds Ratio (95% CI)
First	15 (0.2)	–	40 (0.7)	–
Second	49 (0.3)	1.3 (.7–2.3)	67 (0.4)	0.7 (0.4–0.97)
Third	36 (0.6)	2.4 (1.3–4.3)	57 (0.9)	1.4 (0.9–1.2)
Fourth	31 (2.1)	9.0 (4.8–16.7)	35 (2.4)	3.8 (2.4–6.0)
Fifth	6 (2.3)	9.8 (3.8–25.5)	9 (3.5)	5.6 (2.7–11.6)
Six or more	6 (6.7)	29.8 (11.3–78.7)	8 (9.0)	15.2 (6.9–33.5)

CI, confidence interval.

Silver RM, Landon MB, Rouse DJ, Leveno KJ, Spong CY, Thom EA, et al. Maternal morbidity associated with multiple repeat cesarean deliveries. National Institute of Child Health and Human Development Maternal–Fetal Medicine Units Network. Obstet Gynecol 2006;107:1226–32.

There is also weak quality evidence of a lower risk of neonatal encephalopathy and asphyxia with elective cesarean delivery without labor compared with the combined risks of spontaneous vaginal delivery, operative vaginal delivery, emergency cesarean delivery, and cesarean delivery with labor (9, 10). The incidence of brachial plexus injury is significantly lower for cesarean delivery than vaginal delivery, with the highest incidence for assisted vaginal delivery. The incidence of fetal laceration at the time of cesarean delivery is lower for elective cesarean delivery without labor (0.8%) than unscheduled cesarean delivery (1.4–1.5%) (11). Studies on neonatal mortality and long-term neonatal outcomes lacked statistical power and quality data to assess the effect of the planned delivery route.

Summary of Data

In summary, only five outcome variables have moderate quality evidence regarding delivery route: 1) maternal hemorrhage, 2) maternal length of stay, 3) neonatal respiratory morbidity, 4) subsequent placenta previa or accreta, and 5) subsequent uterine rupture. The remaining outcome assessments are based on weak evidence, which limits the reliability of the results. A potential benefit of cesarean delivery on maternal request as compared with planned vaginal delivery is a decreased risk of hemorrhage for the mother. Potential risks of cesarean delivery on maternal request include a longer maternal hospital stay, an increased risk of respiratory problems for the baby, and greater complications in subsequent pregnancies, including uterine rupture and placental implantation problems.

Other Factors

When a woman desires a cesarean delivery on maternal request, her health care provider should consider her specific risk factors, such as age, body mass index, accuracy of estimated gestational age, reproductive plans, personal values, and cultural context. Critical life experiences (eg, trauma, violence, poor obstetric outcomes) and anxiety about the birth process may prompt her request. If her main concern is a fear of pain in childbirth, then prenatal childbirth education, emotional support in labor, and anesthesia for childbirth should be offered.

Further research is needed to get direct evidence for better counseling in the future. This includes surveys on cesarean delivery on maternal request, modification of birth certificates and Current Procedural Terminology coding to facilitate tracking, prospective cohort studies, database studies, and studies of modifiable risk factors for cesarean delivery on maternal request versus planned vaginal delivery. Short-term and long-term maternal and neonatal outcomes as well as cost need further study.

Conclusions

The available data on cesarean delivery on maternal request compared with planned vaginal delivery is minimal and mostly based on indirect comparisons. Most of the studies of proxy outcomes do not adequately adjust for confounding factors and, thus, must be interpreted cautiously.

Recommendations

- Cesarean delivery on maternal request should not be performed before gestational age of 39 weeks has been accurately determined unless there is documentation of lung maturity.
- Cesarean delivery on maternal request should not be motivated by the unavailability of effective pain management.
- Cesarean delivery on maternal request is not recommended for women desiring several children, given that the risks of placenta previa, placenta accreta, and gravid hysterectomy increase with each cesarean delivery.

References

1. Hamilton BE, Martin JA, Ventura SJ. Births: preliminary data for 2005. Natl Vital Stat Rep 2006;55(11):1–18.

2. National Institutes of Health. NIH State-of-the-Science Conference statement on cesarean delivery on maternal request. NIH Consensus and State-of-the-Science Statements. Bethesda (MD): NIH; 2006. Available at: http://consensus.nih.gov/2006/CesareanStatement_Final053106.pdf. Retrieved July 20, 2007.

3. Hannah ME, Whyte H, Hannah WJ, Hewson S, Amankwah K, Cheng M, et al. Maternal outcomes at 2 years after planned cesarean section versus planned vaginal birth for breech presentation at term: the international randomized Term Breech Trial. Term Breech Trial Collaborative Group. Am J Obstet Gynecol 2004;191:917–27.

4. Hannah ME, Hannah WJ, Hodnett ED, Chalmers B, Kung R, Willan A, et al. Outcomes at 3 months after planned cesarean vs planned vaginal delivery for breech presentation at term: the international randomized Term Breech Trial. Term Breech Trial 3-Month Follow-up Collaborative Group. JAMA 2002;287:1822–31.

5. Rortveit G, Daltveit AK, Hannestad YS, Hunskaar S. Urinary incontinence after vaginal delivery or cesarean section. Norwegian EPINCONT Study. N Engl J Med 2003;348: 900–7.

6. Liu S, Liston RM, Joseph KS, Heaman M, Sauve R, Kramer MS. Maternal mortality and severe morbidity associated with low-risk planned cesarean delivery versus planned vaginal delivery at term. Maternal Health Study Group of the Canadian Perinatal Surveillance System. CMAJ 2007; 176:455–60.

7. Zanardo V, Simbi AK, Franzoi M, Solda G, Salvadori A, Trevisanuto D. Neonatal respiratory morbidity risk and mode of delivery at term: influence of timing of elective caesarean delivery. Acta Paediatr 2004;93:643–7.

8. Morrison JJ, Rennie JM, Milton PJ. Neonatal respiratory morbidity and mode of delivery at term: influence of timing of elective caesarean section. Br J Obstet Gynaecol 1995;102:101–6.

9. Badawi N, Kurinczuk JJ, Keogh JM, Alessandri LM, O'Sullivan F, Burton PR, et al. Intrapartum risk factors for newborn encephalopathy: the Western Australian case-control study. BMJ 1998;317:1554–8.

10. Towner D, Castro MA, Eby-Wilkens E, Gilbert WM. Effect of mode of delivery in nulliparous women on neonatal intracranial injury. N Engl J Med 1999;341:1709–14.

11. van Ham MA, van Dongen PW, Mulder J. Maternal consequences of caesarean section. A retrospective study of intraoperative and postoperative maternal complications of caesarean section during a 10-year period. Eur J Obstet Gynecol Reprod Biol 1997;74:1–6.

Cesarean delivery on maternal request. ACOG Committee Opinion No. 394. American College of Obstetricians and Gynecologists. Obstet Gynecol 2007;110:1501–4.

ISSN 1074-861X

ACOG COMMITTEE OPINION

Number 402 • March 2008

(Replaces No. 273, May 2002)

Antenatal Corticosteroid Therapy for Fetal Maturation

Committee on Obstetric Practice

This document reflects emerging clinical and scientific advances as of the date issued and is subject to change. The information should not be construed as dictating an exclusive course of treatment or procedure to be followed.

ABSTRACT: A single course of corticosteroids is recommended for all pregnant women between 24 and 34 weeks of gestation who are at risk of preterm delivery within 7 days. A single course of antenatal corticosteroids should be administered to women with premature rupture of membranes (PROM) before 32 weeks of gestation to reduce the risks of respiratory distress syndrome, perinatal mortality, and other morbidities. The efficacy of corticosteroid use at 32–33 completed weeks of gestation for preterm PROM is unclear based on available evidence, but treatment may be beneficial, particularly if pulmonary immaturity is documented. No data exist on the efficacy of corticosteroid use before viability, and such use is not recommended at this time. Because of insufficient scientific evidence, repeat corticosteroid courses, including so-called "rescue therapy," should not be used routinely but should be reserved for women enrolled in clinical trials.

The American College of Obstetricians and Gynecologists

Women's Health Care Physicians

In August 2000, the National Institute of Child Health and Human Development and the Office of Medical Applications of Research of the National Institutes of Health reconvened a consensus conference on antenatal steroids, entitled "Consensus Development Conference on Antenatal Corticosteroids Revisited: Repeat Courses," to address the issue of repeated courses of corticosteroids for fetal maturation. The consensus panel from this conference reaffirmed the 1994 consensus panel's recommendation of giving a single course of corticosteroids to all pregnant women between 24 and 34 weeks of gestation who are at risk of preterm delivery within 7 days (1). Because of insufficient scientific evidence, the panel also recommended that repeat corticosteroid courses, including so-called "rescue therapy," should not be routinely used but should be reserved for women enrolled in clinical trials. The American College of Obstetricians and Gynecologists' Committee on Obstetric Practice supports the conclusions of the consensus conferences.

There is no convincing scientific evidence that antenatal corticosteroid therapy increases the risk of neonatal infection, although multiple courses have been associated with fetal adrenal suppression (2). Follow-up studies of children aged 14 years who were exposed to at least one course of corticosteroid treatment indicate there is no apparent risk of adverse neurodevelopmental outcome associated with antenatal corticosteroids (3). In a randomized trial of single versus multiple courses of antenatal corticosteroids, a reduction in birth weight and an increase in the number of infants who were small for gestational age was found, especially after four courses of corticosteroids (4). Although not consistent, six studies found decreased birth weight and head circumference with repeat courses (4–9) and three studies did not (10–12). Recently it has been shown that repeat doses of antenatal corticosteroids are associated with smaller placentas, but treatment does not appear to have an influence on significant histologic placental findings related to placental maturation, infarction, abruptio placentae, necrosis, or fetal hypoxia (13). The 2000 consensus panel concluded that studies regarding the possible benefits and risks of repeat courses of antenatal corticosteroids are limited because of their study design and "methodologic inconsistencies." The 2000 consensus panel noted that, although there is a suggestion of possible benefit from repeated doses (especially in the reduction and severity of respiratory distress), there also are animal and human data that suggest deleterious effects on the fetus regarding cerebral myelination, lung growth, and function of the hypothalamic–pituitary–adrenal axis. Followup of children at 2 years of age exposed to repeat courses of antenatal corticosteroids showed no significant difference in physical or neurocognitive measures (14, 15). Although not statistically significant, the relative risk of cerebral palsy in infants exposed to multiple courses of antenatal corticosteroids (relative risk = 5.7) is of concern and warrants further study (14). Maternal effects include increased infection and suppression of the hypothalamic–pituitary–adrenal axis (6, 16).

Betamethasone and dexamethasone are the most widely studied corticosteroids and have generally been preferred for antenatal treatment to accelerate fetal organ maturation. Both cross the placenta in their active form and have nearly identical biologic activity. Both lack mineralocorticoid activity and have relatively weak immunosuppressive activity with short-term use. Although betamethasone and dexamethasone differ only by a single methyl group, betamethasone has a longer half-life because of its decreased clearance and larger volume of distribution (17). Meta-analyses of randomized trials have shown that, although both agents decrease the frequency of respiratory distress syndrome, only betamethasone decreases neonatal mortality (18). A recent large, uncontrolled retrospective study suggested that betamethasone also may have significant benefit in decreasing the rate of newborn cystic periventricular leukomalacia by approximately 50% in treated women compared with untreated and dexamethasone-treated women (19). The offspring of pregnant mice who were given betamethasone performed neurobehavioral developmental tasks better than the offspring of pregnant mice given dexamethasone (20). Furthermore, betamethasone requires fewer intramuscular injections. Betamethasone use, however, has been associated with a significant transient decrease in fetal movements and heart rate variability (21, 22). In a recent randomized trial of 299 women, investigators found that although both betamethasone and dexamethasone were comparable in reducing neonatal morbidities and mortality, dexamethasone was more effective in reducing the rate of intraventricular hemorrhage (23).

The 2000 consensus panel reviewed all available reports on the safety and efficacy of betamethasone and dexamethasone. It did not find significant scientific evidence to support a recommendation that betamethasone should be used preferentially instead of dexamethasone. Thus, based on this information, the Committee on Obstetric Practice recommends either of the following corticosteroid regimens:

- Two 12-mg doses of betamethasone given intramuscularly 24 hours apart
- Dexamethasone (6 mg) given intramuscularly every 12 hours for four doses

A single course of corticosteroids is recommended for all pregnant women between 24 and 34 weeks of gestation who are at risk of preterm delivery within 7 days (24). A single course of antenatal corticosteroids should be administered to women with premature rupture of membranes (PROM) before 32 weeks of gestation to reduce the risks of respiratory distress syndrome, perinatal mortality, and other morbidities. The efficacy of corticosteroid use at 32–33 completed weeks of gestation for preterm PROM is unclear based on available evidence, but treatment may be beneficial, particularly if pulmonary immaturity is documented. There are no data regarding the efficacy of corticosteroid use before viability, and it is not recommended at this time. Because of insufficient scientific evidence, repeat corticosteroid courses, including so-called "rescue therapy," should not be used routinely but should be reserved for women enrolled in clinical trials.

References

1. Antenatal corticosteroids revisited: repeat courses. NIH Consens Statement 2000;17(2):1–18.

2. Kairalla AB. Hypothalamic-pituitary-adrenal axis function in premature neonates after extensive prenatal treatment with betamethasone: a case history. Am J Perinatol 1992;9: 428–30.

3. Doyle LW, Ford GW, Rickards AL, Kelly EA, Davis NM, Callanan C, et al. Antenatal corticosteroids and outcome at 14 years of age in children with birth weight less than 1501 grams. Pediatrics 2000;106:E2.

4. Wapner RJ, Sorokin Y, Thom EA, Johnson F, Dudley DJ, Spong CY, et al. Single versus weekly courses of antenatal corticosteroids: evaluation of safety and efficacy. National Institute of Child Health and Human Development Maternal Fetal Medicine Units Network. Am J Obstet Gynecol 2006;195:633–42.

5. French NP, Hagan R, Evans SF, Godfrey M, Newnham JP. Repeated antenatal corticosteroids: size at birth and subsequent development. Am J Obstet Gynecol 1999;180:114–21.

6. Abbasi S, Hirsch D, Davis J, Tolosa J, Stouffer N, Debbs R, et al. Effect of single versus multiple courses of antenatal corticosteroids on maternal and neonatal outcome. Am J Obstet Gynecol 2000;182:1243–9.

7. Banks BA, Cnaan A, Morgan MA, Parer JT, Merrill JD, Ballard PL, et al. Multiple courses of antenatal corticosteroids and outcome of premature neonates. North American Thyrotropin-Releasing Hormone Study Group. Am J Obstet Gynecol 1999;181:709–17.

8. Bloom SL, Sheffield JS, McIntire DD, Leveno KJ. Antenatal dexamethasone and decreased birth weight. Obstet Gynecol 2001;97:485–90.

9. Thorp JA, Jones PG, Knox E, Clark RH. Does antenatal corticosteroid therapy affect birth weight and head circumference? Obstet Gynecol 2002;99:101–8.

10. Guinn DA, Atkinson MW, Sullivan L, Lee M, MacGregor S, Parilla BV, et al. Single vs weekly courses of antenatal corticosteroids for women at risk of preterm delivery: a randomized controlled trial. JAMA 2001;286:1581-7.

11. Pratt L, Waschbusch L, Ladd W, Gangnon R, Hendricks SK. Multiple vs. single betamethasone therapy. Neonatal and maternal effects. J Reprod Med 1999;44:257–64.

12. Shelton SD, Boggess KA, Murtha AP, Groff AO, Herbert WN. Repeated fetal betamethasone treatment and birth weight and head circumference. Obstet Gynecol 2001;97:301–4.

13. Sawady J, Mercer BM, Wapner RJ, Zhao Y, Sorokin Y, Johnson F, et al. The National Institute of Child Health and Human Development Maternal-Fetal Medicine Units Network Beneficial Effects of Antenatal Repeated Steroids study: impact of repeated doses of antenatal corticosteroids on placental growth and histologic findings. National Institute of Child Health and Human Development Maternal Fetal Medicine Units Network. Am J Obstet Gynecol 2007;197:281.e1–8.

14. Wapner RJ, Sorokin Y, Mele L, Johnson F, Dudley DJ, Spong CY, et al. Long-term outcomes after repeat doses of antenatal corticosteroids. National Institute of Child Health and Human Development Maternal-Fetal Medicine Units Network. N Engl J Med 2007;357:1190–8.

15. Crowther CA, Doyle LW, Haslam RR, Hiller JE, Harding JE, Robinson JS. Outcomes at 2 years of age after repeat doses of antenatal corticosteroids. ACTORDS Study Group. N Engl J Med 2007;357:1179–89.

16. McKenna DS, Wittber GM, Nagaraja HN, Samuels P. The effects of repeat doses of antenatal corticosteroids on maternal adrenal function. Am J Obstet Gynecol 2000;183:669–73.

17. Fanaroff AA, Hack M. Periventricular leukomalacia prospects for prevention. N Engl J Med 1999;341:1229–31.

18. Ballard PL, Ballard RA. Scientific basis and therapeutic regimens for use of antenatal glucocorticoids. Am J Obstet Gynecol 1995;173:254–62.

19. Baud O, Foix-L'Helias L, Kaminski M, Audibert F, Jarreau PH, Papiernik E, et al. Antenatal glucocorticoid treatment and cystic periventricular leukomalacia in very premature infants. N Engl J Med 1999;341:1190–6.

20. Rayburn WF, Christensen HD, Gonzalez CL. A placebo-controlled comparison between betamethasone and dexamethasone for fetal maturation: differences in neurobehavioral development of mice offspring. Am J Obstet Gynecol 1997;176:842–50; discussion 850–1.

21. Mulder EJ, Derks JB, Visser GH. Antenatal corticosteroid therapy and fetal behaviour: a randomised study of the effects of betamethasone and dexamethasone. Br J Obstet Gynaecol 1997;104:1239–47.

22. Senat MV, Minoui S, Multon O, Fernandez H, Frydman R, Ville Y. Effect of dexamethasone and betamethasone on fetal heart rate variability in preterm labour: a randomised study. Br J Obstet Gynaecol 1998;105:749–55.

23. Elimian A, Garry D, Figueroa R, Spitzer A, Wiencek V, Quirk JG. Antenatal betamethasone compared with dexamethasone (betacode trial): a randomized controlled trial. Obstet Gynecol 2007;110:26–30.

24. Roberts D, Dalziel S. Antenatal corticosteroids for accelerating fetal lung maturation for women at risk of preterm birth. Cochrane Database of Systematic Reviews 2006, Issue 3. Art. No.: CD004454. DOI: 10.1002/14651858.CD004454.pub2.

Antenatal corticosteroid therapy for fetal maturation. ACOG Committee Opinion No. 402. American College of Obstetricians and Gynecologists. Obstet Gynecol 2008;111:805–7.

ISSN 1074-861X

ACOG COMMITTEE OPINION

Number 404 • April 2008

Late-Preterm Infants

Committee on Obstetric Practice

This Committee Opinion was developed with the assistance of William A. Engle, MD, Kay M. Tomashek, MD, Carol Wallman, MSN, and the American Academy of Pediatrics Committee on Fetus and Newborn.

This document reflects emerging clinical and scientific advances as of the date issued and is subject to change. The information should not be construed as dictating an exclusive course of treatment or procedure to be followed.

ABSTRACT: *Late-preterm infants* (defined as infants born between 34% weeks and 36% weeks of gestation) often are mistakenly believed to be as physiologically and metabolically mature as term infants. However, compared with term infants, late-preterm infants are at higher risk than term infants of developing medical complications, resulting in higher rates of infant mortality, higher rates of morbidity before initial hospital discharge, and higher rates of hospital readmission in the first months of life. Preterm delivery should occur only when an accepted maternal or fetal indication for delivery exists. Collaborative counseling by both obstetric and neonatal clinicians about the outcomes of late-preterm births is warranted unless precluded by emergent conditions.

During the past decade, the proportion of all U.S. births that were *late-preterm births* (defined as birth between 34% weeks and 36% weeks of gestation) increased 16% (1). The rate of all *preterm births* (defined as birth at less than 37 weeks of gestation) in the United States increased from 10.9% in 1990 to 12.7% in 2005 (2), an increase of 16.5%. This increase largely was caused by the increase in late-preterm births. Late-preterm infants often are mistakenly believed to be as physiologically and metabolically mature as term infants. However, compared with term infants, late-preterm infants are at higher risk of developing medical complications resulting in higher rates of infant mortality, higher rates of morbidity before initial hospital discharge (3–5), and higher rates of hospital readmission in the first months of life (4–6).

Infant Implications

Late-preterm births make up 71% of all preterm births (1). It is important to limit late-preterm deliveries to those with a clear maternal or fetal indication for delivery. As the number of late-preterm births increases, it is important to understand the unique problems that this growing population of infants may experience.

The American Academy of Pediatrics has published guidelines for the care of late-preterm infants (7). The following sections contain extracts taken from these guidelines.

Summary

During the initial birth hospitalization, late-preterm infants are 4 times more likely than term infants to have at least 1 medical condition diagnosed and 3.5 times more likely to have 2 or more conditions diagnosed (6). Late-preterm infants are more likely than term infants to be diagnosed during the birth hospitalization with temperature instability (6), hypoglycemia (6), respiratory distress (6, 8–11), apnea (12, 13), jaundice (6), and feeding difficulties (6). During the first month after birth, late-preterm infants are also more likely than term infants to develop hyperbilirubinemia (14–17) and to be readmitted for hyperbilirubinemia (18–20) and non–jaundice-related diagnoses such as feeding difficulties and "rule-out sepsis" (18).

In 2002, the neonatal mortality rate (deaths among infants 0–27 days' chronologic age) for late-preterm infants was 4.6 times higher than the rate for term infants (4.1 vs 0.9 per 1000 live births, respectively). This difference in neonatal mortality has widened slightly since 1995, when there was a fourfold difference in rates between late-preterm and term infants (4.8 vs 1.2 per 1000 live births, respectively). The infant mortality rate was also higher among late-preterm infants

The American College of Obstetricians and Gynecologists
Women's Health Care Physicians

than term infants in 2002 (7.7 vs 2.5 per 1000 live births, respectively). This threefold difference has remained relatively constant since 1995, at which time the infant mortality rate was 9.3 per 1000 live births among late-preterm infants and 3.1 per 1000 live births among term infants.

Pulmonary Function

After birth, infants with fetal lung structure and immature functional capacity are at greatest risk of respiratory distress, need for oxygen and positive-pressure ventilation, and admission for intensive care (6, 9, 21, 22). From 34% through 36% weeks' gestation, terminal respiratory units of the lung evolve from alveolar saccules lined with both cuboidal type II and flat type I epithelial cells (terminal sac period) to mature alveoli lined primarily with extremely thin type I epithelial cells (alveolar period) (23, 24). During the alveolar period, pulmonary capillaries also begin to bulge into the space of each terminal sac, and adult pool sizes of surfactant are attained (25). Functionally, this immature lung structure may be associated with delayed intrapulmonary fluid absorption, surfactant insufficiency, and inefficient gas exchange (8, 26).

Apnea occurs more frequently among late-preterm infants than term infants. The incidence of apnea in late-preterm infants is reported to be between 4% and 7% (12, 21, 27, 28) compared with less than 1% to 2% at term (12, 29). The predisposition to apnea in late-preterm infants is associated with several underlying factors including increased susceptibility to hypoxic respiratory depression, decreased central chemosensitivity to carbon dioxide, immature pulmonary irritant receptors, increased respiratory inhibition sensitivity to laryngeal stimulation, and decreased upper airway dilator muscle tone (12, 13, 21, 30, 31).

Cardiac Function

It is generally believed that structural and functional immaturity restricts the amount of cardiovascular reserve that is available during times of stress (32, 33). Immature cardiovascular function also may complicate recovery of the late-preterm infant with respiratory distress because of delayed ductus arteriosus closure and persistent pulmonary hypertension (34).

Cold Response

Late-preterm infants have less white adipose tissue for insulation, and they cannot generate heat from brown adipose tissue as effectively as infants born at term. In addition, late-preterm infants are likely to lose heat more readily than term infants, because they have a larger ratio of surface area to weight and are smaller in size.

Hypoglycemia

The incidence of hypoglycemia is inversely proportional to gestational age. Preterm infants are at increased risk of developing hypoglycemia after birth, because they have immature hepatic glycogenolysis and adipose tissue lipolysis, hormonal dysregulation, and deficient hepatic gluconeogenesis and ketogenesis. Blood glucose concentrations among preterm infants typically decrease to a nadir 1 to 2 hours after birth and remain low until metabolic pathways can compensate or exogenous sources of glucose are provided (35, 36). Immature glucose regulation likely occurs in late-preterm infants, because hypoglycemia that requires glucose infusion during the initial birth hospitalization occurs more frequently than in term infants (6).

Jaundice

Jaundice and hyperbilirubinemia occur more commonly and are more prolonged among late-preterm infants than term infants, because late-preterm infants have delayed maturation and a lower concentration of uridine diphosphoglucuronate glucuronosyltransferase (14, 37). Late-preterm infants are 2 times more likely than term infants to have significantly elevated bilirubin concentrations and higher concentrations 5 and 7 days after birth (14). Late-preterm infants also have immature gastrointestinal function (38, 39) and feeding difficulties that predispose them to an increase in enterohepatic circulation, decreased stool frequency, dehydration, and hyperbilirubinemia (15, 19, 20, 40–46). Feeding during the birth hospitalization may be transiently successful but not sustained after discharge. Feeding difficulties in late-preterm infants that are associated with relatively low oromotor tone, function, and neural maturation also predispose these infants to dehydration and hyperbilirubinemia (45–48).

Obstetric Implications

Because of the aforementioned increase in rates of morbidity and mortality of late-preterm infants, preterm delivery should only occur when an accepted maternal or fetal indication for delivery exists. Examples may include nonreassuring fetal status or a maternal condition that is likely to be improved by delivery. Collaborative counseling by both obstetric and neonatal clinicians about the outcomes of late-preterm births is warranted unless precluded by emergent conditions.

References

1. Davidoff MJ, Dias T, Damus K, Russell R, Bettegowda R, Dolans, et al. Changes in the gestational age distribution among U.S. singleton births: impact on rates of late preterm birth, 1992 to 2002. Semin Perinatol 2006;30:8–15.

2. Hamilton BE, Martin JA, Ventura SJ. Births: preliminary data for 2005. Natl Vital Stat Rep 2006;55(11):1–18.

3. Kramer MS, Demissie K, Yang H, Platt RW, Sauve R, Liston R. The contribution of mild and moderate preterm birth to infant mortality. Fetal and Infant Health Study Group of the Canadian Perinatal surveillance System. JAMA 2000;284: 843–9.

4. Shapiro-Mendoza CK, Tomashek KM, Kotelchuck M, Barfield W, Weiss J, Evans S. Risk factors for neonatal morbidity and mortality among "healthy," late preterm newborns. Semin Perinatol 2006;30:54–60.

5. Tomashek KM, Shapiro-Mendoza CK, Weiss J, Kotelchuck M, Barfield W, Evans S, et al. Early discharge among late preterm and term newborns and risk of neonatal morbidity. Semin Perinatol 2006;30:61–8.

6. Wang ML, Dorer DJ, Fleming MP, Catlin EA. Clinical outcomes of near-term infants. Pediatrics 2004;114:372–6.

7. Engle WA, Tomashek KM, Wallman C. "Late preterm" infants: a population at risk. Committee on Fetus and Newborn. Pediatrics 2007;120:1390–1401.

8. Escobar GJ, Clark RH, Greene JD. Short-term outcomes of infants born at 35 and 36 weeks gestation: we need to ask more questions. Semin Perinatol 2006;30:28–33.

9. Rubaltelli FF, Bonafe L, Tangucci M, Spagnolo A, Dani C. Epidemiology of neonatal acute respiratory disorders. A multicenter study of incidence and fatality rates of neonatal acute respiratory disorders according to gestational age, maternal age, pregnancy complications and type of delivery. Italian Group of Neonatal Pneumology. Biol Neonate 1998;74:7–15.

10. Gilbert WM, Nesbitt TS, Danielsen B. The cost of prematurity: quantification by gestational age and birth weight. Obstet Gynecol 2003;102:488–92.

11. Dani C, Reali MF, Bertini G, Wiechmann L, Spagnolo A, Tangucci M, et al. Risk factors for the development of respiratory distress syndrome and transient tachypnoea in newborn infants. Italian Group of Neonatal Pneumology. Eur Respir J 1999;14:155–9.

12. Henderson-Smart DJ. The effect of gestational age on the incidence and duration of recurrent apnoea in newborn babies. Aust Paediatr J 1981;17:273–6.

13. Merchant JR, Worwa C, Porter S, Coleman JM, deRegnier RA. Respiratory instability of term and near-term healthy newborn infants in car safety seats. Pediatrics 2001;108: 647–52.

14. Sarici SU, Serdar MA, Korkmaz A, Erdem G, Oran O, Tekinalp G, et al. Incidence, course, and prediction of hyperbilirubinemia in near-term and term newborns. Pediatrics 2004;113:775–80.

15. Newman TB, Escobar GJ, Gonzales VM, Armstrong MA, Gardner MN, Folck BF. Frequency of neonatal bilirubin testing and hyperbilirubinemia in a large health maintenance organization [published erratum appears in Pediatrics 2001;1:126]. Pediatrics 1999;104:1198–203.

16. Newman TB, Liljestrand P, Escobar GJ. Infants with bilirubin levels of 30 mg/dL or more in a large managed care organization. Pediatrics 2003;111:1303–11.

17. Chou SC, Palmer RH, Ezhuthachan S, Newman C, Pradell-Boyd B, Maisels MJ, et al. Management of hyperbilirubinemia in newborns: measuring performance by using a benchmarking model. Pediatrics 2003;112:1264–73.

18. Escobar GJ, Greene JD, Hulac P, Kincannon E, Bischoff K, Gardner MN, at al. Rehospitalisation after birth hospitalisation: patterns among infants of all gestations. Arch Dis Child 2005;90:125–31.

19. Bhutani VK, Johnson LH, Maisels MJ, Newman TB, Phibbs C, Stark AR, et al. Kernicterus: epidemiological strategies for its prevention through systems-based approaches. J Perinatol 2004;24:650–62.

20. Brown AK, Damus K, Kim MH, King K, Harper R, Campbell D, et al. Factors relating to readmission of term and near-term neonates in the first two weeks of life. Early Discharge Survey Group of the Health Professional Advisory Board of the Greater New York Chapter of the March of Dimes. J Perinat Med 1999;27:263–75.

21. Arnon S, Dolfin T, Litmanovitz I, Regev R, Bauer S, Fejgin M. Preterm labour at 34–36 weeks of gestation: should it be arrested? Paediatr Perinat Epidemiol 2001;15:252–6.

22. Avery ME, Mead J. Surface properties in relation to atelectasis and hyaline membrane disease. AMA J Dis Child 1959; 97:517–23.

23. Jobe AH. The respiratory system. Part 1: lung development and maturation. In: Martin RJ, Fanaroff AA, Walsh MC, editors. Fanaroff and Martin's neonatal-perinatal medicine: diseases of the fetus and infant. 8th ed. Philadelphia (PA): Mosby Elsevier; 2006. p. 1069–1194.

24. Post M. Lung development: pulmonary structure and function. In: Gluckman PD, Heymann MA, editors. Pediatrics and perinatology: the scientific basis. 2nd ed. New York (NY): Oxford University Press; 1996. p. 797–800.

25. Hawgood S. Alveolar region: pulmonary structure and function. In: Gluckman PD, Heymann MA, editors. Pediatrics and perinatology: the scientific basis. 2nd ed. New York (NY): Oxford University Press; 1996. p. 814–9.

26. Jain L, Eaton DC. Physiology of fetal lung fluid clearance and the effect of labor. Semin Perinatol 2006;30:34–43.

27. Hunt CE. Ontogeny of autonomic regulation in late preterm infants born at 34–37 weeks postmenstrual age. Semin Perinatol 2006;30:73–76.

28. Henderson-Smart DJ, Pettigrew AG, Campbell DJ. Clinical apnea and brain-stem neural function in preterm infants. N Engl J Med 1983;308:353–7.

29. Ramanathan R, Corwin MJ, Hunt CE, Lister G, Tinsley LR, Baird T, et al. Cardiorespiratory events recorded on home monitors: comparison of healthy infants with those at increased risk for SIDS. Collaborative Home Infant Monitoring Evaluation (CHIME) Study Group. JAMA 2001;285:2199–207.

30. Curzi-Dascalova L, Christova-Gueorguieva E. Respiratory pauses in normal prematurely born infants. A comparison with full-term newborns. Biol Neonate 1983;44:325–32.

31. Miller MJ, Fanaroff AA, Martin RJ. The respiratory system. Part 5: respiratory disorders in preterm and term infants. In: Martin RJ, Fanaroff AA, Walsh MC, editors. Fanaroff and Martin's neonatal-perinatal medicine: diseases of the fetus

and infant. 8th ed. Philadelphia (PA): Mosby Elsevier; 2006. p. 1122–46.

32. Lee LA, Kimball TR, Daniels SR, Khoury P, Meyer RA. Left ventricular mechanics in the preterm infant and their effect on the measurement of cardiac performance. J Pediatr 1992;120:114–19.

33. Zahka KG. The cardiovascular system. Part 4: principles of neonatal cardiovascular hemodynamics. In: Martin RJ, Fanaroff AA, Walsh MC, editors. Fanaroff and Martin's neonatal-perinatal medicine: diseases of the fetus and infant. 8th ed. Philadelphia (PA): Mosby Elsevier; 2006. p. 1211–15.

34. Randala M, Eronen M, Andersson S, Pohjavuori M, Pesonen E. Pulmonary artery pressure in term and preterm neonates. Acta Paediatr 1996;85:1344–47.

35. Stanley CA, Pallotto EK. Disorders of carbohydrate metabolism. In: Taeusch HW, Ballard RA, Gleason CA, editors. Avery's disease of the newborn. 8th ed. Philadelphia (PA): Elsevier Saunders; 2005. p. 1410–22.

36. Kalhan SC, Parimi PS. Metabolic and endocrine disorders. Part 1: disorders of carbohydrate metabolism. In: Martin RJ, Fanaroff AA, Walsh MC, editors. Fanaroff and Martin's neonatal-perinatal medicine: diseases of the fetus and infant. 8th ed. Philadelphia (PA): Mosby Elsevier; 2006. p. 1467–91.

37. Kawade N, Onishi S. The prenatal and postnatal development of UDP-glucuronyltransferase activity towards bilirubin and the effect of premature birth on this activity in the human liver. Biochem J 1981;196:257–60.

38. Berseth CL. Developmental anatomy and physiology of the gastrointestinal tract. In: Taeusch HW, Ballard RA, Gleason CA, editors. Avery's diseases of the newborn. 8th ed. Philadelphia (PA): Elsevier Saunders; 2005. p. 1071–85.

39. Al Tawil Y, Berseth CL. Gestational and postnatal maturation of duodenal motor responses to intragastric feeding. J Pediatr 1996;129:374–81.

40. Hall RT, Simon S, Smith MT. Readmission of breastfed infants in the first 2 weeks of life. J Perinatol 2000;20: 432–7.

41. Maisels MJ, Kring E. Length of stay, jaundice, and hospital readmission. Pediatrics 1998;101:995–8.

42. Maisels MJ, Newman TB. Jaundice in full-term and near-term babies who leave the hospital within 36 hours. The pediatrician's nemesis. Clin Perinatol 1998;25:295–302.

43. Soskolne EI, Schumacher R, Fyock C, Young ML, Schork A. The effect of early discharge and other factors on readmission rates of newborns. Arch Pediatr Adolesc Med 1996;150:373–9.

44. Escobar GJ, Joffe S, Gardner MN, Armstrong MA, Folck BF, Carpenter DM. Rehospitalization in the first two weeks after discharge from the neonatal intensive care unit. Pediatrics 1999;104:e2.

45. Johnson D, Jin Y, Truman C. Early discharge of Alberta mothers post-delivery and the relationship to potentially preventable newborn readmissions. Can J Public Health 2002;93:276–80.

46. Geiger AM, Petitti DB, Yao JF. Rehospitalisation for neonatal jaundice: risk factors and outcomes. Paediatr Perinat Epidemiol 2001;15:352–8.

47. Kinney HC. The near-term (late preterm) human brain and risk for periventricular leukomalacia: a review. Semin Perinatol 2006;30:81–8.

48. Escobar GJ, Gonzales V, Armstrong MA, Folck B, Xiong B, Newman TB. Rehospitalization for neonatal dehydration: a nested case-control study. Arch Pediatr Adolesc Med 2002; 156:155–61.

Late-preterm infants. ACOG Committee Opinion No. 404. American College of Obstetricians and Gynecologists. Obstet Gynecol 2008; 111:1029–32.

ISSN 1074-861X

ACOG COMMITTEE OPINION

Number 418 • September 2008

(Replaces No. 304, November 2004)

Prenatal and Perinatal Human Immunodeficiency Virus Testing: Expanded Recommendations

Committee on Obstetric Practice

This document reflects emerging clinical and scientific advances as of the date issued and is subject to change. The information should not be construed as dictating an exclusive course of treatment or procedure to be followed.

ABSTRACT: Early identification and treatment of all pregnant women with human immunodeficiency virus (HIV) is the best way to prevent neonatal disease and improve the woman's health. Human immunodeficiency virus screening is recommended for all pregnant women after they are notified that they will be tested for HIV infection as part of the routine panel of prenatal blood tests unless they decline the test (ie, opt-out screening). Repeat testing in the third trimester, or rapid HIV testing at labor and delivery as indicated or both also are recommended as additional strategies to further reduce the rate of perinatal HIV transmission. The American College of Obstetricians and Gynecologists makes the following recommendations: obstetrician–gynecologists should follow opt-out prenatal HIV screening where legally possible; repeat conventional or rapid HIV testing in the third trimester is recommended for women in areas with high HIV prevalence, women known to be at high risk for acquiring HIV infection, and women who declined testing earlier in pregnancy; rapid HIV testing should be used in labor for women with undocumented HIV status following opt-out screening; and if a rapid HIV test result in labor is positive, immediate initiation of antiretroviral prophylaxis should be recommended without waiting for the results of the confirmatory test.

The American College of Obstetricians and Gynecologists
Women's Health Care Physicians

The Centers for Disease Control and Prevention (CDC) estimates that 40,000 new cases of human immunodeficiency virus (HIV) infection still occur in the United States each year (1). This figure includes approximately 138 infants infected via mother-to-child (vertical) transmission (2). Antiretroviral medications given to women with HIV perinatally and to their newborns in the first weeks of life reduce the vertical transmission rate from 25% to 2% or less (3–6). Even instituting maternal prophylaxis during labor and delivery, or neonatal prophylaxis within 24–48 hours of delivery, or both can substantially decrease rates of infection in infants (4). A retrospective review of HIV-exposed infants in New York State showed a transmission rate of approximately 10% when zidovudine prophylaxis was begun intrapartum or if given to newborns within 48 hours of life. There is no significant reduction of neonatal transmission if therapy is

started after 3 days of life (4). Early identification and treatment of pregnant women and prophylactic treatment of newborns in the first hours of life are essential to prevent neonatal disease.

Prenatal Human Immunodeficiency Virus Testing

All pregnant women should be screened for HIV infection as early as possible during each pregnancy after they are notified that HIV screening is recommended for all pregnant patients and that they will receive an HIV test as part of the routine panel of prenatal tests unless they decline (opt-out screening). No woman should be tested without her knowledge; however, no additional process or written documentation of informed consent beyond what is required for other routine prenatal tests is required for HIV testing. Pregnant women should be provided with oral or written information about HIV (1, 7) that includes an explanation of HIV infection, a description of interventions that can reduce HIV transmission from mother to infant, the meanings of positive and negative test results, and the opportunity to ask questions and decline testing (1). If a patient declines HIV testing, this should be documented in the medical record and should not affect access to care. Women who decline an HIV test because they have had a previous negative test result should be informed of the importance of retesting during each pregnancy (1). The American College of Obstetricians and Gynecologists, the American Academy of Pediatrics (7), and the CDC (1, 8) recommend opt-out HIV screening for pregnant women. Since the release of CDC recommendations in September 2006 (1), some states have changed their state laws and regulations to opt-out screening. Obstetrician–gynecologists should be aware of and comply with their states' legal requirements for perinatal HIV screening. Legal requirements for perinatal HIV testing may be verified by contacting state or local public health departments. The National HIV/AIDS Clinicians' Consultation Center at the University of California–San Francisco maintains an online compendium of state HIV testing laws that can be a useful resource (see Resources). The Centers for Disease Control and Prevention recommend that jurisdictions with barriers to routine prenatal screening using opt-out screening consider addressing them (9).

Perinatal Human Immunodeficiency Virus Testing

The conventional HIV testing algorithm, which may take up to 2 weeks to complete if a result is positive, begins with a screening test, the enzyme-linked immunosorbent assay (ELISA) that detects antibodies to HIV; if the results are positive, it is followed by a confirmatory test, either a Western blot or an immunofluorescence assay (IFA). A positive ELISA test result is not diagnostic of HIV infection unless confirmed by the Western blot or IFA. The sensitivity and specificity of ELISA with a confirmatory Western blot test are greater than 99%. The false-positive rate for ELISA with a confirmatory Western blot test is 1 in 59,000 tests. If the ELISA test result is positive and the Western blot or IFA test result is negative, the patient is not infected and repeat testing is not indicated.

If the ELISA test result is repeatedly positive and the Western blot result contains some but not all of the viral bands required to make a definitive diagnosis, the test result is labeled indeterminate. Most patients with indeterminate test results are not infected with HIV. However, consultation with a health care provider well versed in HIV infection is recommended. This specialist may suggest viral load testing or repeat testing later in pregnancy to rule out the possibility of recent infection.

If the screening (eg, ELISA) and confirmatory test (eg, Western blot or IFA) results are both positive, the patient should be given her results in person. The impli-

cations of HIV infection and vertical transmission should be discussed with the patient. Additional laboratory evaluation, including CD4 count, HIV viral load, resistance testing, hepatitis C virus antibody, hepatitis B surface antigen, complete blood count with platelet count, and baseline chemistries with liver function tests, will be useful before prescribing antiretroviral prophylaxis.

A rapid HIV test is an HIV screening test with results available within hours. Obstetrician–gynecologists may use rapid testing as their standard outpatient test and should also use rapid testing in labor and delivery (see details as follows regarding labor and delivery). A negative rapid test result is definitive. A positive rapid test result is not definitive and must be confirmed with a supplemental test, such as a Western blot or IFA test. Rapid test results usually will be available during the same clinical visit that the specimen (eg blood, or oral swab) is collected. Health care providers who use these tests must be prepared to provide counseling to pregnant women who receive positive rapid test results the same day that the specimen is collected. Pregnant women with positive rapid test results should be counseled regarding the meaning of these preliminary positive test results and the need for confirmatory testing. As with conventional HIV testing, consultation with a health care provider well versed in HIV infection is recommended. To code for rapid testing, the modifier 92 is added to the basic HIV testing Current Procedural Terminology (CPT®)* code 86701-86703) (10). If the results of the rapid test and the confirmatory test are discrepant, both tests should be repeated and consultation with an infectious disease specialist is recommended.

Any woman who arrives at a labor and delivery facility with undocumented HIV status should be screened with a rapid HIV test unless she declines (opt-out screening) in order to provide an opportunity to begin prophylaxis of previously undiagnosed infection before delivery (1). Data from several studies indicate that 40–85% of infants infected with HIV are born to women whose HIV infection is unknown to their obstetric provider before delivery (11–14). If a rapid test is used in labor and HIV antibodies are detected, immediate initiation of antiretroviral prophylaxis should be recommended without waiting for the results of the confirmatory test to further reduce possible transmission to the infant. All antiretroviral prophylaxis should be discontinued if the confirmatory test result is negative (11). Recommendations for the use of antiretroviral medications in pregnant women infected with HIV are available at www.aidsinfo.nih.gov and are updated frequently.

The rapid HIV antibody screening tests, which are approved by the U.S. Food and Drug Administration, all have sensitivity and specificity equal to or greater than

---

*Current Procedural Terminology (CPT)® is copyright 2008 by American Medical Association. All rights reserved. No fee schedules, basic units, relative values, or related listings are included in CPT. The AMA assumes no liability for the data contained herein. CPT® is a trademark of the American Medical Association.

99% (15). As with all screening tests, the likelihood of a false-positive result is higher in populations with low HIV prevalence when compared with populations with high HIV prevalence. Additionally, at present it is not known how the false-positive rate for rapid testing will compare with the false-positive rate for conventional testing.

If the rapid HIV test result at labor and delivery is positive, the obstetric provider should take the following steps:

1. Tell the woman she may have HIV infection and that her neonate also may be exposed

2. Explain that the rapid test result is preliminary and that false-positive results are possible

3. Assure the woman that a second test is being done right away to confirm the positive rapid test result

4. Immediate initiation of antiretroviral prophylaxis should be recommended without waiting for the results of the confirmatory test to reduce the risk of transmission to the infant

5. Once the woman gives birth, discontinue maternal antiretroviral therapy pending receipt of confirmatory test results

6. Tell the woman that she should postpone breast-feeding until the confirmatory result is available because she should not breast-feed if she is infected with HIV

7. Inform pediatric care providers (depending on state requirements) of positive maternal test results so that they may institute the appropriate neonatal prophylaxis

Repeat Human Immunodeficiency Virus Testing in the Third Trimester

Repeat testing in the third trimester should be considered in jurisdictions with elevated HIV or AIDS incidence and in health care facilities in which prenatal screening identifies at least one HIV-infected pregnant woman per 1,000 women screened (1). Additionally, although physicians need to be aware of and follow their states' perinatal HIV screening requirements, repeat testing in the third trimester, preferably before 36 weeks of gestation, is recommended for pregnant women at high risk for acquiring HIV. Criteria for repeat testing can include (1):

- Have been diagnosed with another sexually transmitted disease in the last year

- Injection drug use or the exchange of sex for money or drugs

- A new or more than one sex partner during this pregnancy or a sex partner(s) known to be HIV-positive or at high risk

Women who are candidates for third-trimester testing, including those who declined testing earlier in pregnancy, should be given a conventional or rapid HIV test rather than waiting to receive a rapid test at labor and delivery (as allowed by state laws and regulations).

Recommendations

Given the enormous advances in the prevention of perinatal transmission of HIV, it is clear that early identification and treatment of all pregnant women with HIV is the best way to prevent neonatal disease and also may improve the women's health. Therefore, the American College of Obstetricians and Gynecologists makes the following recommendations:

- Screen all pregnant women for HIV as early as possible during each pregnancy following opt-out prenatal HIV screening where legally possible

- Repeat HIV testing in the third trimester is recommended for women in areas with high HIV prevalence, women known to be at high risk for acquiring HIV infection, and women who declined testing earlier in pregnancy

- Use conventional or rapid HIV testing for women who are candidates for third-trimester testing

- Use rapid HIV testing in labor for women with undocumented HIV status following opt-out screening

- If a rapid HIV test result in labor is positive, immediate initiation of antiretroviral prophylaxis should be recommended without waiting for the results of the confirmatory test

Resources

AIDS*info*
PO Box 6303
Rockville, MD 20849-6303
1-800-448-0440
www.aidsinfo.nih.gov

The American College of Obstetricians and Gynecologists
409 12th Street SW, PO Box 96920
Washington, DC 20090-6920
800-673-8444 or (202) 638-5577
www.acog.org
Perinatal HIV page: www.acog.org/goto/HIV
ACOG Bookstore: www.acog.org/bookstore

Centers for Disease Control and Prevention
1600 Clifton Road NE
Atlanta, GA 30333
(404) 639-3311 or 800-232-4636
www.cdc.gov
HIV/AIDS page: www.cdc.gov/hiv

National AIDS Hotline: 800-342-AIDS (2437) (English);
800-344-7432 (Spanish); 800-243-7889 (TTY, deaf access)
www.cdc.gov/hiv

National HIV/AIDS Clinicians' Consultation Center
UCSF Department of Family and Community Medicine at
San Francisco General Hospital
1001 Potrero Ave., Bldg. 20, Ward 22
San Francisco, CA 94110
(415) 206-8700
Perinatal HIV Hotline: 1-888-448-8765
www.nccc.ucsf.edu

References

1. Branson BM, Handsfield HH, Lampe MA, Janssen RS, Taylor AW, Lyss SB, et al. Revised recommendations for HIV testing of adults, adolescents, and pregnant women in health-care settings. MMWR Recomm Rep 2006;55(RR-14):1–17; quiz CE1-4.

2. McKenna MT, Hu X. Recent trends in the incidence and morbidity that are associated with perinatal human immunodeficiency virus infection in the United States. Am J Obstet Gynecol 2007;197(suppl):S10–6.

3. Recommendations of the U.S. Public Health Service Task Force on the use of zidovudine to reduce perinatal transmission of human immunodeficiency virus. MMWR Recomm Rep 1994;43(RR-11):1–20.

4. Wade NA, Birkhead GS, Warren BL, Charbonneau TT, French PT, Wang L, et al. Abbreviated regimens of zidovudine prophylaxis and perinatal transmission of the human immunodeficiency virus. N Engl J Med 1998;339:1409–14.

5. Mofenson LM, Lambert JS, Stiehm ER, Bethel J, Meyer WA 3rd, Whitehouse J, et al. Risk factors for perinatal transmission of human immunodeficiency virus type 1 in women treated with zidovudine. Pediatric AIDS Clinical Trials Group Study 185 Team. N Engl J Med 1999;341:385–93.

6. Garcia PM, Kalish LA, Pitt J, Minkoff H, Quinn TC, Burchett SK, et al. Maternal levels of plasma human immunodeficiency virus type 1 RNA and the risk of perinatal transmission. Women and Infants Transmission Study Group. N Engl J Med 1999;341:394–402.

7. American Academy of Pediatrics, American College of Obstetricians and Gynecologists. Joint statement on human immunodeficiency virus screening. Elk Grove Village (IL): AAP; Washington (DC): ACOG; 1999; Reaffirmed 2006.

8. Advancing HIV prevention: new strategies for a changing epidemic—United States, 2003. Centers for Disease Control and Prevention (CDC). MMWR Morb Mortal Wkly Rep 2003;52:329–32.

9. Gerberding JL, Jaffe HW. Routine prenatal testing – the opt-out approach. Atlanta (GA): Centers for Disease Control and Prevention; 2003. Available at: http://www.cdc.gov/ hiv/topics/perinatal/resources/other/dear_colleague-2003.htm. Retrieved June 10, 2008.

10. American Medical Association. Current procedural terminology: CPT® 2008. Standard ed. Chicago (IL): AMA; 2007.

11. Centers for Disease Control and Prevention. Rapid HIV-1 Antibody Testing during Labor and Delivery for Women of Unknown HIV Status: A Practical Guide and Model Protocol. Atlanta (GA): CDC; 2004. Available at: http:// www.cdc.gov/hiv/topics/testing/resources/guidelines/ rt-labor&delivery.htm. Retrieved June 10, 2008.

12. Peters V, Liu KL, Dominguez K, Frederick T, Melville S, Hsu HW, et al. Missed opportunities for perinatal HIV prevention among HIV-exposed infants born 1996-2000, pediatric spectrum of HIV disease cohort. Pediatrics 2003;111: 1186–91.

13. Gross E, Burr CK. HIV counseling and testing in pregnancy. N J Med 2003;100:21–6; quiz 67–8.

14. Paul SM, Grimes-Dennis J, Burr CK, DiFerdinando GT. Rapid diagnostic testing for HIV. Clinical implications. N J Med 2002;99:20–4; quiz 24–6.

15. Centers for Disease Control and Prevention. FDA-approved rapid HIV antibody screening tests. Atlanta (GA): CDC; 2008. Available at: http://www.cdc.gov/hiv/topics/testing/ rapid/rt-comparison.htm. Retrieved June 10, 2008.

Prenatal and perinatal human immunodeficiency virus testing: expanded recommendations. ACOG Committee Opinion No. 418. American College of Obstetricians and Gynecologists. Obstet Gynecol 2008;112:739–42.

ISSN 1074-861X

ACOG COMMITTEE OPINION

Number 419 • October 2008   *(Replaces No. 291, November 2003)*

Use of Progesterone to Reduce Preterm Birth

Committee on Obstetric Practice

This document reflects emerging clinical and scientific advances as of the date issued and is subject to change. The information should not be construed as dictating an exclusive course of treatment or procedure to be followed.

ABSTRACT: Preterm birth affects 12% of all births in the United States. Recent studies support the hypothesis that progesterone supplementation reduces preterm birth in a select group of women. Despite the apparent benefits of progesterone, the ideal progesterone formulation is unknown. The American College of Obstetricians and Gynecologists' Committee on Obstetric Practice and the Society for Maternal Fetal Medicine believe that further studies are needed to evaluate the optimal preparation, dosage, route of administration, and other indications for the use of progesterone for the prevention of preterm delivery. Based on current knowledge, it is important to offer progesterone for pregnancy prolongation to only women with a documented history of a previous spontaneous birth at less than 37 weeks of gestation.

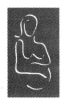

The Society for
Maternal Fetal Medicine
Publications Committee

The American College of Obstetricians and Gynecologists

Women's Health Care Physicians

Preterm birth affects 12% of all births in the United States. This statistic has led multiple investigators to identify those women at greatest risk (eg, those with prior preterm delivery, multiple gestation, short cervical length, maternal weight less than 50 kg, bleeding, and those of African American race). Recent randomized trials comparing progesterone with placebo have been conducted using several groups at high risk and low risk for preterm delivery. The purpose of this Committee Opinion is to review these results.

A large randomized placebo-controlled trial investigating the use of 17α-hydroxy-progesterone caproate ("17P") therapy (250 mg administered intramuscularly) for the prevention of preterm birth in a select, high-risk group of women (with a documented history of a previous spontaneous singleton preterm birth at less than 37 weeks of gestation) was conducted for the National Institute of Child Health and Human Development (NICHD) Maternal-Fetal Medicine Units Network (1). A total of 459 women with a history of previous spontaneous singleton births at less than 37 weeks of gestation were enrolled between 16 weeks and 20 weeks of gestation. Of note, the mean gestational age of their previous preterm deliveries was 30.7 weeks. They were ran-

domly assigned to receive weekly intramuscular injections of 17α-hydroxyprogesterone caproate (n = 306) or placebo (n = 153) from enrollment to 37 weeks of gestation or delivery. The study was stopped early when results showed a significant protection against recurrent preterm birth for all races of women who received 17α-hydroxyprogesterone caproate. This study demonstrated significant reductions in preterm and early preterm birth, low birth-weight, as well as significant reductions in infant complications (intraventricular hemorrhage, necrotizing enterocolitis, neonatal intensive care unit admissions, and the need for supplemental oxygen therapy) with progesterone therapy (Table 1). Four-year follow-up found no adverse health outcomes of surviving children (2).

In a randomized placebo-controlled trial of supplemental vaginal progesterone (100 mg daily) in 142 women at high risk for preterm birth (more than 90% of whom had a previous spontaneous singleton preterm birth) the authors found that for delivery at less than 34 weeks of gestation, the preterm birth rate was significantly lower among women receiving progesterone than among those receiving placebo (2.7% versus 18.6%) (3). The results of this study and the NICHD trial support the hypothesis that proges-

Table 1. Rates of Preterm Labor With Progesterone Therapy or Placebo

Gestation	Placebo Group (n = 153)	Progesterone Group (n = 306)	Relative Risk	Confidence Interval	P
Less than 37 weeks	54.9%	36.3%	0.66	0.54–0.81	.001
Less than 35 weeks	30.7%	20.6%	0.67	0.48–0.93	.0165
Less than 32 weeks	19.6%	11.4%	0.58	0.37–0.91	.0180

Data from Meis PJ, Klebanoff M, Thom E, Dombrowski MP, Sibai B, Moawad AH, et al. Prevention of recurrent preterm delivery by 17 alpha-hydroxyprogesterone caproate. N Engl J Med 2003;348:2379–85.

terone supplementation reduces preterm birth in women at risk for preterm birth, with a prior preterm birth.

The effectiveness of progesterone supplementation has been evaluated in several other high-risk groups for preterm delivery, with conflicting results. A randomized trial of 17α-hydroxyprogesterone caproate in 661 women with twin gestations found no benefit of progesterone supplementation for the prevention of preterm delivery (4). A randomized trial of 659 women with a history of spontaneous preterm delivery randomized and treated between 18 weeks and 23 weeks of gestation with 90 mg of natural progesterone vaginal gel or placebo found no improvement in preterm birth at less than 37 weeks, less than 35 weeks or less than 32 weeks of gestation. (5). Another randomized trial evaluated asymptomatic women with a short cervix and singleton and twin gestations. Of 24,620 women screened with endovaginal ultrasonography between 20 weeks and 25 weeks of gestation, 413 women had a cervical length less than 15 mm (1.5%) and of those women, 250 were randomized (1:1) to daily vaginal progesterone (200 mg micronized progesterone capsules) or placebo from 24 weeks to 34 weeks of gestation. Of note, 15% of the study population had a history of a prior preterm delivery and 10% of the study population had a twin gestation. Overall, progesterone therapy significantly reduced the rate of spontaneous preterm birth at less than 34 weeks of gestation (19.2% versus 34.3%) [6].

Despite the apparent benefits of progesterone in some situations, the ideal formulation is unknown. The 17α-hydroxyprogesterone caproate used in the NICHD trial was specially formulated for the trial and is not currently commercially available. Although the initial trial (3) used 100 mg vaginal suppositories and demonstrated pregnancy prolongation with treatment, vaginal progesterone gel was not beneficial in reducing preterm birth in women with a history of spontaneous preterm delivery randomized and treated between 18 weeks and 23 weeks of gestation (5). Micronized progesterone capsules (200 mg vaginally daily) were used in the trial of progesterone for asymptomatic women with a very short cervix (less than 15 mm), and appeared to be effective for this indication (6). Whether the differences seen in efficacy of the recently studied vaginal preparations reflects differences in dosages (100 mg versus 200 mg), variation in absorp-

tion and bioavailability with different preparations (gel versus capsule versus suppository), or differences in study populations remain to be elucidated. Progesterone has not been studied as a supplemental treatment to cervical cerclage for suspected cervical insufficiency, as a preventive agent for asymptomatic women with a positive cervicovaginal fetal fibronectin screen result, as a tocolytic agent, or as a therapeutic agent after tocolysis, and it should not be used at this time for these indications alone.

Progesterone supplementation for the prevention of recurrent preterm birth should be offered to women with a singleton pregnancy and a prior spontaneous preterm birth due to spontaneous preterm labor or premature rupture of membranes. Current evidence does not support the routine use of progesterone in women with multiple gestations. Progesterone supplementation for asymptomatic women with an incidentally identified very short cervical length (less than 15 mm) may be considered; however, routine cervical length screening is not recommended. The American College of Obstetricians and Gynecologists' Committee on Obstetric Practice and the Society for Maternal Fetal Medicine believe that further studies are needed to determine if there are other indications for progesterone therapy for the prevention of preterm delivery.

References

1. Meis PJ, Klebanoff M, Thom E, Dombrowski MP, Sibai B, Moawad AH, et al. Prevention of recurrent preterm delivery by 17 alpha-hydroxyprogesterone caproate. National Institute of Child Health and Human Development Maternal-Fetal Medicine Units Network [published erratum appears in N Engl J Med 2003;349:1299]. N Engl J Med 2003;348:2379–85.

2. Northen AT, Norman GS, Anderson K, Moseley L, Divito M, Cotroneo M, et al. Follow-up of children exposed in utero to 17 alpha-hydroxyprogesterone caproate compared with placebo. National Institute of Child Health and Human Development (NICHD) Maternal-Fetal Medicine Units (MFMU) Network. Obstet Gynecol 2007;110: 865–72.

3. da Fonseca EB, Bittar RE, Carvalho MH, Zugaib M. Prophylactic administration of progesterone by vaginal suppository to reduce the incidence of spontaneous preterm birth in women at increased risk: a randomized placebo-controlled double-blind study. Am J Obstet Gynecol 2003;188:419–24.

4. Rouse DJ, Caritis SN, Peaceman AM, Sciscione A, Thom EA, Spong CY, et al. A trial of 17 alpha-hydroxyprogesterone caproate to prevent prematurity in twins. National Institute of Child Health and Human Development Maternal-Fetal Medicine Units Network. N Engl J Med 2007;357:454–61.

5. O'Brien JM, Adair CD, Lewis DF, Hall DR, Defranco EA, Fusey S, et al. Progesterone vaginal gel for the reduction of recurrent preterm birth: primary results from a randomized, double-blind, placebo-controlled trial. Ultrasound Obstet Gynecol 2007;30:687–96.

6. da Fonseca EB, Celik E, Parra M, Singh M, Nicolaides KH. Progesterone and the risk of preterm birth among women with a short cervix. N Engl J Med 2007;357:462–9.

Use of progesterone to reduce preterm birth. ACOG Committee Opinion No. 419. American College of Obstetricians and Gynecologists. Obstet Gynecol 2008;112:963–5.

ISSN 1074-861X

ACOG COMMITTEE OPINION

Number 421 • November 2008   *(Replaces Practice Bulletin No. 47, October 2003)*

Antibiotic Prophylaxis for Infective Endocarditis

Committee on Obstetric Practice

This document reflects emerging clinical and scientific advances as of the date issued and is subject to change. The information should not be construed as dictating an exclusive course of treatment or procedure to be followed.

ABSTRACT: The recommendations for endocarditis prophylaxis from the American Heart Association have changed for three main reasons: 1) most cases of endocarditis are not attributable to an invasive procedure but rather are the result of randomly occurring bacteremia from routine daily activities; 2) prophylaxis may only prevent a small number of cases of infective endocarditis in women undergoing genitourinary procedures; and 3) the risk of antibiotic associated adverse events exceeds the benefit, if any, from prophylactic antibiotic therapy. The specific changes pertinent to the obstetrician–gynecologist are discussed.

The recommendations for endocarditis prophylaxis from the American Heart Association have changed for three main reasons: 1) most cases of endocarditis are not attributable to an invasive procedure but rather are the result of randomly occurring bacteremia from routine daily activities; 2) prophylaxis may only prevent a small number of cases of infective endocarditis in women undergoing genitourinary procedures; and 3) the risk of antibiotic associated adverse events exceeds the benefit, if any, from prophylactic antibiotic therapy (1). The specific changes pertinent to the obstetrician–gynecologist are discussed as follows.

Delivery

Infective endocarditis prophylaxis is no longer recommended for vaginal or cesarean delivery in the absence of infection, regardless of the type of maternal cardiac lesion. Mitral valve prolapse is no longer considered a lesion that ever needs infective endocarditis prophylaxis. Only cardiac conditions associated with the highest risk of adverse outcome from endocarditis are appropriate for any infective endocarditis prophylaxis (see box). In patients with one of these conditions and who have an established infection that could cause bacteremia, such as chorioamnionitis or pyelonephritis, the underlying infection should be treated in the usual fashion and the treatment should include a regimen effective for infective endocarditis prophylaxis (Table 1). Prophylaxis should be given intravenously.

Dental Procedures

The American Heart Association recommends that only those women with the cardiac conditions associated with the highest risk of adverse outcome from endocarditis (see box) receive infective endocarditis prophylaxis for certain dental procedures. Specifically, prophylaxis should be provided for all dental procedures that include manipulation of the gingival tissue or periapical region of the teeth or oral mucosa. Prophylaxis is not required in the following circumstances: injecting anesthetic into noninfected tissue, general dental cleaning, cavity filling, performing radiography, placing or adjusting orthodontic appliances, or when there is bleeding from trauma to lips and oral mucosa.

The American College of Obstetricians and Gynecologists
Women's Health Care Physicians

Table 1. Antibiotic Prophylaxis Appropriate for Infective Endocarditis

Treatment	Antibiotic	Regimen (preferably 30–60 min before procedure)
Intravenous therapy	Ampicillin or	2 g intravenously
	Cefazolin or ceftriaxone[†]	1 g intravenously
Allergic to penicillin or ampicillin*	Cefazolin or ceftriaxone[†] or clindamycin[†]	1 g intravenously[†] 600 mg intravenously[†]
Oral	Amoxicillin	2 g

*Cephalosporins should not be used in patients with a significant sensitivity to penicillins.

[†]This regimen does not cover enterococcus. Vancomycin can be used if enterococcus is of concern.

Cardiac Conditions for Which Prophylaxis for Deliveries Associated with Infection, or Certain Dental Procedures, is Reasonable

- Prosthetic cardiac valve or prosthetic material used for cardiac valve repair
- Previous infective endocarditis
- Congenital heart disease (CHD)*
  - Unrepaired cyanotic CHD, including palliative shunts and conduits
  - Completely repaired CHD with prosthetic material or device whether placed by surgery or catheter intervention, during the first 6 months after procedure[†]
  - Repaired CHD with residual defects at the site or adjacent to the site of a prosthetic patch or prosthetic device (which inhibit endothelialization)

*Except for the conditions listed, antibiotic prophylaxis is no longer recommended for any other form of CHD.

[†]Prophylaxis is reasonable because endothelialization of prosthetic material occurs within 6 months after the procedure.

Reference

1. Wilson W, Taubert KA, Gewitz M, Lockhart PB, Baddour LM, Levison M, et al. Prevention of infective endocarditis: guidelines from the American Heart Association: a guideline from the American Heart Association Rheumatic Fever, Endocarditis, and Kawasaki Disease Committee, Council on Cardiovascular Disease in the Young, and the Council on Clinical Cardiology, Council on Cardiovascular Surgery and Anesthesia, and the Quality of Care and Outcomes Research Interdisciplinary Working Group [published erratum appears in Circulation 2007;116:e376-7]. Circulation 2007;116:1736–54.

Antibiotic prophylaxis for infective endocarditis. ACOG Committee Opinion No. 421. American College of Obstetricians and Gynecologists. Obstet Gynecol 2008;112:1193–4.

ISSN 1074-861X

COMMITTEE ON PROFESSIONAL LIABILITY

COMMITTEE ON PROFESSIONAL LIABILITY

ACOG COMMITTEE OPINION

Number 380 • October 2007

Disclosure and Discussion of Adverse Events

Committee on Patient Safety and Quality Improvement

Committee on Professional Liability

Disclosure and discussion of adverse events. ACOG Committee Opinion No. 380. American College of Obstetricians and Gynecologists. Obstet Gynecol 2007;110:957–8.

ISSN 1074-861X

The American College of Obstetricians and Gynecologists

Women's Health Care Physicians

ABSTRACT: Disclosure and discussion of adverse events in health care is desired by patients and championed by safety experts and policy makers. Improving the disclosure process through policies, programmatic training, and accessible resources will enhance patient satisfaction, strengthen the physician–patient relationship, and most importantly, promote a higher quality of health care.

Adverse outcomes, preventable or otherwise, are an uncomfortable reality of medical care. The Institute of Medicine proposes a multifaceted approach toward reducing and managing adverse events, including the establishment of a national focus on patient safety, the creation of a mandatory reporting system, raising standards and expectations for safety improvements at the national level, and creating safety systems in health care organizations (1). Despite continuing efforts to prevent their occurrence, adverse events may happen even in the absence of medical error. Thus, there is a need for health care providers and institutions to understand how to best disclose and discuss these adverse events with patients and their families. The American College of Obstetricians and Gynecologists (ACOG) supports these efforts and seeks to assist members in understanding the value of disclosure and discussion in the face of preventable and nonpreventable adverse events and to provide guidance for such conversations.

The call for health care organizations to develop processes for disclosure is broad-based. Patient advocacy groups, patient safety experts, ethicists, policy makers, accrediting organizations, and physician groups all advocate the adoption of policies related to the disclosure and discussion of unanticipated adverse events. When adverse events occur, providers should engage the patient and family in discussions about the event(s), including expressions of sympathy.

The Joint Commission requires that accredited hospitals tell patients of unantic-

ipated adverse events. According to the Joint Commission Standard RI.2.90, "patients and, when appropriate, their families are informed about the events of care, treatment, and services that have been provided." Further, "the responsible licensed independent practitioner or his or her designee informs the patient (and when appropriate, the family) about those unanticipated outcomes of care, treatment, and services" (2). Similar statements are in the ethics code of the American Medical Association, which states that in cases in which "a patient suffers significant medical complications that may have resulted from a physician's mistake . . . the physician is ethically required to inform the patient of the facts necessary to ensure understanding of what has occurred"(3).

It is important to remember the difference between expressions of sympathy (acknowledgement of suffering) and apology (accountability for suffering). Expressions of sympathy are always appropriate. The appropriateness of an apology, however, will vary from case to case. When considering whether an apology is appropriate, the physician may wish to seek advice from the hospital's risk manager and the physician's liability carrier. It is also important to be knowledgeable about the state's laws on apology and disclosure because these laws vary and may have an effect on the way in which the disclosure is conducted.

Physicians have an ethical obligation to communicate honestly with patients. Disclosing information about unanticipated adverse events likely has benefits for both parties through a strengthened physician–patient relationship and a promotion of trust. Studies show that in the event of an adverse outcome, patients expect and want full disclosure of the event(s), an acknowledgement of responsibility, an understanding of what happened, expressions of sympathy, and discussion of what is being done to prevent recurrence(s) (4, 5). Additionally, disclosure of adverse events can be important for the physician's personal healing.

Barriers to full disclosure are many, including shame, lack of training in how to disclose, and fear of lawsuits (6, 7, 8). Based on surveys, it appears that patients want and expect timely and honest disclosure of adverse events and that patients are more likely to sue if they perceive that such disclosure was absent (9, 10). In studies of patients who sued their health care providers for adverse perinatal events, 43% were driven by a suspicion of a cover-up or by the desire for revenge (11).

Several organizations have reported on the success of their disclosure programs. One of the oldest programs advocating full disclosure of medical errors, the Veterans Affairs Medical Center in Lexington, Kentucky, reported that their facility's liability payments were moderate and comparable to similar institutions despite a proactive disclosure policy that might be anticipated to increase litigation (12). The University of Michigan Health System reported a 50% reduction in legal fees and actions since implementing a policy encouraging disclosure and apology in 2001 (13, 14).

A number of health care organizations, insurance carriers, and states have developed programs to educate physicians about disclosure. Examples include the University of Michigan Hospitals and Health Centers "Guidelines on How to Disclose Errors" and "When Things Go Wrong: Responding to Adverse Events," a consensus statement of the Harvard Hospitals (15). These can provide valuable guidance and education about the specifics of disclosure and apology. COPIC, a professional liability carrier for academic and community physicians in Colorado, provides its physicians with a training program and ongoing support in error disclosure entitled "The 3Rs Program" for Recognize, Respond, and Resolve unanticipated medical events (16).

Health care institutions should have written policies that address the timing, content, communication, and documentation of disclosure. Once policies are developed, health care organizations should educate their providers on the policies and consider the need for additional resources and training such as disclosure coaching, mediation, and emotional support for health care workers involved in harmful medical errors (7, 17). Individual physicians and physician practice groups may contact their local hospitals, liability carriers, specialty organizations, or medical societies for disclosure assistance training and resources available to them.

REFERENCES

1. Institute of Medicine. To err is human: building a safer health system. Washington, DC: National Academy Press; 2000.

2. Joint Commission on Accreditation of Healthcare Organizations. Comprehensive accreditation manual for hospitals: CAMH. Oakbrook Terrace (IL): JCAHO; 2006.

3. American Medical Association. Code of medical ethics of the American Medical Association: current opinions with annotations. 2006–2007 ed. Chicago (IL): AMA; 2006.

4. Gallagher TH, Waterman AD, Ebers AG, Fraser VJ, Levinson W. Patients' and physicians' attitudes regarding the disclosure of medical errors. JAMA 2003;289:1001–7.

5. Mazor KM, Simon SR, Yood RA, Martinson BC, Gunter MJ, Reed GW, et al. Health plan members' views about disclosure of medical errors. Ann Intern Med 2004;140:409–18.

6. Finkelstein D, Wu AW, Holtzman NA, Smith MK. When a physician harms a patient by a medical error: ethical, legal, and risk-management considerations. J Clin Ethics 1997;8:330.

7. Goldberg RM, Kuhn G, Andrew LB, Thomas HA Jr. Coping with medical mistakes and errors in judgment. Ann Emerg Med 2002;39:287–92.

8. Mello MM, Studdert DM, DesRoches CM, Peugh J, Zapert K, Brennan TA, et al. Caring for patients in a malpractice crisis: physician satisfaction and quality of care. Health Aff (Millwood) 2004;23(4):42–53.

9. Vincent C, Young M, Phillips A. Why do people sue doctors? A study of patients and relatives taking legal action. Lancet 1994;343:1609–13.

10. Beckman HB, Markakis KM, Suchman AL, Frankel RM. The doctor–patient relationship and malpractice. Lessons from plaintiff depositions. Arch Intern Med 1994;154:1365–70.

11. Hickson GB, Clayton EW, Githens PB, Sloan FA. Factors that prompted families to file medical malpractice claims following perinatal injuries. JAMA 1992;267:1359–63.

12. Kraman SS, Hamm G. Risk management: extreme honesty may be the best policy. Ann Intern Med 1999;131:963–7.

13. Gallagher TH, Levinson W. Disclosing harmful medical errors to patients: a time for professional action. Arch Intern Med 2005;165:1819–24.

14. Orlovsky C. Proposed legislation encourages hospital disclosure initiatives. Glen Carbon (IL): The Sorry Works! Coalition; 2005. Available at: http://www.sorryworks.net/media40.phtml. Retrieved March 5, 2007.

15. Massachusetts Coalition for the Prevention of Medical Errors. When things go wrong: responding to adverse events: a consensus statement of the Harvard Hospitals. Burlington (MA): MAC; 2006. Available at: http://www.macoalition.org/documents/respondingToAdverseEvents.pdf. Retrieved March 5, 2007.

16. 3Rs program. Denver (CO): Copic Companies. Available at: http://www.callcopic.com/home/what-we-offer/coveages/medical-professional-liability-insurance-co/physicians-medical-practices/special-programs/3rs-program. Retrieved March 5, 2007.

17. Liebman CB, Hyman CS. A mediation skills model to manage disclosure of errors and adverse events to patients. Health Aff (Millwood) 2004;23(4):22–32.

ACOG COMMITTEE OPINION

Number 406 • May 2008   (Replaces No. 309, February 2005)

Coping With the Stress of Medical Professional Liability Litigation

Committee on Professional Liability

This document provides risk management information that is current as of the date issued and is subject to change. This document does not define a standard of care nor should it be interpreted as legal advice.

ABSTRACT: Obstetrician–gynecologists should recognize that being a defendant in a medical professional liability lawsuit can be one of life's most stressful experiences. Coping with the stress of medical professional liability litigation is an ongoing, complex process in which physicians often must struggle to regain a sense of personal identity and professional mastery, as well as control of their clinical practices. Open communication with family members will assist in reducing emotional isolation and self-blame; however, legal and clinical aspects of a case must be kept confidential. Peer support and individual professional counseling can be of great benefit. Rapid intervention facilitates healthier coping strategies and can restore a sense of equilibrium and self-esteem during an unpredictable time.

The American College of Obstetricians and Gynecologists

Women's Health Care Physicians

The American College of Obstetricians and Gynecologists (ACOG) has long been concerned about the psychologic and emotional impact of medical professional liability litigation on physicians, especially because 89.2% of ACOG Fellows have been sued at least once in their careers (1). Defendant physicians may experience a wide range of distressing emotions and increased stress, which can disrupt their personal lives and the lives of their families, their relationships with patients, and their medical practices. Because a medical professional liability case in obstetrics and gynecology usually takes several years to resolve, this stressful period can seem interminable for all involved.

Common responses to medical liability litigation include feelings of shock, outrage, denial, anxiety, guilt, shame, and despair. Coping with medical professional liability litigation is an ongoing, complex process in which physicians often must struggle to regain a sense of personal identity and professional mastery as well as control of their clinical practices.

Claims managers and defense attorneys often advise physicians not to speak to anyone regarding any aspect of the medical liability case. Nevertheless, physicians often need to express their emotional responses to being sued. Literal adherence to the advice

to "speak to no one" can result in isolation, increased stress, and dysfunctional behavior. Guidance on interventions for impaired or dysfunctional physician behavior is addressed elsewhere (2). Such behavior may jeopardize family relationships and also may affect the physician's ability to function professionally and to represent himself or herself appropriately and effectively during a trial. Therefore, the physician is encouraged to inform family members of the lawsuit, the allegations, the potential for publicity, and any expected testimony, while maintaining confidentiality. Children should be told about the lawsuit and their questions honestly answered, commensurate with their age and ability to understand the information. Open communication with family members will assist in reducing emotional isolation and self-blame (3).

Certainly, legal and clinical aspects of a case must be kept confidential. An exception to this rule, however, might be made in the context of professional counseling. Any clinical aspects of a medical professional liability case that are discussed in counseling should be disclosed within the confines of a formal counselor–patient relationship to ensure the confidentiality privilege. State laws determine whether confidentiality can be maintained if the counselor is other than a physician or member of the clergy. Moreover, confidentiality may be lost if third parties are present.

Obstetrician–gynecologists should recognize that being a defendant in a medical professional liability lawsuit can be one of life's most stressful experiences. Although negative emotions in response to a lawsuit are normal, physicians may need help from professionals or peers to cope with this stress. Residents, as young physicians in training, may be particularly vulnerable to the psychologic and emotional upheaval that often occurs when named in a medical liability claim. State or local medical societies and medical liability insurance carriers often sponsor support groups for defendant physicians and their families. Support mechanisms for residents also may be available through residency program directors, department chairs, departments of risk management, or mentors. In the absence of such services, individual professional counseling can be of great benefit. Rapid intervention facilitates healthier coping strategies and can restore a sense of equilibrium and self-esteem during an unpredictable time.

References

1. Wilson N, Strunk AL. Overview of the 2006 ACOG Survey on Professional Liability. ACOG Clin Rev 2007;12(2):1, 13–16.

2. American College of Obstetricians and Gynecologists. Guidelines for women's health care: a resource manual. 3rd ed. Washington, DC: ACOG; 2007.

3. Charles SC, Frish PR. Adverse events, stress, and litigation: a physician's guide. New York (NY): Oxford University Press; 2005.

Bibliography

Brazeau CM. Coping with the stress of being sued. Fam Pract Manag 2001;8(5):41–4.

Charles SC. How to handle the stress of litigation. Clin Plast Surg 1999;26:69–77, vii.

Charles SC. Medical liability litigation as a disruptive life event. Bull Am Coll Surg 2005;90(12):17–23.

Hutchison JR, Hutchison S. The toughest part of being sued. Med Econ 1995;72(23):36–7, 41–4, 48, passim.

Page L. On the defensive. A physician's confidence can shatter in the wake of a lawsuit. Mod Healthc 2004;34:51, 54.

Physician Litigation Stress Resource Center. St. Joseph (MI): PLSRC; 2007. Available at: http://www.physicianlitigationstress.org. Retrieved November 14, 2007.

Settel KM. The impact of malpractice litigation on physicians. Forum 1998;19(4):13–5.

Weiss GG. You've been sued. There's help. Med Econ 2003; 80(3):56, 59–60.

Coping with the stress of medical professional liability litigation. ACOG Committee Opinion No. 406. American College of Obstetricians and Gynecologists. Obstet Gynecol 2008;111:1257–8.

COMMITTEE ON PATIENT SAFETY
AND QUALITY IMPROVEMENT

Committee on Patient Safety and Quality Improvement

ACOG COMMITTEE OPINION

Number 366 • May 2007

Disruptive Behavior

Committee on Patient Safety and Quality Improvement

This document reflects emerging concepts on patient safety and is subject to change. The information should not be construed as dictating an exclusive course of treatment or procedure to be followed.

ABSTRACT: Disruptive behavior may have a negative effect on patient care. Consequently, it is important that a systematic process be in place to discourage, identify, and remedy episodes of disruptive behavior.

A growing number of organizations recognize that disruptive behavior may compromise patient care. Numerous reports of disruptive physician behavior in the media and literature demonstrate its effect on patient care and other staff. The AMA Report of the Council on Ethical and Judicial Affairs defines disruptive behavior as "a style of interaction...that interferes with patient care...[and] that tends to cause distress among other staff and affect overall morale within the work environment, undermining productivity and possibly leading to high staff turnover or even resulting in ineffective or substandard care." (1) Several types of behavior can create distress or negatively affect morale in the work environment. Example behaviors include:

- Profane or disrespectful language
- Yelling at or insulting others
- Throwing instruments, charts, or other objects
- Bullying or demeaning behavior
- Criticizing other caregivers in front of patients or other staff
- Sexual comments or innuendo (2)

Yelling, insulting others, or a refusal to carry out duties are among the most common types of behaviors reported. The targets of such behavior are often co-workers with less power than the offending individual as exemplified by the relationships between staff physicians and nurses, residents, or medical students (3). A consequence of this type of behavior is corruption of teamwork.

Best estimates suggest that a small number of physicians (3–5%) are responsible for most of the reported disruptive behavior (3). Although relatively few physicians exhibit these behaviors, 95% of physician executives reported knowing of "disturbing, disruptive and potentially dangerous behaviors on a regular basis" (4). A recent study concluded that many disruptive physicians began to show evidence of such behavior as medical students (5), highlighting the potential importance of recognizing behavioral patterns early in career development.

Ultimately, disruptive behavior may have a negative effect on patient safety and quality of care by causing others to avoid the disruptive physician. Staff may refrain from asking for help or clarification and hesitate to make suggestions about care to the disruptive physician. Additionally, patients who witness the behavior may lose confidence in the health care provider as well as the institution.

Several factors contribute to a reluctance to systematically confront disruptive behavior, including financial concerns such as physician referrals and fear of retribution (eg, lawsuit for antitrust or defamation of character) (6). Therefore, institutions should develop a multifaceted approach for dealing with disruptive behavior. It is essential that administration fully support and show commitment to addressing disruptive behavior.

The American College of Obstetricians and Gynecologists
Women's Health Care Physicians

An effective approach would include the following components (2).

Establishing a Code of Conduct

Institutions should consider establishing a code of conduct that stipulates behavioral standards and the consequences for failure to comply. Specific examples of unacceptable behavior should be included to provide guidance for leadership, employees, and staff in determining what constitutes disruptive behavior. If a formal mechanism is adopted, at appointment and reappointment, each medical staff member should acknowledge acceptance of both the behavioral standards and the consequences of failure to comply, as detailed in the code of conduct, consistent with provisions contained in the medical staff bylaws. A training program about the code and attendant behavioral expectations may be included as part of this approach.

Instituting a Monitoring and Reporting System

A monitoring system may be considered. Systematic review could include regular surveys of staff, focus groups, peer and team member evaluations, and direct observation to detect incidents of disruptive behavior (2). Implementing a confidential system for reporting also could include routine confidential evaluations and formal analysis of complaints by patients, co-workers, or others. These evaluations should be provided in a confidential manner to the appropriate administrative individual, such as the chair of the department of obstetrics and gynecology or the chief of staff for resolution. The individual in question should be notified and given an opportunity to respond to the complaint.

Resolution

Any complaints should be handled in a confidential manner with interventions designed to assist in behavioral change whenever possible. Complaint resolution should be consistent with medical staff, departmental, or other institutional policies and procedures. Appropriate steps should be taken to resolve the problem. Disciplinary actions should be appropriate to the type of infraction and frequency of behavior, including any mitigating factors. Each institution should establish thresholds for taking action that depend on the severity of the behavior. Some actions may merit zero tolerance. All attempts to address disruptive behavior should be clearly and thoroughly documented. The department chair should be informed of individuals with persistent problem behaviors and responsible for establishing an appropriate response. The response may include some or all of the following steps:

- Face-to-face meeting with the physician exhibiting disruptive behavior

- A follow-up meeting (if the problem is still unresolved), resulting in a behavioral contract setting forth any disciplinary actions that may be taken if disruptive behavior persists

- Formal counseling

- Administrative hearing

- Summary suspension for egregious behavior

Assessment and treatment programs that are tailored to the individual should be made available as necessary. Special attention should be given to the possibility of substance abuse or psychiatric diagnosis, which can contribute to disruptive behavior. At least initially, these programs should attempt to enable the individual to continue or resume practice.

Conclusion

Disruptive physician behavior creates a difficult working environment for all staff and threatens the quality of patient care and, ultimately, patient safety. Colleagues often find confronting these individuals difficult. Therefore, it is important that clear standards of behavior are established and all staff are informed of such standards, as well as the consequences of persistent disruptive behavior. Confidential reporting systems, as well as assistance programs for the offending physician, should be established.

References

1. American Medical Association. Physicians with disruptive behavior. In: Code of medical ethics: current opinions and annotations. Chicago (IL): AMA: 2006. p. 279–80.

2. Porto G, Lauve R. Disruptive clinician: a persistent threat to patient safety. Patient Saf Qual Healthc 2006;144: 107–15.

3. Leape LL, Fromson JA. Problem doctors: is there a system-level solution? Ann Intern Med 2006;144:107–115.

4. Weber DO. For safety's sake disruptive behavior must be tamed. Physician Exec 2004;30:16–7.

5. Papadakis MA, Teherani A, Banach MA, Knettler TR, Rattner SL, Stern DT, et al. Disciplinary action by medical boards and prior behavior in medical school. N Engl J Med 2005;353:2673–82.

6. ECRI. Disruptive practitioner behavior. HRC Risk Analysis Supplement A. Plymouth Meeting (PA): ECRI; 2006.

Disruptive behavior. ACOG Committee Opinion No. 366. American College of Obstetricians and Gynecologists. Obstet Gynecol 2007; 109:1261–2.

ISSN 1074-861X

ACOG COMMITTEE OPINION

Number 367 • June 2007

Communication Strategies for Patient Handoffs

Committee on
Patient Safety and
Quality Improvement

This document reflects emerging concepts on patient safety and is subject to change. The information should not be construed as dictating an exclusive course of treatment or procedure to be followed.

ABSTRACT: Handoff communication, which includes up-to-date information regarding patient care, treatment and service, condition, and any recent or anticipated changes, should be interactive to allow for discussion between the giver and receiver of patient information. It requires a process for verification of the received information, including read-back or other methods as appropriate.

Accurate communication of information about a patient from one physician to another is a critical element of patient care and safety; it is also one of the least studied and taught elements of patient care that physicians use on a daily basis. In its 1999 publication, "To Err is Human: Building a Safer Health System," the Institute of Medicine estimated that between 44,000 and 98,000 patients die each year in U.S. hospitals because of injuries that result from errors (1). One of the leading causes of these errors is a breakdown in communication. Ineffective communication was cited as the root cause of 66% of all reported sentinel events from 1995 to 2004 and accounted for 85% of sentinel events related to maternal death and injury in 2005 (2). This breakdown in communication may occur between health care providers at every level of the health care system. Physician-to-physician handoff of patient information is one of the most important factors to focus on to prevent discontinuity of care, eliminate preventable errors, and provide a safer patient environment.

Communication is the process by which information is exchanged between individuals, groups, and organizations. In order to be effective, communication should be complete, clear, concise, and timely. Barriers to effective communication include factors such as lack of time, hierarchies, defensiveness, varying communication styles, distraction, fatigue, conflict, and workload.

A *handoff* may be described as the transfer of patient information and knowledge along with authority and responsibility from one physician or team of physicians to another physician or provider. The Joint Commission requires implementation of a standardized approach to handoff communications (National Patient Safety Goal [NPSG] 2E) (3). Properly executed handoffs are interactive and include the opportunity for questions and answers. A handoff may occur during the transfer of care in any of several circumstances, including from one on-call physician to another, from the office physician to the hospital laborist or vice versa, or from the generalist obstetrician–gynecologist to the intensivist. It also may occur between the attending physician and a resident or between the attending physician and nursing staff. Every important aspect of the patient's condition and circumstance must be accurately communicated and acknowledged from one party to the other for a safe and effective handoff to occur. Communication at the time of the handoff should result in a clear understanding by each provider about who is responsible for which aspects of the patient's care. Unacknowledged messages, such as voice mail, do not constitute an acceptable form of handoff.

Patient handoffs can be improved. Addressing aspects such as physical environment, confidentiality, language, organizational culture, communication method, and documentation are key to improving the process.

Physical Environment

The physical environment in which the transfer takes place may hinder effective

The American College of Obstetricians and Gynecologists
Women's Health Care Physicians

communication. For example, a noisy nursing station is a less desirable setting for communicating handoff information than a quiet conference room located away from other distractions. Having discussions in an environment without distractions will enhance communication during handoffs. Clinical acuity of the patient's condition must be considered in deciding the circumstances, the setting, and the content of the handoff.

Confidentiality

Care must be taken to maintain patient confidentiality by allowing only those involved with her care to hear or view protected health care information. Physicians must be aware of and comply with Health Insurance Portability and Accountability Act (HIPAA) regulations.

Language

Language differences may interfere with the accurate transfer of information. Using standardized medical terminology avoids errors in communication that may occur when colloquialisms are used. Awareness of cultural and gender differences in communication style is an important factor in how handoffs may be presented and received.

Organizational Culture

The hierarchy of personnel, particularly in teaching settings, also may inhibit the transfer of important information about the patient. When information about the patient's care is being conveyed, a first-year resident should be made to feel as comfortable talking with the senior attending physician as with another resident. Every member of the health care team that is present should be encouraged to participate in and contribute to the transfer of information without reluctance.

Communication Method

The method of communication may be a significant barrier to the effective transfer of vital information. Structured forms of communication, such as the Situation-Background-Assessment-Recommendation (SBAR) technique, should be considered. Communication may be verbal, written, or both (4). The Joint Commission NPSG 2A requires that the person receiving a verbal or phone order or test result "read back" the complete order or test result for verification (3). Verbal communication includes a face-to-face conversation or a telephone call. Face-to-face exchange of information is generally the preferred form of verbal communication because it allows direct interaction among those present. Not only may questions be asked and answered, but further nonverbal information may be expressed by body language and facial expression. Written communication may assist the person handing off the patient in organizing his or her thoughts and presenting important details. It also allows the receiving party to have a paper- or computer-generated hard copy of information for reference. Written communica-

tion, however, lacks the subjective interpersonal aspect of verbal communication. The most effective handoff of patient information includes both verbal and written components.

Documentation

The written component of the handoff may be produced by hand or by computer using an electronic medical record (EMR). One of the main advantages of an EMR is that it eliminates illegibility. Illegible handwriting has been shown to be a major contributor to errors in patient care. This issue is being addressed by many different groups, including the Joint Commission. Although there is no universally accepted protocol for all of the information that a written handoff should contain, there are several key elements that should be present in any transfer of patient care. These include pertinent demographic information, a brief history and the results of a physical examination, an active problem list, medications and allergies, pending test results, ongoing or anticipated therapy, and any other critical information. Such information as code status, psychosocial status, family issues, and long-term care issues also may be included as circumstances warrant.

Conclusion

Providing a safer health care environment for patients must become the hallmark of future health care. By improving the process for transferring information that occurs during physician handoffs, the care that patients receive will be optimized and ideally should be seamless. Studies are currently underway to determine the most effective methods to perform and teach the transfer of patient information. Physicians must strive to improve their communication skills, not only with each other, but also when interacting with other members of the health care team. Awareness of the importance and challenges of effective communication and implementation of effective communication processes, especially as it relates to handoffs, will decrease errors that result in adverse events and provide a safer patient environment.

References

1. Institute of Medicine (US). To err is human: building a safer health system. Washington, DC: The Institute; 1999.

2. Joint Commission on Accreditation of Healthcare Organizations. Sentinel event statistics. Oakbrook Terrace (IL): JCAHO; 2006. Available at: http://www.jointcommission. org/sentinel events/statistics. Retrieved February 15, 2007.

3. Joint Commission on Accreditation of Healthcare Organizations. Comprehensive accreditation manual for hospitals: CAMH. Oakbrook Terrace (IL): JCAHO; 2006.

4. Institute for Healthcare Improvement. SBAR technique for communication: a situational briefing model. Cambridge (MA): IHI; 2006. Available at: http://www.ihi.org/IHI/ Topics/PatientSafety/SafetyGeneral/Tools/SBARTechniquef orCommunicationASituationalBriefingModel.htm. Retrieved February 15, 2007.

Additional Resources

JCAHO's 2006 National Patient Safety Goals: handoffs are biggest challenge. Hosp Peer Rev 2005;30:89–93.

Solet DJ, Norvell JM, Rutan GH, Frankel RM. Lost in translation: challenges and opportunities in physician-to-physician communication during patient handoffs. Acad Med 2005;80:1094

Focus on five: strategies to improve hand-off communication: implementing a process to resolve questions. Jt Comm Perspect Pat Saf 2005;5(7):11.

Communication strategies for patient handoffs. ACOG Committee Opinion No. 367. American College of Obstetricians and Gynecologists. Obstet Gynecol 2007;109:1503–5.

ISSN 1074-861X

ACOG COMMITTEE OPINION

Number 398 • February 2008

Fatigue and Patient Safety

**Committee on
Patient Safety and
Quality Improvement**

This document reflects emerging concepts on patient safety and is subject to change. The information should not be construed as dictating an exclusive course of treatment or procedure to be followed.

ABSTRACT: It has long been recognized that fatigue can affect human cognitive and physical function. Although there are limited published data on the effects of fatigue on health care providers, including full-time practicing physicians, there is increasing awareness within the patient safety movement that fatigue, even partial sleep deprivation, impairs performance. Most of the current literature reviews resident function after recent work reform changes. However, the information available from many studies in health care and other occupations can be applied to the work habits of practicing obstetrician–gynecologists.

**The American College
of Obstetricians
and Gynecologists**
*Women's Health Care
Physicians*

A safe and effective health care system must be structured to minimize error and confusion. Individuals who are tired are more likely to make mistakes. Reducing fatigue may improve patient care and safety as well as reduce the risk of adverse outcomes, improve health care provider's satisfaction, and increase communication. One of the most significant limitations in evaluating fatigue is the absence of an available metric for measuring accurately fatigue and its subsequent effect on patient care.

Physicians are expected to offer safe and effective care to their patients. Maturity as a clinician requires recognition that medicine is a human endeavor. As individuals develop their clinical skills, they become aware of their own unique strengths and weaknesses. Professionals regularly seek consultations when a problem exceeds their experience or expertise. Seeking assistance when one is fatigued is beginning to be seen in a similar light. Fatigue may greatly affect health care provider's skills and abilities, communication, and possibly outcomes. Because of a lack of research on the subject, there are no current guidelines placing any limits on the volume of deliveries and procedures performed by a single individual or the length of time one may be on call and still perform procedures. Each physician must recognize his or her limitations caused by fatigue that can occur from an excessively busy practice and impose limits. External factors not related to the practice of medicine also must be considered. Physicians at all stages in their careers need to be cognizant of the demands

placed on them professionally and personally and should strive to achieve a balance that will not lead to excessive fatigue or overcommitment.

The National Sleep Foundation (www.sleepfoundation.org) recommends 8 hours of sleep per night for an adult (1). The average American adult sleeps only approximately 7 hours per night. Sleep deprivation can be caused by insufficient sleep, fragmented sleep, or both. Although there is wide variation in sleep needs, individuals do not get accustomed to less sleep than their biologic requirement. One cannot store up sleep. Recovery from a period of insufficient sleep requires at least two or three full nights of adequate uninterrupted sleep (1).

A number of uncontrolled studies have looked at the effect of sleep restriction on cognitive function (2–4). One small study compared reaction times and performance on a driving simulator between residents who had ingested alcohol but were rested and residents who were on a call rotation every fourth night and found a correlation. Emergency department physicians who were rested have been compared with others on sequential night call. The disruption of sleep produced by shift work had a significant impact on both visual memory and cognitive performance (5, 6).

Several reviews of the literature show that even a single night of missed sleep measurably affects cognitive performance. When adults do not sleep at least 5 hours per night, language and numeric skills, retention of information, short-term memory, and concentration all decline on standardized testing. Speed of performance may be affected more than accuracy. For example, surgeons operated more slowly in simulated procedures when sleep deprived; emergency department physicians took longer to intubate a mannequin (7–10).

In other industries, fatigue often is invoked as a cause of error and accident. The National Transportation Safety Board rates excessive sleepiness as the second leading cause of driving accidents in the United States (11). A recent study by the Federal Railroad Administration showed that human factor errors are responsible for almost 40% of all train accidents over the past 5 years and that fatigue played a role in approximately 25% of the accidents (12). However, there is no clear evidence in health care that restricting work hours improves patient outcome. Several potential explanations for this exist. In the residency setting, work-hour restriction often has been achieved through a night-float system, which has not been shown to decrease fatigue. Repeated episodes of night work may result in accumulating sleep debt as physicians find themselves unable to rest during the day. Even a single night of complete sleep loss can require up to 3 days for recovery. Thus, any resident schedule of every fourth night or more frequent call schedules, regardless of total hours worked, may result in reduced acuity and function. Reduced hours may not be enough to show reduced fatigue or improved outcomes. Further, supervision of residents by other caregivers may intercept incipient errors (6, 13).

The inability to document improved outcome after residency work-hour reform does not mean that fatigue can safely be ignored by practicing physicians. Memory consolidation and insight formation require sleep. Sleep-deprived adults tend to exhibit impaired complex problem solving and to continue with solutions that do not work (14). The need for sleep, like the need for food, can affect decision making. Fatigue may drive people to avoid work responsibilities to address sleep deprivation. Safe and effective care requires mindful communication between the patient and the physician and between the physician and other caregivers. Mood may be even more affected by sleep deprivation than cognitive or motor performance and may have a significant impact on a physician's ability to communicate effectively (9).

Although the implication of the studies mentioned is that quality of care may be enhanced by increased physician rest, there is no current evidence that proves this premise. We should continue to study and consider the potential benefit of limiting physician call schedules balanced against loss of continuity of care.

It would be prudent to consider adapting, when feasible, the following guidelines from the National Highway Traffic Safety Administration to medical work (11):

- Structure work to take advantage of circadian influences.

- Recognize that the drive to sleep is very strong between 2 AM and 9 AM, and especially between 3 AM and 5 AM. Avoid unnecessary work at that time.
- Sleep when sleepy.
- Provide for backup during times impairment is likely.
- After working a night shift, go immediately to sleep to maximize sleep length.
- Apply good sleep habits. The sleep environment should be quiet and dark. It should have adequate ventilation and a comfortable temperature to allow daytime sleep.
- Recognize behavioral changes such as irritability that may indicate dangerous levels of fatigue.
- Use naps strategically. A 2-hour nap before a night shift will help prevent sleepiness. If a 2-hour nap cannot be scheduled, then sleep no more than 45 minutes to avoid deep sleep and subsequent difficulty with arousal.

Each practicing physician and every group should review their work habits with these principles in mind. Even though there may be some economic impact of changing schedules to accommodate avoidance of fatigue, patient care and safety must take priority over economic concerns. A balance needs to be found between reducing work hours and providing appropriate continuity of care for individual patients.

Each provider should consider the following questions:

- Should I work a half day or a full clinic day after a night on call (or work at all)?
- Should I perform surgery if I have been awake most of the previous night or should the procedure be rescheduled?
- What back-up system is available if I recognize a worrisome level of fatigue?
- What adjustments should be made to my call schedule to avoid a worrisome level of fatigue?

Because physicians may not easily be able to assess the degree of their own fatigue, it also may be prudent for groups or departments to develop processes that provide backup care when physician fatigue may diminish the quality of care. Physicians should consider postponing tasks that can be performed more safely at a later time. Departments and groups also should recognize that fatigue may arise from obligations outside the workplace. Some departments have systems that encourage collaboration between practices when a provider has not had a sufficient period of uninterrupted sleep.

There is no question that the human factor of fatigue can affect performance. Because of the issues of patient safety, fatigue should be addressed by all practitioners, and efforts should be made to adjust workloads, work hours, and time commitments to avoid fatigue when caring for patients. Physicians should not fear economic or other penalties for requesting assistance.

Additional research on the effects of fatigue on experienced practicing obstetrician–gynecologists is necessary before specific national guidelines that are evidence based can be promulgated to improve overall patient safety and care. In the meantime, practicing physicians should evaluate the effects that fatigue has on their professional and personal lives.

References

1. Malik SW, Kaplan J. Sleep deprivation. Prim Care 2005; 32:475–90.

2. Arnedt JT, Owens J, Crouch M, Stahl J, Carskadon MA. Neurobehavioral performance of residents after heavy night call vs after alcohol ingestion. JAMA 2005;294:1025–33.

3. Dawson D, Reid K. Fatigue, alcohol and performance impairment. Nature 1997;388:235.

4. Australian Transport Safety Bureau. Development of measures of fatigue: using an alcohol comparison to validate the effects of fatigue on performance. Road Safety Research Report CR 189. Canberra: ATSB; 2000. Available at: http://www.atsb.gov.au/publications/2000/pdf/Fatig_Alc.pdf. Retrieved September 4, 2007.

5. Rollinson DC, Rathlev NK, Moss M, Killiany R, Sassower KC, Auerbach S, et al. The effects of consecutive night shifts on neuropsychological performance of interns in the emergency department: a pilot study. Ann Emerg Med 2003; 41:400–6.

6. Dula DJ, Dula NL, Hamrick C, Wood GC. The effect of working serial night shifts on the cognitive functioning of emergency physicians. Ann Emerg Med 2001;38:152–5.

7. Pilcher JJ, Huffcutt AI. Effects of sleep deprivation on performance: a meta-analysis. Sleep 1996;19:318–26.

8. Jha AK, Duncan BW, Bates DW. Fatigue, sleepiness, and medical errors. In: Agency for Healthcare Research and Quality. Making health care safer: a critical analysis of patient safety practices. Evidence Report/Technology Assessment No. 43. Rockville (MD): AHRQ; 2001. p. 523–37. Available at: http://www.ahrq.gov/clinic/ptsafety/chap46a.htm. Retrieved August 27, 2007.

9. Friedman WA. Resident duty hours in American neurosurgery. Neurosurgery 2004;54:925–31; discussion 931–3.

10. Smith-Coggins R, Rosekind MR, Hurd S, Buccino KR. Relationship of day versus night sleep to physician performance and mood. Ann Emerg Med 1994;24:928–34.

11. National Transportation Safety Board. Factors that affect fatigue in heavy truck accidents. NTSB Report No. NTSB/SS-95/01. Washington, DC: NTSB; 1995.

12. Federal Railroad Administration. The railroad fatigue risk management program at the federal railroad administration: past, present and future. Washington, DC: FRA; 2006. Available at: http://www.fra.dot.gov/downloads/safety/fatiguewhitepaper112706.pdf. Retrieved September 4, 2007.

13. Kuhn G. Circadian rhythm, shift work, and emergency medicine. Ann Emerg Med 2001;37:88–98.

14. Ellenbogen JM. Cognitive benefits of sleep and their loss due to sleep deprivation. Neurology 2005;64:E25–7.

Fatigue and patient safety. ACOG Committee Opinion No. 398. American College of Obstetricians and Gynecologists. Obstet Gynecol 2008;111:471–3.

ISSN 1074-861X

ACOG COMMITTEE OPINION

Number 400 • March 2008

Technologic Advances to Reduce Medication-Related Errors

Committee on Patient Safety and Quality Improvement

This document reflects emerging concepts on patient safety and is subject to change. The information should not be construed as dictating an exclusive course of treatment or procedure to be followed.

ABSTRACT: The Institute of Medicine estimates that up to 7,000 individuals die each year as a result of medication errors. Despite the significant national attention medical errors are receiving, they continue to pervade the U.S. health care system. Medication-related errors consistently rank at the top of all medical errors, accounting for thousands of deaths annually in the United States. Many new technologies are available that, when integrated into the various medication-related processes, can significantly reduce the incidence of preventable medication errors. Practicing obstetrician–gynecologists should be familiar with these technologies and the evidence supporting their use.

A report by the Institute of Medicine (IOM) on medication-related errors suggests that despite the attention and progress in patient safety since the book *To Err is Human: Building a Safer Health System* was published in 2000 (1), medication-related errors consistently rank at the top of all medical errors (2). Errors are common at every step of the medication administration process. In hospitals, errors occur most frequently when medication is prescribed and administered. There is at least one medication error per hospital patient per day (2), but not all errors result in injury. Studies indicate, however, that 400,000 preventable drug-related injuries occur each year in hospitals (2). It is estimated that preventable drug-related injuries in hospitals resulted in at least $3.5 billion in additional medical costs in 2007 (2).

Human factors inherently limit the safety of health care processes. These factors include fatigue, inattention, memory lapse, ignorance, failure to communicate, use of poorly designed equipment, noisy working conditions, and numerous other personal and environmental factors. Leading patient safety organizations universally have focused on improving practices involving medication administration and have endorsed automated systems technology to reduce harmful medication-related errors. The Committee on Patient Safety and Quality Improvement considers three of these automated systems to have potential relevance to practicing obstetrician–gynecologists: 1) computerized physician order entry, 2) bar coding, and 3) intravenous infusion technology; ie, "smart pumps" (Table 1).

The American College of Obstetricians and Gynecologists

Women's Health Care Physicians

Table 1. Summary of Automated System Technologies for Medication Error Reduction

	Computerized Order Entry	Bar Coding	Smart Pumps
Medication Process Affected	Ordering Transcription	Dispensing Administration	Administration
Estimated time to implementation	18–36 months	6+ months	3+ months
Strength of supporting evidence*	Good	Fair	Fair

*Harris RP, Helfand M, Woolf SH, Lohr KN, Mulrow CD, Teutsch SM, et al. Current methods of the US Preventive Services Task Force: a review of the process. Methods Work Group, Third US Preventive Services Task Force. Am J Prev Med 2001;20(suppl):21–35.

Computerized Physician Order Entry

Computerized physician order entry refers to a computer-based system of ordering medications, laboratory tests, diagnostic tests, and consultations. Practitioners directly enter orders into a computer system that ensures standardized, legible, and complete orders. To maximize its benefits, computerized physician order entry should be linked to some form of a clinical decision support system. A clinical decision support system is an "active knowledge system that uses two or more items of patient data to generate case-specific advice" (3). The system typically is designed to integrate a medical knowledge base, patient data, and an inference engine to generate case-specific advice. Computerized physician order entry has been evaluated and endorsed by the IOM, Agency for Healthcare Research and Quality, The Leapfrog Group, National Quality Forum, Institute for Safe Medication Practices, and the American Hospital Association (2, 4, 5).

Benefits

Computerized physician order entry is a useful tool for preventing medication-related errors as follows:

- Eliminates adverse drug events related to illegible handwriting and decimal point errors
- Improves processes when linked to a clinical decision support system by including defaults for drug dosages, routes, and frequencies; alerting health care professionals to drug–drug and drug–allergy interactions; screening for drug dosage according to patient age, weight, or renal function; and reducing problems with look-alike or sound-alike drugs, duplicate therapies, and dosage calculations
- Eliminates transcription errors, if implemented with an electronic medication administration record
- Standardizes care by incorporating approved order sets that improve compliance with evidence-based best practices
- Improves efficiency of care delivery by reducing calls, turnaround time, and data re-entry
- Reduces costs by alerting physicians to charges associated with diagnostic tests and medications

It also should be noted that although e-prescribing is a function usually found within computerized physician order entry systems and embedded in many, if not all, electronic medical records, there also are freestanding e-prescribing solutions that are very inexpensive to implement. These programs are Web accessible and can be used with existing office computers or wireless personal digital assistants. These systems can contribute to patient safety by reducing the chances that illegible prescriptions or improper unsafe dosages are accidentally written. In addition, the direct transmission of a prescription to the pharmacy, and the formulary checks many systems can perform, have the potential to reduce phone calls from pharmacists requesting clarification.

Brigham and Women's Hospital recently reported significant return on investment with its internally developed and implemented computerized physician order entry system. Brigham and Women's Hospital spent $11.8 million to develop, implement, and operate the system between 1993 and 2002. Over 10 years, Brigham and Women's Hospital saved $28.5 million, including cumulative net savings of $16.7 million and net operating budget savings of $9.5 million, given the institutional 80% prospective reimbursement rate (6). Other organizations have documented similar improvements:

- In 1995, Latter Day Saints Hospital in Salt Lake City experienced a 70% reduction in antibiotic-related adverse drug events and drug costs with further reductions in length of stay and overall hospital costs after implementation of a computerized physician order entry system with a clinical decision support system (7).
- In 2000, Ohio State University Medical Center reported reductions in medication turnaround time (64%), radiologic procedure completion time (43%), and laboratory result reporting time (25%) (8).

Limitations

The computerized physician order entry system primarily is beneficial during the ordering and transcription processes. Errors still can occur if physicians override system alerts and they can occur during the administration steps.

Bar Coding for Medication Administration

Bar coding refers to methods of encoding data for fast and accurate electronic readability. Barcodes are a series of alternating bars and spaces representing encoded information that can be read by electronic readers. The U.S. Food and Drug Administration (FDA) requires bar coding on most prescription drugs, certain over-the-counter drugs, and blood and blood components intended for transfusion.

Benefits

In order to achieve reductions in dispensing errors, all administered medications should have bar codes. The use of bar coding also can help prevent medication-related medical errors in the following ways:

- Adds automation to help ensure the traditional "five rights" (right patient, right medication, right dosage, right route, and right time) of medication administration
- Streamlines nurse workflow if bar coding is implemented with an electronic medication administration record. The medication record immediately is updated in the hospital information system, ensuring accuracy and saving nurses time in the charting process.

Positive outcomes have been reported from the use of bar coding. In 1994, the medication-related error rate was reduced by 71% at the North Colorado Medical Center (9). In 2001, at Veterans Administration's Colmery-O'Neill Medical Center, the overall medication-related error rate was reduced from 22 incidents per 100,000 units dispensed to 3 incidents per 100,000 units dispensed, an 86% reduction (10).

Limitations

When the bar-code rule was fully implemented in 2006, FDA estimated that it would help prevent nearly 500,000 adverse drug events and transfusion errors in 20 years. The economic benefit of reducing health care costs, patient pain and suffering, and lost work time is estimated at $93 billion over the same period (11–14). However, no national standard has been established for the medication bar-code format. It is estimated that less than 50% of all available medications are currently bar coded at the unit-dose level.

Intravenous Infusion Technology: "Smart Pumps"

Approximately 38% of adverse drug events occur during the administration steps with only 2% intercepted before the event occurs (15). Advances with smart pumps now offer programmable limits and other safety mechanisms beyond the standard free-flow protection, which can reduce risks of dosage errors. A smart pump is a parenteral infusion pump equipped with intravenous medication error-prevention software that alerts operators or interrupts the infusion process when a pump setting is programmed outside of preconfigured limits. Smart pumps are designed to recognize prescription errors, dosage misinterpretations, and keypad programming errors (16, 17).

Benefits

Smart pumps have the following features that work to reduce the rates of medication-related errors:

- Smart pumps incorporate dose error reduction systems, a safety feature that warns users when a programmed dose falls outside predefined limits.
- Dose limits can be set for minimal and maximal limits and may be categorized as soft or hard alerts.
- An event tracking log captures programming details, and data can be exported to a spreadsheet for analysis and performance improvement.

Positive outcomes have been reported with the use of smart pumps. Pooled analysis of aggregated tracking data from seven hospitals (average size, 350 beds) demonstrated that one potentially life-threatening intravenous medication-related error was averted every 2.6 days using smart pumps (18). At the Nebraska Medical Center, over 8 months, 157 infusions were reprogrammed; 17 infusions (11%) involved potentially fatal errors (19).

Limitations

As with computerized physician order entry and bar coding, smart pumps alone will not prevent all medication-related errors. For example, dose error reduction systems will not detect that a wrong patient, medication, or time has been selected unless bar-coding technology also is incorporated.

Global Challenges

Major challenges are involved in implementing automated system technology. Listed as follows are challenges that can significantly affect their adoption, or effectiveness, or both:

- Lack of definitive standards and clear state-of-the-art products with responsive, intuitive user interfaces
- Cost to implement
- Involvement of clinicians early in system design and integration into health care processes
- Clinician resistance to change and fears regarding loss of control over clinical care and how data will be used
- Clinician "workarounds" that intentionally bypass safety features

Studies have shown that physician acceptance of a clinical decision support system is significantly improved if they trust the system to help them take better care of their patients, remind them of something they may have forgotten, or provide them with information that was previously unavailable (20).

Conclusion

In 2001, the IOM Committee on Quality Health Care in America indicated that "Healthcare has safety and quality problems because it relies on outmoded systems of work. Poor designs set the workforce up to fail, regardless of how hard they try. If we want safer, higher-quality care, we will need to have redesigned systems of care, including the use of information technology to support clinical and administrative processes (21)."

It is clear from review of available evidence that automated health care technologies hold perhaps the greatest potential for dramatically reducing the incidence of harm related to medical errors and, in particular, medication-related errors. The evidence supporting the efficacy of these technologies ranges from good (computerized physician order entry systems) to fair (bar coding and smart pumps). Equally clear is the fact that the impact of these technologies depends on the speed with which national standards emerge and the success with which they are integrated into well-designed care processes.

References

1. Institute of Medicine (US). To err is human: building a safer health system. Washington, DC: National Academies Press; 2000.

2. Institute of Medicine (US). Preventing medication errors. Washington, DC: National Academies Press; 2007.

3. Wyatt J, Spiegelhalter D. Field trials of medical decision-aids: potential problems and solutions. Proc Annu Symp Comput Appl Med Care 1991;1991:3–7.

4. Kaushal R, Bates DW. Computerized physician order entry (CPOE) with clinical decision support systems (CDSSs). In: Agency for Healthcare Research and Quality. Making health care safer: a critical analysis of patient safety practices. Evidence Report/Technology Assessment No. 43. Rockville (MD): AHRQ; 2001. p. 59–69.

5. National Quality Forum. Safe practices for better healthcare 2006 update: a consensus report. Washington, DC: NQF; 2006.

6. Kaushal R, Jha AK, Franz C, Glaser J, Shetty KD, Jaggi T, et al. Return on investment for a computerized physician order entry system. Brigham and Women's Hospital CPOE Working Group. J Am Med Inform Assoc 2006;13:261–6.

7. Evans RS, Pestotnik SL, Classen DC, Clemmer TP, Weaver LK, Orme JF Jr, et al. A computer-assisted management program for antibiotics and other antiinfective agents. N Engl J Med 1998;338:232–8.

8. Mekhjian HS, Kumar RR, Kuehn L, Bentley TD, Teater P, Thomas A, et al. Immediate benefits realized following implementation of physician order entry at an academic medical center. J Am Med Inform Assoc 2002;9:529–39.

9. Puckett F. Medication-management component of a point-of-care information system. Am J Health Syst Pharm 1995;52:1305–9.

10. Johnson CL, Carlson RA, Tucker CL, Willette C. Using BCMA software to improve patient safety in Veterans Administration Medical Centers. J Healthc Inf Manag 2002;16:46–51.

11. Bar code label requirement for human drug products and biological products. Final rule. Food and Drug Administration, HHS. Fed Regist 2004;69:9119–71.

12. Bar code label requirements. 21 CFR §201.25 (2007).

13. Bar code label requirements. 21 CFR §610.67 (2007).

14. Container label. 21 CFR §606.121 (2007).

15. Bates DW, Cullen DJ, Laird N, Petersen LA, Small SD, Servi D, et al. Incidence of adverse drug events and potential adverse drug events. Implications for prevention. ADE Prevention Study Group. JAMA 1995;274:29–34.

16. FAQs for the Joint Commission's 2007 national patient safety goals. (Updated 1/07). Oakbrook Terrace (IL): JC; 2007. Available at http://www.jointcommission.org/NR/rdonlyres/B423198E-8EB1-468C-B01E-DBB0324B5C60/0/07_NPSG_FAQs_3.pdf. Retrieved November 27, 2007.

17. The Joint Commission. Sentinel event statistics - June 30, 2007. Oakbrook Terrace (IL): JC; 2007. Available at: http://www.jointcommission.org/SentinelEvents/Statistics. Retrieved October 24, 2007.

18. Fields M, Peterman J. Intravenous medication safety system averts high-risk medication errors and provides actionable data. Nurs Adm Q 2005;29:78–87.

19. Malashock CM, Shull SS, Gould DA. Effect of smart infusion pumps on medication errors related to infusion device programming. Hosp Pharm 2004;39:460–9.

20. Sittig DF, Krall MA, Dykstra RH, Russell A, Chin HL. A survey of factors affecting clinician acceptance of clinical decision support. BMC Med Inform Decis Mak 2006;6:6.

21. Institute of Medicine (US). Crossing the quality chasm: a new health system for the 21st century. Washington, DC: National Academies Press; 2001.

Technologic advances to reduce medication-related errors. ACOG Committee Opinion No. 400. American College of Obstetricians and Gynecologists. Obstet Gynecol 2008;111:795–8.

ISSN 1074-861X

PRACTICE BULLETINS — OBSTETRICS

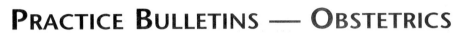

PRACTICE BULLETINS — OBSTETRICS

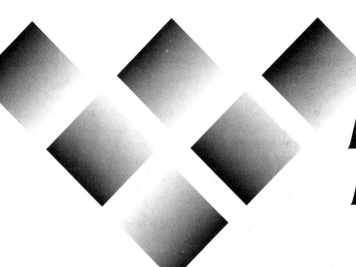

ACOG PRACTICE BULLETIN

CLINICAL MANAGEMENT GUIDELINES FOR OBSTETRICIAN–GYNECOLOGISTS

NUMBER 77, JANUARY 2007

Replaces Practice Bulletin Number 27, May 2001, and Committee Opinion Number 296, July 2004

This Practice Bulletin was developed by the ACOG Committee on Practice Bulletins—Obstetrics, the ACOG Committee on Genetics, and the Society for Maternal–Fetal Medicine Publications Committee with the assistance of Ray Bahado-Singh, MD, and Deborah Driscoll, MD. The information is designed to aid practitioners in making decisions about appropriate obstetric and gynecologic care. These guidelines should not be construed as dictating an exclusive course of treatment or procedure. Variations in practice may be warranted based on the needs of the individual patient, resources, and limitations unique to the institution or type of practice.

Reaffirmed 2008

The Society for
Maternal-Fetal Medicine

Screening for Fetal Chromosomal Abnormalities

In the past decade, numerous markers and strategies for Down syndrome screening have been developed. Algorithms that combine ultrasound and serum markers in the first and second trimesters have been evaluated. Furthermore, the practice of using age cutoffs to determine whether women should be offered screening or invasive diagnostic testing has been challenged. The purpose of this document is to 1) present and evaluate the best available evidence for the use of ultrasonographic and serum markers for selected aneuploidy screening in pregnancy and 2) offer practical recommendations for implementing Down syndrome screening in practice.

Background

Historically, maternal age 35 years or older at the time of delivery has been used to identify women at highest risk of having a child with Down syndrome, and these women have been offered genetic counseling and amniocentesis or chorionic villus sampling (CVS). Biochemical serum screening for Down syndrome in women younger than 35 years was introduced in 1984, when an association between low maternal serum alpha-fetoprotein (AFP) levels and Down syndrome was reported (1). In the 1990s, human chorionic gonadotropin (hCG) and unconjugated estriol were used in combination with maternal serum AFP to improve the detection rates for Down syndrome and trisomy 18. The average maternal serum AFP level in Down syndrome pregnancies is reduced to 0.74 multiples of the median (MoM) observed in euploid pregnancies (2). Intact hCG is increased in affected pregnancies, with an average level of 2.06 MoM, whereas unconjugated estriol is reduced to an average level of 0.75 MoM (2). When the levels of all three markers (triple test) are used to modify the maternal age-related Down syndrome risk, the detection rate for Down syndrome is approximately 70%; approximately 5% of all pregnancies will have a positive screen result. Typically, the levels of all three markers are reduced when the fetus has trisomy 18. Adding inhibin A to the triple test (quadruple screen) improves the detection rate for Down syndrome to approximately 80%. The median value of the maternal inhibin A level is increased at 1.77 MoM in Down syndrome pregnancies (3), but inhibin A is not used in the calculation of risk for trisomy 18. Screening with biochemical markers, ultrasonography, or both is being offered increasingly to the entire pregnant population to provide a more accurate estimate of individual Down syndrome risk. Higher sensitivity or detection rates (defined as the percentage of Down syndrome pregnancies identified with a positive test result) at low false-positive rates have led to increased use of screening and a decline in the number of amniocenteses performed.

Studies done in the early and mid-1990s revealed a strong association between the size of a fluid collection at the back of the fetal neck in the first trimester, referred to as "nuchal translucency," and the risk of trisomy 21 (4). An increase in nuchal translucency is now widely recognized to be an early presenting feature of a broad range of fetal chromosomal, genetic, and structural abnormalities. However, considerable variability in the detection rates for Down syndrome among the early studies of nuchal translucency measurement limited the practical utility of the test (5). Now guidelines for the systematic measurement of nuchal translucency have been standardized (6). Specific training for a standardized method of measurement and ongoing audits of examination quality are recommended for screening programs that include nuchal translucency measurement (7). Other first-trimester ultrasonographic markers such as nonvisualization of the nasal bone and tricuspid regurgitation are being evaluated for their potential as screening tests for Down syndrome, but their clinical usefulness remains uncertain.

A significant breakthrough in first-trimester screening for Down syndrome was achieved when large studies in the United States and the United Kingdom demonstrated that, when expressing the nuchal translucency measurement as an MoM, it could be combined with two first-trimester serum analytes, free β-hCG and pregnancy-associated plasma protein A (PAPP-A). The average level of free β-hCG in first-trimester Down syndrome pregnancies is elevated to 1.98 MoM (8), and the average level of PAPP-A, a glycoprotein that, like hCG, is produced by the trophoblast, is reduced to approximately 0.43 MoM (9). Maternal serum analytes, PAPP-A, and hCG or free β-hCG are effective for screening in the first

trimester, whereas AFP, unconjugated estriol, and inhibin A are useful only in the second trimester.

Several approaches to Down syndrome screening in the first and second trimesters have been evaluated and are described in this document (Table 1). Not all strategies include nuchal translucency measurement because this screening approach is not available in all regions due to the need for specialized training to obtain it, and this measurement might not be obtained successfully in an individual patient.

Table 1. Down Syndrome Screening Tests and Detection Rates (5% Positive Screen Rate)

Screening Test	Detection Rate (%)
First Trimester	
NT measurement	64–70*
NT measurement, PAPP-A, free or total β-hCG†	82–87*
Second trimester	
Triple screen (MSAFP, hCG, unconjugated estriol)	69*
Quadruple screen (MSAFP, hCG, unconjugated estriol, inhibin A)	81*
First Plus Second Trimester	
Integrated (NT, PAPP-A, quad screen)	94–96*
Serum integrated (PAPP-A, quad screen)	85–88*
Stepwise sequential	95*
First-trimester test result:	
Positive: diagnostic test offered	
Negative: second-trimester test offered	
Final: risk assessment incorporates first and second results	
Contingent sequential	88–94%‡
First-trimester test result:	
Positive: diagnostic test offered	
Negative: no further testing	
Intermediate: second-trimester test offered	
Final: risk assessment incorporates first and second results	

Abbreviations: hCG, human chorionic gonadotropin; MSAFP, maternal serum alpha-fetoprotein; NT, nuchal translucency; PAPP-A, pregnancy-associated plasma protein A; quad, quadruple.

*From the FASTER trial (Malone F, Canick JA, Ball RH, Nyberg DA, Comstock CH, Buckowski R, et al. First-trimester or second-trimester screening, or both, for Down's syndrome. First- and Second-Trimester Evaluation of Risk (FASTER) Research Consortium. N Engl J Med 2005;353:2001–11.)

†Also referred to as combined first-trimester screen

‡Modeled predicted detection rates (Cuckle H, Benn P, Wright D. Down syndrome screening in the first and/or second trimester: model predicted performance using meta-analysis parameters. Semin Perinatol 2005;29:252–7.)

Clinical Considerations and Recommendations

▶ *Should all patients be counseled about screening for aneuploidy?*

Ideally, all women should be offered aneuploidy screening before 20 weeks of gestation, regardless of maternal age. It is not practical to have patients choose from among the large array of screening strategies that might be used. Before deciding which strategy or strategies to offer patients, review the evidence presented in this document, identify which tests are available in your area, and determine which strategy or strategies will best meet the needs of your patients. The options for women who are first seen during the second trimester are limited to quadruple (or "quad") screening and ultrasound examination. A strategy that incorporates both first- and second-trimester screening should be offered to women who seek prenatal care in the first trimester.

Regardless of which screening tests you decide to offer your patients, information about the detection and false-positive rates, advantages, disadvantages, and limitations, as well as the risks and benefits of diagnostic procedures, should be available to patients so that they can make informed decisions. Patients may decline Down syndrome screening because they would not use the information in deciding whether to have a diagnostic test or because they wish to avoid the chance of a false-positive screening test result. The choice of screening test depends on many factors, including gestational age at first prenatal visit, number of fetuses, previous obstetric history, family history, availability of nuchal translucency measurement, test sensitivity and limitations, risk of invasive diagnostic procedures, desire for early test results, and options for earlier termination. Some patients may benefit from a more extensive discussion with a genetics professional or a maternal–fetal medicine specialist, especially if there is a family history of a chromosome abnormality, genetic disorder, or congenital malformation.

▶ *What are the advantages and disadvantages of screening for aneuploidy compared with diagnostic testing?*

Screening for aneuploidy identifies a population of women whose fetuses are at increased risk for Down syndrome, trisomy 18, or trisomy 13. If women who have had a positive screening test result choose to undergo a diagnostic procedure, such as CVS or amniocentesis, there is a higher chance of identifying an affected fetus than there would be if the diagnostic test was performed in an unscreened population. Fewer invasive procedures will be required to identify an aneuploid fetus in patients who have screening, thus resulting in a decreased number of procedure-related losses of normal fetuses.

The main disadvantage of screening approaches for the detection of aneuploidies is that not all affected fetuses will be detected. Although the currently available approaches have relatively high detection rates (sensitivity) at low screen positive rates, women should understand that screening provides an individual risk assessment but is not diagnostic and thus will not detect all chromosomal abnormalities. Counseling should be provided regarding the specific detection rates and false-positive rates of the screening strategy or strategies they are considering.

In comparison with the sensitivity of screening, the main advantage of invasive diagnostic testing is that all autosomal trisomies will be detected. Diagnostic testing also will reliably detect sex chromosome aneuploidies, large deletions or duplications of chromosomes, and chromosomal mosaicism. However, in an unscreened population, more invasive procedures will be performed for each affected fetus identified, resulting in a greater loss of normal fetuses when compared with a screened population. Patients informed of the risks, particularly those at increased risk of having an aneuploid fetus, may opt to have diagnostic testing without first having screening.

▶ *How are aneuploidy screening test results interpreted?*

Laboratories that report screening test results generally provide the clinician with numerical information regarding the patient's age-related risk and a revised risk assessment based on age, the serum analyte levels, and nuchal translucency measurement if available. Communicating a numerical risk assessment after screening enables women and their partners to balance the risk and the consequences of having a child with the particular problem against the risk and consequences of an invasive diagnostic test. Because this decision involves personal values, it is preferable to provide patients with their numerical risk determined by the screening test, rather than a positive versus negative screening result using an arbitrary cutoff. It is often useful to contrast this risk with the general population risk and their age-related risk before screening.

Screening test results may be reported as screen positive or screen negative based on fixed cutoff values. The use of fixed cutoffs in clinical studies is of value because they provide a basis for comparison of sensitivity (detection rates), false-positive rates, and acceptability to patients within various study groups or between different studies. Often these fixed cutoffs have been arbitrarily selected at levels that are comparable with the risk for women at certain ages and seem to provide an appropriate balance against the risk of pregnancy loss as the result of an invasive diagnostic test. Fixed screening cutoffs also are useful in public policy considerations when the benefits, risks, and costs in a population are being considered.

▶ *Is nuchal translucency measurement alone a sensitive screening test for aneuploidy in the first trimester?*

Despite the relatively high detection rate using nuchal translucency measurement alone, recent trials in the United States and the United Kingdom demonstrate improved detection of Down syndrome at lower false-positive rates when nuchal translucency measurement is combined with biochemical markers. Nuchal translucency measurements may be useful in the evaluation of multifetal gestations, for which serum screening is not as accurate (twins) or is unavailable (triplets or higher), compared with a singleton gestation.

Use of standardized techniques for measuring nuchal translucency has resulted in higher detection rates for Down syndrome, trisomy 18, trisomy 13, and Turner's syndrome. The optimal time to schedule nuchal translucency measurement appears to be 12–13 weeks of gestation, although the measurement is valid from 10 4/7 to 13 6/7 weeks. Training is required to learn standardized techniques for measuring nuchal translucency, and specific guidelines for measuring it must be adhered to in order to maintain the detection rate. This has resulted in Down syndrome detection rates of 72% at a screen-positive rate of 5% in an unselected population (10). In addition, 74.8% of trisomy 18 cases, 72% of trisomy 13 cases, 87% of Turner's syndrome cases, 59% of triploidy cases, and 55% of other significant chromosomal defects were detected. A recent review of prospective first-trimester screening studies performed in the past 10 years, which included 871 Down syndrome cases, reported a Down syndrome detection rate with nuchal translucency measurement alone of 76.8%, with a screen-positive rate of 4.2% (11). Among first-trimester fetuses with increased nuchal translucency measurement, approximately one third will have chromosome defects. Down syndrome accounts for approximately 50% of these chromosomal disorders (10).

▶ *What is the sensitivity of first-trimester screening?*

Several large, multicenter trials have shown that, in the first trimester, a combination of nuchal translucency measurement, serum markers (PAPP-A and free or total β-hCG), and maternal age is a very effective screening test for Down syndrome (Table 2). This approach has been called combined screening. The detection rates for first-trimester Down syndrome screening are comparable to the second-trimester quadruple screen for women younger than 35 years at the time of delivery. For older women (35 years or older), the detection rate is approxi-

Table 2. Combined First-Trimester Screening Prospective Study Outcomes*

Study	Patients	Down Syndrome Cases	Detection Rate† (%)
BUN‡	8,216	61	79
FASTER§	33,557	84	83
SURUSS¶	47,053	101	83
OSCAR#	15,030	82	90
Total	103,856	328	84

*First-trimester detection rate (DR) at 5% of false-positive rate (FPR)

†95% CI: 79.7–87.0%

‡Wapner RJ, Thom EA, Simpson JL, Pergament E, Silver R, Filkins K, et al. First-trimester screening for trisomies 21 and 18. First Trimester Maternal Serum Biochemistry and Fetal Nuchal Translucency Screening (BUN) Study Group. N Engl J Med 2003;349:1405–13.

§Malone FD, Wald NJ, Canick JA, Ball RH, Nyberg DA, Comstock CH, et al. First- and second-trimester evaluation of risk (FASTER) trial: principal results of the NICHD multicenter Down syndrome screening study [abstract]. Am J Obstet Gynecol 2003;189:(suppl 1):s56.

¶Wald NJ, Rodeck C, Hackshaw AK, Walters J, Chitty L, Mackinson AM. First and second trimester antenatal screening for Down's syndrome: the results of the Serum, Urine and Ultrasound Screening Study (SURUSS) [published erratum appears in J Med Screen 2006;13:51–2]. J Med Screen 2003;10:56–104.

#Spencer K, Spencer CE, Power M, Dawson C, Nicolaides KH. Screening for chromosomal abnormalities in the first trimester using ultrasound and maternal serum biochemistry in a one-stop clinic: a review of three years prospective experience. BJOG 2003;110:281–6.

Reprinted from: Wapner RJ. First trimester screening: the BUN study. Semin Perinatol 2005;29:236–9. With permission from Elsevier.

mately 90%, but at a higher screen-positive rate (approximately 16–22%) (12, 13). For women of all ages, 90% of trisomy 18 cases are detected at a 2% screen-positive rate (13).

▶ *What is the advantage of first-trimester screening?*

The advantage of first-trimester screening is that women who present for prenatal care before 14 weeks of gestation can have information sooner. If the woman is found to be at an increased risk of fetal aneuploidy, she can be offered genetic counseling and CVS, if the procedure is available. Alternatively, she may choose to have a second-trimester amniocentesis.

▶ *Should first- and second-trimester screening tests be performed independently?*

When first-trimester and second-trimester screening tests are performed during the pregnancy and interpreted independently, there is a high Down syndrome detection rate (94–98%); however, the false-positive rates are additive, leading to many more unnecessary invasive procedures (11–17%) (12, 14). For this reason, women who have had first-trimester screening for aneuploidy should not undergo independent second-trimester serum screening in the same pregnancy. Instead, women who want a higher detection rate can have an integrated or a sequential screening test, which combines both first- and second-trimester screening results.

▶ *What is integrated screening?*

The "integrated" approach to screening uses both the first-trimester and second-trimester markers to adjust a woman's age-related risk of having a child with Down syndrome (15). The results are reported only after both first- and second-trimester screening tests are completed. In the FASTER (First- and Second-Trimester Evaluation of Risk) trial, the detection rate was 94–96% at a 5% screen-positive rate (12). Similar results were achieved in the SURUSS (Serum, Urine, and Ultrasound Screening Study) trial (16). Further refinements in interpretation may result in additional sensitivity and reduction of screen-positive rates.

Integrated screening also can be performed using only first- and second-trimester serum markers, without incorporating a nuchal translucency measurement. In the FASTER trial, the serum integrated screen resulted in an 85–88% detection rate (12). This approach is ideal for patients without access to nuchal translucency measurement or for whom reliable measurement cannot be obtained. A recent prospective trial of serum-only integrated screening in a population with limited access to

CVS reported acceptance of this screening algorithm by most patients surveyed (17).

▶ *What are the advantages and disadvantages of having an integrated first- and second-trimester Down syndrome screening test (first- and second-trimester markers analyzed together [integrated], with only one result given in the second trimester)?*

Integrated screening best meets the goal of screening by providing the highest sensitivity with the lowest false-positive rate. The lower false-positive rate results in fewer invasive tests and thus fewer procedure-related losses of normal pregnancies (12, 18). Although some patients value early screening, others are willing to wait several weeks if doing so results in an improved detection rate and less chance that they will need an invasive diagnostic test (19). Concerns about integrated screening include possible patient anxiety generated by having to wait 3–4 weeks between initiation and completion of the screening and the loss of the opportunity to consider CVS if the first-trimester screening indicates a high risk of aneuploidy (20). The possibility that patients might fail to complete the second-trimester portion of the screening test after performing the first-trimester component is another potential disadvantage because the patient would be left with no screening results.

▶ *Is there an advantage to using a sequential screening test for Down syndrome?*

Sequential screening approaches that obviate some of the disadvantages of integrated screening have been developed. With this strategy, the patient is informed of the first-trimester screening result. Those at highest risk might opt for an early diagnostic procedure and those at lower risk can still take advantage of the higher detection rate achieved with additional second-trimester screening.

Two strategies have been proposed: "stepwise sequential screening" and "contingent sequential screening." In the stepwise model, women determined to be at high risk (Down syndrome risk above a predetermined cutoff) after the first-trimester screen are offered genetic counseling and the option of invasive diagnostic testing, and women below the cutoff are offered second-trimester screening. Contingent sequential screening has been proposed as a model, but large clinical trials using this approach have not yet been published. The contingent model classifies pregnancy risk as high, intermediate, or low on the basis of the first-trimester screen results; women at high risk would be offered CVS, and those at low risk would have no further screening or testing. Only women at intermediate risk would be offered second-trimester screening. Hence, fewer women would go on to second-trimester screening. In both the stepwise and contingent models, the patients at highest risk identified by first-trimester screening are offered an early diagnostic procedure. Both first- and second-trimester results are used to calculate a final risk for aneuploidy in patients at lower risk. The sequential approach takes advantage of the higher detection rate achieved by incorporating the first- and second-trimester results with only a marginal increase in the false-positive rate. Theoretically, the contingent approach should maintain high detection rates with low false-positive rates while reducing the number of second-trimester tests performed.

▶ *What subsequent evaluation should be offered after first-trimester screening?*

Women found to have an increased risk of aneuploidy with first-trimester screening should be offered genetic counseling and diagnostic testing by CVS or a second-trimester genetic amniocentesis. Neural tube defect screening should be offered in the second trimester to patients who elected to have only first-trimester screening for aneuploidy or who have had a normal result from CVS. Neural tube defect screening may include second-trimester serum AFP screening or ultrasonography. Patients who have a fetal nuchal translucency measurement of 3.5 mm or greater in the first trimester, despite a negative result on an aneuploidy screen, normal fetal chromosomes, or both, should be offered a targeted ultrasound examination, fetal echocardiogram, or both, because such fetuses are at a significant risk for nonchromosomal anomalies, including congenital heart defects, abdominal wall defects, diaphragmatic hernias, and genetic syndromes (21–25).

Patients with abnormal first-trimester serum markers or an increased nuchal translucency measurement also may be at increased risk for an adverse pregnancy outcome such as spontaneous fetal loss before 24 weeks of gestation, fetal demise, low birth weight, or preterm birth (26, 27). At the present time, there are no data indicating whether or not fetal surveillance in the third trimester will be helpful in the care of these patients.

The significance of ultrasonographic markers identified by a second-trimester ultrasound examination in a patient who has had a negative first-trimester screening test result is unknown. A variety of ultrasound findings have been associated with Down syndrome. A major anomaly, such as a cardiac defect, deserves further evaluation. More subtle findings ("soft markers"), such as pyelectasis, shortened femur or humerus, or echogenic bowel individually, do not significantly increase the risk of Down syndrome. However, these findings should be considered in the context of the screening results, patient's age, and history.

▶ *Are there other first-trimester ultrasonographic markers that are useful for Down syndrome screening?*

Several other first-trimester ultrasonographic markers, including nonvisualized nasal bone, tricuspid regurgitation, crown–rump length, femur and humeral length, head and trunk volumes, and umbilical cord diameters, have been evaluated as potential markers for aneuploidy in the first trimester. Studies in high-risk first-trimester populations indicate a high rate of nonvisualization of the nasal bone in fetuses with Down syndrome. Three European studies reported a 66.7–80% Down syndrome detection rate at a 0.2–1.4% false-positive rate (28–30). The value of nasal bone assessment as a Down syndrome screening test in the general population is controversial. A first-trimester study performed in the United States did not find the test to be useful (12). In addition, there are considerable ethnic differences in the prevalence of absent nasal bone; absence of the nasal bone in a euploid fetus is found in only 2.8% of Caucasians, compared with 6.8% of Asians and 10.4% of Afro-Caribbeans (31). It has been suggested that standardization of nasal bone assessment (32), along with extensive teaching and quality control programs, should be developed before this technique is used in the general population (33). Strategies restricting assessment of nasal bone to a subset of pregnant women at the highest risk after first-trimester combined screening, rather than the entire population, appear to be more practical and are being investigated.

▶ *What are the benefits and limitations of second-trimester ultrasound examination as a screening test for Down syndrome?*

Individual second-trimester ultrasonographic markers, such as echogenic bowel, intracardiac echogenic focus, and dilated renal pelvis, have a low sensitivity and specificity for Down syndrome particularly when used to screen a low-risk population (34). Studies indicate that the highest detection rate is achieved with systematic combination of ultrasonographic markers and gross anomalies, such as thick nuchal fold or cardiac defects (35, 36). Studies done in high-risk populations have reported detection rates of approximately 50–75% in the second trimester. However, the false-positive rates are high (eg, a 21.9% false-positive rate for a 100% Down syndrome detection rate) (37). One group has reported that if no abnormal ultrasonographic markers are identified after a carefully performed scan at a specialized center with skilled ultrasonographers, the a priori risk of Down syndrome in a high-risk patient (advanced maternal age, abnormal serum screen) may be reduced by 82–88% (38). Because the RADIUS (Routine Antenatal Diagnostic Imaging With Ultrasound) trial (39) and others showed that even major fetal anomalies are frequently missed by ultrasound examination, the disadvantages of relying solely on ultrasonography for Down syndrome screening should be considered carefully. Combining second-trimester ultrasonographic and biochemical markers is a relatively new development that has been shown to be a feasible method to improve Down syndrome screening performance over either ultrasonography or second-trimester serum markers by themselves (40), provided that the ultrasound examination is performed as part of a specific screening protocol (37).

A major limitation of the use of second-trimester ultrasonographic markers has been the lack of standardization in measurements and definitions of what constitutes abnormal findings. This has contributed to variability in the diagnostic performance reported by different groups. Recent prospective studies that used specific criteria to define abnormal markers in large groups of unselected patients in the United States confirm a statistically significant increase in the frequency of individual ultrasonographic markers in Down syndrome compared with normal second-trimester cases (41, 42). At this time, risk adjustment based on second-trimester ultrasonographic markers should be limited to centers with ultrasonographic expertise and centers engaged in clinical research to develop a standardized approach to evaluating these markers. However, an abnormal second-trimester ultrasound finding identifying a major congenital anomaly significantly increases the risk of aneuploidy and warrants further counseling and the offer of a diagnostic procedure.

▶ How does screening for aneuploidy differ in multifetal gestations?

Serum screening tests are not as sensitive in twin or triplet gestations, in part because data from multiple gestations that include an aneuploid fetus is so scarce that expected analyte levels must be estimated by mathematical modeling. In addition, analytes from both the normal and the affected fetuses enter the maternal serum and are in effect averaged together, thus masking the abnormal levels of the affected fetus. In monochorionic twin pregnancies, the median nuchal translucency values are larger in 38% of twin pairs destined to develop severe twin–twin transfusion syndrome (43). Furthermore, counseling is more complex because women must consider a different set of options in the event that only one of the fetuses is affected. Nuchal translucency screening in the first trimester with the option of a CVS and earlier

selective reduction may be desirable for some women. Experience is limited with triplet gestations, but studies suggest that nuchal translucency measurement is feasible. Until further studies are done, however, risk assessment in multiple gestations should be performed judiciously, and patients who are at increased risk of aneuploidy should be counseled regarding diagnostic testing.

▶ Should invasive diagnostic testing for aneuploidy be available to all women?

All women, regardless of age, should have the option of invasive testing. A woman's decision to have an amniocentesis or CVS is based on many factors, including the risk that the fetus will have a chromosomal abnormality, the risk of pregnancy loss from an invasive procedure, and the consequences of having an affected child if diagnostic testing is not done. Studies that have evaluated women's preferences have shown that women weigh these potential outcomes differently. The decision to offer invasive testing should take into account these preferences and should not be solely age based. The differences between screening and diagnostic testing should be discussed with all women. Thus, maternal age of 35 years alone should no longer be used as a cutoff to determine who is offered screening versus who is offered invasive testing.

▶ With so many Down syndrome screening tests available, how do I decide which tests to offer?

The goal is to offer screening tests with high detection rates and low false-positive rates that also provide patients with the diagnostic options they might want to consider. Ideally, patients seen early in pregnancy should be offered aneuploidy screening that combines first- and second-trimester testing (integrated or sequential). The screening strategy chosen will depend on availability of CVS and of personnel trained in nuchal translucency measurement in the area. When CVS is not available, it makes sense to offer integrated screening to patients who present in the first trimester in order to take advantage of the improved detection rate and low false-positive rate and to offer second-trimester screening to patients who present after 13⅚ weeks. If nuchal translucency measurement is not available or cannot be obtained in an individual patient, a reasonable approach is to offer serum integrated screening to patients who present early and second-trimester screening to those who present later. In areas where every screening strategy is possible, it is reasonable to choose two screening strategies for the practice, such as sequential screening for patients who present for prenatal care before 14 weeks of gestation (because it provides them with a first-trimester risk assessment and the option of waiting until the second trimester for an adjusted risk assessment that includes their second-trimester serum results), and second-trimester serum screening for patients who present after 13⅙ weeks of gestation. In some instances, patients who would consider first-trimester termination of pregnancy but not second-trimester termination of pregnancy may want only first-trimester screening.

Summary of Recommendations and Conclusions

The following recommendations are based on good and consistent scientific evidence (Level A):

▶ First-trimester screening using both nuchal translucency measurement and biochemical markers is an effective screening test for Down syndrome in the general population. At the same false-positive rates, this screening strategy results in a higher Down syndrome detection rate than does the second-trimester maternal serum triple screen and is comparable to the quadruple screen.

▶ Measurement of nuchal translucency alone is less effective for first-trimester screening than is the combined test (nuchal translucency measurement and biochemical markers).

▶ Women found to have increased risk of aneuploidy with first-trimester screening should be offered genetic counseling and the option of CVS or second-trimester amniocentesis.

▶ Specific training, standardization, use of appropriate ultrasound equipment, and ongoing quality assessment are important to achieve optimal nuchal translucency measurement for Down syndrome risk assessment, and this procedure should be limited to centers and individuals meeting these criteria.

▶ Neural tube defect screening should be offered in the second trimester to women who elect only first-trimester screening for aneuploidy.

The following recommendations are based on limited or inconsistent scientific evidence (Level B):

▶ Screening and invasive diagnostic testing for aneuploidy should be available to all women who present for prenatal care before 20 weeks of gestation regardless of maternal age. Women should be counseled regarding the differences between screening and invasive diagnostic testing.

▶ Integrated first- and second-trimester screening is more sensitive with lower false-positive rates than first-trimester screening alone.

▶ Serum integrated screening is a useful option in pregnancies where nuchal translucency measurement is not available or cannot be obtained.

▶ An abnormal finding on second-trimester ultrasound examination identifying a major congenital anomaly significantly increases the risk of aneuploidy and warrants further counseling and the offer of a diagnostic procedure.

▶ Patients who have a fetal nuchal translucency measurement of 3.5 mm or higher in the first trimester, despite a negative aneuploidy screen, or normal fetal chromosomes, should be offered a targeted ultrasound examination, fetal echocardiogram, or both.

▶ Down syndrome risk assessment in multiple gestation using first- or second-trimester serum analytes is less accurate than in singleton pregnancies.

▶ First-trimester nuchal translucency screening for Down syndrome is feasible in twin or triplet gestation but has lower sensitivity than first-trimester screening in singleton pregnancies.

The following recommendations are based primarily on consensus and expert opinion (Level C):

▶ After first-trimester screening, subsequent second-trimester Down syndrome screening is not indicated unless it is being performed as a component of the integrated test, stepwise sequential, or contingent sequential test.

▶ Subtle second-trimester ultrasonographic markers should be interpreted in the context of a patient's age, history, and serum screening results.

Proposed Performance Measure

Percentage of patients with documentation of discussion regarding Down syndrome screening

---

Glossary

Aneuploidy: In this condition there is an extra or missing chromosome.

Screen-positive rate: percentage of the population with a positive screening test result. This includes true positives and false positives.

Nuchal translucency measurement: Accumulated fluid behind the fetal neck is measured in a standardized way.

References

1. Merkatz IR, Nitowsky HM, Macri JN, Johnson WE. An association between low maternal serum alpha-fetoprotein and fetal chromosomal abnormalities. Am J Obstet Gynecol 1984;148:886–94. (Level II-2)

2. Wald NJ, Kennard A, Hackshaw A, McGuire A. Antenatal screening for Down's syndrome. Health Technol Assess 1998;2:i–iv,1–112. (Level III)

3. Spencer K, Wallace EM, Ritoe S. Second-trimester dimeric inhibin-A in Down's syndrome screening. Prenat Diagn 1996;16:1101–10. (Level II-3)

4. Nicolaides KH, Snijders RJ, Gosden CM, Berry C, Campbell S. Ultrasonographically detectable markers of fetal chromosomal abnormalities. Lancet 1992;340:704–7. (Level III)

5. Malone FD, Berkowitz RL, Canick JA, D'Alton ME. First-trimester screening for aneuploidy: research or standard of care? Am J Obstet Gynecol 2000;182:490–6. (Level III)

6. Nicolaides KH, Heath V, Liao AW. The 11-14 week scan. Baillieres Best Pract Res Clin Obstet Gynaecol 2000;14:581–94. (Level III)

7. Snijders RJ, Thom EA, Zachary JM, Platt LD, Greene N, Jacson LG, et al. First-trimester trisomy screening: nuchal translucency measurement training and quality assurance to correct and unify technique. Ultrasound Obstet Gynecol 2002;19:353–9. (Level III)

8. Cuckle H. Biochemical screening for Down syndrome. Eur J Obstet Gynecol Reprod Biol 2000;92:97–101. (Level III)

9. Spencer K, Souter V, Tul N, Snijders R, Nicolaides KH. A screening program for trisomy 21 at 10-14 weeks using fetal nuchal translucency, maternal serum free beta-human chorionic gonadotropin and pregnancy-associated plasma protein-A. Ultrasound Obstet Gynecol 1999;13:231–7. (Level II-3)

10. Snijders RJ, Noble P, Sebire N, Souka A, Nicolaides KH. UK multicentre project on assessment of risk of trisomy 21 by maternal age and fetal nuchal-translucency thickness at 10-14 weeks of gestation. Fetal Medicine Foundation First Trimester Screening Group. Lancet 1998;352:343–6. (Level III)

11. Nicolaides KH. Nuchal translucency and other first-trimester sonographic markers of chromosomal abnormalities. Am J Obstet Gynecol 2004;191:45–67. (Level III)

12. Malone F, Canick JA, Ball RH, Nyberg DA, Comstock CH, Buckowski R, et al. First-trimester or second-trimester screening, or both, for Down's syndrome. First-and Second-Trimester Evaluation of Risk (FASTER) Research Consortium. N Engl J Med 2005;353:2001–11. (Level II-2)

13. Wapner R, Thom E, Simpson JL, Pergament E, Silver R, Filkins K, et al. First-trimester screening for trisomies 21 and 18. First Trimester Maternal Serum Biochemistry and Fetal Nuchal Translucency Screening (BUN) Study Group. N Engl J Med 2003;349:1405–13. (Level II-3)

14. Platt LD, Greene N, Johnson A, Zachary J, Thom E, Krantz D, et al. Sequential pathways of testing after first

trimester screening for trisomy 21. First Trimester Maternal Serum Biochemistry and Fetal Nuchal Translucency Screening (BUN) Study Group. Obstet Gynecol 2004;104:661–6. (Level II-3)

15. Wald NJ, Watt HC, Hackshaw AK. Integrated screening for Down's syndrome on the basis of tests performed during the first and second trimesters. N Engl J Med 1999;341:461–7. (Level III)

16. Wald NJ, Rodeck C, Hackshaw AK, Walters J, Chitty L, Mackinson AM. First and second trimester antenatal screening for Down's syndrome: the results of the Serum, Urine and Ultrasound Screening Study (SURUSS) [published erratum appears in J Med Screen 2006;13:51–2]. J Med Screen 2003;10:56–104 (Level II-2)

17. Palomaki GE, Knight GJ, Neveux LM, Pandian R, Haddow JE. Maternal serum invasive trophoblast antigen and first-trimester Down syndrome screening. Clin Chem 2005;51:1499–504. (Level II-3)

18. Wald NJ, Rodeck C, Hackshaw AK, Rudnicka A. SURUSS in perspective. BJOG 2004;111:521–31. (Level II-2)

19. Bishop AJ, Marteau TM, Armstrong D, Chitty LS, Longworth L, Buxton MJ, et al. Women and health care professionals' preferences for Down's syndrome screening tests: a conjoint analysis study. BJOG 2004;111:775–9. (Level III)

20. Copel JA, Bahado-Singh RO. Prenatal screening for Down's syndrome—a search for the family's values. N Engl J Med 1999;341:521–2. (Level III)

21. Makrydimas G, Sotiriadis A, Huggon IC, Simpson J, Sharland G, Carvalho JS, et al. Nuchal translucency and fetal cardiac defects: a pooled analysis of major fetal echocardiography centers. Am J Obstet Gynecol 2005;192:89–95. (Level II-3)

22. Bahado-Singh RO, Wapner R, Thom E, Zachary J, Platt L, Mahoney MJ, et al. Elevated first-trimester nuchal translucency increases the risk of congenital heart defects. First Trimester Maternal Serum Biochemistry and Fetal Nuchal Translucency Screening Study Group. Am J Obstet Gynecol 2005;192:1357–61. (Level II-3)

23. Hyett J, Perdu M, Sharland G, Snijders R, Nicolaides KH. Using fetal nuchal translucency to screen for major congenital cardiac defects at 10-14 weeks of gestation: population based cohort study. BMJ 1999;318:81–5. (Level II-3)

24. Souka AP, Von Kaisenberg CS, Hyett JA, Sonek JD, Nicolaides KH. Increased nuchal translucency with normal karyotype [published erratum appears in Am J Obstet Gynecol 2005;192:2096]. Am J Obstet Gynecol 2005;192:1005–21. (Level III)

25. Comstock CH, Malone FD, Ball RH, Nyberg DA, Saade GR, Berkowitz RL, et al. Is there a nuchal translucency millimeter measurement above which there is no added benefit from first trimester serum screening? FASTER Research Consortium. Am J Obstet Gynecol 2006;195:843–7. (Level III)

26. Dugoff L, Hobbins JC, Malone FD, Porter TF, Luthy D, Comstock CH, et al. First-trimester maternal serum PAPP-A and free-beta subunit human chorionic gonadotropin concentrations and nuchal translucency are associ-

ated with obstetric complications: a population-based screening study (the FASTER Trial). Am J Obstet Gynecol 2004;191:1446–51. (Level II-3)

27. Smith GC, Shah I, Crossley JA, Aitken DA, Pell JP, Nelson SM, et al. Pregnancy-associated plasma protein A and alpha-fetoprotein and prediction of adverse perinatal outcome. Obstet Gynecol 2006;107:161–6. (Level II-2)

28. Zoppi MA, Ibba RM, Axiana C, Floris M, Manca F, Monni G. Absence of fetal nasal bone and aneuploides at first-trimester nuchal translucency screening in unselected pregnancies. Prenat Diagn 2003;23:496–500. (Level III)

29. Orlandi F, Bilardo CM, Campogrande M, Krantz D, Hallahan T, Rossi C, et al. Measurement of nasal bone length at 11-14 weeks of pregnancy and its potential role in Down syndrome risk assessment. Ultrasound Obstet Gynecol 2003;22:36–9. (Level II-3)

30. Viora E, Masturzo B, Errante G, Sciarrone A, Bastonero S, Campogrande M. Ultrasound evaluation of fetal nasal bone at 11 to 14 weeks in a consecutive series of 1906 fetuses. Prenat Diagn 2003;23:784–7. (Level II-3)

31. Cicero S, Longo D, Rembouskos G, Sacchini C, Nicolaides KH. Absent nasal bone at 11-14 weeks of gestation and chromosomal defects. Ultrasound Obstet Gynecol 2003;22:31–5. (Level III)

32. Sonek JD. Nasal bone evaluation with ultrasonography: a marker for fetal aneuploidy. Ultrasound Obstet Gynecol 2003;22:11–5. (Level III)

33. Senat MV, Bernard JP, Boulvain M, Ville Y. Intra- and interoperator variability in fetal nasal bone assessment at 11-14 weeks of gestation. Ultrasound Obstet Gynecol 2003;22:138–41. (Level III)

34. Smith-Bindman R, Hosmer W, Feldstein V, Deeks J, Goldberg J. Second-trimester ultrasound to detect fetuses with Down syndrome. JAMA 2001;285:1044–55. (Meta-analysis)

35. Vintzileos AM, Campbell WA, Rodis JF, Guzman ER, Smulian JC, Knuppel RA. The use of second-trimester genetic sonogram in guiding clinical management of patients at increased risk for fetal trisomy 21. Obstet Gynecol 1996;87:948–52. (Level II-3)

36. Bromley B, Benacerraf BR. The genetic sonogram scoring index. Semin Perinatol 2003;27:124–9. (Level III)

37. Bahado-Singh RO, Oz U, Mendilicioglu I, Mahoney M. The mid-trimester genetic sonogram. Semin Perinatol 2005;29:209–14. (Level III)

38. Yeo L, Vintzileos AM. The use of genetic sonography to reduce the need for amniocentesis in women at high risk of Down syndrome. Semin Perinatol 2003;27;152–9. (Level III)

39. Ewigman BG, Crane JP, Frigoletto FD, LeFevre ML, Bain RP, McNellis D. Effect of prenatal ultrasound screening on perinatal outcome. RADIUS Study Group. N Engl J Med 1993;329:821–7. (Level I)

40. Benn PA, Kaminsky LM, Ying J, Borgida AF, Egan JF. Combined second-trimester biochemical and ultrasound screening for Down syndrome. Obstet Gynecol 2002; 100:1168–76. (Level II-3)

41. Schluter PJ, Pritchard B. Mid trimester sonographic findings for the prediction of Down syndrome in a sonographically screened population. Am J Obstet Gynecol 2005;192:10–6. (Level II-2)

42. Benacerraf BR. The role of the second trimester genetic sonogram in screening for fetal Down syndrome. Semin Perinatol 2005;29:386–94. (Level III)

43. Sebire NJ, D'Ercole C, Hughes K, Carvalho M, Nicolaides KH. Increased nuchal translucency thickness at 10–14 weeks of gestation as a predictor of severe twin-to-twin transfusion syndrome. Ultrasound Obstet Gynecol 1997;10:86–9. (Level II-3)

The MEDLINE database, the Cochrane Library, and the American College of Obstetricians and Gynecologists' own internal resources and documents were used to conduct a literature search to locate relevant articles published between January 1985 and September 2006. The search was restricted to articles published in the English language. Priority was given to articles reporting results of original research, although review articles and commentaries also were consulted. Abstracts of research presented at symposia and scientific conferences were not considered adequate for inclusion in this document. Guidelines published by organizations or institutions such as the National Institutes of Health and ACOG were reviewed, and additional studies were located by reviewing bibliographies of identified articles. When reliable research was not available, expert opinions from obstetrician–gynecologists were used.

Studies were reviewed and evaluated for quality according to the method outlined by the U.S. Preventive Services Task Force:

I   Evidence obtained from at least one properly designed randomized controlled trial.

II-1   Evidence obtained from well-designed controlled trials without randomization.

II-2   Evidence obtained from well-designed cohort or case–control analytic studies, preferably from more than one center or research group.

II-3   Evidence obtained from multiple time series with or without the intervention. Dramatic results in uncontrolled experiments also could be regarded as this type of evidence.

III   Opinions of respected authorities, based on clinical experience, descriptive studies, or reports of expert committees.

Based on the highest level of evidence found in the data, recommendations are provided and graded according to the following categories:

Level A—Recommendations are based on good and consistent scientific evidence.

Level B—Recommendations are based on limited or inconsistent scientific evidence.

Level C—Recommendations are based primarily on consensus and expert opinion.

ISSN 1099-3630

The American College of Obstetricians and Gynecologists
409 12th Street, SW, PO Box 96920, Washington, DC 20090-6920

Screening for fetal chromosomal abnormalities. ACOG Practice Bulletin No. 77. American College of Obstetricians and Gynecologists. Obstet Gynecol 2007;109:217–27.

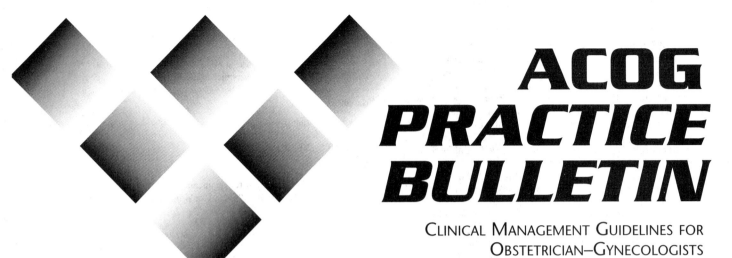

ACOG PRACTICE BULLETIN

CLINICAL MANAGEMENT GUIDELINES FOR
OBSTETRICIAN–GYNECOLOGISTS

NUMBER 78, JANUARY 2007

(Replaces Practice Bulletin Number 64, July 2005)

Hemoglobinopathies in Pregnancy

This Practice Bulletin was developed by the ACOG Committee on Practice Bulletins—Obstetrics with the assistance of John Williams III, MD. The information is designed to aid practitioners in making decisions about appropriate obstetric and gynecologic care. These guidelines should not be construed as dictating an exclusive course of treatment or procedure. Variations in practice may be warranted based on the needs of the individual patient, resources, and limitations unique to the institution or type of practice.

Reaffirmed 2008

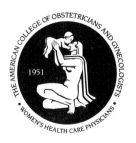

The hemoglobinopathies are a heterogeneous group of single-gene disorders that includes the structural hemoglobin variants and the thalassemias. More than 270 million people worldwide are heterozygous carriers of hereditary disorders of hemoglobin, and at least 300,000 affected homozygotes or compound heterozygotes are born each year (1). The purpose of this document is to review the most common hemoglobinopathies and to provide recommendations for screening and clinical management of hemoglobinopathies during pregnancy.

Background

Hemoglobin Structure

Hemoglobin consists of four interlocking polypeptide chains, each of which has an attached heme molecule. The polypeptide chains are called alpha (α), beta (β), gamma (γ), delta (δ), epsilon (ϵ), and zeta (ζ). Adult hemoglobins consist of two α-chains and either two β-chains (hemoglobin A), two γ-chains (hemoglobin F), or two δ-chains (hemoglobin A_2). Hemoglobin F (fetal hemoglobin, Hb F) is the primary hemoglobin of the fetus from 12 to 24 weeks of gestation. In the third trimester, production of Hb F decreases as production of β-chains and Hb A begins. The genes that code for α-globin chains are located on the short arm of chromosome 16, and the β-globin gene is located on the short arm of chromosome 11.

Sickle Cell Disease

Sickle cell disease refers to a group of autosomal recessive disorders involving abnormal hemoglobin (hemoglobin S). Hemoglobin S differs from the normal Hb A because of a single nucleotide substitution of thymine for adenine in the β-globin gene; this alteration causes a substitution of valine for glutamic acid in the number six position of the β-globin polypeptide. Asymptomatic individuals with heterozygous Hb S genotypes (carriers) are said to have sickle cell trait. The most severe form of the disease, Hb SS (homozygous Hb S), is called sickle cell anemia.

Sickle cell disorders are found not only in patients who have the hemoglobin genotype SS, but also in those who have Hb S and one other abnormality of β-globin structure or β-globin production. The most common of these are Hb SC disease and Hb S/β-thalassemia. In Hb C, the same nucleotide involved in the Hb S mutation is altered with the substitution of adenine for guanine, which results in the amino acid substitution of lysine for glutamic acid. This and other abnormal hemoglobins, when inherited with Hb S, may cause clinically significant vasoocclusive phenomena and hemolytic anemia similar to Hb SS.

Sickle cell disease occurs most commonly in people of African origin. Approximately 1 in 12 African Americans has sickle cell trait (2). One in every 300 African-American newborns has some form of sickle cell disease, and approximately 1 in 600 has sickle cell anemia. Hemoglobin S also is found in high frequency in other populations such as Greeks, Italians (particularly Sicilians), Turks, Arabs, Southern Iranians, and Asian Indians (3).

The classical clinical feature of patients with sickle cell disease is seen under conditions of decreased oxygen tension, in which the red blood cells become distorted into various shapes, some of which resemble sickles. The distorted red cells lead to increased viscosity, hemolysis, and anemia and a further decrease in oxygenation. When sickling occurs within small blood vessels, it can cause "logjams" that can interrupt blood supply to vital organs (vasoocclusive crisis). Repeated vasoocclusive crises result in widespread microvascular obstruction with interruption of normal perfusion and function of several organs, including the spleen, lungs, kidneys, heart, and brain. Adults with Hb SS are functionally asplenic, having undergone autosplenectomy by adolescence. Absence of the spleen contributes to the increased incidence and severity of infection in patients with sickle cell disease.

The most significant threat to patients with sickle cell disease is acute chest syndrome. Chest syndrome is characterized by a pulmonary infiltrate with fever that leads to hypoxemia and acidosis. The infiltrates are not infectious in origin but rather are due to vasoocclusion from sickling or embolization of marrow from long bones affected by sickling (4).

The diagnosis of hemoglobinopathies, including sickle cell disorders, is made by hemoglobin electrophoresis. In the homozygous form, nearly all the hemoglobin is Hb S with small amounts of Hb A_2 and Hb F. Heterozygous sickle cell trait (Hb AS) is identified by a larger percentage of Hb A and an asymptomatic course. Solubility tests (Sickledex) alone are inadequate for diagnosis of sickle cell disorders because they cannot distinguish between the heterozygous AS and homozygous SS genotypes. In addition, they fail to detect other pathologic variants such as Hb C trait, β-thalassemia trait, Hb E trait, Hb B trait, and Hb D trait.

The Thalassemias

The thalassemias represent a wide spectrum of hematologic disorders that are characterized by a reduced synthesis of globin chains, resulting in microcytic anemia. Thalassemias are classified according to the globin chain affected, with the most common types being α-thalassemia and β-thalassemia. Many different molecular mechanisms lead to thalassemia in populations from different areas of the world (5).

Alpha-Thalassemia

Alpha-thalassemia usually results from a gene deletion of two or more copies of the four α-globin genes. Deletion of one α-globin gene (α-/αα) is clinically unrecognizable, and laboratory testing yields normal results. Deletion of two α-globin genes causes α-thalassemia trait, a mild asymptomatic microcytic anemia. The deletions can be on the same chromosome or in *cis* (αα/--), or on each chromosome or in *trans* (α-/α-). Individuals with these chromosomal abnormalities are referred to as carriers and are at an increased risk for having a child with a more severe form of thalassemia caused by deletions of three or four copies of the α-globin gene (α-thalassemia major). The possible genetic combinations are summarized in Table 1.

Alpha-thalassemia trait (α-thalassemia minor) is common among individuals of Southeast Asian, African, and West Indian descent. It also is common in individuals with Mediterranean ancestry. Individuals with Southeast Asian ancestry are more likely to carry two gene deletions in *cis* or on the same chromosome (--/αα) and are at an increased risk for offspring with Hb Bart's or Hb H disease. Hemoglobin H disease, which is caused by the deletion of three α-globin genes, usually is associated with mild to moderate hemolytic anemia. Alpha-thalassemia major (Hb Bart's) results in the absence of α-globin (--/--); this is associated with hydrops fetalis, intrauterine death, and preeclampsia (3).

In individuals of African descent, α-thalassemia usually is due to a deletion of a single α-globin gene on each chromosome 16 (α-/α-). This is in contrast to the common Asian genotype, which is a deletion of both α-globin genes on one chromosome 16 (*cis*) (αα/--). Hemoglobin Bart's disease does not typically develop in fetuses of α-thalassemia carriers of African origin.

Because Hb S results from an abnormality of the β-chain, both heterozygous (AS) and homozygous (SS)

Table 1. Classification of Alpha-Thalassemias

Number of Globin Genes	Genotype	Description	Clinical Features
4	αα/αα	Normal	Normal
3	α-/αα	Heterozygous α⁺-thalassemia	Asymptomatic
2	α-/α-	Homozygous α⁺-thalassemia	Mild anemia
	αα/--	Heterozygous α°-thalassemia	
1	α-/--	α⁺-Thalassemia/ α°-thalassemia	Hb H disease hemolytic anemia
0	--/--	Homozygous α°-thalassemia	Hb Bart's disease hydrops fetalis

forms can be inherited with heterozygous or homozygous α⁺-thalassemia. In individuals with sickle cell trait (Hb AS), α-thalassemia lowers the proportion of Hb S, and in those with Hb SS, it lessens the severity of sickle cell disease.

Alpha-thalassemia also may occur as a result of a gene mutation. In this case, the genes are present but not functioning normally. This may result from mutation in the stop codon leading to synthesis of a longer and unstable α-chain (Hb Constant Spring), from substitutions impairing αβ dimer formation (Hb Qong Sze), and from point substitutions in the poly A region at the 3' end of the gene (α^TSaudi).

Beta-Thalassemia

Beta-thalassemia is caused by a mutation in the β-globin gene that causes deficient or absent β-chain production, which results in absence of Hb A. Classification of β-thalassemias is based on a description of the molecular mutation or by clinical manifestations. Individuals who are heterozygous for this mutation have β-thalassemia minor. Those who are homozygous have β-thalassemia major (Cooley's anemia) or a milder form called thalassemia intermedia. Beta-thalassemia major is characterized by severe anemia with resultant extramedullary erythropoesis, delayed sexual development, and poor growth. Elevated levels of Hb F in individuals with β-thalassemia major partially compensate for the absence of Hb A; however, death usually occurs by age 10 years unless treatment is begun early with periodic blood transfusions. With transfusion, the severe anemia is reversed and extramedullary erythropoesis is suppressed. In homozygotes with the less severe β⁺-thalassemia mutations, often referred to as β-thalassemia intermedia, variable but decreased amounts of β-chains

are produced and, as a result, variable amounts of Hb A are produced. The genes for Hb S and β-thalassemia usually behave as alleles, with only one gene inherited from each parent. The expression of the resulting Hb S/β-thalassemia is determined by the type of β-thalassemia mutation (6).

Beta-thalassemia minor, common in individuals of Mediterranean, Asian, Middle Eastern, Hispanic, and West Indian descent, varies in severity of disease. Depending on the amount of β-chain production, it usually is associated with asymptomatic mild anemia. Beta-thalassemia minor often occurs in association with Hb S. In the most severe form, no normal β-globin chains are produced. This results in a clinically severe syndrome called sickle cell–β⁰-thalassemia, in which no Hb A is produced.

Clinical Considerations and Recommendations

▶ *Who should be screened for hemoglobinopathies and how should this be accomplished?*

Genetic screening can identify couples at risk for offspring with hemoglobinopathies and allow them to make informed decisions regarding reproduction and prenatal diagnosis (3). Individuals of African, Southeast Asian, and Mediterranean ancestry are at a higher risk for being carriers of hemoglobinopathies and should be offered carrier screening. Ethnic groups considered to be at low risk for hemoglobinopathies include northern Europeans, Japanese, Native Americans, Inuit (Eskimo), and Koreans. If both parents are determined to be carriers, genetic counseling is recommended. It should be noted that ethnicity is not always a good predictor of risk because individuals from at-risk groups may marry outside their ethnic group (3).

A combination of laboratory tests may be required to provide the information necessary to counsel couples who are carriers of one of the thalassemias or sickle cell disease (Fig. 1). To ensure accurate hemoglobin identification, which is essential for genetic counseling, a complete blood count (CBC) is the appropriate initial laboratory test for individuals of non-African descent. In individuals of African descent, a hemoglobin electrophoresis should be performed in addition to a CBC. Several tests, including solubility testing such as a test for the presence of Hb S (Sickledex), isoelectric focusing, and high-performance liquid chromatography (HPLC), have been used for primary screening. However, solubility tests alone are inadequate for screening and fail to identify important transmissible hemoglobin gene abnormalities affecting fetal outcome (eg, Hb C trait, β-thal-assemia trait, Hb E trait, Hb B trait, Hb D trait). Many individuals with these genotypes are asymptomatic, but if their partners have the sickle cell trait or other hemoglobinopathies, they may produce offspring with more seri-

ous hemoglobinopathies, such as Hb S/β-thalassemia and Hb SC disease. Solubility testing may be valuable, however, for rapid screening for sickling when this information is critical for immediate patient care.

Determination of mean corpuscular volume (MCV) is recommended for patients who are at risk for α- or β-thalassemia. Patients who have a low MCV (less than 80 fL) may have one of the thalassemia traits and are candidates for hemoglobin electrophoresis. These individuals also may have iron deficiency anemia, and measurement of serum ferretin levels is recommended. Beta-thalassemia is associated with elevated Hb F and elevated Hb A_2 levels (more than 3.5%). Neither hemoglobin electrophoresis nor solubility testing can identify individuals with α-thalassemia trait; only molecular genetic testing can identify this condition. If the MCV is below normal, iron deficiency anemia has been excluded, and the hemoglobin electrophoresis is not consistent with β-thalassemia trait (ie, there is no elevation of Hb A_2 or Hb F), then DNA-based testing should be used to detect α-globin gene deletions characteristic of α-thalassemia.

The hematologic features of some of the common hemoglobinopathies are shown in Table 2. If both part-

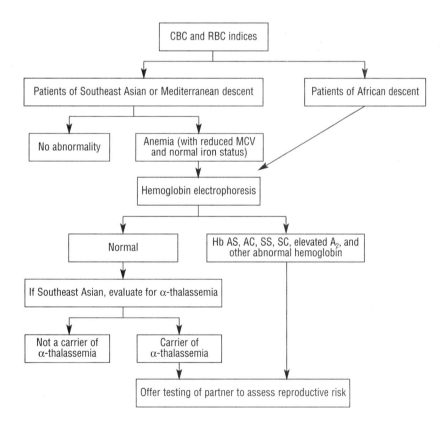

Figure 1. Specialized antepartum evaluation for hematologic assessment of patients of African, Southeast Asian, or Mediterranean descent. Patients of Southeast Asian or Mediterranean descent should undergo electrophoresis if their blood test results reveal anemia. Abbreviations: CBC, complete blood count; Hb, hemoglobin; MCV, mean corpuscular volume; RBC, red blood cell.

Table 2. Hematologic Features of Main Hemoglobinopathies

Disorder	Heterozygous State	Homozygous State	DNA Analysis
α^+ Thalassemia (-α)	0–2% Hb Bart's at birth	5–10% Hb Bart's in the neonatal period, low MCV	S. blot: α-gene probe, abnormal band with Bam H1
α^o Thalassemia (--)	5–10% Hb Bart's in the neonatal period, low MCV, normal Hb A$_2$	Hb Bart's hydrops fetalis	S. blot or PCR: absence of: α-gene band in homozygote
β^o Thalassemia	Low MCH & MCV, Hb A$_2$ 3.5–7.0%	Thalassemia major: Hb F 98% Hb A$_2$ 2%	PCR, ASO – dot blot, S. blot β-gene probe
β^+ Thalassemia (severe)	Low MCH & MCV, Hb A$_2$ 3.5–7.0%	Thalassemia major: Hb F 70–95%	PCR, ASO – dot blot, S. blot β-gene probe
β^+ Thalassemia (mild)	Low MCH & MCV, Hb A$_2$ 3.5–7.0%	Thalassemia intermedia: Hb F 20–40%	PCR, ASO – dot blot, S. blot β-gene probe
Hb S	Hb A, Hb S, Hb A$_2$	Hb S, Hb F (1–15%), Hb A$_2$	PCR: Dde 1 digestion PCR, ASO – dot blot
Hb S/β-Thalassemia	—	If β^o thalassemia, severe sickle cell anemia; if β^+ thalassemia, less severe	PCR: Dde 1 digestion PCR, ASO – dot blot
Hb E/β-Thalassemia	—	Thalassemia major or intermedia: Hb E 60–70%, Hb F 30–40%	PCR: Hb E by Mnl 1 digestion

Abbreviations: ASO, allele specific oligonucleotide; Hb, hemoglobin; MCH, mean corpuscular hemoglobin; MCV, mean corpuscular volume; PCR, polymerase chain reaction; S. blot, Southern blot.

Modified from Milunsky, Aubrey, MB.B.Ch., D.Sc., F.R.C.P., F.A.C.M.G., D.C.H., ed. Genetic Disorders and the Fetus, fifth edition: Diagnosis, Prevention, and Treatment. pp. 665, Table 19.1. © 2004 Aubrey Milunsky. Reprinted with permission of The Johns Hopkins University Press.

ners are identified as carriers of a gene for abnormal hemoglobins, genetic counseling is recommended.

▶ *For couples with an increased risk for having an affected offspring, what methods are available for genetic diagnosis of the fetus or embryo?*

Couples at risk for having a child with a hemoglobinopathy may benefit from genetic counseling to review the natural history of these disorders, prospects for treatment and cure, their risk, availability of prenatal genetic testing, and reproductive options. Prenatal diagnostic testing for the single mutation responsible for sickle cell disease is widely available. Testing for α- and β-thalassemia is possible if the mutations and deletions have been previously identified in both parents. These DNA-based tests can be performed using chorionic villi obtained by chorionic villus sampling (CVS) at 10–12 weeks of gestation or using cultured amniotic fluid cells obtained by amniocentesis after 15 weeks of gestation. For some couples, preimplantation genetic diagnosis in combination with in vitro fertilization may be a desirable alternative to avoid termination of an affected pregnancy. Preimplantation genetic diagnosis has been successfully performed for sickle cell disease and most cases of β-thalassemia.

Although the advances in prenatal diagnosis of hemoglobinopathies have been impressive, use of the technology has been somewhat limited because of ethical, social, and cultural concerns. Prenatal diagnosis is most commonly requested by families who have had a child with sickle cell disease and who wish to be certain that their next child is not affected. In many respects, these families are "self-counseled." The difficulty in counseling families who have not had an affected child lies in the variable severity of the disease and the inability to predict its course (6). One investigator found that nearly 70% of families in whom prenatal diagnosis confirmed that the fetus was affected with Hb SS elected to continue the pregnancy (7).

▶ *How is sickle cell disease in pregnancy managed?*

Pregnancy in women with sickle cell disease is associated with an increased risk of morbidity and mortality because of the combination of underlying hemolytic anemia and multiorgan dysfunction associated with this disorder. Morbidity and mortality have decreased markedly over the past 3 decades because of improvements in general medical care for patients with sickle cell disease, improvements in transfusion medicine, and advancements in neonatal care (8, 9). In spite of the decline in maternal and perinatal mortality rates, however, pregnancy is still a significant clinical risk for many patients with sickle cell disease. The magnitude of the risk varies with genotype and severity of anemia. When compared with Hb AA patients, women with Hb SS have increased risk for maternal complications, such as preterm labor, premature rupture of membranes, antepartum hospitalization, and postpartum infection. In addition, patients with Hb SS are at higher risk for fetal complications, such as intrauterine growth restriction (IUGR), low birth weight, and preterm delivery (9, 10). Patients with Hb SC disease also are at risk for the aforementioned complications but to a lesser extent than patients with Hb SS disease (10).

Pregnant patients with sickle cell disease need increased prenatal folic acid supplementation. The standard 1 mg of folate in prenatal vitamins is not adequate for patients with hemoglobinopathies; 4 mg per day of folic acid should be prescribed because of the continual turnover of red blood cells.

Routine cesarean delivery for women with sickle cell disease is not indicated and should be performed only for obstetric indications. Epidural analgesia usually is well tolerated as long as care is taken to avoid hypotension and hypoxemia. Pregnant patients should, if possible, be cared for at institutions that are able to manage both the complications of sickle cell disease and high-risk pregnancies. They also should have regular prenatal care by or in consultation with obstetricians who are experienced in the management of sickle cell disease.

The most common cause of recurrent morbidity in Hb SS disease is painful crisis. If possible, precipitating factors, such as cold environment, heavy physical exertion, dehydration, and stress, should be avoided. Hydroxyurea has been shown to reduce the frequency of painful crises in nonpregnant patients with severe sickle cell disease (11). However, the use of hydroxyurea is not recommended during pregnancy because it is teratogenic.

Painful crises in pregnancy as well as in the nonpregnant patient are managed with rapid assessment of the level of pain and prompt administration of analgesia. Pain, respiratory rate, and level of sedation should be assessed until pain is controlled. Opiates can be given orally or parenterally by the intravenous, intramuscular, or subcutaneous route. Oxygen should be given if the O_2 saturation is less than 95% by pulse oximetry. The initial clinical assessment also should focus on detection of serious medical complications requiring specific therapy, such as acute chest syndrome (fever tachypnea, chest pain, and hypoxia), infection, dehydration, severe anemia, cholecystitis, and hypersplenism. A multidisciplinary approach should be used involving obstetricians, hematologists, and anesthesiologists (12). Painful crises in the third trimester may have a prolonged course and may not resolve until after delivery.

▶ *What is the role of transfusion or prophylactic exchange transfusion for pregnancies complicated by sickle cell anemia?*

Controversy exists regarding the role of prophylactic blood transfusion in the management of sickle cell disease in pregnancy (13–15). By limiting transfusion to situations in which it is clinically indicated, patients are not subjected to the increased risk for alloimmunization (16), viral infections, and iron overload. Major complications (eg, worsening anemia; intrapartum complications such as hemorrhage, septicemia, and cesarean delivery; painful crisis; and chest syndrome) may require intervention with an exchange transfusion. There is no consensus regarding the exact hematocrit value below which transfusion should be considered. However, when a transfusion is clinically indicated in the patient with sickle cell disease, the objective is to lower the percentage of Hb S to approximately 40% while simultaneously raising the total hemoglobin concentration to about 10 g/dL. Hemoglobin levels and the percentage of Hb S should be monitored serially during the remainder of the pregnancy to determine the need for subsequent transfusions.

Prophylactic exchange transfusion was first proposed by Ricks in 1965, who recommended exchange transfusion 4–6 weeks before the delivery date (17). Preliminary results appeared to show a benefit in that all women and infants survived (18). Subsequently, several studies have shown improvement in maternal and fetal outcome with prophylactic transfusion (15, 19). However, the evidence is not conclusive that transfusion is responsible for the improvement; similar improvement has been observed in programs that do not use prophylactic transfusion. In the only randomized controlled trial published to date, prophylactic transfusion was associated with a decreased risk for painful crisis and severe anemia, but no difference was observed for pregnancy outcome (14). It appears from the available evidence that the reduction in morbidity and mortality of sickle cell disease in pregnancy is attributable to improvements in general management of pregnancy rather than prophylactic transfusion per se.

▶ *Is fetal surveillance useful in pregnancies complicated by sickle cell anemia?*

Pregnancies in women with sickle cell disease are at increased risk for spontaneous abortion, preterm labor, IUGR, and stillbirth (20). For this reason, a plan for serial ultrasound examinations and antepartum fetal testing is reasonable. Published data on antenatal fetal surveillance in women with sickle cell disease are limited. In a retrospective review of 58 pregnancies in women with sickle cell disease undergoing prophylactic transfusion, no patients had a nonreactive nonstress test result or positive contraction stress test result (21). All pregnancy outcomes were normal. The investigators concluded that placental reserve and fetal reactivity were uncompromised and that these tests were as sensitive for assessment of fetal well-being in women with sickle cell disease as for women with other indications for antenatal testing.

Because patients with sickle cell crisis usually require narcotics for pain control, the results of abnormal antepartum testing should be interpreted with caution. One small study has shown that nonstress test results and biophysical profiles may be abnormal during an episode of crisis but revert back to normal with resolution of the episode (22). The clinical significance of this is unclear.

▶ *How is thalassemia in pregnancy managed?*

The course of pregnancy in women with the α-thalassemia trait is not significantly different from that of women with normal hemoglobin. Pregnancy in women with Hb H disease has been reported, and with the exception of mild to moderate chronic anemia, outcomes have been favorable. However, the number of reports is too few to draw definite conclusions regarding pregnancy outcome in all women with Hb H disease (23).

Until recently, pregnancy in women with β-thalassemia major was extremely rare. Initially, this was because delay of growth and sexual development and early death in untreated patients prevented reproduction. After the introduction of transfusion therapy in the 1960s, pregnancy was still uncommon because of infertility (secondary to hypothalamic dysfunction and anovulation caused by hemosiderin deposition). Since the introduction of hypertransfusion and iron chelation therapy with deferoxamine in the late 1970s, several reports and case series have documented favorable pregnancy outcomes in women with β-thalassemia major (24, 25). Pregnancy in women with β-thalassemia major is recommended only for those with normal cardiac function who have had prolonged hypertransfusion therapy to maintain hemoglobin levels at 10 g/dL and iron chelation therapy with deferoxamine (25). During pregnancy, hemoglobin levels should be maintained at or near 10 g/dL with transfusions. Deferoxamine usually is discontinued because the safety of iron chelation therapy during pregnancy has not been established. Fetal growth should be monitored with serial ultrasonography. In cases in which fetal growth is suboptimal, patients should have fetal surveillance. The mode of delivery should be individualized, with cesarean delivery reserved for obstetric indications.

Beta-thalassemia minor usually causes mild asymptomatic anemia. In the absence of documented iron deficiency, replacement beyond prophylactic doses of iron is not indicated. Studies involving fairly small numbers of patients suggest that pregnancy outcome is favorable in women with β-thalassemia minor. A study of 261 pregnant women with β-thalassemia minor found a significantly higher rate of IUGR and oligohydramnios than is found in nonthalassemic patients (26). No differences were noted in perinatal outcomes such as low Apgar scores, congenital malformations, or perinatal mortality (26).

Summary of Recommendations and Conclusions

The following recommendations are based on good and consistent scientific evidence (Level A):

▶ Individuals of African, Southeast Asian, and Mediterranean descent are at increased risk for being carriers of hemoglobinopathies and should be offered carrier screening and, if both parents are determined to be carriers, genetic counseling.

▶ A complete blood count and hemoglobin electrophoresis are appropriate laboratory tests for screening for hemoglobinopathies. Solubility tests alone are inadequate for screening because they fail to identify important transmissible hemoglobin gene abnormalities affecting fetal outcome.

▶ Couples at risk for having a child with sickle cell disease or thalassemia should be offered genetic counseling to review prenatal testing and reproduction options. Prenatal diagnosis of hemoglobinopathies is best accomplished by DNA analysis of cultured amniocytes or chorionic villi.

References

1. Angastiniotis M, Modell B. Global epidemiology of hemoglobin disorders. Ann N Y Acad Sci 1998;850:251–69. (Level II-3)

2. Motulsky AG. Frequency of sickling disorders in U.S. blacks. N Engl J Med 1973;288:31–3. (Level III)

3. Davies SC, Cronin E, Gill M, Greengross P, Hickman M, Normand C. Screening for sickle cell disease and thalassemia: a systematic review with supplementary research. Health Technol Assess 2000;4:i–v, 1–99. (Level III)

4. Duffy TP. Hematologic aspects of pregnancy. In: Burrow GN, Duffy TP, Copel JA, editors. Medical complications

during pregnancy. 6th ed. Philadelphia (PA): Elsevier Saunders; 2004. p. 69–86. (Level III)

5. Kazazian HH Jr. The thalassemia syndromes: molecular basis and prenatal diagnosis in 1990. Semin Hematol 1990;27:209–28. (Level III)

6. Serjeant GR, Serjeant BE. Sickle cell disease. 3rd ed. New York (NY): Oxford University Press; 2001. (Level III)

7. Alter BP. Prenatal diagnosis of hematologic diseases, 1986 update. Acta Haematol 1987;78:137–41. (Level II-3)

8. Smith JA, Espeland M, Bellevue R, Bonds D, Brown AK, Koshy M. Pregnancy in sickle cell disease: experience of the Cooperative Study of Sickle Cell Disease. Obstet Gynecol 1996;87:199–204. (Level II-2)

9. Sun PM, Wilburn W, Raynor BD, Jamieson D. Sickle cell disease in pregnancy: twenty years of experience at Grady Memorial Hospital, Atlanta, Georgia. Am J Obstet Gynecol 2001;184:1127–30. (Level II-2)

10. Powars DR, Sandhu M, Niland-Weiss J, Johnson C, Bruce S, Manning PR. Pregnancy in sickle cell disease. Obstet Gynecol 1986;67:217–28. (Level II-3)

11. Charache S. Mechanism of action on hydroxyurea in the management of sickle cell anemia in adults. Semin Hematol 1997;34(suppl 3):15–21. (Level I)

12. Rees DC, Olujohungbe AD, Parker NE, Stephens AD, Telfer P, Wright J. Guidelines for the management of the acute painful crisis in sickle cell disease. British Committee for Standards in Haematology General Haematology Task Force by the Sickle Cell Working Party. Br J Haematol 2003;120:744–52. (Level III)

13. Tuck SM, James CE, Brewster EM, Pearson TC, Studd JW. Prophylactic blood transfusion in maternal sickle cell syndromes. Br J Obstet Gynaecol 1987;94:121–5. (Level III)

14. Koshy M, Burd L, Wallace D, Moawad A, Baron J. Prophylactic red-cell transfusions in pregnant patients with sickle cell disease. A randomized cooperative study. N Engl J Med 1988;319:1447–52. (Level I)

15. Morrison JC, Schneider JM, Whybrew WD, Bucovaz ET, Menzel DM. Prophylactic transfusions in pregnant patients with sickle cell hemoglobinopathies: benefit versus risk. Obstet Gynecol 1980;56:274–80. (Level III)

16. Brumfield CG, Huddleston JF, DuBois LB, Harris BA Jr. A delayed hemolytic transfusion reaction after partial exchange transfusion for sickle cell disease in pregnancy: a case report and review of literature. Obstet Gynecol 1984;63(suppl):13s–15s. (Level III)

17. Ricks P Jr. Exchange transfusion in sickle cell anemia in pregnancy. Obstet Gynecol 1965;25:117–9. (Level III)

18. Ricks P Jr. Further experience with exchange transfusion in sickle cell anemia in pregnancy. Am J Obstet Gynecol 1968;100:1087–90. (Level III)

19. Morrison JC, Wiser WL. The use of prophylactic partial exchange transfusion in pregnancies associated with sickle cell hemoglobinopathies. Obstet Gynecol 1976;48:516–20. (Level III)

20. Serjeant GR, Loy LL, Crowther M, Hambleton IR, Thame M. Outcome of pregnancy in homozygous sickle cell disease. Obstet Gynecol 2004;103:1278–85. (Level II–2)

21. Morrison JC, Blake PG, McCoy C, Martin JN Jr, Wiser WL. Fetal health assessment in pregnancies complicated by sickle hemoglobinopathies. Obstet Gynecol 1983;61: 22–4. (Level III)

22. Anyaegbunam A, Morel MI, Merkatz IR. Antepartum fetal surveillance tests during sickle cell crisis. Am J Obstet Gynecol 1991;165:1081–3. (Level II-2)

23. Ong HC, White JC, Sinnathuray TA. Haemoglobin H disease and pregnancy in a Malaysian woman. Acta Haematol 1977;58:229–33. (Level III)

24. Jensen CE, Tuck SM, Wonke B. Fertility in beta thalassemia major: a report of 16 pregnancies, preconceptual evaluation and a review of the literature. Br J Obstet Gynaecol 1995;102:625–9. (Level III)

25. Aessopos A, Karabatsos F, Farmakis D, Katsantoni A, Hatziliami A, Youssef J, et al. Pregnancy in patients with well-treated beta-thalassemia: outcome for mothers and newborn infants. Am J Obstet Gynecol 1999;180:360–5. (Level III)

26. Sheiner E, Levy A, Yerushalmi R, Katz M. Beta-thalassemia minor during pregnancy. Obstet Gynecol 2004;103: 1273–7. (Level II-2)

The MEDLINE database, the Cochrane Library, and ACOG's own internal resources and documents were used to conduct a literature search to locate relevant articles published between January 1985 and March 2005. The search was restricted to articles published in the English language. Priority was given to articles reporting results of original research, although review articles and commentaries also were consulted. Abstracts of research presented at symposia and scientific conferences were not considered adequate for inclusion in this document. Guidelines published by organizations or institutions such as the National Institutes of Health and the American College of Obstetricians and Gynecologists were reviewed, and additional studies were located by reviewing bibliographies of identified articles. When reliable research was not available, expert opinions from obstetrician–gynecologists were used.

Studies were reviewed and evaluated for quality according to the method outlined by the U.S. Preventive Services Task Force:

I   Evidence obtained from at least one properly designed randomized controlled trial.

II-1   Evidence obtained from well-designed controlled trials without randomization.

II-2   Evidence obtained from well-designed cohort or case–control analytic studies, preferably from more than one center or research group.

II-3   Evidence obtained from multiple time series with or without the intervention. Dramatic results in uncontrolled experiments also could be regarded as this type of evidence.

III   Opinions of respected authorities, based on clinical experience, descriptive studies, or reports of expert committees.

Based on the highest level of evidence found in the data, recommendations are provided and graded according to the following categories:

Level A—Recommendations are based on good and consistent scientific evidence.

Level B—Recommendations are based on limited or inconsistent scientific evidence.

Level C—Recommendations are based primarily on consensus and expert opinion.

ISSN 1099-3630

The American College of
Obstetricians and Gynecologists
409 12th Street, SW
PO Box 96920
Washington, DC 20090-6920

Hemoglobinopathies in pregnancy. ACOG Practice Bulletin No. 78. American College of Obstetricians and Gynecologists. Obstet Gynecol 2007;109:229–37.

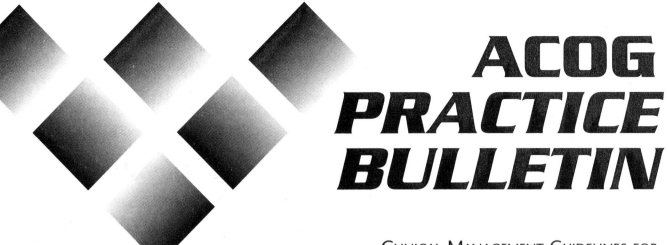

ACOG PRACTICE BULLETIN

CLINICAL MANAGEMENT GUIDELINES FOR
OBSTETRICIAN–GYNECOLOGISTS

NUMBER 80, APRIL 2007

(Replaces Practice Bulletin Number 1, June 1998)

This Practice Bulletin was developed by the ACOG Committee on Practice Bulletins— Obstetrics with the assistance of Brian Mercer, MD. The information is designed to aid practitioners in making decisions about appropriate obstetric and gynecologic care. These guidelines should not be construed as dictating an exclusive course of treatment or procedure. Variations in practice may be warranted based on the needs of the individual patient, resources, and limitations unique to the institution or type of practice.

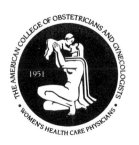

Premature Rupture of Membranes

Preterm delivery occurs in approximately 12% of all births in the United States and is a major factor contributing to perinatal morbidity and mortality (1, 2). Despite extensive research in this area, the rate of preterm birth has increased by 38% since 1981 (3). Premature rupture of membranes (PROM) is a complication in approximately one third of preterm births. It typically is associated with brief latency between membrane rupture and delivery, increased potential for perinatal infection, and in utero umbilical cord compression. Because of this, both PROM at and before term can lead to significant perinatal morbidity and mortality. There is some controversy over the optimal approaches to clinical assessment and treatment of women with term and preterm PROM. Management hinges on knowledge of gestational age and evaluation of the relative risks of preterm birth versus intrauterine infection, abruptio placentae, and cord accident that could occur with expectant management. The purpose of this document is to review the current understanding of this condition and to provide management guidelines that have been validated by appropriately conducted outcome-based research. Additional guidelines on the basis of consensus and expert opinion also are presented.

Background

The definition of PROM is rupture of membranes before the onset of labor. Membrane rupture that occurs before 37 weeks of gestation is referred to as preterm PROM. Although term PROM results from the normal physiologic process of progressive membrane weakening, preterm PROM can result from a wide array of pathologic mechanisms acting individually or in concert (4). The gestational age and fetal status at membrane rupture have significant implications in the etiology and consequences of PROM. Management may be dictated by the presence of overt intrauterine infection, advanced labor, or fetal compromise. When such factors are not present, especially with preterm PROM, obstetric management may have a significant impact on maternal and infant outcomes. An accurate assessment of gestational age and knowledge of the maternal, fetal, and neonatal risks are essential to appropriate evaluation, counseling, and care of patients with PROM.

Etiology

Membrane rupture may occur for a variety of reasons. At term, weakening of the membranes may result from physiologic changes combined with shearing forces created by uterine contractions (5–8). Intraamniotic infection has been shown to be commonly associated with preterm PROM, especially if preterm PROM occurs at earlier gestational ages (9). In addition, factors such as low socioeconomic status, second- and third-trimester bleeding, low body mass index (calculated as weight in kilograms divided by the square of height in meters) less than 19.8, nutritional deficiencies of copper and ascorbic acid, connective tissue disorders (eg, Ehlers–Danlos syndrome), maternal cigarette smoking, cervical conization or cerclage, pulmonary disease in pregnancy, uterine overdistention, and amniocentesis have been linked to the occurrence of preterm PROM (10–19). The risk of recurrence for preterm PROM is between 16% and 32% (20, 21). In addition, women with a previous preterm birth (especially if it is due to PROM), those with a short cervical length (less than 25 mm) in the second trimester, and women with preterm labor or symptomatic contractions in the current pregnancy are at increased risk for PROM (12, 22). Although each of these risk factors can act individually or in concert to cause PROM, in many cases PROM will occur in the absence of recognized risk factors. As a result, it has been difficult to identify effective treatment strategies for the prevention of PROM. Recent studies have suggested progesterone therapy to reduce the risk of recurrent spontaneous preterm birth resulting from preterm labor or PROM (23, 24). However, because most cases of PROM occur in women without identifiable risk factors, the mainstay of care has been treatment after membrane rupture occurs.

Term Premature Rupture of Membranes

At term, PROM complicates approximately 8% of pregnancies and generally is followed by the prompt onset of spontaneous labor and delivery. In a large randomized trial, half of women with PROM who were managed expectantly gave birth within 5 hours, and 95% gave birth within 28 hours of membrane rupture (25). The most significant maternal risk of term PROM is intrauterine infection, a risk that increases with the duration of membrane rupture (25–29). Fetal risks associated with term PROM include umbilical cord compression and ascending infection.

Leakage of Fluid After Amniocentesis

When leakage of amniotic fluid occurs after amniocentesis, the outcome is better than after spontaneous preterm PROM. In studies involving women who had second-trimester amniocentesis for prenatal diagnosis of genetic disorders, the risk of PROM was 1–1.2%, and the attributable risk of pregnancy loss was 0.06% (30). In most patients, the membranes reseal with restoration of normal amniotic fluid volume (31, 32).

Preterm Premature Rupture of Membranes

Regardless of obstetric management or clinical presentation, birth within 1 week is the most likely outcome for any patient with preterm PROM in the absence of adjunctive treatments. The earlier in gestation that PROM occurs, the greater is the latency period. With expectant management, 2.8–13% of women can anticipate cessation of fluid leakage and possible restoration of normal amniotic fluid volume (28, 32).

Of women with preterm PROM, clinically evident intraamniotic infection occurs in 13–60%, and postpartum infection occurs in 2–13% (33–37). The incidence of infection increases with decreasing gestational age at membrane rupture (38, 39) and increases with digital vaginal examination (40). Fetal malpresentation is increased with preterm PROM. Abruptio placentae affects 4–12% of pregnancies with preterm PROM (41, 42). However, serious maternal sequelae are uncommon (35, 43).

The most significant risks to the fetus after preterm PROM are complications of prematurity. At all gestational ages before term, respiratory distress has been reported to be the most common complication of preterm birth (4, 44). Other serious forms of morbidity, including neonatal infections, intraventricular hemorrhage, and necrotizing enterocolitis, also are associated with prematurity, but these are less common nearer to term. Preterm PROM and exposure to intrauterine inflammation have been associated with an increased risk of neurodevelopmental impairment (9, 45). Early gestational age at membrane rupture also has been associated with an increased risk of neonatal white matter damage (P <.001), after controlling for corticosteroid administration, latency interval, gestational age at delivery, and birth weight (46). However, no data exist that suggest immediate delivery after presentation with PROM will avert these risks. The presence of maternal infection poses the additional risk of neonatal infection. Infection, cord accident, and other factors contribute to the 1–2% risk of antenatal fetal demise after preterm PROM (43).

Previable Premature Rupture of Membranes

The fetal survival rate subsequent to PROM at 24–26 weeks of gestation has been reported to be approximately 57% (47). A recent systematic review of 201 cases from 11 studies revealed a 21% perinatal survival rate after expectant management of PROM before viability (48). Survival data may vary by institution. Most studies of second-trimester and previable PROM have been retrospective and have included only those patients appropriate for and accepting of expectant management, potentially exaggerating latency and improving apparent outcomes.

A small number of patients with previable PROM will have an extended latency period. In a review of 12 studies evaluating patients with second-trimester PROM, the mean latency period ranged from 10.6 to 21.5 days (47), with 57% of patients giving birth within 1 week and 22% remaining pregnant for 1 month or more. The incidence of stillbirth subsequent to PROM at 16–28 weeks of gestation ranges from 3.8% to 22% (11, 33, 49) compared with 0–2% at 30–36 weeks of gestation (50, 51). This increased rate of death may be explained by increased susceptibility of the umbilical cord to compression or of the fetus to hypoxia and intrauterine infection. Alternatively, this finding may reflect the lack of intervention for fetal compromise before viability.

Significant maternal complications occurring after second trimester and previable PROM have been reported to include intraamniotic infection, endometritis, abruptio placentae, retained placenta, and postpartum hemorrhage. Maternal sepsis is a rare but serious complication reported in approximately 1% of cases, and isolated maternal deaths due to infection have been reported in this setting (52). Outcomes of survivors of preterm PROM depend on the gestational age, presence of infection, length of latency, and other maternal and fetal complications.

A variety of conditions associated with fetal lung compression or oligohydramnios or both can result in pulmonary hypoplasia. Reported risks of pulmonary hypoplasia after PROM at 16–26 weeks of gestation vary from less than 1% to 27% (37, 52). Lethal pulmonary hypoplasia rarely occurs with membrane rupture subsequent to 24 weeks of gestation, presumably because alveolar growth adequate to support postnatal development already has occurred (53, 54). Early second-trimester membrane rupture, severe oligohydramnios, and duration of membrane rupture longer than 14 days are primary determinants of the risk of pulmonary hypoplasia (55, 56). Prolonged oligohydramnios also is associated with in utero deformation, including abnormal facies (ie, low-set ears and epicanthal folds) and limb contractures and other positioning abnormalities.

Clinical Considerations and Recommendations

▶ *How is premature rupture of membranes diagnosed?*

Most cases of PROM can be diagnosed on the basis of the patient's history and physical examination. Examination should be performed in a manner that minimizes the risk of introducing infection, particularly before term. Because digital cervical examinations increase the risk of infection and add little information to that available with speculum examination, digital examinations should be avoided unless the patient is in active labor or imminent delivery is planned (40, 57–59). Sterile speculum examination provides an opportunity to inspect for cervicitis and umbilical cord or fetal prolapse, assess cervical dilatation and effacement, and obtain cultures as appropriate.

The diagnosis of membrane rupture is confirmed by the visualization of fluid passing from the cervical canal. If the diagnosis remains in question, the pH of the vaginal sidewalls or from fluid in the posterior vaginal fornix can be assessed. The pH of the vaginal secretions is generally 4.5–6.0, whereas amniotic fluid usually has a pH of 7.1–7.3. False-positive results may occur in the presence of blood or semen contamination, alkaline antiseptics, or bacterial vaginosis. Alternatively, false-negative results may occur with prolonged leakage and minimal residual fluid. Additional information can be obtained by swabbing the posterior fornix (avoiding cervical mucus) and allowing the vaginal fluid to dry on a microscope slide. The presence of arborization (ferning) under microscopic visualization further suggests membrane rupture.

Ultrasound examination of amniotic fluid volume may be a useful adjunct in documenting oligohydramnios, but is not diagnostic. When the clinical history or physical examination is unclear, membrane rupture can be diagnosed unequivocally with ultrasonographically guided transabdominal instillation of indigo carmine dye (1 mL in 9 mL of sterile normal saline), followed by observation for passage of blue fluid from the vagina.

▶ *What does the initial management involve once PROM has been confirmed?*

In all patients with PROM, gestational age, fetal presentation, and well-being should be determined. At any gestational age, a patient with evident intrauterine infection, abruptio placentae, or evidence of fetal compromise is best cared for by expeditious delivery. In the absence of an indication for immediate delivery, swabs for diagnosis of *Chlamydia trachomatis* and *Neisseria gonorrhoeae* may be obtained from the cervix, if appropriate. The need for group B streptococcal intrapartum prophylaxis should be determined if preterm PROM occurs (60).

In patients with preterm PROM, electronic fetal heart rate monitoring and uterine activity monitoring offer the opportunity to identify occult umbilical cord compression and to evaluate for asymptomatic contractions. In one study, variable decelerations occurred in 32% of women with preterm PROM (61). Biophysical profile test scores of 6 or less within 24 hours of delivery also have been demonstrated to correlate with positive amniotic fluid cultures and perinatal infection. At least eight studies have confirmed this association (62). Most of these studies have included daily fetal assessment after preterm PROM. An abnormal test result should lead to reassessment of the clinical circumstances and may lead to a decision to proceed to delivery. It is important to remember that heart rate testing at less than 32 weeks of gestation may not yield a reactive result in an immature but otherwise healthy fetus. However, once a reactive result has been achieved, a subsequently nonreactive test should be considered suspicious. Consensus has not been reached among experts on the optimal frequency of and modality of fetal testing in the face of PROM.

▶ *What is the optimal method of initial management for a patient with PROM at term?*

Fetal heart rate monitoring should be used to assess fetal status. Dating criteria should be reviewed to assign gestational age because virtually all aspects of subsequent care will hinge on that information. Because optimal results are seen with 4 hours between group B streptococcal prophylaxis and birth, when the decision to deliver is made, group B streptococcal prophylaxis should be given based on prior culture results or risk factors if cultures have not been previously performed (60).

The largest randomized study to date found that oxytocin induction reduced the time interval between PROM and delivery as well as the frequencies of chorioamnionitis, postpartum febrile morbidity, and neonatal antibiotic treatments, without increasing cesarean deliveries or neonatal infections (25). These data suggest that for women with PROM at term, labor should be induced at the time of presentation, generally with oxytocin infusion, to reduce the risk of chorioamnionitis. An adequate time for the latent phase of labor to progress should be allowed.

▶ *When is delivery recommended for the preterm fetus in the presence of premature rupture of membranes?*

The decision to deliver is based on gestational age and fetal status (Table 1), and the time considered optimal may vary among institutions. At 32–33 completed weeks of gestation, the risk of severe complications of prematurity is low if fetal pulmonary maturity is evident by amniotic fluid samples collected vaginally or by amniocentesis (51). Therefore, labor induction may be considered if pulmonary maturity has been documented. If pulmonary maturity cannot be established, expectant management may be beneficial. The efficacy of corticosteroid use at 32–33 completed weeks of gestation has not been specifically addressed for women with PROM but has been recommended by some experts.

Because of the increased risk of chorioamnionitis (63, 64), and because antenatal corticosteroids are not recommended after 34 weeks of gestation to accelerate fetal pulmonary maturity, delivery is recommended when PROM occurs at or beyond 34 weeks of gestation. The patient who experiences PROM between 24 weeks and 31 completed weeks of gestation should be cared for expectantly if no maternal or fetal contraindications exist until 33 completed weeks of gestation. Prophylaxis using antibiotics to prolong latency and a single course of antenatal corticosteroids can help reduce the risks of infection and gestational age-dependent neonatal morbidity.

▶ *What general approaches are used in cases of preterm PROM managed expectantly?*

Expectant management of preterm PROM generally consists of modified bed rest to enhance reaccumulation of amniotic fluid and complete pelvic rest. Patients should be assessed periodically for evidence of infection, abruptio placentae, umbilical cord compression, fetal wellbeing, and labor. There is no consensus on the frequency of assessment that is optimal, but an acceptable strategy would include periodic ultrasound monitoring of amniotic fluid volume and fetal heart rate monitoring. In a

Table 1. Management of Premature Rupture of Membranes Chronologically

Gestational Age	Management
Term (37 weeks or more)	• Proceed to delivery, usually by induction of labor • Group B streptococcal prophylaxis recommended
Near term (34 weeks to 36 completed weeks)	• Same as for term
Preterm (32 weeks to 33 completed weeks)	• Expectant management, unless fetal pulmonary maturity is documented • Group B streptococcal prophylaxis recommended • Corticosteroid—no consensus, but some experts recommend • Antibiotics recommended to prolong latency if there are no contraindications
Preterm (24 weeks to 31 completed weeks)	• Expectant management • Group B streptococcal prophylaxis recommended • Single-course corticosteroid use recommended • Tocolytics—no consensus • Antibiotics recommended to prolong latency if there are no contraindications
Less than 24 weeks*	• Patient counseling • Expectant management or induction of labor • Group B streptococcal prophylaxis is not recommended • Corticosteroids are not recommended • Antibiotics—there are incomplete data on use in prolonging latency

*The combination of birthweight, gestational age, and sex provide the best estimate of chances of survival and should be considered in individual cases.

patient with preterm PROM, a temperature exceeding 38.0°C (100.4°F) may indicate infection, although some investigators have suggested that fever, with additional factors such as uterine tenderness and maternal or fetal tachycardia, is a more accurate indicator of maternal infection (34, 65). Leukocyte counts are nonspecific when there is no clinical evidence of infection, especially if antenatal corticosteroids have been administered.

Low initial amniotic fluid volume (amniotic fluid index less than 5 cm or maximum vertical fluid pocket less than 2 cm) has been associated with shorter latency to delivery and an increased risk of neonatal morbidity, including respiratory distress syndrome (RDS), but not with increased maternal or neonatal infection after PROM (66). However, the predictive value of a low amniotic fluid volume for adverse outcomes is poor. Several investigators have evaluated the utility of endovaginal ultrasound assessment of cervical length for prediction of latency during expectant management of PROM remote from term. Some experts have suggested a short cervical length after PROM to be associated with shorter latency (67–69). In the most recent study, the likelihood of delivery within 7 days was 83% if the initial cervical length was 1–10 mm (versus 18% for cervical length more than 30 mm); however, the number of

women in these categories was small (N = 24 and 17, respectively) (67). Although the combination of clinical and ultrasound markers may yield improved predictive models in the future, initial amniotic fluid volume determination and cervical length generally should not be used in isolation to direct management of PROM.

▶ *Should tocolytics be considered for patients with preterm PROM?*

Use of prophylactic tocolysis after preterm PROM has been shown to prolong latency in the short term (70–72), whereas the use of therapeutic tocolysis (ie, instituting tocolysis only after contractions have ensued) has not been shown to prolong latency (73). A retrospective study compared the use of aggressive tocolysis (84% of antepartum days) with limited tocolysis as needed for contractions only during the first 48 hours (7% of antepartum days). Aggressive therapy was found not to be associated with significantly longer latency to delivery (3.8 versus 4.5 days, *P* = .16) (74). However, a recent retrospective study compared the prolonged use of tocolysis for longer than 48 hours plus antibiotics and steroids with gestational age-matched infants not treated for PROM. The investigators concluded that chorioamnionitis and a latency of greater than 1 week achieved by prolonged use of tocolysis lessens the advantages of extended gestational age and decreased predischarge neonatal morbidity (75).

The effect of tocolysis to permit antibiotic and antenatal corticosteroid administration in the patient with preterm PROM who is having contractions has yet to be conclusively evaluated; therefore, specific recommendations for or against tocolysis administration cannot be made. As detailed as follows, use of both antibiotics and antenatal corticosteroids improves outcome in patients with preterm PROM who are being treated expectantly.

▶ *Should antenatal corticosteroids be administered to patients with preterm PROM?*

The impact of antenatal corticosteroid administration after preterm PROM on neonatal outcomes has been evaluated in a number of clinical trials. Multivariate analysis of prospective observational trials also has suggested a benefit of antenatal corticosteroid use regardless of membrane rupture (76), and the National Institutes of Health Consensus Development Panel has recommended a single course of antenatal corticosteroids for women with PROM before 32 weeks of gestation in the absence of intraamniotic infection (77, 78). Several meta-analyses have addressed this issue (79–82). Early reviews resulted in conflicting conclusions regarding the impact of antenatal steroids on the occurrence of RDS. Two more recent meta-analyses suggest that steroid therapy significantly reduces the risks of RDS, intraventricular hemorrhage, and necrotizing enterocolitis without increasing the risks of maternal or neonatal infection regardless of gestational age (82, 83). The risk of infection from corticosteroid use at 32–33 completed weeks of gestation is unclear, but based on available evidence, their use has been recommended by some experts, particularly if pulmonary immaturity is documented. Studies of the combined use of corticosteroids and prophylactic antibiotics after preterm PROM suggest significant reductions in RDS, perinatal mortality, and other morbidities with no evident increase in perinatal infections after steroid administration (84, 85).

▶ *Should antibiotics be administered to patients with preterm PROM?*

The issue of adjunctive antibiotic therapy to treat or prevent ascending decidual infection in order to prolong pregnancy and reduce neonatal infections and gestational age-dependent morbidity has been widely studied (43, 86, 87). In the most recent meta-analysis, investigators suggested prophylactic antibiotic administration to delay delivery and reduce major markers of neonatal morbidity, but suggested that amoxicillin–clavulanic acid be avoided because of the increased risk of neonatal necrotizing enterocolitis (87).

Two large, multicenter clinical trials have adequate power to evaluate the utility of adjunctive antibiotics in this setting (65, 88). The National Institutes of Child Health and Human Development Maternal Fetal Medicine Research Units (NICHD-MFMU) Research Network found that the combination of initial intravenous therapy (48 hours) with ampicillin and erythromycin, followed by oral therapy of limited duration (5 days) with amoxicillin and enteric-coated erythromycin-base at 24–32 weeks of gestation, decreased the likelihood of chorioamnionitis and delivery for up to 3 weeks, as well as the number of infants with one or more major morbidities (defined as death, RDS, early sepsis, severe intraventricular hemorrhage, or severe necrotizing enterocolitis) (65). In addition, therapy reduced the likelihood of individual gestational age–dependent morbidities, including RDS, stage 3–4 necrotizing enterocolitis, patent ductus arteriosus, and chronic lung disease. Neonatal sepsis and pneumonia were less frequent in the antibiotic group for those who were not carriers of group B streptococci. (Group B streptococci carriers in both study arms received ampicillin for 1 week and then again during labor.)

A second large multicenter trial that examined the use of oral antibiotic therapy with erythromycin, amoxicillin–clavulanic acid, or both for up to 10 days after preterm PROM before 37 weeks of gestation found that oral erythromycin therapy 1) prolonged pregnancy only briefly (not significant at 7 days), 2) reduced the need for supplemental oxygen, and 3) reduced the frequency of positive blood cultures with no improvement in the primary outcome (one or more outcomes of death, chronic lung disease, or major cerebral abnormality on ultrasonography) (88). Oral amoxicillin–clavulanic acid reduced delivery within 7 days and reduced the need for supplemental oxygen but was associated with an increased risk of necrotizing enterocolitis (1.9% versus 0.5%, $P = .001$) without preventing other neonatal morbidities. The finding of increased necrotizing enterocolitis with oral amoxicillin–clavulanic acid differs from the NICHD-MFMU trial finding of reduced stage 2 or 3 necrotizing enterocolitis with amoxicillin–erythromycin therapy in a higher risk population, and review of the current literature does not reveal a consistent pattern regarding an increased risk with broad-spectrum antibiotic therapy. Several recent studies have attempted to determine whether a shorter duration of antibiotic therapy is adequate after preterm PROM, but these studies are of inadequate size and power to demonstrate equivalent effectiveness against infant morbidity (89, 90).

Based on available information, a 7-day course of parenteral and oral therapy with ampicillin or amoxicillin and erythromycin is recommended during expectant management of preterm PROM remote from term to prolong pregnancy and to reduce infectious and gestational age-dependent neonatal morbidity. Use of the combination of oral erythromycin and extended-spectrum ampicillin–clavulanic acid in women near term does not appear to be beneficial, may be harmful, and is not recommended. Antibiotic administration to prolong latency must be distinguished from well-established protocols directed at prevention of group B streptococcal infection in term and preterm patients (60). The prophylactic antibiotic regimen would appropriately treat group B streptococcal infections during expectant management of preterm PROM remote from term. However, women with PROM and a viable fetus, who are known carriers of group B streptococci and those who give birth before carrier status can be delineated, should receive intrapartum prophylaxis to prevent vertical transmission regardless of earlier treatments.

▶ Can preterm PROM be managed with home care?

Generally, hospitalization for bed rest and pelvic rest is indicated after preterm PROM once viability is reached. Recognizing that latency is frequently brief, that intrauterine and fetal infection may occur suddenly, and that the fetus is at risk for umbilical cord compression, ongoing surveillance of both the woman and her fetus is recommended once the limit of potential viability has been reached.

For a woman with preterm PROM and a viable fetus, the safety of expectant management at home has not been established. One clinical trial of discharge after preterm PROM suggested that relatively few patients will be eligible for discharge to home care (91). Only 67 of 349 women (18%) were eligible for antepartum home care after 72 hours (negative cervical cultures and no evident labor, intrauterine infection, or fetal compromise). There were no identifiable differences in latency or in the incidences of intraamniotic infection, variable decelerations, or cesarean delivery. Infant outcomes were similar, but the power of this study to identify differences in these outcomes was low. Although the potential for a reduction in health care costs with antepartum discharge is enticing, it is important to ensure that such management will not be associated with increased risks and costs related to perinatal morbidity and mortality. Any cost savings from antenatal discharge may be rapidly lost with a small increase in the stay in the neonatal intensive care unit.

▶ How should a patient with preterm PROM and a cervical cerclage be treated?

There are no prospective studies available with which to guide the care of women with preterm PROM and a cervical cerclage in situ. Retrospective studies have found that removal of cerclage after PROM is associated with similar pregnancy outcomes to those with PROM but no cerclage (92, 93). Cerclage retention after preterm PROM has been associated with trends toward increased maternal infectious morbidity (94–96), reaching statistical significance in one evaluation (97), and with only brief pregnancy prolongation. One study found increased infant mortality and sepsis-related death when the cerclage was left in place after PROM (94). One study found significant pregnancy prolongation with cerclage retention by comparing differing practices at two institutions; however, this could reflect population or practice differences at these institutions (95). Because the available studies are small and nonrandomized, the optimal timing of cerclage removal is unclear. However, no controlled study has found cerclage retention after PROM to improve neonatal outcomes. The risks and benefits of short-term cerclage retention pending completion of antenatal corticosteroid therapy to enhance fetal maturation have not been evaluated.

▶ What is the optimal treatment for a patient with preterm PROM and herpes simplex virus infection?

Neonatal herpes simplex virus infection usually results from maternal–fetal transmission during the delivery process. Neonatal infection occurs in 34–80% of infants delivered in the setting of primary maternal infection, and in 1–5% with secondary infections (98, 99). Based on a small case series of women with active genital herpes infection in 1971, totaling just 36 patients, it has been believed that latency of more than 4–6 hours after membrane rupture is associated with an increased risk of neonatal infection (100, 101). However, a more recent case series of 29 women treated expectantly with active recurrent herpes simplex virus lesions and PROM before 32 weeks of gestation found none of the infants developed neonatal herpes infection (102). Latency from membrane rupture to delivery ranged from 1 to 35 days, and cesarean delivery was performed if active lesions were present at the time of delivery. These data suggest that the risk of prematurity should be weighed against the potential risk of neonatal herpes simplex virus in considering expectant management of PROM complicated by recurrent maternal herpes simplex virus infection. Prophylactic treatment with antiviral agents (eg, acyclovir) may be considered.

▶ *How does care differ for patients with PROM that occurs before the threshold of potential neonatal viability?*

Women presenting with PROM before potential viability should be counseled regarding the impact of immediate delivery and the potential risks and benefits of expectant management. Counseling should include a realistic appraisal of neonatal outcomes, including the availability of obstetric monitoring and neonatal intensive care facilities. Because of advances in perinatal care, morbidity and mortality rates continue to improve rapidly (43, 44, 103). An attempt should be made to provide parents with the most up-to-date information possible.

Although no evidence or consensus of opinion exists regarding the benefit of an initial period of inpatient observation in these patients, this approach may include strict bed and pelvic rest to enhance the opportunity for resealing, as well as early identification of infection and abruptio placentae if expectant management is pursued. In addition to clinical follow-up, it may be useful to instruct patients to abstain from intercourse, limit their activities, and monitor their temperatures.

Typically, women with previable PROM who have been cared for as outpatients are readmitted to the hospital for bed rest and observation for infection, abruptio placentae, labor, and nonreassuring fetal heart rate patterns once the pregnancy has reached the limit of viability. Administration of antenatal corticosteroids for fetal maturation is appropriate at this time given that early delivery remains likely.

Summary of Recommendations and Conclusions

The following recommendations and conclusions are based on good and consistent scientific evidence (Level A):

▶ For women with PROM at term, labor should be induced at the time of presentation, generally with oxytocin infusion, to reduce the risk chorioamnionitis.

▶ Patients with PROM before 32 weeks of gestation should be cared for expectantly until 33 completed weeks of gestation if no maternal or fetal contraindications exist.

▶ A 48-hour course of intravenous ampicillin and erythromycin followed by 5 days of amoxicillin and erythromycin is recommended during expectant management of preterm PROM remote from term to prolong pregnancy and to reduce infectious and gestational age–dependent neonatal morbidity.

▶ All women with PROM and a viable fetus, including those known to be carriers of group B streptococci and those who give birth before carrier status can be delineated, should receive intrapartum chemoprophylaxis to prevent vertical transmission of group B streptococci regardless of earlier treatments.

▶ A single course of antenatal corticosteroids should be administered to women with PROM before 32 weeks of gestation to reduce the risks of RDS, perinatal mortality, and other morbidities.

The following recommendations and conclusions are based on limited and inconsistent scientific evidence (Level B):

▶ Delivery is recommended when PROM occurs at or beyond 34 weeks of gestation.

▶ With PROM at 32–33 completed weeks of gestation, labor induction may be considered if fetal pulmonary maturity has been documented.

▶ Digital cervical examinations should be avoided in patients with PROM unless they are in active labor or imminent delivery is anticipated.

The following recommendations and conclusions are based primarily on consensus and expert opinion (Level C):

▶ A specific recommendation for or against tocolysis administration cannot be made.

▶ The efficacy of corticosteroid use at 32–33 completed weeks is unclear based on available evidence, but treatment may be beneficial particularly if pulmonary immaturity is documented.

▶ For a woman with preterm PROM and a viable fetus, the safety of expectant management at home has not been established.

Proposed Performance Measure

The percentage of patients with PROM and a viable fetus who are known group B streptococci carriers or whose status as a carrier is unknown who receive intrapartum group B streptococcal prophylaxis

References

1. Goldenberg RL, Rouse DJ. Prevention of premature birth. N Engl J Med 1998;339:313–20. (Level III)

2. Mathews TJ, Mac Dorman MF. Infant mortality statistics from the 2003 period linked birth/infant death data set. Natl Vital Stat Rep 2006;54(16):1–29. (Level II-3)

3. Martin JA, Hamilton BE, Sutton PD, Ventura SJ, Menacker F, Kirmeyer S. Births: final data for 2004. Natl Vital Stat Rep 2006;5(1):1–101. (Level II-3)

4. Mercer BM. Preterm premature rupture of the membranes. Obstet Gynecol 2003;101:178–93. (Level III)

5. Lavery JP, Miller CE, Knight RD. The effect of labor on the rheologic response of chorioamniotic membranes. Obstet Gynecol 1982;60:87–92. (Level II-3)

6. McLaren J, Taylor DJ, Bell SC. Increased incidence of apoptosis in non-labour-affected cytotrophoblast cells in term fetal membranes overlying the cervix. Hum Reprod 1999;14:2895–900. (Level II-3)

7. El Khwad M, Stetzer B, Moore RM, Kumar D, Mercer B, Arikat S, et al. Term human fetal membranes have a weak zone overlying the lower uterine pole and cervix before onset of labor. Biol Reprod 2005;72:720–6. (Level II-3)

8. Moore RM, Mansour JM, Redline RW, Mercer BM, Moore JJ. The physiology of fetal membrane rupture: insight gained from the determination of physical properties. Placenta 2006;27:1037–51. (Level II-3).

9. Yoon BH, Romero R, Park JS, Kim CJ, Kim SH, Choi JH, et al. Fetal exposure to an intra-amniotic inflammation and the development of cerebral palsy at the age of three years. Am J Obstet Gynecol 2000;182:675–81. (Level II-3)

10. Harger JH, Hsing AW, Tuomala RE, Gibbs RS, Mead PB, Eschenbach DA, et al. Risk factors for preterm premature rupture of fetal membranes: a multicenter case-control study. Am J Obstet Gynecol 1990;163:130–7. (Level II-2)

11. Taylor J, Garite TJ. Premature rupture of membranes before fetal viability. Obstet Gynecol 1984;64:615–20. (Level II-3)

12. Mercer BM, Goldenberg RL, Meis PJ, Moawad AH, Shellhaas C, Das A, et al. The Preterm Prediction Study: prediction of preterm premature rupture of membranes using clinical findings and ancillary testing. The National Institute of Child Health and Human Development Maternal–Fetal Medicine Units Network. Am J Obstet Gynecol 2000;183:738–45. (Level II-2)

13. Minkoff H, Grunebaum AN, Schwarz RH, Feldman J, Cummings M, Crombleholme W, et al. Risk factors for prematurity and premature rupture of membranes: a prospective study of the vaginal flora in pregnancy. Am J Obstet Gynecol 1984;150:965–72. (Level II-2)

14. Naeye RL. Factors that predispose to premature rupture of the fetal membranes. Obstet Gynecol 1982;60:93–8. (Level II-3)

15. Naeye RL, Peters EC. Causes and consequences of premature rupture of fetal membranes. Lancet 1980;1:192–4. (Level II-3)

16. Charles D, Edwards WR. Infectious complications of cervical cerclage. Am J Obstet Gynecol 1981;141:1065–71. (Level II-3)

17. Hadley CB, Main DM, Gabbe SG. Risk factors for preterm premature rupture of the fetal membranes. Am J Perinatol 1990;7:374–9. (Level II-2)

18. Siega-Riz AM, Promislow JH, Savitz DA, Thorp JM Jr, McDonald T. Vitamin C intake and the risk of preterm delivery. Am J Obstet Gynecol 2003;189:519–25. (Level II-2)

19. Gold RB, Goyert GL, Schwartz DB, Evans MI, Seabolt LA. Conservative management of second-trimester postamniocentesis fluid leakage. Obstet Gynecol 1989;74:745–7. (Level II-3)

20. Lee T, Carpenter M, Heber WW, Silver HM. Preterm premature rupture of membranes: risks of recurrent complications in the next pregnancy among a population-based sample of gravid women. Am J Obstet Gynecol 2003;188:209–13. (Level II-2)

21. Asrat T, Lewis DF, Garite TJ, Major CA, Nageotte MP, Towers CV, et al. Rate of recurrence of preterm premature rupture of membranes in consecutive pregnancies. Am J Obstet Gynecol 1991;165:1111–5. (Level III)

22. Guinn DA, Goldenberg RL, Hauth JC, Andrews WW, Thom E, Romero R. Risk factors for the development of preterm premature rupture of the membranes after arrest of preterm labor. Am J Obstet Gynecol 1995;173:1310–5. (Level II-2)

23. Meis PJ, Klebanoff M, Thom E, Dombrowski MP, Sibai B, Moawad AH, et al. Prevention of recurrent preterm delivery by 17 alpha-hydroxyprogesterone caproate. National Institute of Child Health and Human Development Maternal-Fetal Medicine Units Network [published erratum appears in N Engl J Med 2003;349:1299]. N Engl J Med 2003;348:2379–85. (Level I)

24. da Fonseca EB, Bittar RE, Carvalho MH, Zugaib M. Prophylactic administration of progesterone by vaginal suppository to reduce the incidence of spontaneous preterm birth in women at increased risk: a randomized placebo-controlled double-blind study. Am J Obstet Gynecol 2003;188:419–24. (Level I)

25. Hannah ME, Ohlsson A, Farine D, Hewson SA, Hodnett ED, Myhr TL, et al. Induction of labor compared with expectant management for prelabor rupture of the membranes at term. TERMPROM Study Group. N Engl J Med 1996;334:1005–10. (Level I)

26. Wagner MV, Chin VP, Peters CJ, Drexler B, Newman LA. A comparison of early and delayed induction of labor with spontaneous rupture of membranes at term. Obstet Gynecol 1989;74:93–7. (Level II-1)

27. Guise JM, Duff P, Christian JS. Management of term patients with premature rupture of membranes and an unfavorable cervix. Am J Perinatol 1992;9:56–60. (Level II-2)

28. Johnson JW, Egerman RS, Moorhead J. Cases with ruptured membranes that "reseal." Am J Obstet Gynecol 1990;163:1024–30; discussion 1030–2. (Level II-2)

29. Novak-Antolic Z, Pajntar M, Verdenik I. Rupture of the membranes and postpartum infection. Eur J Obstet Gynecol Reprod Biol 1997;71:141–6. (Level II-3)

30. Eddleman K, Malone F, Sullivan L, Dukes K, Berkowitz R, Kharbutli Y, et al. Pregnancy loss rates after midtrimester amniocentesis. Obstet Gynecol 2006;108:1067–72. (Level II-2)

31. Borgida AF, Mills AA, Feldman DM, Rodis JF, Egan JF. Outcome of pregnancies complicated by ruptured membranes after genetic amniocentesis. Am J Obstet Gynecol 2000;183:937–9. (Level II-3)

32. Gold RB, Goyert GL, Schwartz DB, Evans MI, Seabolt LA. Conservative management of second trimester postamniocentesis fluid leakage. Obstet Gynecol 1989;74:745–7. (Level II-3).

33. Mercer BM. Management of premature rupture of membranes before 26 weeks' gestation. Obstet Gynecol Clin North Am 1992;19:339–51. (Level III)

34. Beydoun SN, Yasin SY. Premature rupture of the membranes before 28 weeks: conservative management. Am J Obstet Gynecol 1986;155:471–9. (Level II-3)

35. Garite TJ, Freeman RK. Chorioamnionitis in the preterm gestation. Obstet Gynecol 1982;59:539–45. (Level II-3)

36. Simpson GF, Harbert GM Jr. Use of beta-methasone in management of preterm gestation with premature rupture of membranes. Obstet Gynecol 1985;66:168–75. (Level II-2)

37. Vergani P, Ghidini A, Locatelli A, Cavallone M, Ciarla I, Cappellini A. Risk factors for pulmonary hypoplasia in second-trimester premature rupture of membranes. Am J Obstet Gynecol 1994;170:1359–64. (Level II-3)

38. Hillier SL, Martius J, Krohn M, Kiviat N, Holmes KK, Eschenbach DA. A case-control study of chorioamnionic infection and histologic chorioamnionitis in prematurity. N Engl J Med 1988;319:972–8. (Level II-2)

39. Morales WJ. The effect of chorioamnionitis on the developmental outcome of preterm infants at one year. Obstet Gynecol 1987;70:183–6. (Level II-3)

40. Alexander JM, Mercer BM, Miodovnik M, Thurnau GR, Goldenberg RL, Das AF, et al. The impact of digital cervical examination on expectantly managed preterm rupture of membranes. Am J Obstet Gynecol 2000;183(4):1003–7. (Level II-3)

41. Ananth CV, Savitz DA, Williams MA. Placental abruption and its association with hypertension and prolonged rupture of membranes: a methodologic review and meta-analysis. Obstet Gynecol 1996;88:309–18. (Meta-analysis)

42. Gonen R, Hannah ME, Milligan JE. Does prolonged preterm premature rupture of the membranes predispose to abruptio placentae? Obstet Gynecol 1989;74:347–50. (Level II-2)

43. Mercer BM, Arheart KL. Antimicrobial therapy in expectant management of preterm premature rupture of membranes [published erratum appears in Lancet 1996;347:410]. Lancet 1995;346:1271–9. (Meta-analysis)

44. Lemons JA, Bauer CR, Oh W, Korones SB, Papile LA, Stoll BJ, et al. Very low birth weight outcomes of the National Institute of Child Health and Human Development Neonatal Research Network, January 1995 through December 1996. NICHD Neonatal Research Network. Pediatrics 2001;107:E1. (Level II-2)

45. Spinillo A, Capuzzo E, Stronati M, Ometto A, Orcesi S, Fazzi E. Effect of preterm premature rupture of membranes on neurodevelopmental outcome: follow up at two years of age. Br J Obstet Gynaecol 1995;102:882–7. (Level II-3)

46. Locatelli A, Ghidini A, Paterlini G, Patane L, Doria V, Zorloni C, et al. Gestational age at preterm premature rupture of membranes: a risk factor for neonatal white matter damage. Am J Obstet Gynecol 2005;193:947–51. (Level II-3)

47. Schucker JL, Mercer BM. Midtrimester premature rupture of the membranes. Semin Perinatol 1996;20:389–400. (Level III)

48. Dewan H, Morris JM. A systematic review of pregnancy outcome following preterm premature rupture of membranes at a previable gestational age. Aust N Z J Obstet Gynaecol 2001;41:389–94. (Meta-analysis)

49. Bengtson JM, VanMarter LJ, Barss VA, Greene MF, Tuomala RE, Epstein MF. Pregnancy outcome after premature rupture of the membranes at or before 26 weeks' gestation. Obstet Gynecol 1989;73:921–7. (Level II-3)

50. Cox SM, Leveno KJ. Intentional delivery versus expectant management with preterm ruptured membranes at 30–34 weeks' gestation. Obstet Gynecol 1995;86:875–9. (Level I)

51. Mercer BM, Crocker LG, Boe NM, Sibai BM. Induction versus expectant management in premature rupture of the membranes with mature amniotic fluid at 32 to 36 weeks: a randomized trial. Am J Obstet Gynecol 1993;169:775–82. (Level I)

52. Moretti M, Sibai BM. Maternal and perinatal outcome of expectant management of premature rupture of the membranes in the midtrimester. Am J Obstet Gynecol 1988;159:390–6. (Level II-3)

53. Rotschild A, Ling EW, Puterman ML, Farquharson D. Neonatal outcome after prolonged preterm rupture of the membranes. Am J Obstet Gynecol 1990;162:46–52. (Level II-3)

54. van Eyck J, van der Mooren K, Wladimiroff JW. Ductus arteriosus flow velocity modulation by fetal breathing movements as a measure of fetal lung development. Am J Obstet Gynecol 1990;163:558–66. (Level II-3)

55. Winn HN, Chen M, Amon E, Leet TL, Shumway JB, Mostello D. Neonatal pulmonary hypoplasia and perinatal mortality in patients with midtrimester rupture of amniotic membranes—a critical analysis. Am J Obstet Gynecol 2000;182:1638–44. (Level II-2)

56. Shumway J, Al-Malt A, Amon E, Cohlan B, Amini S, Abboud M, et al. Impact of oligohydramnios on maternal and perinatal outcomes of spontaneous premature rupture of the membranes at 18–28 weeks. J Matern Fetal Med 1999;8:20–3. (Level II-2)

57. Munson LA, Graham A, Koos BJ, Valenzuela GJ. Is there a need for digital examination in patients with spontaneous rupture of the membranes? Am J Obstet Gynecol 1985;153:562–3. (Level II-3)

58. Brown CL, Ludwiczak MH, Blanco JD, Hirsch CE. Cervical dilation: accuracy of visual and digital examinations. Obstet Gynecol 1993;81:215–6. (Level II-2)

59. Lewis DF, Major CA, Towers CV, Asrat T, Harding JA, Garite TJ. Effects of digital vaginal examinations on latency period in preterm premature rupture of membranes. Obstet Gynecol 1992;80:630–4. (Level II-3)

60. American College of Obstetricians and Gynecologists. Prevention of early-onset group B streptococcal disease in newborns. ACOG Committee Opinion No. 289. Obstet Gynecol 2002;100:1405–12. (Level III)

61. Smith CV, Greenspoon J, Phelan JP, Platt LD. Clinical utility of the nonstress test in the conservative management of women with preterm spontaneous premature rupture of the membranes. J Reprod Med 1987;32:1–4. (Level II-3)

62. Hanley ML, Vintzileos AM. Biophysical testing in premature rupture of the membranes. Semin Perinatol 1996; 20:418–25. (Level III)

63. Naef RW 3rd, Allbert JR, Ross EL, Weber BM, Martin RW, Morrison JC. Premature rupture of membranes at 34 to 37 weeks' gestation: aggressive versus conservative management. Am J Obstet Gynecol 1998;178:126–30. (Level I)

64. Neerhof MG, Cravello C, Haney EI, Silver RK. Timing of labor induction after premature rupture of membranes between 32 and 36 weeks' gestation. Am J Obstet Gynecol 1999;180:349–52. (Level II-3)

65. Mercer BM, Miodovnik M, Thurnau GR, Goldenberg RL, Das AF, Ramsey RD, et al. Antibiotic therapy for reduction of infant morbidity after preterm premature rupture of the membranes. A randomized controlled trial. National Institute of Child Health and Human Development Maternal–Fetal Medicine Units Network. JAMA 1997; 278:989–95. (Level I)

66. Mercer BM, Rabello YA, Thurnau GR, Miodovnik M, Goldenberg RL, Das AF, et al. The NICHD-MFMU antibiotic treatment of preterm PROM study: impact of initial amniotic fluid volume on pregnancy outcome. NICHD-MFMU Network. Am J Obstet Gynecol 2006; 194:438–45. (Level II-2)

67. Tsoi E, Fuchs I, Henrich W, Dudenhausen JW, Nicolaides KH. Sonographic measurement of cervical length in preterm prelabor amniorrhexis. Ultrasound Obstet Gynecol 2004;24:550–3. (Level II-3)

68. Rizzo G, Capponi A, Angelini E, Vlachopoulou A, Grassi C, Romanini C. The value of transvaginal ultrasonographic examination of the uterine cervix in predicting preterm delivery in patients with preterm premature rupture of membranes. Ultrasound Obstet Gynecol 1998;11:23–9. (Level II-2)

69. Carlan SJ, Richmond LB, O'Brien WF. Randomized trial of endovaginal ultrasound in preterm premature rupture of membranes. Obstet Gynecol 1997;89:458–61. (Level I)

70. Christensen KK, Ingemarsson I, Leideman T, Solum H, Svenningsen N. Effect of ritodrine on labor after premature rupture of the membranes. Obstet Gynecol 1980;55: 187–90. (Level I)

71. Levy DL, Warsof SL. Oral ritodrine and preterm premature rupture of membranes. Obstet Gynecol 1985;66: 621–3. (Level II-1)

72. Weiner CP, Renk K, Klugman M. The therapeutic efficacy and cost-effectiveness of aggressive tocolysis for premature labor associated with premature rupture of the membranes [published erratum appears in Am J Obstet Gynecol 1991;165:785]. Am J Obstet Gynecol 1988;159: 216–22. (Level I)

73. Garite TJ, Keegan KA, Freeman RK, Nageotte MP. A randomized trial of ritodrine tocolysis versus expectant management in patients with premature rupture of membranes at 25 to 30 weeks of gestation. Am J Obstet Gynecol 1987;157:388–93. (Level II-1)

74. Combs CA, McCune M, Clark R, Fishman A. Aggressive tocolysis does not prolong pregnancy or reduce neonatal morbidity after preterm premature rupture of the membranes. Am J Obstet Gynecol 2004;190:1723–8; discussion 1728–31. (Level I)

75. Wolfensberger A, Zimmermann R, von Mandach U. Neonatal mortality and morbidity after aggressive long-term tocolysis for preterm premature rupture of the membranes. Fetal Diagn Ther 2006;21:366–73. (Level II-2)

76. Wright LL, Verter J, Younes N, Stevenson D, Fanaroff AA, Shankaran S, et al. Antenatal corticosteroid administration and neonatal outcome in very low birth weight infants: the NICHD Neonatal Research Network. Am J Obstet Gynecol 1995;173:269–74. (Level II-3)

77. Antenatal corticosteroids revisited: repeat courses— National Institutes of Health Consensus Development Conference Statement, August 17–18, 2000. National Institutes of Health Consensus Development Panel. Obstet Gynecol 2001;98:144–50. (Level III)

78. Antenatal corticosteroid therapy for fetal maturation. ACOG Committee Opinion No. 273. American College of Obstetricians and Gynecologists. Obstet Gynecol 2002; 99:871–3. (Level III)

79. Ohlsson A. Treatments of preterm premature rupture of the membranes: a meta-analysis. Am J Obstet Gynecol 1989;160:890–906. (Meta-analysis)

80. Crowley PA. Antenatal corticosteroid therapy: a meta-analysis of the randomized trials, 1972 to 1994. Am J Obstet Gynecol 1995;173:322–35. (Meta-analysis)

81. Lovett SM, Weiss JD, Diogo MJ, Williams PT, Garite TJ. A prospective, double-blind, randomized, controlled clinical trial of ampicillin-sulbactam for preterm premature rupture of membranes in women receiving antenatal corticosteroid therapy. Am J Obstet Gynecol 1997;176: 1030–8. (Level I)

82. Roberts D, Dalziel S. Antenatal corticosteroids for accelerating fetal lung maturation for women at risk of preterm birth. Cochrane Database of Systematic Reviews 2006, Issue 3. Art. No.: CD004454. DOI: 10.1002/14651858. CD004454.pub2. (Meta-analysis)

83. Harding JE, Pang J, Knight DB, Liggins GC. Do antenatal corticosteroids help in the setting of preterm rupture of membranes? Am J Obstet Gynecol 2001;184:131–9. (Meta-analysis)

84. Lewis DF, Brody K, Edwards MS, Brouillette RM, Burlison S, London SN. Preterm premature ruptured membranes: a randomized trial of steroids after treatment with antibiotics. Obstet Gynecol 1996;88:801–5. (Level I)

85. Pattinson RC, Makin JD, Funk M, Delport SD, Macdonald AP, Norman K, et al. The use of dexamethasone in women with preterm premature rupture of membranes—a multicentre, double-blind, placebo-controlled, randomised trial. Dexiprom Study Group. S Afr Med J 1999;89:865–70. (Level I)

86. Egarter C, Leitich H, Karas H, Wieser F, Husslein P, Kaider A, et al. Antibiotic treatment in premature rupture of membranes and neonatal morbidity: a metaanalysis. Am J Obstet Gynecol 1996;174:589–97. (Meta-analysis)

87. Kenyon S, Boulvain M, Neilson J. Antibiotics for preterm rupture of membranes. Cochrane Database of Systematic Reviews 2003, Issue 2. Art No.: CD001058. DOI: 10.1002/14651858.CD001058. (Meta-analysis)

88. Kenyon SL, Taylor DJ, Tarnow-Mordi W. Broad spectrum antibiotics for preterm, prelabor rupture of fetal membranes: the ORACLE I randomized trial. ORACLE Collaborative Group [published erratum appears in Lancet 2001;358:156]. Lancet 2001;357:979–88. (Level I)

89. Lewis DF, Adair CD, Robichaux AG, Jaekle RK, Moore JA, Evans AT, et al. Antibiotic therapy in preterm premature rupture of membranes: are seven days necessary? A preliminary, randomized clinical trial. Am J Obstet Gynecol 2003;188:1413–6; discussion 1416–7. (Level I)

90. Segel SY, Miles AM, Clothier B, Parry S, Macones GA. Duration of antibiotic therapy after preterm premature rupture of fetal membranes. Am J Obstet Gynecol 2003;189:799–802. (Level I)

91. Carlan SJ, O'Brien WF, Parsons MT, Lense JJ. Preterm premature rupture of membranes: a randomized study of home versus hospital management. Obstet Gynecol 1993;81:61–4. (Level I)

92. Blickstein I, Katz Z, Lancet M, Molgilner BM. The outcome of pregnancies complicated by preterm rupture of the membranes with and without cerclage. Int J Gynaecol Obstet 1989;28:237–42. (Level II-3)

93. Yeast JD, Garite TR. The role of cervical cerclage in the management of preterm premature rupture of the membranes. Am J Obstet Gynecol 1988;158:106–10. (Level II-3)

94. Ludmir J, Bader T, Chen L, Lindenbaum C, Wong G. Poor perinatal outcome associated with retained cerclage in patients with premature rupture of membranes. Obstet Gynecol 1994;84:823–6. (Level II-3)

95. Jenkins TM, Berghella V, Shlossman PA, McIntyre CJ, Maas BD, Pollock MA, et al. Timing of cerclage removal after preterm premature rupture of membranes: maternal and neonatal outcomes. Am J Obstet Gynecol 2000;183:847–52. (Level II-3)

96. McElrath TF, Norwitz ER, Lieberman ES, Heffner LJ. Perinatal outcome after preterm premature rupture of membranes with in situ cervical cerclage. Am J Obstet Gynecol 2002;187:1147–52. (Level II-3)

97. Kuhn RJ, Pepperell RJ. Cervical ligation: a review of 242 pregnancies. Aust N Z J Obstet Gynecol 1977;17:79–83. (Level II-3)

98. Chuang T. Neonatal herpes: incidence, prevention, and consequences. Am J Prev Med 1988;4:47–53. (Level III)

99. Amstey MS. Management of pregnancy complicated by genital herpes virus infection. Obstet Gynecol 1971;37:515–20. (Level II-3)

100. Nahmias AJ, Josey WE, Naib ZM, Freeman MG, Fernandez RJ, Wheeler JH. Perinatal risk associated with maternal genital herpes simplex virus infection. Am J Obstet Gynecol 1971;110:825–37. (Level II-3)

101. Gibbs RS, Amstey MS, Lezotte DC. Role of cesarean delivery in preventing neonatal herpes virus infection. JAMA 1993;270:94–5. (Level III)

102. Major CA, Towers CV, Lewis DF, Garite TJ. Expectant management of preterm premature rupture of membranes complicated by active recurrent genital herpes. Am J Obstet Gynecol 2003;188:1551–4; discussion 1554–5. (Level II-3)

103. Perinatal care at the threshold of viability. ACOG Practice Bulletin No. 38. American College of Obstetricians and Gynecologists. Obstet Gynecol 2002;100:617–24. (Level III)

The MEDLINE database, the Cochrane Library, and ACOG's own internal resources and documents were used to conduct a literature search to locate relevant articles published between January 1985 and November 2006. The search was restricted to articles published in the English language. Priority was given to articles reporting results of original research, although review articles and commentaries also were consulted. Abstracts of research presented at symposia and scientific conferences were not considered adequate for inclusion in this document. Guidelines published by organizations or institutions such as the National Institutes of Health and the American College of Obstetricians and Gynecologists were reviewed, and additional studies were located by reviewing bibliographies of identified articles. When reliable research was not available, expert opinions from obstetrician–gynecologists were used.

Studies were reviewed and evaluated for quality according to the method outlined by the U.S. Preventive Services Task Force:

I   Evidence obtained from at least one properly designed randomized controlled trial.

II-1   Evidence obtained from well-designed controlled trials without randomization.

II-2   Evidence obtained from well-designed cohort or case–control analytic studies, preferably from more than one center or research group.

II-3   Evidence obtained from multiple time series with or without the intervention. Dramatic results in uncontrolled experiments also could be regarded as this type of evidence.

III   Opinions of respected authorities, based on clinical experience, descriptive studies, or reports of expert committees.

Based on the highest level of evidence found in the data, recommendations are provided and graded according to the following categories:

Level A—Recommendations are based on good and consistent scientific evidence.

Level B—Recommendations are based on limited or inconsistent scientific evidence.

Level C—Recommendations are based primarily on consensus and expert opinion.

ISSN 1099-3630

The American College of Obstetricians and Gynecologists
409 12th Street, SW, PO Box 96920, Washington, DC 20090-6920

Premature rupture of membranes. ACOG Practice Bulletin No. 80. American College of Obstetricians and Gynecologists. Obstet Gynecol 2007;109:1007–19.

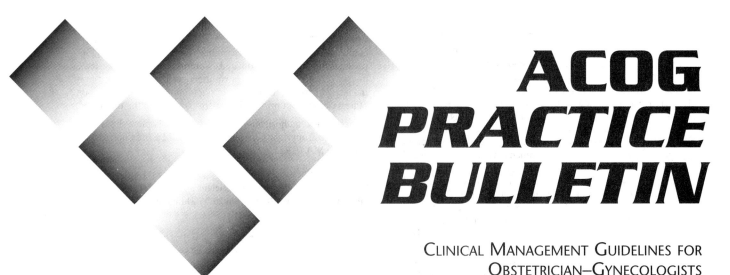

CLINICAL MANAGEMENT GUIDELINES FOR
OBSTETRICIAN–GYNECOLOGISTS

NUMBER 82, JUNE 2007

(Replaces Practice Bulletin Number 8, October 1999)

Management of Herpes in Pregnancy

This Practice Bulletin was developed by the ACOG Committee on Practice Bulletins—Obstetrics with the assistance of Lisa Hollier, MD. The information is designed to aid practitioners in making decisions about appropriate obstetric and gynecologic care. These guidelines should not be construed as dictating an exclusive course of treatment or procedure. Variations in practice may be warranted based on the needs of the individual patient, resources, and limitations unique to the institution or type of practice.

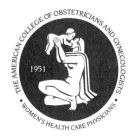

Genital herpes simplex virus (HSV) infection during pregnancy poses a risk to the developing fetus and newborn. Genital herpes infection occurs in one in five women in the United States. Because many women of childbearing age are infected or are becoming infected with HSV, the risk of maternal transmission of this virus to the fetus or newborn is a major health concern. The purpose of this document is to outline the spectrum of maternal and neonatal infection, including risks of transmission, and provide management guidelines supported by appropriately conducted outcome-based research. Additional guidelines based on consensus and expert opinion also are presented to permit a review of most clinical aspects of HSV.

Background

Etiology

Herpes simplex virus is a double-stranded DNA virus that can be differentiated into HSV type 1 (HSV-1) and HSV type 2 (HSV-2) based on the glycoproteins in the lipid bilayer envelope. Glycoprotein G2 is associated with HSV-2, and glycoprotein G1 is associated with HSV-1. Herpes simplex virus type 1 is the primary etiologic agent of herpes labialis, gingivostomatitis, and keratoconjunctivitis. Most genital infections with HSV are caused by HSV-2, but genital HSV-1 infections are becoming increasingly common, particularly among adolescent and young women (1).

Herpes simplex virus is transmitted from person to person through direct contact. Infection is initiated when the virus contacts mucosa or abraded skin. The incubation period after acquisition of HSV-1 or HSV-2 ranges from 2 days to 12 days. Herpes simplex virus then replicates in the epidermis and dermis, with resulting cellular destruction and inflammation. During the initial infection, the virus gains access to the sensory neurons, and then the infection becomes latent in the sensory ganglia. Reactivation of viral replication occurs and may manifest clinically as recurrent ulcerative lesions or subclinically as asymptomatic viral shedding. Both the cellular and humoral immune systems play an important role in controlling this viral infection (2).

Herpes virus has a characteristic protein coat, and each of the viral types has identifiable proteins. Type-specific antibodies to the viral proteins develop within the first several weeks of infection and persist. Antibodies to HSV can be detected by most assays within 2–3 weeks after infection with the virus (3).

Genital infection with HSV is a primary infection when HSV-1 or HSV-2 is detected in individuals with no evidence of antibodies to either viral type in the serum. An outbreak is considered a nonprimary first episode when one viral type is detected in an individual with serologic evidence of past infection with the other viral type. Recurrent episodes are characterized by isolation of HSV-1 or HSV-2 in the presence of antibodies of the same serotype.

Incidence

Herpes simplex virus infection of the genital tract is one of the most common sexually transmitted infections. The true incidence of genital HSV infection is not known because it is not a reportable disease. It is estimated that approximately 45 million adolescent and adult Americans have been infected with HSV-2 (4). In a large, national serologic study, it was found that approximately 26% of women had serologic evidence of HSV-2 infection (4). It should be emphasized that serologic studies of HSV-2 underestimate the prevalence of genital herpes because HSV-1 also causes genital disease.

Most individuals who are infected with HSV are unaware that they have contracted the virus. Only approximately 5–15% of infected individuals report recognition of their infection (4, 5). The increasing burden of infection has important implications for health care providers. The number of initial visits to physicians' offices as a result of genital HSV infection increased from approximately 75,000 per year in 1978 to nearly 270,000 per year in 2004 (6). Risk factors for HSV infection include female gender, duration of sexual activity, minority ethnicity, previous genital infection, family income, and number of sex partners (4, 7).

Whereas HSV-2 is virtually always a genital pathogen, HSV-1 is increasingly recognized as the etiologic agent of genital herpes infection. Up to 80% of new genital infections among all women may be caused by HSV-1 (8, 9). This increase in initial infections with HSV-1 is particularly pronounced in the adolescent and young adult populations. In these populations, genital infection with HSV-1 may have surpassed new genital infection with HSV-2 (1).

Among women with serologic test results that indicate susceptibility to HSV infection, the incidence of new HSV-1 or HSV-2 infection during pregnancy is approximately 2% (10). Approximately 10% of women who are HSV-2 seronegative have partners who are seropositive and are at risk for transmission of HSV-2 during the pregnancy (11). Consistent with nonpregnant patients, most new infections in pregnant patients are asymptomatic (10). The timing of infection is relatively evenly distributed, with approximately one third of women becoming infected in each trimester (10). Among women with recurrent genital HSV, approximately 75% can expect at least one recurrence during pregnancy, and approximately 14% of patients will have prodromal symptoms or clinical recurrence at delivery (12, 13).

Neonatal herpes usually is acquired during the intrapartum period through exposure to the virus in the genital tract, although in utero and postnatal infections are rare but can occur. Approximately 80% of infected infants are born to mothers with no reported history of HSV infection (14). Although the actual incidence is unknown because neonatal herpes infection is not a reportable disease, estimates suggest that approximately 1,200–1,500 cases occur each year in the United States (15). Approximately one third to one half of cases of neonatal herpes are caused by HSV-1 (15, 16). Neonatal HSV infections can be classified as disseminated disease (25%); central nervous system disease (30%); and disease limited to the skin, eyes, or mouth (45%) (14). Mortality has decreased substantially over the past two decades, decreasing to 30% for disseminated disease and 4% for central nervous system disease. Approximately 20% of survivors of neonatal herpes have long-term neurologic sequelae (17).

Clinical Considerations and Recommendations

▶ *How can the diagnosis of herpes simplex virus be established?*

All suspected herpes virus infections should be confirmed through viral or serological testing. A diagnosis of genital herpes based on the clinical presentation alone has a sensitivity of 40% and specificity of 99% and a false-positive rate of 20% (18). The tests used to confirm the presence of HSV infection can be divided into two basic groups: 1) viral detection techniques and 2) antibody detection techniques. Primary viral DNA testing techniques are viral culture and HSV antigen detection by polymerase chain reaction (PCR). The antibody detection techniques include the use of both laboratory-based and point-of-care serologic tests to detect the presence of antibodies to either HSV-1 or HSV-2. With viral detection techniques, negative results do not rule out the presence of infection. The diagnosis of HSV should be confirmed either serologically or with viral culture.

Isolation of HSV in cell culture is the preferred virologic test for patients who seek medical treatment for genital ulcers or other mucocutaneous lesions and allows differentiation of the type of virus (HSV-1 versus HSV-2) (18). The sensitivity of this test is limited because of several issues related to sampling and transportation of the specimen (19). Primary lesions are more likely than recurrent lesions to yield positive cultures (80% versus 40% of patients, respectively) (20, 21). Additionally, as the lesions heal, they are less likely to be culture positive (21). Thus, a positive genital culture provides conclusive evidence of genital HSV infection; however, a negative result does not exclude the presence of infection. When a genital specimen is collected for HSV culture, the vesicles should be unroofed, if present, and vesicular fluid should be collected.

Polymerase chain reaction techniques involve the amplification of particular sequences of DNA or RNA before detection and can thus detect evidence of viral DNA at low concentrations. Because of the increased sensitivity of PCR, unroofing vesicles is unnecessary. In one very large study, PCR results were three to five times more likely to be positive than were cultures (19). Cultures were more likely to be positive at increasing concentrations of virus, as demonstrated by a linear relationship between the proportion of positive cultures and copy numbers of HSV DNA in samples. Polymerase chain reaction techniques are commercially available and can differentiate between HSV-1 and HSV-2. Polymerase chain reaction provides increased sensitivity over culture (19, 20, 22) and may ultimately replace culture as the standard of care for diagnosis. Presently, however, there are no interlaboratory standards that ensure that identical specimens processed in different laboratories will yield identical results. Additionally, the PCR tests are not U.S. Food and Drug Administration (FDA) approved for clinical testing of genital specimens (18).

For patients who do not present with active lesions or whose lesions have negative culture or PCR test results, accurate type-specific serologic assays that accurately distinguish between HSV-1 and HSV-2 antibodies are now commercially available. Currently, there are several FDA-approved type-specific tests, and others are under development (see box). The sensitivity of these assays varies from 93–100% and specificity from 93–98% (23). The predictive value of a positive test result is influenced by the prevalence of the disease in

---

U.S. Food and Drug Administration-Approved Type-Specific Tests

Laboratory-based assays
- HerpeSelect-1 and 2 ELISA IgG
- HerpeSelect 1 and 2 Immunoblot IgG
- Captia HSV-1 and 2 ELISA

Rapid tests (formerly known as the POCkit test)
- BiokitHSV-2 Rapid Test
- Sure-Vue HSV-2

---

the population tested. In a high-risk population, the positive predictive value for the ELISA test results was 80–94% (24, 25). Repeat testing, using a different type-specific assay, has been shown to increase the positive predictive value of a single test result, and this may be especially important in populations with low HSV prevalence (24).

Because HSV-2 is an uncommon cause of oral infection, detection of HSV-2 antibodies is virtually diagnostic of genital HSV infection (26). Conversely, detection of HSV-1 antibodies alone may represent orolabial infection or may be indicative of genital infection. Correlation with direct viral identification techniques and the patient's symptoms is important.

▶ *How can primary herpes simplex virus infection be distinguished from a nonprimary first episode during pregnancy?*

It is not possible to distinguish primary from nonprimary herpes simplex virus infection on the basis of clinical findings alone (27). Diagnosis is based on the combination of positive viral detection and negative serologic test results or evidence of seroconversion.

A primary outbreak in the first trimester of pregnancy has been associated with neonatal chorioretinitis, microcephaly, and skin lesions in rare cases (28). Although HSV has been associated with an increased risk for spontaneous abortion, recent studies do not support such a risk (29).

▶ *How should a primary outbreak be managed in pregnancy?*

At the time of the initial outbreak, antiviral treatment may be administered orally to pregnant women to reduce the duration and the severity of the symptoms as well as reduce the duration of viral shedding (Table 1) (30). In patients who have severe disease, oral treatment can be

Table 1. Recommended Doses of Antiviral Medications for Herpes in Pregnancy

Indication	Acyclovir	Valacyclovir
Primary or first-episode infection	400 mg orally, three times daily, for 7–10* days	1 g orally, twice daily, for 7–10* days
Symptomatic recurrent episode	400 mg orally, three times daily, for 5 days or 800 mg orally, twice daily, for 5 days	500 mg orally, twice daily, for 3 days or 1 g orally, daily, for 5 days
Daily suppression	400 mg orally, three times daily, from 36 weeks estimated gestational age until delivery	500 mg orally, twice daily, from 36 weeks estimated gestational age until delivery
Severe or disseminated disease	5–10 mg/kg, intravenously, every 8 hours for 2–7 days, then oral therapy for primary infection to complete 10 days	

*Treatment may be extended if healing is incomplete after 10 days.

Adapted from Sexually transmitted diseases treatment guidelines, 2006 [published erratum appears in MMWR Recomm Rep 2006;55:997]. Centers for Disease Control and Prevention. MMWR Recomm Rep 2006;55(RR–11):1–94.

extended for more than 10 days if lesions are incompletely healed at that time (18).

Acyclovir may be administered intravenously to pregnant women with severe genital HSV infection or with disseminated herpetic infections. Case reports have associated significant improvement in expected survival with acyclovir treatment in cases of pregnant women with disseminated HSV, herpes pneumonitis, herpes hepatitis, and herpes encephalitis (31–33).

Primary genital herpes infection during pregnancy constitutes a higher risk for perinatal transmission than does recurrent infection. The risk of vertical transmission to the neonate when a primary outbreak occurs at the time of delivery is approximately 30–60% (10, 15). Several factors likely contribute to the increased risk. First, when women have acquired infection near the time of delivery, there is likely reduced transplacental passage of protective HSV-2 specific antibodies. Higher titers of neutralizing antibodies in the neonate have been associated with a reduced risk of neonatal infection (34). Second, neonatal exposure to the virus in the genital tract may be increased. The genital viral shedding in women with primary infection is of higher concentration and longer duration than shedding that occurs with recurrent episodes. Women with primary herpes that is untreated have a mean duration of viral shedding of 15 days (30). In addition, cervical shedding was detected by viral culture in 90% of women with primary infection (30).

Data regarding interventions to reduce vertical transmission in the specific setting of primary herpes are limited. One randomized trial of acyclovir versus placebo given from 36 weeks of gestation until delivery to women with their first episode of genital herpes infection during pregnancy found a significant reduction in clinical recurrences at delivery (35). The number of cesarean

deliveries for clinical herpes recurrences was reduced; however, the total number of cesarean deliveries in the treatment and placebo groups was similar. The number of deliveries was insufficient to evaluate efficacy of antiviral treatment to prevent neonatal herpes. Evidence of the effectiveness of cesarean delivery before labor for the prevention of vertical transmission is lacking.

▶ *How should recurrent herpes simplex virus infection in pregnant women be managed?*

All women should be asked early in pregnancy about symptoms of genital herpes, including prodromal symptoms. Women with a history of herpes should be examined for external herpetic lesions when they present for evaluation in labor and delivery (6).

Among women with recurrent lesions at the time of delivery, the rate of transmission with a vaginal delivery is only 3% (36). For women with a history of recurrent disease and no visible lesions at delivery, the transmission risk has been estimated to be 2/10,000 (15, 36). The low risk is in part attributed to the presence and transplacental passage of antiherpes antibodies (15, 34, 36). Cesarean delivery is not indicated in women with a history of HSV in the absence of active genital lesions or prodromes.

The efficacy of suppressive therapy during pregnancy to prevent recurrences near term has been evaluated in numerous studies (13, 35, 37–41). Because many of the individual trials were small, a recent systematic review of randomized controlled trials was performed to assess the effectiveness of acyclovir suppression therapy given to prevent a clinical recurrence at delivery, cesarean delivery for recurrent genital herpes, and the detection of HSV at delivery (42). The risk of recurrence at delivery was reduced by 75%, and the rate of cesarean delivery for recurrent genital herpes was reduced by 40% for women who received suppression therapy after 36 weeks of gestation. Viral detection at delivery using culture or PCR was reduced by 90% among treated women, but shedding was not completely eliminated (in one trial, virus was detected in one woman receiving acyclovir) (13). There were no cases of neonatal herpes in any of the studies. Several trials demonstrating similar efficacy of valacyclovir have been published since the meta-analysis (12, 43). Women with active recurrent genital herpes should be offered suppressive viral therapy at or beyond 36 weeks of gestation. The doses of antiviral medication used in the randomized trials in pregnancy are higher than the corresponding doses in nonpregnant women. (Table 1.) Although neutropenia is a recognized, transient complication of acyclovir treatment of neonatal HSV infection, it has not been reported following maternal suppressive therapy (17). The acyclovir concentrations at which neutropenia occurred were approximately 5–30 times higher than were observed in umbilical vein plasma in a pharmacokinetic study of valacyclovir in pregnancy (44).

▶ *What medications are available for treatment of herpes simplex virus infection during pregnancy?*

There are three antiviral agents that are commonly used to treat HSV infections. Acyclovir, famciclovir, and valacyclovir are all FDA pregnancy category B medications. These drugs are all approved for the treatment of primary genital herpes, the treatment of episodes of recurrent disease, and the daily treatment for suppression of outbreaks of recurrent genital herpes.

Acyclovir is a nucleoside analogue that enters virally infected cells and acts specifically to inhibit the viral thymidine kinase and, thus, DNA replication. The bioavailability of oral acyclovir is approximately 20%, which necessitates more frequent dosage intervals (45). Valacyclovir is a prodrug of acyclovir and is rapidly converted to acyclovir after metabolism in the liver. The bioavailability of acyclovir after doses with valacyclovir is approximately 54% (46). This is three to five times higher than achieved with oral acyclovir and, at a dose of 1 gm, approximates levels achieved with intravenous doses of acyclovir. The pharmacokinetics of both drugs have been evaluated in pregnancy. After doses of acyclovir and valacyclovir, there was evidence of acyclovir concentration in the amniotic fluid but no evidence of preferential fetal drug accumulation (44, 47). Famciclovir also is a prodrug that is rapidly transformed into penciclovir in the body. The bioavailability of the active drug from an oral dose is approximately 77%, so the dosage interval is less frequent than with acyclovir (48). There are no published data on the use of famciclovir in pregnancy.

Development of viral resistance to acyclovir has not been a problem in immunocompetent patients. In two large, laboratory-based studies, a very low prevalence of acyclovir resistance in viruses isolated from immunocompetent patients has been estimated (0.3–0.6%), whereas acyclovir-resistant HSV infections occur more commonly among patients who are immunocompromised (6–7%) (49, 50).

There are no documented increases in adverse fetal effects because of medication exposure (39, 50, 51). The manufacturer of acyclovir and valacyclovir, in cooperation with the Centers for Disease Control and Prevention, maintained a registry for exposure to these drugs during pregnancy through 1999. More than 700 infants reported were exposed to acyclovir during the first trimester, and there was no increase in adverse fetal or neonatal effects, although the safety has not been definitely established (18). There are insufficient data on valacyclovir and famciclovir exposure in the pregnancy registry for analyses (52). Topical therapy offers limited benefit and should be discouraged.

▶ *Is there a role for routine screening for genital herpes during pregnancy or at delivery?*

In the past, screening referred to the use of a viral detection method, most commonly culture, to assess whether viral shedding was present. Asymptomatic shedding during the antepartum period does not predict asymptomatic shedding at delivery (53, 54). Thus, routine antepartum genital HSV cultures in asymptomatic patients with recurrent disease are not recommended.

With the advent of serologic tests that can reliably detect disease in asymptomatic patients, screening now refers to the detection of HSV infection. Maternal HSV screening has been proposed to reduce neonatal herpes by identifying women infected (seropositive) with genital herpes and offering suppressive antiviral therapy near term. It also may identify susceptible women (seronegative) whose partners could be offered screening, allowing for counseling of at-risk couples about strategies to reduce the possibility of new maternal infection during pregnancy. Several analyses have evaluated the cost-effectiveness of various screening protocols for pregnant patients to reduce the incidence of neonatal HSV infection (55–59). The results from these analyses are highly variable—estimates of the cost to prevent one case of neonatal herpes range from $200,000 to $4,000,000.

A number of factors influence these cost estimates, including the costs of testing and counseling, effectiveness of antiviral therapy, the probability of lesions or shedding at delivery in asymptomatic women in whom HSV has been diagnosed only by the screening test, and the likelihood of neonatal herpes with vaginal delivery (54, 55). Currently, there is no evidence of cost-effectiveness of screening strategies from clinical trials or well-designed cohort studies in pregnancy. Whereas screening may be beneficial in particular populations or couples, routine HSV screening of pregnant women is not recommended.

▶ *When should cesarean delivery be performed to prevent perinatal herpes simplex virus transmissions?*

Cesarean delivery is indicated in women with active genital lesions or prodromal symptoms, such as vulvar pain or burning at delivery, because these symptoms may indicate an impending outbreak. The incidence of neonatal disease is low when there is recurrent maternal disease, but cesarean delivery is recommended because of the potentially serious nature of the disease. In a large cohort study, women who had given birth by cesarean delivery were much less likely to transmit HSV infection to their infants (15). Among women with HSV detected at delivery, neonatal herpes occurred in 1.2% of infants delivered by cesarean delivery compared with 7.7% of infants delivered vaginally (15).

Cesarean delivery does not completely prevent vertical transmission to the neonate. Transmission has been documented in the setting of cesarean delivery performed before membrane rupture (14, 60). Cesarean delivery is not recommended for women with a history of HSV infection but no active genital disease during labor (61).

▶ *Is cesarean delivery recommended for women with recurrent herpes simplex virus lesions on the back, thigh, or buttock?*

Cesarean delivery is not recommended for women with nongenital lesions. These lesions may be covered with an occlusive dressing, and the patient then can give birth vaginally. However, women with lesions elsewhere also may have cervical lesions and should be examined.

The risk of transmission among women with recurrent HSV at the time of labor is low, estimated to be less than 1% (18, 62). As with other women with recurrent herpes, the low risk is probably related to preexisting maternal type-specific antibodies. Thus, the risk of neonatal HSV associated with vaginal delivery in a woman with recurrent HSV and nongenital lesions would appear to be very low.

▶ *In a patient with active herpes simplex virus genital infection and ruptured membranes, should cesarean delivery be performed to prevent perinatal transmission?*

In patients with active HSV infection and ruptured membranes at or near term, a cesarean delivery should be performed as soon as the necessary personnel and equipment can be readied. There is no evidence that there is a duration of rupture of membranes beyond which the fetus does not benefit from cesarean delivery (63). At any time after rupture of membranes, cesarean delivery is recommended.

▶ *How should a woman with active herpes simplex virus and preterm premature rupture of membranes be managed?*

In a patient with preterm premature rupture of membranes and active HSV, the risks of prematurity should be weighed against the risk of neonatal HSV disease in considering expectant management. In pregnancies remote from term, especially in women with recurrent disease, there is increasing support for continuing the pregnancy to gain benefit from time and use of corticosteroids (64, 65). There is no consensus on the gestational age at which the risks of prematurity outweigh the risks of HSV. When expectant management is elected, treatment with an antiviral agent may be considered. The decision to use corticosteroids should be based on the balance between the risk of pulmonary immaturity and the risk of neonatal herpes.

▶ *Are invasive procedures contraindicated in pregnant women with herpes simplex virus?*

In women with a history of recurrent HSV, transabdominal invasive procedures, such as chorionic villus sampling, amniocentesis, and percutaneous umbilical cord blood sampling, may be performed even when genital lesions are present. Because cervical shedding is associated with genital recurrences, it seems reasonable to delay transcervical procedures until lesions appear to have resolved.

Invasive monitoring, such as fetal scalp electrodes, is a risk factor for transmission of HSV, increasing the risk of neonatal infection approximately six times compared with externally monitored patients (15). However, if there are indications for fetal scalp monitoring, it is reasonable in a woman who has a history of recurrent HSV and no active lesions.

▶ *Should women with active herpes simplex virus breastfeed or handle their infants?*

Unless there is a lesion on the breast, breastfeeding is not contraindicated. To prevent postnatal transmission, mothers with herpetic lesions on any part of the body should be advised to take special consideration of hand-washing. Postnatally acquired disease can be as lethal as that acquired during delivery. Oropharyngeal or cutaneous lesions can be an effective source of virus for transmission to the newborn. Because the herpes virus is transmitted through direct contact (eg, hand-to-mouth), neonatal infection may be acquired from family members other than the mother and from sites other than the genital tract (66, 67). Most strains of HSV responsible for nosocomial neonatal disease are HSV-1 rather than HSV-2. Mothers with active lesions should use caution when handling their babies.

Valacyclovir appears to be safe for breastfeeding mothers. Although acyclovir was found in the breast milk in concentrations that were higher than the maternal serum, the amount of acyclovir in the breast milk was only 2% of that used for therapeutic doses in neonates (68).

Summary of Recommendations and Conclusions

The following recommendations and conclusions are based on limited or inconsistent scientific evidence (Level B):

▶ Women with active recurrent genital herpes should be offered suppressive viral therapy at or beyond 36 weeks of gestation.

▶ Cesarean delivery is indicated in women with active genital lesions or prodromal symptoms, such as vulvar pain or burning at delivery, because these symptoms may indicate an impending outbreak.

The following recommendations and conclusions are based primarily on consensus and expert opinion (Level C):

▶ In women with premature rupture of membranes, there is no consensus on the gestational age at which the risks of prematurity outweigh the risks of HSV.

▶ Cesarean delivery is not recommended for women with a history of HSV infection but no active genital disease during labor.

▶ Routine antepartum genital HSV cultures in asymptomatic patients with recurrent disease are not recommended.

▶ Routine HSV screening of pregnant women is not recommended

Proposed Performance Measure

The percentage of pregnant women who have been asked about their history of herpes

References

1. Roberts CM, Pfister JR, Spear SJ. Increasing proportion of herpes simplex virus type 1 as a cause of genital herpes infection in college students. Sex Transm Dis 2003; 30:797–800. (Level II-3)

2. Pertel PE, Spear PG. Biology of herpesviruses. In Holmes KK, Mardh PA, Sparling PF, Lemon SM, Stamm WE, Piot P, et al editors. Sexually transmitted diseases. 3rd ed. New York (NY): McGraw-Hill 1999. p.269–83. (Level III)

3. Brown ZA, Gardella C, Wald A, Morrow RA, Corey L. Genital herpes complicating pregnancy [published erratum appears in Obstet Gynecol 2006;107:428]. Obstet Gynecol 2005;106:845–56. (Level III)

4. Fleming DT, McQuillan GM, Johnson RE, Nahmias AJ, Aral SO, Lee FK. Herpes simplex virus type 2 in the United States, 1976 to 1994. N Engl J Med 1997;337: 1105–11. (Level II-3)

5. Leone P, Fleming DT, Gilsenan AW, Li L, Justus S. Seroprevalence of herpes simplex virus-2 in suburban primary care offices in the United States. Sex Transm Dis 2004;31:311–6. (Level II-2)

6. Centers for Disease Control and Prevention. Sexually transmitted disease surveillance 2004. Atlanta (GA): CDC; 2005. Available at: http://www.cdc.gov/std/stats/04pdf/2004SurveillanceAll.pdf. Retrieved November 29, 2006. (Level II-2)

7. Mertz GJ, Benedetti J, Ashley R, Selke SA, Corey L. Risk factors for the sexual transmission of genital herpes. Ann Intern Med 1992;116:197–202. (Level II-3)

8. Lafferty WE, Downey L, Celum C, Wald A. Herpes simplex virus type 1 as a cause of genital herpes: impact on surveillance and prevention. J Infect Dis 2000;181: 1454–7. (Level II-3)

9. Nilsen A, Myrmel H. Changing trends in genital herpes simplex virus infection in Bergen, Norway. Acta Obstet Gynecol Scand 2000;79:693–6. (Level II-3)

10. Brown ZA, Selke S, Zeh J, Kopelman J, Maslow A, Ashley RL, et al. The acquisition of herpes simplex virus during pregnancy. N Engl J Med 1997;337:509–15. (Level II-2)

11. Gardella C, Brown Z, Wald A, Selke S, Zeh J, Morrow RA, et al. Risk factors for herpes simplex virus transmission to pregnant women: a couples study. Am J Obstet Gynecol 2005;193:1891–9. (Level II-2)

12. Sheffield JS, Hill JB, Hollier LM, Laibl VR, Roberts SW, Sanchez PJ, et al. Valacyclovir prophylaxis to prevent recurrent herpes at delivery: a randomized clinical trial [published erratum appears in Obstet Gynecol 2006; 108:695]. Obstet Gynecol 2006;108:141–7. (Level I)

13. Watts DH, Brown ZA, Money D, Selke S, Huang ML, Sacks SL, et al. A double-blind, randomized, placebo-controlled trial of acyclovir in late pregnancy for the reduction of herpes simplex virus shedding and cesarean delivery. Am J Obstet Gynecol 2003;188:836–43. (Level I)

14. Whitley RJ, Corey L, Arvin A, Lakeman FD, Sumaya CV, Wright PF, et al. Changing presentation of herpes simplex virus infection in neonates. J Infect Dis 1988;158:109–116. (Level II-3)

15. Brown ZA, Wald A, Morrow RA, Selke S, Zeh J, Corey L. Effect of serologic status and cesarean delivery on transmission rates of herpes simplex virus from mother to infant. JAMA 2003;289:203–9. (Level II-2)

16. Whitley R, Arvin A, Prober C, Burchett S, Corey L, Powell D, et al. A controlled trial comparing vidarabine with acyclovir in neonatal herpes simplex virus infection. Infectious Diseases Collaborative Antiviral Study Group. N Engl J Med 1991;324:444–9. (Level I)

17. Kimberlin DW, Lin CY, Jacobs RF, Powell DA, Corey L, Gruber WC, et al. Safety and efficacy of high-dose intravenous acyclovir in the management of neonatal herpes simplex virus infections. National Institute of Allergy and Infectious Diseases Collaborative Antiviral Study Group. Pediatrics 2001;108:230–8. (Level II-3)

18. Sexually transmitted diseases treatment guidelines, 2006 [published erratum appears in MMWR Recomm Rep 2006;55:997]. Centers for Disease Control and Prevention. MMWR Recomm Rep 2006;55(RR-11):1–94. (Level III)

19. Wald A, Huang ML, Carrell D, Selke S, Corey L. Polymerase chain reaction for detection of herpes simplex virus (HSV) DNA on mucosal surfaces: comparison with HSV isolation in cell culture. J Infect Dis 2003;188:1345–51. (Level II-3)

20. Moseley RC, Corey L, Benjamin D, Winter C, Remington ML. Comparison of viral isolation, direct immunofluorescence, and indirect immunoperoxidase techniques for detection of genital herpes simplex virus infection. J Clin Microbiol 1981;13:913–8. (Level II-2)

21. Cone RW, Hobson AC, Palmer J, Remington M, Corey L. Extended duration of herpes simplex virus DNA in genital lesions detected by the polymerase chain reaction. J Infect Dis 1991;164:757–60. (Level II-3)

22. Slomka MJ, Emery L, Munday PE, Moulsdale M, Brown DW. A comparison of PCR with virus isolation and direct antigen detection for diagnosis and typing of genital herpes. J Med Virol 1998;55:177–83. (Level II-3)

23. Ashley RL. Performance and use of HSV type-specific serology test kits. Herpes 2002;9:38–45. (Level III)

24. Morrow RA, Friedrich D, Meier A, Corey L. Use of "biokit HSV-2 Rapid Assay" to improve the positive predictive value of Focus HerpeSelect HSV-2 ELISA. BMC Infect Dis 2005;5:84–90. (Level II-3)

25. Turner KR, Wong EH, Kent CK, Klausner JD. Serologic herpes testing in the real world: validation of new type-specific serologic herpes simplex virus tests in a public health laboratory. Sex Transm Dis 2002;29:422–5. (Level II-3)

26. Wald A, Ericsson M, Krantz E, Selke S, Corey L. Oral shedding of herpes simplex virus type 2 [published erratum appears in Sex Transm Infect 2004;80:546]. Sex Transm Infect 2004;80:272–6. (Level II-2)

27. Hensleigh PA, Andrews WW, Brown Z, Greenspoon J, Yasukawa L, Prober CG. Genital herpes during pregnancy: inability to distinguish primary and recurrent infections clinically. Obstet Gynecol 1997;89:891–5. (Level II-2)

28. Hutto C, Arvin A, Jacobs R, Steele R, Stagno S, Lyrene R, et al. Intrauterine herpes simplex virus infections. J Pediatr 1987;110:97–101. (Level II-3)

29. Ratanajamit C, Vinther Skriver M, Jepsen P, Chongsuvivatwong V, Olsen J, Sorensen HT. Adverse pregnancy outcome in women exposed to acyclovir during pregnancy: a population-based observational study. Scand J Infect Dis 2003;35:255–9. (Level II-2)

30. Bryson YJ, Dillon M, Lovett M, Acuna G, Taylor S, Cherry JD, et al. Treatment of first episodes of genital herpes simplex virus infection with oral acyclovir. A randomized double-blind controlled trial in normal subjects. N Engl J Med 1983;308:916–21. (Level I)

31. Young EJ, Chafizadeh E, Oliveira VL, Genta RM. Disseminated herpesvirus infection during pregnancy. Clin Infect Dis 1996;22:51–8. (Level III)

32. Grover L, Kane J, Kravitz J, Cruz A. Systemic acyclovir in pregnancy: a case report. Obstet Gynecol 1985;65:284–7. (Level III)

33. Lagrew DC Jr, Furlow TG, Hager WD, Yarrish RL. Disseminated herpes simplex virus infection in pregnancy. Successful treatment with acyclovir. JAMA 1984;252:2058–9. (Level III)

34. Prober CG, Sullender WM, Yasukawa LL, Au DS, Yeager AS, Arvin AM. Low risk of herpes simplex virus infections in neonates exposed to the virus at the time of vaginal delivery to mothers with recurrent genital herpes simplex virus infections. N Engl J Med 1987;316:240–4. (Level II-3)

35. Scott LL, Sanchez PJ, Jackson GL, Zeray F, Wendel GD Jr. Acyclovir suppression to prevent cesarean delivery after first-episode genital herpes. Obstet Gynecol 1996;87:69–73. (Level I)

36. Brown ZA, Benedetti J, Ashley R, Burchett S, Selke S, Berry S, et al. Neonatal herpes simplex virus infection in relation to asymptomatic maternal infection at the time of labor. N Engl J Med 1991;324:1247–52. (Level II-2)

37. Braig S, Luton D, Sibony O, Edlinger C, Boissinot C, Blot P, et al. Acyclovir prophylaxis in late pregnancy prevents recurrent genital herpes and viral shedding. Eur J Obstet Gynecol Reprod Biol 2001;96:55–8. (Level I)

38. Brocklehurst P, Kinghorn G, Carney O, Helsen K, Ross E, Ellis E, et al. A randomised placebo controlled trial of suppressive acyclovir in late pregnancy in women with recurrent genital herpes infection. Br J Obstet Gynaecol 1998;105:275–80. (Level I)

39. Scott LL, Hollier LM, McIntire D, Sanchez PJ, Jackson GL, Wendel GD Jr. Acyclovir suppression to prevent clinical recurrences at delivery after first episode genital

herpes in pregnancy: an open-label trial. Infect Dis Obstet Gynecol 2001;9:75–80. (Level II-2)

40. Scott LL, Hollier LM, McIntire D, Sanchez PJ, Jackson GL, Wendel GD Jr. Acyclovir suppression to prevent recurrent genital herpes at delivery. Infect Dis Obstet Gynecol 2002;10:71–7. (Level I)

41. Stray-Pedersen B. Acyclovir in late pregnancy to prevent neonatal herpes simples [letter]. Lancet 1990;336:756. (Level I)

42. Sheffield JS, Hollier LM, Hill JB, Stuart GS, Wendel GD. Acyclovir prophylaxis to prevent herpes simplex virus recurrence at delivery: a systematic review. Obstet Gynecol 2003;102:1396–403. (Level I)

43. Andrews WW, Kimberlin DF, Whitley R, Cliver S, Ramsey PS, Deeter R. Valacyclovir therapy to reduce recurrent genital herpes in pregnant women. Am J Obstet Gynecol 2006;194:774–81. (Level I)

44. Kimberlin DF, Weller S, Whitley RJ, Andrews WW, Hauth JC, Lakeman F, et al. Pharmacokinetics of oral valacyclovir and acyclovir in late pregnancy. Am J Obstet Gynecol 1998:179:846–51. (Level II-3)

45. de Miranda P, Blum MR. Pharmacokinetics of acyclovir after intravenous and oral administration. J Antimicrob Chemother 1983;12(suppl B):29–37. (Level II-3)

46. Soul-Lawton J, Seaber E, On N, Wootton R, Rolan P, Posner J. Absolute bioavailability and metabolic disposition of valaciclovir, the L-valyl ester of acyclovir, following oral administration to humans. Antimicrob Agents Chemother 1995;39:2759–2764. (Level II-3)

47. Frenkel LM, Brown ZA, Bryson YJ, Corey L, Unadkat JD, Hensleigh PA, et al. Pharmacokinetics of acyclovir in the term human pregnancy and neonate. Am J Obstet Gynecol 1991;164:569–76. (Level II-2)

48. Pue MA, Benet LZ. Pharmacokinetics of famciclovir in man. Antiviral Chem Chemother 1993;4(suppl 1):47–55. (Level II-3)

49. Christophers J, Clayton J, Craske J, Ward R, Collins P, Trowbridge M, et al. Survey of resistance of herpes simplex virus to acyclovir in northwest England. Antimicrob Agents Chemother 1998;42:868–72. (Level II-2)

50. Stranska R, Schuurman R, Nienhuis E, Goedegebuure IW, Polman M, Weel JF, et al. Survey of acyclovir-resistant herpes simplex virus in the Netherlands: prevalence and characterization. J Clin Virol 2005;32:7–18. (Level II-2)

51. Stone KM, Reiff-Eldridge R, White AD, Cordero JF, Brown Z, Alexander ER, et al. Pregnancy outcomes following systemic prenatal acyclovir exposure: conclusions from the international acyclovir pregnancy registry, 1984–1999. Birth Defects Res A Clin Mol Teratol 2004;70:201–7. (Level II-2)

52. Pregnancy outcomes following systemic prenatal acyclovir exposure - June 1, 1984–June 30, 1993. Centers for Disease Control and Prevention. MMWR Morb Mortal Wkly Rep 1993;42:806–9. (Level III)

53. Wittek AE, Yeager AS, Au DS, Hensleigh PA. Asymptomatic shedding of herpes simplex virus from the cervix and lesion site during pregnancy. Correlation of antepartum shedding with shedding at delivery. Am J Dis Child 1984;138:439–42. (Level II-3)

54. Arvin AM, Hensleigh PA, Prober CG, Au DS, Yasukawa LL, Wittek AE, et al. Failure of antepartum maternal cultures to predict the infant's risk of exposure to herpes simplex virus at delivery. N Engl J Med 1986;315:796–800. (Level II-3)

55. Cleary KL, Pare E, Stamilio D, Macones GA. Type-specific screening for asymptomatic herpes infection in pregnancy: a decision analysis. BJOG 2005;112:731–6. (Decision analysis)

56. Thung SF, Grobman WA. The cost-effectiveness of routine antenatal screening for maternal herpes simplex virus-1 and -2 antibodies. Am J Obstet Gynecol 2005;192(2):483–8. (Cost-effectiveness analysis)

57. Baker D, Brown Z, Hollier LM, Wendel GD Jr, Hulme L, Griffiths DA, et al. Cost-effectiveness of herpes simplex virus type 2 serologic testing and antiviral therapy in pregnancy. Am J Obstet Gynecol 2004;191:2074–84. (Cost-effectiveness analysis)

58. Barnabas RV, Carabin H, Garnett GP. The potential role of suppressive therapy for sex partners in the prevention of neonatal herpes: a health economic analysis. Sex Transm Infect 2002;78:425–9. (Cost-effectiveness analysis)

59. Rouse DJ, Stringer JS. An appraisal of screening for maternal type-specific herpes simplex virus antibodies to prevent neonatal herpes. Am J Obstet Gynecol 2000; 183:400–6. (Cost analysis)

60. Peng J, Krause PJ, Kresch M. Neonatal herpes simplex virus infection after cesarean section with intact amniotic membranes. J Perinatol 1996;16:397–9. (Level III)

61. Roberts SW, Cox SM, Dax J, Wendel GD Jr, Leveno KJ. Genital herpes during pregnancy: no lesions, no cesarean. Obstet Gynecol 1995;85:261–4. (Level II-2)

62. Kerkering K, Gardella C, Selke S, Krantz E, Corey L, Wald A. Isolation of herpes simplex virus from the genital tract during symptomatic recurrence on the buttocks. Obstet Gynecol 2006;108:947–52. (Level II-2)

63. Nahmias AJ, Josey WE, Naib ZM, Freeman MG, Fernandez RJ, Wheeler JH. Perinatal risk associated with maternal genital herpes simplex virus infection. Am J Obstet Gynecol 1971;110:825–37. (Level II-3)

64. Majors CA, Towers CV Lewis DF, Garite TJ. Expectant management of preterm premature rupture of membranes complicated by active recurrent genital herpes. Am J Obstet Gynecol 2003;188:1551–4;discussion 1554–5. (Level II-3)

65. Effect of corticosteroids for fetal maturation on perinatal outcomes, February 28–March 2, 1994. National Institutes of Health. Consensus Development Conference Statement. Am J Obstet Gynecol 1995;173:246–52. (Level III)

66. Douglas J, Schmidt O, Corey L. Acquisition of neonatal HSV-1 infection from a paternal source contact. J Pediatr 1983;103:908–10. (Level III)

67. Hammerberg O, Watts J, Chernesky M, Luchsinger I, Rawls W. An outbreak of herpes simplex virus type 1 in an intensive care nursery. Pediatr Infect Dis 1983;2: 290–4. (Level III)

68. Sheffield JS, Fish DN, Hollier LM, Cadematori S, Nobles BJ, Wendel GD Jr. Acyclovir concentrations in human breast milk after valacyclovir administration. Am J Obstet Gynecol 2002;186:100–2. (Level II-2)

The MEDLINE database, the Cochrane Library, and ACOG's own internal resources and documents were used to conduct a literature search to locate relevant articles published between January 1985 and October 2006. The search was restricted to articles published in the English language. Priority was given to articles reporting results of original research, although review articles and commentaries also were consulted. Abstracts of research presented at symposia and scientific conferences were not considered adequate for inclusion in this document. Guidelines published by organizations or institutions such as the National Institutes of Health and the American College of Obstetricians and Gynecologists were reviewed, and additional studies were located by reviewing bibliographies of identified articles. When reliable research was not available, expert opinions from obstetrician–gynecologists were used.

Studies were reviewed and evaluated for quality according to the method outlined by the U.S. Preventive Services Task Force:

I   Evidence obtained from at least one properly designed randomized controlled trial.

II-1 Evidence obtained from well-designed controlled trials without randomization.

II-2 Evidence obtained from well-designed cohort or case–control analytic studies, preferably from more than one center or research group.

II-3 Evidence obtained from multiple time series with or without the intervention. Dramatic results in uncontrolled experiments also could be regarded as this type of evidence.

III   Opinions of respected authorities, based on clinical experience, descriptive studies, or reports of expert committees.

Based on the highest level of evidence found in the data, recommendations are provided and graded according to the following categories:

Level A—Recommendations are based on good and consistent scientific evidence.

Level B—Recommendations are based on limited or inconsistent scientific evidence.

Level C—Recommendations are based primarily on consensus and expert opinion.

ISSN 1099-3630

The American College of Obstetricians and Gynecologists
409 12th Street, SW, PO Box 96920, Washington, DC 20090-6920

Management of herpes in pregnancy. ACOG Practice Bulletin No. 82. American College of Obstetricians and Gynecologists. Obstet Gynecol 2007;109:1489–98.

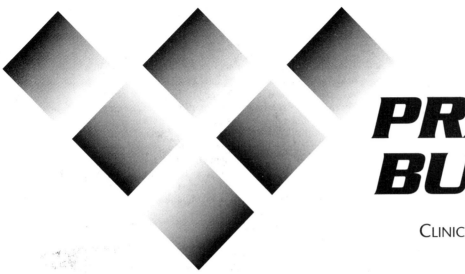

ACOG PRACTICE BULLETIN

CLINICAL MANAGEMENT GUIDELINES FOR
OBSTETRICIAN–GYNECOLOGISTS
NUMBER 86, OCTOBER 2007

(Replaces Educational Bulletin Number 248, July 1998)

This Practice Bulletin was developed by the ACOG Committee on Practice Bulletins—Obstetrics with the assistance of Neil S. Silverman, MD. The information is designed to aid practitioners in making decisions about appropriate obstetric and gynecologic care. These guidelines should not be construed as dictating an exclusive course of treatment or procedure. Variations in practice may be warranted based on the needs of the individual patient, resources, and limitations unique to the institution or type of practice.

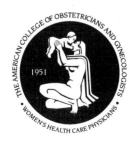

Viral Hepatitis in Pregnancy

Viral hepatitis is one of the most common and potentially serious infections that can occur in pregnant women. Six forms of viral hepatitis have now been identified, two of which, hepatitis A and hepatitis B, can be prevented effectively through vaccination. The purpose of this document is to describe the specific subtypes of hepatitis, their implications during pregnancy, the risk of perinatal transmission, and issues related to both treatment and prevention of infection.

Background

Hepatitis A

The hepatitis A virus is a small (27 nm) RNA virus that produces either symptomatic or asymptomatic infection in humans after an average incubation period of 28 days (range, 15–50 days). Hepatitis A virus (HAV) replicates within the liver and is excreted in bile, with highest viral concentrations late in the incubation period in the feces; this represents the window of greatest infectivity.

In the prevaccine era, approximately one third of cases of acute hepatitis in the United States were attributable to HAV infection. Person-to-person transmission through fecal–oral contamination is the primary means of HAV infection in the United States, most often in household and extended family settings (1). Because children usually have asymptomatic or unrecognized infection, they can play a key role in infecting others. Studies have demonstrated that up to 40% of adults without an identifiable source of infection had close contact with a child younger than 6 years (2), which underscores the importance of primary HAV prevention within families of women of reproductive age.

Poor hygiene and poor sanitation can result in common-source outbreaks of HAV infection. Food also can be contaminated after cooking, as commonly occurs in outbreaks associated with HAV-infected food handlers whose hygiene practices are substandard (3). Depending on conditions, HAV can be stable in the environment for months. Heating foods to above 185°F for 1 minute or disinfecting surfaces with a dilute solution of household bleach can inactivate the virus.

Serious complications of HAV infection are uncommon; the overall case–fatality ratio among reported cases is less than 1%, but reaches 2% among adults older than 50 years. Hepatitis A does not lead to chronic infection, although 10–15% of symptomatic individuals can have prolonged or relapsing disease lasting up to 6 months (4).

Hepatitis B

Hepatitis B is caused by a small DNA virus. The intact virus is termed the Dane particle. Hepatitis B virus (HBV) contains three principal antigens. Hepatitis B surface antigen (HBsAg) is present on the surface of the virus and circulates freely in the serum in spherical and filamentous forms. The middle portion of the Dane particle contains hepatitis B core antigen (HBcAg). The core antigen is present only in hepatocytes and does not circulate in the serum. Hepatitis B e antigen (HBeAg) is encoded by the same portion of the viral genome that codes for the core antigen. The presence of HBeAg indicates an extremely high viral inoculum and active virus replication.

Hepatitis B virus is transmitted by parenteral and sexual contact. Although HBsAg has been detected in a variety of body fluids, only serum, semen, and saliva have been proved to be infectious (5, 6). The virus is relatively stable in the environment, can be viable for up to 7 days on surfaces at room temperature, and may cause transmission via surfaces at concentrations of only 10^2–10^3 virions per milliliter, even if there is no visible blood (7). Individuals at greatest risk of becoming infected are those who have multiple sexual partners, inject drugs percutaneously, or have sexual partners who engage in these risk-taking behaviors. Sexual contact is an efficient mechanism for spreading the virus. Approximately 25% of the frequent sexual contacts of infected individuals will themselves become infected (8).

All blood donors are screened routinely for HBsAg. Transmission of HBV by transfusion of blood or blood products is rare as a result of both donor screening and blood banking viral inactivation procedures. Recently, it has been estimated that the risk of transfusion-attributable HBV infection is 1 per 137,000 transfused units of screened blood (9, 10). In contrast, however, HBV transmission has been reported via patient-to-patient use of institution-based fingerstick devices for blood sampling, such as blood glucose meters (11). Appropriate attention to hygiene and universal precautions is critical within households and institutions using such devices (12).

The mortality associated with acute hepatitis B is approximately 1%. Of adult patients who become infected, 85–90% experience complete resolution of their physical findings and develop protective levels of the antibody. The other 10–15% of patients become chronically infected. They continue to have detectable serum levels of HBsAg but are asymptomatic, and most have no biochemical evidence of hepatic dysfunction. In a small subgroup (15–30%) of those chronically infected, viral replication continues and is manifested by persistence of the e antigen and active viral DNA synthesis. These individuals risk subsequent development of chronic or persistent hepatitis and cirrhosis, and approximately 4,000–5,000 die annually of complications of chronic liver disease, including hepatocellular carcinoma (12, 13).

Hepatitis C

At least six distinct hepatitis C virus (HCV) genotypes have been identified, with broad geographic variation and widely ranging prognoses for both disease progression and response to therapy (14). Among presumably low-risk volunteer blood donors in developed countries, rates of HCV seropositivity of 0.5–1.4% have been reported. Groups at higher risk for HCV infection include patients in sexually transmitted disease (STD) clinics (seroprevalence, 1.5–6.2%), hemophiliacs (64–86%), and intravenous drug users (56–86%) (15–17).

The principal risk factors for HCV transmission have been transfusion of blood products and use of intravenous drugs. At least 90% of cases of posttransfusion hepatitis have been traceable to HCV, usually within 5–10 weeks of the transfusion. Mass screening of the blood supply for HCV has markedly decreased the risk of HCV infection to less than 1 per 1,000,000 screened units of blood. Because the risk of HCV infection from blood transfusions has decreased, the number of HCV infections attributable to drug use has significantly increased, from 20% to at least 60% (18).

Acute HCV infection occurs after an incubation period of 30–60 days. Asymptomatic infection occurs in 75% of patients, and at least 50% of infected individuals progress to chronic infection, regardless of the mode of acquisition or severity of initial infection. Chronic HCV infection also has been associated with an increased risk of developing both B-cell lymphomas and cryoglobulinemia. Although at least 20% of chronic HCV infections lead to chronic active hepatitis or cirrhosis, whether a link to hepatocellular carcinoma exists is controversial and may vary by geographic region (19). Hepatitis C and HIV share common transmission routes, and concomitant infection has been reported to accelerate the progression and severity of hepatic injury (18).

Hepatitis D

Hepatitis D virus (HDV) is an incomplete viral particle that causes disease only in the presence of HBV, from which it acquires a viral envelope consisting entirely of excess HBsAg produced by HBV. Infection with HDV occurs either simultaneously with HBV infection (coinfection) or may be acquired after HBV (superinfection). Transmission is primarily through blood; approximately 20–25% of chronic HBV carriers also have evidence of HDV infection (20, 21).

Chronic hepatitis D produces severe disease more often than other forms of chronic hepatitis. Of patients with chronic hepatitis D, 70–80% ultimately develop cirrhosis and portal hypertension, 15% of whom develop an unusually rapid progression to cirrhosis within 2 years of the initial onset of acute illness. Mortality as a result of hepatic failure approaches 25%. In contrast, only 15–30% of patients with chronic hepatitis B virus infection develop cirrhosis and portal hypertension, and the disease progression typically is much slower (21).

Hepatitis E

The epidemiologic features of hepatitis E virus (HEV) are similar to those of hepatitis A. The disease has been reported only rarely in the United States, and the highest rates of infection occur in regions of the developing world where inadequate sanitation promotes transmission of the virus. Hepatitis E is primarily a waterborne disease; epidemics have been reported in areas where fecal contamination of drinking water is common. The ingestion of raw or undercooked shellfish also has been a source of sporadic cases of HEV infection in endemic areas (22).

In general, HEV produces a self-limited viral infection followed by recovery; the incubation period is 3–8 weeks, with a mean of 40 days. Among pregnant women, however, a higher risk of fulminant hepatitis E has been reported in a number of small series, with maternal mortality rates as high as 20% after infection in the third trimester (22, 23). In one report, HEV infection in women coinfected with HIV resulted in a 100% mortality rate (24).

Vaccinations

Hepatitis A

The hepatitis A vaccination is indicated for adults in groups at increased risk for hepatitis A or its adverse consequences (25). Medical indications include persons with chronic liver disease and persons who receive clotting factor concentrates. Behavioral risk populations are men who have sex with men and persons who use illegal drugs. Occupational risks include persons working with HAV-infected primates or with HAV in a research laboratory setting. Other indications are persons traveling to or working in countries that have high or intermediate endemicity of hepatitis A (a list of countries is available

at http://www.cdc.gov/travel/diseases.htm) and any person who would like to obtain immunity.

The hepatitis A vaccine is available as both a single-antigen vaccine and as a combination vaccine (containing both HAV and HBV antigens). Both vaccines use inactivated HAV, and the HBV component is a recombinant protein nonviral antigen. There are two HAV vaccines available that are given in two doses, either 6–12 months apart or 6–18 months apart. The combination vaccine is given in three doses at 0, 1, and 6 months. The HAV vaccine is 94–100% immunogenic after the first dose (26) and is highly effective in both reducing disease incidence and interrupting ongoing epidemics (27, 28). Immune globulin remains available for postexposure prophylaxis, although primary vaccine-based prevention is preferred. Hepatitis A vaccination should still be administered in addition to immune globulin even in the context of postexposure prevention. Studies of HAV vaccine alone have shown protection against infection in a limited series (29), although no trials comparing the vaccine with immune globulin have been conducted to date. This strategy of administering HAV vaccine alone for postexposure prophylaxis in individuals younger than 40 years has recently been proposed by some experts.

Hepatitis B

All individuals with risk factors, particularly health care workers, should be vaccinated against HBV infection. Other groups at increased risk include hemodialysis patients, injection drug users, persons with more than one sexual partner during the past 3 months or in whom an STD has been diagnosed recently, clients and staff in centers for the developmentally delayed, and international travelers who will be in high or intermediate prevalence areas for HBV infection (list of countries at http://www.cdc.gov/travel/yellowBookCh4-HepB.aspx#333) (30).

In general, prevaccination testing is not recommended. It may be cost-effective to screen for the antibody to HBV in women who belong to groups with a high risk of infection in order to avoid vaccinating adults who have had or currently have hepatitis B infection. In most other low-risk groups, antibody screening before vaccination probably is not indicated.

Two single antigen vaccines for hepatitis B virus have been developed (Table 1). Currently available vaccines are prepared from yeast cultures by using recombinant DNA technology. They are highly immunogenic and result in seroconversion in more than 95% of recipients. There is one combination vaccine available for adults at risk of both hepatitis A and B virus infection (Twinrix); it contains recombinant HBsAg and inactivated hepatitis A virus. The dosage of the hepatitis A component in the combination

Table 1. Recommended Dosages and Schedules of Single-Antigen Hepatitis B Vaccines

Vaccine	Age Group	Dose	Volume	No. of Doses	Schedule*
Engerix-B[†] (GlaxoSmithKline)	0–19 y	10 mcg	0.5 mL	3	Infants: birth, age 1–4, 6–18 mo Alternative for older children: 0, 1–2, 4 mo
	20 y and older	20 mcg	1.0 mL	3	0, 1, 6 mo
Recombivax HB[‡] (Merck & Co.)	0–19 y	5 mcg	0.5 mL	3	Infants: birth, age 1–4, 6–18 mo Alternative for older children: 0, 1–2, 4 mo
	11–15 y	10 mcg	1.0 mL	2	0, 4–6 mo
	20 y and older	10 mcg	1.0 mL	3	0, 1, 6 mo

*The schedule for hepatitis B vaccination is flexible and varies. Consult the Advisory Committee on Immunization Practices (ACIP) statements on hepatitis B (12/2005 and 12/2006) or the package insert for details.

[†]For adult dialysis patients, the Engerix-B dose required is 40 mcg/2.0 mL (use the adult 20 mcg/mL formulation) on a schedule of 0, 1, 2, and 6 months.

[‡]For Recombivax HB, a special formulation for dialysis patients is available. The dose is 40 mcg/1.0 mL and it is given on a schedule of 0, 1, and 6 months.

Immunization Action Coalition. Hepatitis A & B vaccines: be sure your patient gets the correct dose! St. Paul (MN): IAC; 2005. Available at: http://www.immunize.org/catg.d/2081ab.pdf. Retrieved July 20, 2007.

vaccine is lower than that in the single-antigen hepatitis A vaccine, allowing it to be administered in a three-dose schedule (0, 1, and 6 months) instead of the two-dose schedule used for the single-antigen vaccine. An accelerated schedule (0, 7, 21–30 days, followed by a booster dose at 12 months) is an option when a rapid immune response is needed for an occupational or behavioral imminent risk for hepatitis A and B or for international travel (31).

The vaccine should be administered into the deltoid muscle. Intragluteal and intradermal injections result in lower rates of seroconversion. Pregnancy is not a contraindication to vaccination. In fact, susceptible pregnant women who are at risk for HBV infection should be specifically targeted for vaccination (32).

Unvaccinated individuals or persons known not to have responded to a complete hepatitis B vaccine series and who have been exposed to HBV through a discrete, identifiable exposure to blood or to body fluids that contain blood should receive passive immunization with hepatitis B immune globulin (HBIG) and start the immunization series. Immunoprophylaxis should be administered as soon as possible after exposure (preferably within 24 hours). For sexual exposures, HBIG should not be administered more than 14 days after exposure (8).

Clinical Considerations and Recommendations

▶ *What are the clinical manifestations of hepatitis?*

The usual subjective symptoms in patients with acute viral hepatitis are malaise, fatigue, anorexia, nausea, and right upper quadrant or epigastric pain. Typical physical findings include jaundice, upper abdominal tenderness, and hepatomegaly, although many cases of hepatitis are anicteric. The patient's urine usually is darkened, and the stool may be gray or acholic. In cases of fulminant hepatitis, signs of coagulopathy and encephalopathy may be present.

In patients with hepatitis A or E, clinical manifestations usually are related temporally to recent travel to an endemic area or exposure to an infected person. Similarly, infections with hepatitis B, C, or D typically ensue after parenteral exposure to contaminated blood or sexual contact with an infected partner. The evolution of acute clinical illness in patients with hepatitis D often follows a biphasic course. In the initial phase of infection, patients with hepatitis D are indistinguishable from individuals with acute hepatitis B. Two to four weeks after apparent resolution of symptoms, patients typically have a relapse, which usually is of a milder nature and is associated with a second episode of elevation in serum transaminases. At this time serologic assay results for hepatitis D virus usually are positive.

As noted previously, in some patients with acute hepatitis B, C, or D, symptomatic infection resolves, and some become chronic carriers of viral infection. Although most viral hepatitis carriers initially are asymptomatic, up to one third subsequently develop chronic active or persistent hepatitis or cirrhosis. Once cirrhosis ensues, patients have the typical signs of end-stage liver disease, such as jaundice, muscle wasting, ascites, spider angioma, palmar erythema, and, ultimately, hepatic encephalopathy. Hepatitis C is the leading cause of chronic liver disease in the United States, whereas hepatitis B virus is the leading cause worldwide (13, 18).

▶ *How is acute hepatitis managed in pregnant women?*

Patients with acute hepatitis should be hospitalized if they have encephalopathy, coagulopathy, or severe debilitation. Nutritional needs should be addressed within the context of the severity of the disease. Fluid and electrolyte abnormalities should be corrected. If a coagulopathy is present, administration of erythrocytes, platelets, and clotting factors such as fresh frozen plasma or cryoprecipitate may be necessary. Activity should be limited, and the patient should be protected from upper abdominal trauma (32).

Women who are less severely ill may be treated as outpatients. They should reduce their level of activity, avoid upper abdominal trauma, and maintain good nutrition. Infected women also should avoid intimate contact with household members and sexual partners until these individuals receive appropriate prophylaxis (32).

General Tests

Coincident with the onset of symptoms, patients with acute hepatitis usually have a marked increase in the serum concentration of alanine aminotransferase (ALT, previously known as serum glutamate pyruvate transaminase) and aspartate aminotransferase (AST, previously known as serum glutamic oxaloacetic transaminase). In addition, the serum bilirubin concentration often is increased. In patients who are moderately to severely ill, coagulation abnormalities and hyperammonemia also

may be present (18). Although liver biopsy is rarely indicated in pregnancy, viral hepatitis may be distinguished histologically from other causes of hepatic injury by its characteristic pattern of extensive hepatocellular injury and inflammatory infiltrate. Initial evaluation of the patient with suspected viral hepatitis should include specific tests.

Specific Tests

If hepatitis is suspected based on the initial evaluation and general tests, the type of virus is determined through laboratory analysis.

Hepatitis A

The diagnosis of acute hepatitis A is confirmed by detecting specific immunoglobulin M (IgM) antibodies to the virus. A chronic carrier state for this infection does not exist, but immunoglobulin G (IgG) antibodies to hepatitis A virus will persist in patients with either previous infection or prior vaccination (32, 33).

Hepatitis B

The appearance of HBsAg predates clinical symptoms by 4 weeks on average and remains detectable for 1–6 weeks (Fig. 1). The chronic carrier state for HBV is defined by persistence of HBsAg and the absence of hepatitis B surface IgG antibody (anti-HBs), which is the protective antibody that defines immunity (Fig. 2). Titers of anti-HBs (in noncarriers) increase slowly during clin-

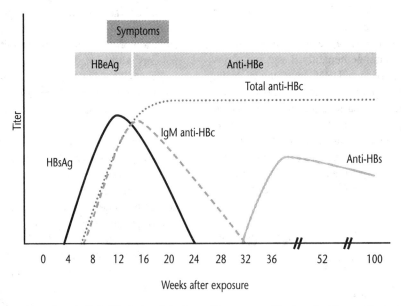

Figure 1. Typical serologic course of acute hepatitis B virus infection with recovery. (Centers for Disease Control and Prevention slide set adapted from Mast EE, Weinbaum CM, Fiore AE, Alter MJ, Bell BP, Finelli L, et al. A comprehensive immunization strategy to eliminate transmission of hepatitis B virus infection in the United States: recommendations of the Advisory Committee on Immunization Practices [ACIP] part II: immunization of adults. MMWR Recomm Rep 2006;55(RR-16):1–33; quiz CE1–4.)

ical recovery and continue to increase for up to 10–12 months after HBsAg has been cleared. In most patients with self-limited acute HBV infection, anti-HBs and HBsAg do not coexist detectably in serum, and anti-HBs is seen only after HBsAg has been cleared. The chronic carrier state usually can be predicted by HBsAg seropositivity for more than 20 weeks (8, 13, 32, 33).

A serologic "window" has been described for HBV infection when, despite clinical symptoms, HBsAg is clearing and undetectable but anti-HBs is not yet detectable either. In this period, HBV infection can still be diagnosed by detection of hepatitis B core IgG antibody (anti-HBc), which appears 3–5 weeks after HBsAg. Hepatitis B core IgG antibody is present only in the context of natural HBV infection and is not a protective antibody. It does not distinguish acute resolving infections from the chronic infection state, which is done only by persistence or clearance of HBsAg. An IgM antibody to the hepatitis B core antigen (IgM anti-HBc) appears during acute or after recent HBV infection and is present for approximately 6 months. In contrast, only anti-HBs becomes detectable in serum of vaccinated individuals. Therefore, the detection of anti-HBs in the absence of HBsAg and anti-HBc distinguishes vaccine-mediated immunity from natural infection-based immunity (where anti-HBc and anti-HBs are both present without HBsAg). Hepatitis B core antigen is not detectable outside of research laboratory assays, and tests for it should not be ordered as part of a "hepatitis B panel" (8, 13, 32, 33). With the variety of HBV-specific antigens and antibodies identified, interpretation of hepatitis B serologies is complex (Table 2).

Hepatitis C

The diagnosis of hepatitis C is confirmed by the identification of the antibody to hepatitis C virus, via a second- or third-generation enzyme immunoassay (ELISA) (34). The antibody may not be present until 6–10 weeks after the onset of clinical illness. Hepatitis C viral RNA can be detected by polymerase chain reaction assay of serum soon after infection, as well as in chronic disease. These other more specific tests for HCV, including HCV-specific RNA testing and genotyping, are available to define the specificity of infection, given that there are small but real false-positive rates associated with antibody testing or screening that vary with prevalence or risk of the disease in the screened populations. Such DNA-based specific testing usually is best interpreted by specialists trained in the treatment of hepatitis, to whom patients with positive serologic antibody test results should be referred (34). A reference table for the interpretation of these tests is available from the Centers for Disease Control and Prevention (Table 3).

Hepatitis D

Laboratory tests that may be used to confirm the diagnosis of acute hepatitis D are the detection of D antigen in hepatic tissue or serum and the identification of the IgM antibody to hepatitis D virus. Hepatitis D antigene-

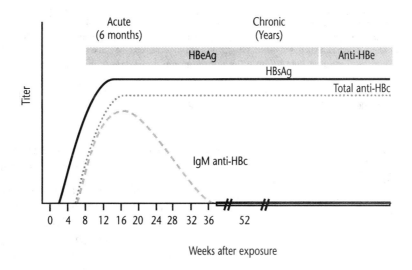

Figure 2. Progression to chronic hepatitis B virus infection: typical serologic course. (Centers for Disease Control and Prevention slide set adapted from Mast EE, Weinbaum CM, Fiore AE, Alter MJ, Bell BP, Finelli L, et al. A comprehensive immunization strategy to eliminate transmission of hepatitis B virus infection in the United States: recommendations of the Advisory Committee on Immunization Practices (ACIP) part II: immunization of adults. MMWR Recomm Rep 2006;55(RR-16):1–33; quiz CE1-4.

Table 2. Interpretation of Hepatitis B Virus (HBV) Testing

Test	Results	Interpretation
HBsAg Anti-HBc Anti-HBs	Negative Negative Negative	Susceptible
HBsAg Anti-HBc Anti-HBs	Negative Positive Positive	Immune due to natural infection
HBsAg Anti-HBc Anti-HBs	Negative Negative Positive	Immune due to hepatitis B vaccination*
HBsAg Anti-HBc IgM anti-HBc Anti-HBs	Positive Positive Positive Negative	Acutely infected
HBsAg Anti-HBc IgM anti-HBc Anti-HBs	Positive Positive Negative Negative	Chronically infected
HBsAg Anti-HBc Anti-HBs	Negative Positive Negative	Four interpretations possible†

*Antibody response (anti-HBs) can be measured quantitatively or qualitatively. A protective antibody response is reported quantitatively as 10 or more milli-international units (10 mIU/mL or less) or qualitatively as positive. Postvaccination testing should be completed 1–2 months after the third vaccine dose for results to be meaningful.

†Four interpretations:

Might be recovering from acute HBV infection

Might be distantly immune and test not sensitive enough to detect very low level of anti-HBs in serum

Might be susceptible with a false-positive anti-HBc

Might be undetectable level of HBsAg present in the serum and the person is actually chronically infected

Definitions

Hepatitis B surface antigen (HBsAg): A serologic marker on the surface of HBV. It can be detected in high levels in serum during acute or chronic hepatitis. The presence of HBsAg indicates that the person is infectious. The body normally produces antibodies to HBsAg as part of the normal immune response to infection.

Hepatitis B surface antibody (anti-HBs): The presence of anti-HBs generally is interpreted as indicating recovery and immunity from HBV infection. Anti-HBs also develops in a person who has been successfully vaccinated against hepatitis B.

Total hepatitis B core antibody (anti-HBc): Appears at the onset of symptoms in acute hepatitis B and persists for life. The presence of anti-HBc indicates previous or ongoing infection with hepatitis B virus (HBV) in an undefined time frame.

IgM antibody to hepatitis B core antigen (IgM anti-HBc): This antibody appears during acute or recent HBV infection and is present for approximately 6 months.

Centers for Disease Control and Prevention. Interpretation of the hepatitis B panel. Atlanta (GA): CDC; 2006. Available at: http://www.cdc.gov/ncidod/diseases/hepatitis/b/Bserology.htm. Retrieved July 11, 2007.

mia usually persists in patients with chronic hepatitis D despite the appearance of the IgG antibody to the virus. Thus, as in hepatitis C and HIV infection, viremia and end-organ damage can continue despite the presence of the antibody to the virus (35).

Hepatitis E

The diagnosis of infection with hepatitis E is documented by the presence of virus-specific antibodies in individuals with risk factors. The primary risk factor is travel exposure (33).

▶ *How are pregnant patients who are presumed chronic hepatitis carriers treated?*

Persons with diagnosed chronic HBV and HCV infection should be referred for evaluation to a physician experienced in the management of chronic liver disease. Diagnosis in the context of pregnancy-specific screening opens the opportunity for individuals who might otherwise have not ever been tested to receive appropriate subspecialty care for counseling and targeted treatment, usually after delivery. Women who are chronic carriers of HBV or HCV should inform sexual, household, and

Table 3. Interpretation of Hepatitis C Virus (HCV) Test Results

Anti-HCV Screening Test Result*	Anti-HCV Supplemental Test Result		Anti-HCV Result	HCV Infection	Additional Testing or Evaluation
	RIBA[†]	HCV RNA			
Negative	Not needed	Not needed	Negative	None	No
Positive	Not done	Not done	Not known	Not known	Supplemental anti-HCV (RIBA) or HCV RNA
Positive	Not done	Negative	Not known	Not known[†]	Supplemental anti-HCV (RIBA)
Positive (high s/co ratios[†‡])	Not done	Not done	Positive	Past/current	Evaluate for chronic infection and liver disease
Positive	Negative	Not needed	Negative	None	No
Positive	Positive	Not done	Positive	Past/current	Evaluate for chronic infection and liver disease
Positive	Positive	Negative	Positive	Past/current[§]	Repeat HCV RNA
Positive	Positive/not done	Positive	Positive	Current	Evaluate for chronic infection and liver disease
Positive	Indeterminate	Not done	Indeterminate	Not known	Test for HCV RNA or repeat anti-HCV testing
Positive	Indeterminate	Positive	Indeterminate	Current	Evaluate for chronic infection and liver disease
Positive	Indeterminate	Negative	Negative	None	No

*EIA, enzyme immunoassay or CIA, enhanced chemiluminescence immunoassay

[†]Recombinant immunoblot assay, a more specific anti-HCV assay viremia.

[‡]Samples with high signal-to-cutoff (s/co) ratios usually more than 95%) confirm positive, but supplemental serologic testing was not performed. Less than 5 of every 100 test results might represent false-positives; more specific testing should be requested, if indicated.

[§]Single negative HCV RNA result cannot determine infection status; patients might have intermittent viremia.

Centers for Disease Control and Prevention. Reference for interpretation of HCV test results. Atlanta (GA): CDC; 2006. Available at: http://www.cdc.gov/ncidod/diseases/hepatitis/resource/PDFs/hcv_graph.pdf. Retrieved July 11, 2007.

needle-sharing contacts of their status and learn about and use methods to prevent or reduce the risk of transmission of infections to others. All HBsAg-positive laboratory results should be reported to the state or local health department in accordance with state requirements for reporting of chronic HBV infection (8, 13).

▶ *How can the risk of vertical transmission of HBV be reduced?*

Because hepatitis B virus is highly pathogenic and infectious, perinatal transmission of infection represents the single largest cause of chronically infected individuals worldwide. Because risk-factor-based prenatal screening protocols have been shown to detect at most 60% of women who are HBV carriers, routine prenatal screening of all pregnant women with HBsAg is recommended

(13). Approximately 10–20% of women who are seropositive for HBsAg alone transmit the virus to their neonates in the absence of neonatal immunoprophylaxis. In women who are seropositive for both HBsAg and HBeAg, the frequency of vertical transmission increases to approximately 90% without neonatal prophylaxis. For adult-acquired HBV infection, the risk of chronic infection and its sequelae is only 5–10%. In contrast, HBV infection acquired perinatally carries an 85–95% risk of persistence and chronic infection, with a 25–30% lifetime risk of serious or fatal liver disease.

In patients with acute hepatitis B, the frequency of vertical transmission also depends on the time during gestation that maternal infection occurs. When it occurs in the first trimester, up to 10% of neonates will be seropositive for HBsAg. In women acutely infected in the third trimester, 80–90% of offspring will be infected (13).

The Centers for Disease Control and Prevention recommends universal active immunization of all infants born in the United States. The immunization schedule for infants of women who have been screened and have negative results should be started preferably before discharge, but by no later than 2 months of age. Preterm infants weighing less than 2,000 g and born to women who are HBsAg negative should have their first vaccine dose delayed until 1 month after birth or hospital discharge (13).

Current guidelines stipulate that infants of women who are HBsAg positive or whose status is unknown at the time of delivery also should receive both HBIG and hepatitis B vaccine within 12 hours of birth given simultaneously at different sites intramuscularly. It should then be followed by two more injections of hepatitis B vaccine in the first 6 months of life. The physician responsible for the care of a newborn delivered of a woman with chronic hepatitis B should be informed of her carrier status so that the appropriate doses of hepatitis B vaccine and HBIG can be given as soon as possible after delivery (13).

Neonatal immunoprophylaxis will not prevent HBV infection in newborns who are already infected in utero; therefore, current research is focusing on the potential efficacy of antepartum treatment of HBV-infected women to lower the risk of such infection, particularly in women who have risk factors for transmission (36–39). In addition, women who did not receive prenatal care will have unknown HBV status at the time of delivery, and these women have been shown to have significantly higher rates of being chronic HBV carriers than women enrolled in prenatal care (40). The combination of passive and active immunization has been particularly effective (85–95% efficacy) in reducing the frequency of perinatal transmission of hepatitis B virus.

▶ How can transmission of other forms of hepatitis be prevented?

Hepatitis C virus seroprevalence rates of 0.6–6.6% have been reported in study cohorts of pregnant women worldwide (41–44). Vertical HCV transmission rates of 2–8% have been demonstrated, with maternal viremia (detectable presence of HCV RNA in blood) an almost uniform prerequisite for transmission (35, 45–47). In pregnancies among HCV-infected mothers who were HCV RNA negative, vertical transmission was rare. Maternal coinfection with HIV significantly increases the risk of vertical HCV transmission to as much as 44% (45, 47). In a recent cohort study, risk factors associated with an increased rate of vertical HCV transmission to include higher maternal HCV viral titer, pro-

longed membrane rupture during labor (6 hours or longer), and use of internal fetal monitoring during labor were reported (48). If duration of membrane rupture and internal fetal monitoring are confirmed to be associated with transmission in further investigations, interventions may be possible to decrease the risk of transmission.

Currently, no preventive measures are available to lower the risk of vertical HCV infection of neonates as there are for HBV. Routine prenatal HCV screening is not recommended; however, women with significant risk factors for infection (see the box) should be offered antibody screening. Testing for HCV RNA should not be used for screening purposes.

Vertical transmission of hepatitis D virus has been documented. Transmission is uncommon, however,

---

Risk Factors Warranting Hepatitis C Screening: CDC Guidelines

Individuals who should be screened routinely:

1. Persons who ever injected illegal drugs (even once)

2. Persons notified that they received blood products before 1987 or from a donor who later tested positive for hepatitis C virus (HCV)

3. Recipients of transfusions or organ transplants, particularly if received before July 1992

4. Persons ever on long-term hemodialysis

5. Persons with persistently elevated alanine aminotransferase (ALT) or other evidence of liver disease

6. Persons seeking evaluation or care for a sexually transmitted infection, including human immunodeficiency virus

Individuals for whom routine testing is of uncertain need:

1. Recipients of tissue transplants (eg, cornea, skin, sperm, ova)

2. Users of intranasal cocaine or other illegal noninjected drugs

3. Persons with a history of tattooing or body piercing

4. Persons with a history of sexually transmitted diseases or multiple sexual partners

5. Long-term steady sex partner of an HCV-infected individual

Centers for Disease Control and Prevention. Recommendations for prevention and control of hepatitis C virus (HCV) infection and HCV-related chronic disease. MMWR 1998;47(RR-19):1–33 and Centers for Disease Control and Prevention. Sexually transmitted diseases treatment guidelines, 2006. MMWR 2006;55(RR-11):1–94.

because the measures used to prevent perinatal infection with hepatitis B virus are almost uniformly effective in preventing infection by hepatitis D. Vertical transmission of HEV has been reported, but information is limited.

▶ *Are there special considerations for intrapartum care in the context of maternal hepatitis infection?*

Between 85% and 95% of cases of perinatal transmission of HBV occur as a consequence of intrapartum exposure of the infant to infected blood and genital tract secretions. The remaining cases result from hematogenous transplacental dissemination and close postnatal contact between the infant and the infected parent. Risk factors for intrauterine HBV infection have been reported to include maternal HBeAg seropositivity, history of threatened preterm labor, higher HBsAg and HBV DNA titers, and the presence of HBV DNA in villous capillary endothelial cells (49). Adequate data regarding the risk of transmission with operative vaginal delivery or internal fetal monitoring are not available to make recommendations.

The route of delivery has not been shown to influence the risk of vertical HCV transmission (35, 50). Cesarean delivery should be performed in HCV-infected women only for obstetric indications.

▶ *What is the safety of invasive prenatal diagnostic procedures for patients with chronic hepatitis?*

The risk of transmission through amniocentesis appears to be low for women who are chronically infected with hepatitis B or hepatitis C, although the number of exposed cases in the literature is small. Of the 115 women reported to be positive for hepatitis B surface-antigen who underwent second-trimester amniocentesis, the rate of neonatal infection was no different than in women who did not have an amniocentesis. All of the infants received hepatitis B vaccination and immunoprophylaxis beginning at birth (50–53). There is only one series of 22 HCV-positive women reported in the literature who underwent second-trimester amniocentesis. No infants in this series were found to be hepatitis C RNA positive on postnatal testing. This group included one woman with hepatitis C RNA-positive amniotic fluid (54). Data are insufficient in the literature to assess the risk of chorionic villus sampling in these women or to estimate the risk of fetal infection among women with anterior placentas, those who are HBe antigen pos-

itive, or those with high hepatitis B or hepatitis C viral loads.

Because of the limited information regarding the risk of invasive procedures in women chronically infected with hepatitis B or hepatitis C, it would be prudent to discuss noninvasive screening options with these women.

▶ *Is breastfeeding contraindicated for infants of women with hepatitis?*

In HAV-infected women, breastfeeding is permissible with appropriate hygienic precautions. Although immune globulin has been administered to newborns in specific situations, the efficacy of this practice has not been established. Breastfeeding is not contraindicated for women who are HBsAg positive at the time of delivery. In addition, breastfeeding is not contraindicated in women chronically infected with HBV if the infant receives HBIG passive prophylaxis and vaccine active prophylaxis (13). There are no data from which to make a recommendation for HBeAg positive patients. In addition, breastfeeding has not been associated with an increased risk of neonatal HCV infection (56–59) and, therefore, is not contraindicated in HCV-infected mothers (58, 59).

Breastfeeding was not detrimental to newborns of HEV-infected women in one recent series of 93 pregnancies. In this cohort, anti-HEV antibody and HEV RNA were present in clostral samples, but at significantly lower levels than in maternal serum (60).

Immunotherapy

▶ *What is the role of specific immunotherapy in the treatment of chronic hepatitis in pregnancy?*

Hepatitis A

Given the nonchronic and usually self-limited course of symptomatic HAV infection, no specific antiviral agent is used for its treatment. The hepatitis A vaccine is not contraindicated during pregnancy. In populations that have expected high rates of previous HAV infection, prevaccination testing may be considered to reduce costs by not vaccinating persons who are already immune. Prevaccination serologic testing may be cost-effective for adults who were born in or lived for extended periods in HAV-endemic areas; adults in certain population groups (Native Americans, Alaska Natives, and Hispanics); and adults in groups with a high prevalence of infection (eg, injection drug users) (25).

Patients who have had close personal or sexual contact with an HAV-infected individual should receive postexposure prophylaxis if they have not been immunized. Immune globulin does not pose a risk to either a pregnant woman or her fetus and should be administered during pregnancy if indicated. Immune globulin provides protection through passive antibody transfer. For postexposure prophylaxis, a single intramuscular dose of 0.02 mL/kg should be administered as soon as possible after contact with the infected individual; this confers protection for up to 3 months at an 80–90% efficacy level. Administration of immune globulin more than 2 weeks after exposure is not effective in preventing or ameliorating the severity of hepatitis A (25). The HAV vaccination series also should be initiated in conjunction with postexposure administration of IgG. Although some studies suggest that HAV vaccine alone also may prevent postexposure infection, no comparative trials have been conducted (29). This strategy of administering HAV vaccine alone for postexposure prophylaxis in individuals younger than 40 years has been proposed by some experts.

Hepatitis B

No specific therapy is available for treatment of acute HBV infection. Persons with chronic HBV infection should be referred for evaluation to a physician experienced in the management of chronic liver disease.

Therapeutic agents have been approved by the FDA for treatment of chronic HBV infection and can achieve sustained suppression of HBV replication and remission of liver disease in some persons (32). One of these agents, the antiviral agent lamivudine, also has been shown to be effective, in combination with other medications, for both the treatment of infections with the human immunodeficiency virus (HIV) and for the interruption of vertical HIV transmission. Recent research has demonstrated potential benefit from lamivudine treatment in decreasing the risk of in utero HBV infection in women who were HBV carriers during the last months of pregnancy (37, 39). Other investigators have studied the use of hepatitis B immune globulin (HBIG) administered to the mother toward the end of pregnancy to achieve similar results (36, 38).

Hepatitis C

Optimal obstetric care of women infected with HCV is limited by the lack of any available prenatal or postnatal pharmacologic or immunologic measures to decrease the risk of vertical transmission. Use of antiretroviral treatment to decrease both maternal viral titers and the risk of neonatal HIV infections (61) raises the question of the potential for comparable treatment of maternal HCV infection, given that maternal HCV titer also has been

associated with an increased risk of transmission (44, 46). Recent advances in combination therapy for HCV infection in nonpregnant adults have made sustained normalization of transaminase levels and clearance of HCV RNA possible, even in individuals with HCV genotypes that have a poorer prognosis (62). More recently, the modification of interferon alfa-2a via a branched-chain polyethylene glycol moiety has produced a compound, peginterferon alfa-2a, with prolonged absorption, slower clearance, and a longer half-life than standard interferon, allowing once-weekly dosing (63). Randomized trials have shown peginterferon to be superior to standard interferon, either alone or in combination with ribavirin, for the treatment of chronic HCV infection in adults (64). Even though the use of ribavirin is contraindicated in pregnancy, interferon has been used safely for the treatment of T-cell leukemias during pregnancy (65, 66), and its potential role as an anti-HCV therapy for both maternal benefit and fetal and neonatal benefit warrants further study.

▶ *How can accidental or occupational exposures to hepatitis virus be managed?*

Accidental exposures are classified as occupational or nonoccupational for management recommendations. Guidelines for postexposure prophylaxis of occupational exposures have been published by the Centers for Disease Control and Prevention (13, 67, 68) and are intended for use in settings in which postvaccination testing is recommended for certain employees and in which programs are available to implement testing and follow-up algorithms. There are also specific guidelines for care of persons with nonoccupational exposure to HBV through exposure to blood or body fluids (13).

All health care workers who may be exposed to blood or blood products should be vaccinated against hepatitis B. The principal mechanism of transmission of HBV from patient to health care workers is through injury from a sharp object that is contaminated with infected blood. Of all the bloodborne transmissible viruses (including HCV and HIV), HBV exists in highest concentrations in blood. Hepatitis B requires much smaller volumes for transmission and, therefore, can be injected without hollow-bore needles or deep penetrating injuries. The risk of infection per injury with HBV-infected blood is 20–30%. Transmission of HBV also has been reported by mucosal contamination from body fluid "splash" exposures.

The risk of health care workers acquiring HCV infection through workplace exposure to infected blood is lower than the risk of acquiring HBV (30%) and higher than the risk of acquiring HIV (0.3%) (68, 69). Standard precautions such as not recapping used needles has been shown to decrease the risk of workplace injury; however, recent research has demonstrated that even practitioners in high-risk subspecialties failed to routinely practice standard universal precautions (69).

Summary of Recommendations and Conclusions

The following recommendations are based on good and consistent scientific evidence (Level A):

▶ Routine prenatal screening of all pregnant women by HBsAg testing is recommended.

▶ Newborns born to hepatitis B carriers should receive combined immunoprophylaxis consisting of HBIG and hepatitis B vaccine within 12 hours of birth.

▶ Hepatitis B infection is a preventable disease, and all at-risk individuals, particularly health care workers, should be vaccinated. All infants should receive the hepatitis B vaccine series as part of the recommended childhood immunization schedule.

▶ Breastfeeding is not contraindicated in women with HAV infection with appropriate hygienic precautions, in those chronically infected with hepatitis B if the infant receives HBIG passive prophylaxis and vaccine active prophylaxis, or in women with HCV infection.

The following recommendations are based on limited or inconsistent scientific evidence (Level B):

▶ Routine prenatal HCV screening is not recommended; however, women with significant risk factors for infection should be offered antibody screening.

▶ Route of delivery has not been shown to influence the risk of vertical HCV transmission, and cesarean delivery should be reserved for obstetric indications in women with HCV infection.

The following recommendations are based primarily on consensus and expert opinion (Level C):

▶ The risk of transmission of hepatitis B associated with amniocentesis is low.

▶ Susceptible pregnant women who are at risk for hepatitis B infections should be specifically targeted for vaccination.

Proposed Performance Measure

Percentage of women receiving prenatal care who are screened for hepatitis B by hepatitis B surface antigen testing

References

1. Bell BP, Shapiro CN, Alter MJ, Moyer LA, Judson FN, Moltram K, et al. The diverse patterns of hepatitis A epidemiology in the United States—implications for vaccination strategies. J Infect Dis 1998;178:1579–84. (Level I)

2. Staes CJ, Schlenker TL, Risk I, Cannon KG, Harris H, Pavia AT, et al. Sources of infection among persons with acute hepatitis A and no identified risk factors during a sustained community-wide outbreak. Pediatrics 2000; 106:e54. (Level II-3)

3. Fiore AE. Hepatitis A transmitted by food. Clin Infect Dis 2004;38:705–15. (Level III)

4. Glikson M, Galun E, Oren R, Tur-Kaspa R, Shouval D. Relapsing hepatitis A: review of 14 cases and literature survey. Medicine 1992;71:14–23. (Level III)

5. Alter HJ, Purcell RH, Gerin JL, London WT, Kaplan PM, McAuliffe VJ, et al. Transmission of hepatitis B to chimpanzees by hepatitis surface antigen-positive saliva and semen. Infect Immun 1977;16:928–33. (Animal)

6. Bancroft WH, Snitbhan R, Scott RM, Tingpalapong M, Watson WT, Tanticharoenyos P, et al. Transmission of hepatitis B virus to gibbons by exposure to human saliva containing hepatitis B surface antigen. J Infect Dis 1977;135:79–85. (Animal)

7. Bond WW, Favero MS, Petersen NJ, Gravelle CR, Ebert JW, Maynard JE. Survival of hepatitis B virus after drying and storage for one week. Lancet 1981;1:550–1. (Level III)

8. Mast EE, Margolis HS, Fiore AE, Brink EW, Goldstein ST, Wang SA, et al. A comprehensive immunization strategy to eliminate transmission of hepatitis B virus infection in the United States: recommendations of the Advisory Committee on Immunization Practices (ACIP) part II: immunization of adults. MMWR 2006;55(RR-16):1–33. (Level III)

9. Stramer SL, Glynn SA, Kleinman SH, Strong DM, Caglioti S, Wright DJ, et al. Detection of HIV-1 and HCV infections among antibody-negative blood donors by nucleic-acid amplification testing. National Heart, Lung, and Blood Institute Nucleic Acid Test Study Group. N Engl J Med 2004;351:760–8. (Level II-3)

10. Schreiber GB, Busch MP, Kleinman SH, Koralitz JJ. The risk of transfusion-transmitted viral infections. The Retrovirus Epidemiology Donor Study. N Engl J Med 1996;334:1685–90. (Level 11-3)

11. American Association of Blood Banks. Transfusion-transmitted diseases. Bethesda (MD): AABB; 2005. Available

at: http://www.aabb.org/content/About_Blood/Facts_About_Blood_and_Blood_Banking/fabloodtrans.htm. Retrieved July 11, 2007. (Level III)

12. Transmission of hepatitis B virus among persons undergoing blood glucose monitoring in long-term-care facilities—Mississippi, North Carolina, and Los Angeles County, California, 2003-2004. Centers for Disease Control and Prevention (CDC). MMWR Morb Mortal Wkly Rep 2005;54:220–3. (Level II-2)

13. Mast EE, Margolis HS, Fiore AE, Brink EW, Goldstein ST, Wang SA, et al. A comprehensive immunization strategy to eliminate transmission of hepatitis B virus infection in the United States: recommendations of the Advisory Committee on Immunization Practices (ACIP) part 1: immunization of infants, children, and adolescents. Advisory Committee on Immunization Practices (ACIP) [published erratum appears in MMWR Morb Mortal Wkly Rep 2006;55:158–9]. MMWR Recomm Rep 2005;54(RR-16):1–31. (Level III)

14. van der Poel CL, Cuypers HT, Reesink HW. Hepatitis C virus six years on. Lancet 1994;344:1475–9. (Level III)

15. Widell A, Hansson BG, Berntorp E, Moestrup T, Johansson HP, Hansson H, et al. Antibody to a hepatitis C virus related protein among patients at high risk for hepatitis B. Scand J Infect Dis 1991;10:19–24. (Level II-3)

16. Brettler DB, Alter HJ, Dienstag JL, Forsberg AD, Levine PH. Prevalence of hepatitis C virus antibody in a cohort of hemophilia patients. Blood 1990;76:254–6. (Level II-3)

17. van den Hoek JA, van Haastrecht HJ, Goudsmit J, de Wolf F, Coutinho RA. Prevalence, incidence, and risk factors of hepatitis C virus infection among drug users in Amsterdam. J Infect Dis 1990;162:823–6. (Level III)

18. Recommendations for prevention and control of hepatitis C (virus HCV) infection and HCV-related chronic disease. Centers for Disease Control and Prevention. MMWR Recomm Rep 1998;47(RR-19):1–39. (Level III)

19. Jeffers LJ, Hasan F, De Medina M, Reddy R, Parker T, Silva M, et al. Prevalence of antibodies to hepatitis C virus among patients with cryptogenic chronic hepatitis and cirrhosis. Hepatology 1992;15:187–90. (Level II-3)

20. Hoofnagle JH. Type D (delta) hepatitis [published erratum in JAMA 1989;261:3552]. JAMA 1989;261:1321–5. (Level III)

21. Drobeniuc J, Hutin YJ, Harpaz R, Favorov M, Meinik A, Iarovoi P, et al. Prevalence of hepatitis B, D and C virus infections among children and pregnant women in Moldova: additional evidence supporting the need for routine hepatitis B vaccination of infants. Epidemiol Infect 1999;123:463–7. (Level II-3)

22. Aggarwal R, Krawczynski K. Hepatitis E: an overview and recent advances in clinical and laboratory research. J Gastroenterol Hepatol 2000;15:9–20. (Level III)

23. Hussaini SH, Skidmore SJ, Richardson P, Sherratt LM, Cooper BT, O'Grady JG. Severe hepatitis E infection during pregnancy. J Viral Hepat 1997;4:51–4. (Level III)

24. Singh S, Mohanty A, Joshi YK, Deka D, Mohanty S, Panda SK. Mother-to-child transmission of hepatitis E virus infection. Indian J Pediatr 2003;70:37–9. (Level III)

25. Fiore AE, Wasley A, Bell BP. Prevention of hepatitis A through active or passive immunization: recommendations of the Advisory Committee on Immunization Practices (ACIP). Advisory Committee on Immunization Practices (ACIP). MMWR Recomm Rep 2006;55(RR-7):1–23. (Level III)

26. Clemens R, Safary A, Hepburn A, Roche C, Stanbury WJ, André FE. Clinical experience with an inactivated hepatitis A vaccine. J Infect Dis 1995;171(suppl 1):S44–9. (Level III)

27. Zamir C, Rishpon S, Zamir D, Leventhal A, Rimon N, Ben-Porath E. Control of a community-wide outbreak of hepatitis A by mass vaccination with inactivated hepatitis A vaccine. Eur J Clin Microbiol Infect Dis 2001;20:185–7. (Level II-3)

28. Hepatitis A vaccination programs in communities with high rates of hepatitis A. Centers for Disease Control and Prevention (CDC). MMWR Morb Mortal Wkly Rep 1997;46:600–3. (Level II-3)

29. Sagliocca L, Amoroso P, Stroffolini T, Adamo B, Tosti ME, Lettieri G, et al. Efficacy of hepatitis A vaccine in prevention of secondary hepatitis A infection: a randomised trial [published erratum appears in Lancet 1999;353:2078]. Lancet 1999;353:1136–9. (Level I)

30. Centers for Disease Control and Prevention. Recommended adult immunization schedule: United States, October 2006–September 2007. Atlanta (GA): CDC, 2006. Available at: http://www.cdc.gov/nip/recs/ adultschedule. pdf. Retrieved May 16, 2007. (Level III)

31. Connor BA, Blatter MM, Beran J, Zou B, Trofa AF. Rapid and sustained immune response against hepatitis A and B achieved with combined vaccine using an accelerated administration schedule. J Trav Med 2007;14:9–15. (Level I)

32. Workowski KA, Berman SM. Sexually transmitted diseases treatment guidelines, 2006. Centers for Disease Control and Prevention [published erratum appears in MMWR Morb Mortal Wkly Rep 2006;55:997]. MMWR Recomm Rep 2006;55(RR-11):1–94. (Level III)

33. American Academy of Pediatrics. Red book: 2006 report of the Committee on Infectious Diseases. 27th ed. Elk Grove Village (IL): AAP; 2006. (Level III)

34. Scott JD, Gretch DR. Molecular diagnostics of hepatitis C virus infection. JAMA 2007;297:724–32. (Level III)

35. Zanetti AR, Tanzi E, Romano L, Zuin G, Minola E, Vecchi L, et al. Prospective study on mother-to-infant transmission of hepatitis C virus. Intervirology 1998;41:208–12. (Level II-2)

36. Li XM, Shi MF, Yang YB, Shi ZJ, Hou HY, Shen HM, et al. Effect of hepatitis B immunoglobulin on interruption of HBV intrauterine infection. World J Gastroenterol 2004;10:3215–7. (Level I)

37. Xu WM, Cui YT, Wang L, Yang H, Liang ZQ, Li XM, et al. Efficacy and safety of lamivudine in late pregnancy for the prevention of mother-child transmission of hepatitis B; a multicentre, randomised, double-blind, placebo-controlled study [abstract]. Hepatology 2004;40(suppl 1):272A–3A. (Level I)

38. Zhu Q, Yu G, Yu H, Lu Q, Gu X, Dong Z, et al. A randomized controlled trial on interruption of HBV transmission in utero. Chinese Med J 2003;116:685–7. (Level I)

39. van Zonneveld M, van Nunen AB, Niesters HG, de Man RA, Schalm SW, Janssen HL. Lamivudine treatment during pregnancy to prevent perinatal transmission of hepatitis B virus infection. J Viral Hepat 2003;10:294–7. (Level II-2)

40. Silverman NS, Darby MJ, Ronkin SL, Wapner RJ. Hepatitis B prevalence in an unregistered prenatal population. Implications for neonatal therapy. JAMA 1991; 266:2852–5. (Level II-3)

41. Silverman NS, Snyder M, Hodinka RL, McGillen P, Knee G. Detection of hepatitis C virus antibodies and specific hepatitis C virus ribonucleic acid sequences in cord bloods from a heterogeneous prenatal population. Am J Obstet Gynecol 1995;173:1396–400. (Level II-3)

42. Bohman VR, Slettler W, Little BB, Wendel GD, Sutor LJ, Cunningham FG. Seroprevalence and risk factors for hepatitis C virus antibody in pregnant women. Obstet Gynecol 1992;80:609–13. (Level II-3)

43. Choy Y, Gittens-Williams L, Apuzzio J, Skurnick J, Zollicoffer C, McGovern PG. Risk factors for hepatitis C infection among sexually transmitted disease-infected, inner city obstetric patients. Infect Dis Obstet Gynecol 2003;11:191–8. (Level II-3)

44. Okamoto M, Nagata I, Murakami J, Kaji S, Iitsuka T, Hoschika T, et al. Prospective reevaluation of risk factors in mother-to-child transmission of hepatitis C virus: high virus load, vaginal delivery, and negative anti-NS4 antibody. J Infect Dis 2000;182:1511–4. (Level II-2)

45. Ferrero S, Lungaro P, Bruzzone BM, Gotta C, Bentivoglio G, Ragni N. Prospective study of mother-to-infant transmission of hepatitis C virus: a 10-year survey. Acta Obstet Gynecol Scand 2003;82:229–34. (Level II-2)

46. Tajiri H, Miyoshi Y, Funada S, Etani Y, Abe J, Onodera T, et al. Prospective study of mother-to-infant transmission of hepatitis C virus. Pediatr Infect Dis J 2001;20:10–4. (Level II-2)

47. Granovsky MO, Minkoff HL, Tess BH, Waters D, Hatzakis A, Devoid DE, et al. Hepatitis C virus infection in the mothers and infants cohort study. Pediatrics 1998;102:355–9. (Level II-2)

48. Mast EE, Hwang LY, Seto DS, Nolte FS, Nainan OV, Wurtzel H, et al. Risk factors for perinatal transmission of hepatitis C virus (HCV) and the natural history of HCV infection acquired in infancy. J Infect Dis 2005;192: 1880–9. (Level II-2)

49. Xu DZ, Yan YP, Choi BC, Xu JQ, Men K, Zhang JX, et al. Risk factors and mechanism of transplacental transmission of hepatitis B virus: a case-control study. J Med Virol 2002;67:20–6. (Level II-2)

50. Towers CV, Asrat T, Rumney P. The presence of hepatitis B surface antigen and deoxyribonucleic acid in amniotic fluid and cord blood. Am J Obstet Gynecol 2001; 184:1514–8; discussion 1518–20. (Level II-2)

51. Alexander JM, Ramus R, Jackson G, Sercely B, Wendel GD Jr. Risk of hepatitis B transmission after amniocentesis in chronic hepatitis B carriers. Infect Dis Obstet Gynecol 1999;7:283–6. (Level III)

52. Grosheide PM, Quartero HW, Schalm SW, Heijtink RA, Christiaens GC. Early invasive prenatal diagnosis in HBsAg-positive women. Prenat Diagn 1994;14:553–8. (Level III)

53. Ko TM, Tseng LH, Chang MH, Chen DS, Hsieh FJ, Chuang SM, et al. Amniocentesis in mothers who are hepatitis B virus carriers does not expose the infant to an increased risk of hepatitis B virus infection. Arch Gynecol Obstet 1994;255:25–30. (Level II-2)

54. Delamare C, Carbonne B, Heim N, Berkane N, Petit JC, Uzan S, et al. Detection of hepatitis C virus RNA (HCV RNA) in amniotic fluid: a prospective study. J Hepatol 1999;31:416–20. (Level II-2)

55. A significant sex—but not elective cesarean section—effect on mother-to-child transmission of hepatitis C virus infection. J Infect Dis 2005;192:1872–9. (Level II-2)

56. Kumar RM, Shahul S. Role of breast-feeding in transmission of hepatitis C virus to infants of HCV-infected mothers. J Hepatol 1009;29:191–7. (Level II-2)

57. Lin HH, Kao JH, Hsu HY, Ni YH, Chang MH, Huang SC, et al. Absence of infection in breast-fed infants born to hepatitis C virus-infected mothers. J Pediatr 1995;126: 589–91. (Level III)

58. American Academy of Pediatrics, American College of Obstetricians and Gynecologists. Breastfeeding handbook for physicians. Elk Grove Village (IL): AAP; Washington, DC: ACOG; 2006. (Level III)

59. Breastfeeding: maternal and infant aspects. ACOG Committee Opinion No. 361. American College of Obstetricians and Gynecologists. Obstet Gynecol 2007; 109:479–80. (Level III)

60. Chibber RM, Usmani MA, Al-Sibai MH. Should HEV infected mothers breast feed? Arch Gynecol Obstet 2004;270:15–20. (Level II-2)

61. Cooper ER, Chaurat M, Mofenson L, Hanson IC, Pitt J, Diaz C, et al. Combination antiretroviral strategies for the treatment of pregnant HIV-1-infected women and prevention of perinatal HIV-1 transmission. Women and Infants' Transmission Study Group. J Acquir Immune Defic Syndr 2002;29:484–94. (Level II-2)

62. Poynard T, Marcellin P, Lee SS, Niederau C, Minuk GS, Ideo G, et al. Randomised trial of interferon alpha2b plus ribavirin for 48 weeks or for 24 weeks versus interferon alpha2b plus placebo for 48 weeks for treatment of chronic infection with hepatitis C virus. International Hepatitis Interventional Therapy Group (IHIT). Lancet 1998;352: 1426–32. (Level I)

63. Lindsay KL, Trepo C, Heintges T, Shiffman ML, Gordon SC, Hoefs JC, et al. A randomized, double-blind trial comparing pegylated interferon alfa-2b to interferon alfa-2b as initial treatment for chronic hepatitis C. Hepatitis Interventional Therapy Group. Hepatology 2001;34: 395–403. (Level I)

64. Fried MW, Shiffman ML, Reddy KR, Smith C, Marinos G, Goncales FL Jr, et al. Peginterferon alfa-2a plus ribavirin for chronic hepatitis C virus infection. N Engl J Med 2002;347:975–82. (Level I)

65. Hiratsuka M, Minakami H, Koshizuka S, Sato I. Administration of interferon-alpha during pregnancy: effects on fetus. J Perinat Med 2000;28:372–6. (Level III)

66. Crump M, Wang XH, Sermer M, Keating A. Successful pregnancy and delivery during alpha-interferon therapy for chronic myeloid leukemia. Am J Hematol 1992;40:238–9. (Level III)

67. Updated U.S. Public Health Service guidelines for the management of occupational exposures to HBV, HCV, and HIV and recommendations for postexposure prophylaxis. Centers for Disease Control and Prevention. MMWR Recomm Rep 2001;50 (RR-11):1–52. (Level III)

68. Panlilio AL, Cardo DM, Grohskopf LA, Heneine W, Ross CS. Updated U.S. Public Health Service guidelines for the management of occupational exposures to HIV and recommendations for postexposure prophylaxis. Centers for Disease Control and Prevention. MMWR Recomm Rep 2005;54 (RR-9): 1–17. (Level III)

69. Baffoy-Fayard N, Maugat S, Sapoval M, Cluzel P, Denys A, Sellier N, et al. Potential exposure to hepatitis C virus through accidental blood contact in interventional radiology. Study Group on Hygiene Practices in Interventional Radiology. J Vasc Interv Radiol 2003;14:173–9. (Level II-3)

The MEDLINE database, the Cochrane Library, and ACOG's own internal resources and documents were used to conduct a literature search to locate relevant articles published between January 1985 and February 2007. The search was restricted to articles published in the English language. Priority was given to articles reporting results of original research, although review articles and commentaries also were consulted. Abstracts of research presented at symposia and scientific conferences were not considered adequate for inclusion in this document. Guidelines published by organizations or institutions such as the National Institutes of Health and the American College of Obstetricians and Gynecologists were reviewed, and additional studies were located by reviewing bibliographies of identified articles. When reliable research was not available, expert opinions from obstetrician–gynecologists were used.

Studies were reviewed and evaluated for quality according to the method outlined by the U.S. Preventive Services Task Force:

I   Evidence obtained from at least one properly designed randomized controlled trial.

II-1   Evidence obtained from well-designed controlled trials without randomization.

II-2   Evidence obtained from well-designed cohort or case–control analytic studies, preferably from more than one center or research group.

II-3   Evidence obtained from multiple time series with or without the intervention. Dramatic results in uncontrolled experiments also could be regarded as this type of evidence.

III   Opinions of respected authorities, based on clinical experience, descriptive studies, or reports of expert committees.

Based on the highest level of evidence found in the data, recommendations are provided and graded according to the following categories:

Level A—Recommendations are based on good and consistent scientific evidence.

Level B—Recommendations are based on limited or inconsistent scientific evidence.

Level C—Recommendations are based primarily on consensus and expert opinion.

ISSN 1099-3630

The American College of Obstetricians and Gynecologists
409 12th Street, SW, PO Box 96920, Washington, DC 20090-6920

Viral hepatitis in pregnancy. ACOG Practice Bulletin No. 86. American College of Obstetricians and Gynecologists. Obstet Gynecol 2007;110:941–55.

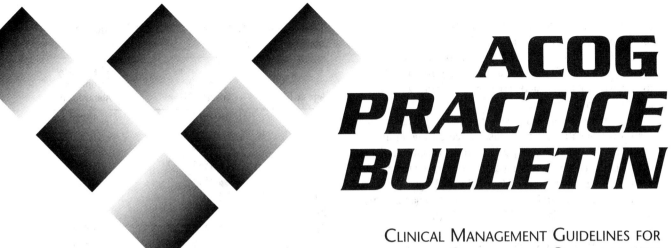

CLINICAL MANAGEMENT GUIDELINES FOR
OBSTETRICIAN–GYNECOLOGISTS
NUMBER 88, DECEMBER 2007

Invasive Prenatal Testing for Aneuploidy

Prenatal diagnosis of fetal chromosomal abnormalities is the most common indication for invasive prenatal testing. The prevalence of chromosomal abnormalities in clinically recognized early pregnancy loss is greater than 50% (1). Fetuses with aneuploidy account for 6–11% of all stillbirths and neonatal deaths (2). Chromosomal abnormalities that are compatible with life but cause considerable morbidity occur in 0.65% of newborns, and structural chromosomal rearrangements that will eventually affect reproduction occur in 0.2% of newborns (3). Consequently, screening and diagnostic programs to detect the most common autosomal trisomies in liveborn infants, including Down syndrome, are well established. The purpose of this document is to provide clinical management guidelines for the prenatal diagnosis of these aneuploidies.

This Practice Bulletin was developed by the ACOG Committee on Practice Bulletins— Obstetrics and the Committee on Genetics with the assistance of James Goldberg, MD. The information is designed to aid practitioners in making decisions about appropriate obstetric and gynecologic care. These guidelines should not be construed as dictating an exclusive course of treatment or procedure. Variations in practice may be warranted based on the needs of the individual patient, resources, and limitations unique to the institution or type of practice.

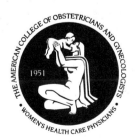

Background

There are many strategies available to screen for chromosomal abnormalities (4). These incorporate maternal age and a variety of first- and second-trimester ultrasound and biochemical markers that include nuchal translucency measurement and pregnancy-associated plasma protein A, human chorionic gonadotropin, alpha-fetoprotein, estriol, and inhibin levels. All of these approaches provide an adjusted risk for Down syndrome and trisomy 18. Whereas these risk figures provide a more accurate risk for Down syndrome and trisomy 18 than maternal age alone, they do not exclude the possibility of an affected fetus because the test sensitivity is less than 100%, so not all fetuses can be identified. Studies have shown that many factors influence a woman's decision to undergo an invasive procedure (5). These include feelings about having a child in whom a chromosomal abnormality has been diagnosed and feelings about the loss of a normal child as a result of the diagnostic procedure.

Down syndrome and other trisomies are primarily the result of meiotic nondisjunction, which increases with maternal age. Women contemplating screening versus diagnostic testing for aneuploidy may find it helpful to compare their adjusted risk after screening with their age-related risk (Table 1).

Fetuses with aneuploidy may have major anatomic malformations that often are discovered during an ultrasound examination that is performed for another indication. Abnormalities involving a major organ or structure, with a few notable exceptions, or the finding of two or more minor structural abnormalities in the same fetus indicate increased risk of fetal aneuploidy (6, 7) (Table 2). There are genetic and nongenetic causes of structural anomalies. If an aneuploidy is suspected, only a cytogenetic analysis of fetal cells can provide a definitive diagnosis. In some cases, a fetal karyotype will be sufficient but, in other situations, adjunct testing such as fluorescence in situ hybridization or other genetic testing may be required to detect chromosomal microdeletions or duplications or to further characterize marker chromosomes or chromosomal rearrangements.

Amniocentesis

Traditional genetic amniocentesis usually is offered between 15 weeks and 20 weeks of gestation. Many large, multicenter studies have confirmed the safety of genetic amniocentesis as well as its cytogenetic diagnostic accuracy (greater than 99%) (8). All of the large collaborative studies in which the risk of amniocentesis was evaluated were performed before the use of high-resolution concurrent ultrasonography. In more recent studies, it is suggested that the procedure-related loss rate is as low as 1 in 300–500 and may be even lower with experienced individuals or centers (9, 10). Complications, which occur infrequently, include transient vaginal spotting or amniotic fluid leakage in approximately 1–2% of all cases and chorioamnionitis in less than 1 in 1,000 cases. The perinatal survival rate in cases of amniotic fluid leakage after midtrimester amniocentesis is greater than 90% (11). Needle injuries to the fetus have been reported but are very rare when amniocentesis is performed under continuous ultrasound guidance. Amniotic fluid cell culture failure occurs in 0.1% of samples. In several studies, it has been confirmed that the incidence of pregnancy loss, blood-contaminated specimens, leaking of amniotic fluid, and the need for more than one needle puncture are related to the experience of the operator, the use of small-gauge needles, and ultrasound guidance (12–14).

Early amniocentesis performed from 11 weeks to 13 weeks of gestation has been widely studied, and the tech-

Table 1. Risk Table for Chromosomal Abnormalities By Maternal Age at Term

Age at Term	Risk for Trisomy 21[†]	Risk for Any Chromosome Abnormality[‡]
15*	1:1578	1:454
16*	1:1572	1:475
17*	1:1565	1:499
18*	1:1556	1:525
19*	1:1544	1:555
20	1:1480	1:525
21	1:1460	1:525
22	1:1440	1:499
23	1:1420	1:499
24	1:1380	1:475
25	1:1340	1:475
26	1:1290	1:475
27	1:1220	1:454
28	1:1140	1:434
29	1:1050	1:416
30	1:940	1:384
31	1:820	1:384
32	1:700	1:322
33	1:570	1:285
34	1:456	1:243
35	1:353	1:178
36	1:267	1:148
37	1:199	1:122
38	1:148	1:104
39	1:111	1:80
40	1:85	1:62
41	1:67	1:48
42	1:54	1:38
43	1:45	1:30
44	1:39	1:23
45	1:35	1:18
46	1:31	1:14
47	1:29	1:10
48	1:27	1:8
49	1:26	1:6
50	1:25	§

*Data from Cuckle HS, Wald NJ, Thompson SG. Estimating a woman's risk of having a pregnancy associated with Down's syndrome using her age and serum alpha-fetoprotein level. Br J Obstet Gynaecol 1987;94:387–402.

[†]Data from Morris JK, Wald NJ, Mutton DE, Alberman E. Comparison of models of maternal age-specific risk for Down syndrome live births. Prenat Diagn 2003;23:252–8.

[‡]Risk for any chromosomal abnormality includes the risk for trisomy 21 and trisomy 18 in addition to trisomy 13, 47,XXY, 47,XYY, Turner syndrome genotype, and other clinically significant abnormalities, 47,XXX not included. Data from Hook EB. Rates of chromosome abnormalities at different maternal ages. Obstet Gynecol 1981;58:282–5.

§Data not available

Table 2. Aneuploid Risk of Major Anomalies

Structural Defect	Population Incidence	Aneuploidy Risk	Most Common Aneuploidy
Cystic hygroma	1/120 EU–1/6,000 B	60–75%	45X (80%); 21,18,13,XXY
Hydrops	1/1,500–4,000 B	30–80%*	13,21,18,45X
Hydrocephalus	3–8/10,000 LB	3–8%	13,18, triploidy
Hydranencephaly	2/1,000 IA	Minimal	
Holoprosencephaly	1/16,000 LB	40–60%	13,18,18p-
Cardiac defects	7–9/1,000 LB	5–30%	21,18,13,22,8,9
Complete atrioventricular canal		40–70%	21
Diaphragmatic hernia	1/3,500–4,000 LB	20–25%	13,18,21,45X
Omphalocele	1/5,800 LB	30–40%	13,18
Gastroschisis	1/10,000–15,000 LB	Minimal	
Duodenal atresia	1/10,000 LB	20–30%	21
Bladder outlet obstruction	1–2/1,000 LB	20–25%	13,18
Facial cleft	1/700 LB	1%	13,18, deletions
Limb reduction	4–6/10,000 LB	8%	18
Club foot	1.2/1,000 LB	6%	18,13,4p-,18q-
Single umbilical artery	1%	Minimal	

Abbreviations: B, birth; EU, early ultrasonography; LB, livebirth; IA, infant autopsy

*30% if diagnosed at 24 weeks of gestation or later; 80% if diagnosed at 17 weeks of gestation or earlier

Data from Shipp TD, Benacerraf BR. The significance of prenatally identified isolated clubfoot: is amniocentesis indicated? Am J Obstet Gynecol 1998;178:600–602 and Nyberg DA, Crane JP. Chromosome abnormalities. In: Nyberg DA, Mahony BS, Pretorius DH. Diagnostic ultrasound of fetal anomalies: text and atlas. Chicago (IL): Year Book Medical; 1990. p. 676–724.

nique is similar to traditional amniocentesis (15–17); however, performing early amniocentesis results in significantly higher rates of pregnancy loss and complication than performing traditional amniocentesis. In a multicenter randomized trial, the spontaneous pregnancy loss rate after early amniocentesis was 2.5%, compared with 0.7% with traditional amniocentesis (18). The overall incidence of talipes was 1.4% after the early procedure, compared with 0.1% (the same as the background rate) after traditional amniocentesis, and membrane rupture was more likely after the early procedure. Significantly more amniotic fluid culture failures occurred after the early procedure, necessitating an additional invasive procedure for diagnosis. For these reasons, early amniocentesis (at less than 14 weeks of gestation) should not be performed.

Chorionic Villus Sampling

Chorionic villus sampling (CVS) generally is performed after 9 completed weeks of gestation. Placental villi may be obtained through transcervical or transabdominal access to the placenta. There is no difference in fetal loss

rates after transcervical or transabdominal CVS (8). The primary advantage of CVS over amniocentesis is that results are available earlier in pregnancy, which provides reassurance for parents when results are normal and, when results are abnormal, may allow for earlier and safer methods of pregnancy termination.

The overall pregnancy loss rate after CVS is greater than the rate after midtrimester amniocentesis because of the increased background rate of spontaneous pregnancy loss between 9 weeks and 16 weeks of gestation. Although recent data are limited, the procedure-related pregnancy loss rate for CVS appears to approach, and may be the same as, the rate for midtrimester amniocentesis (19–22).

In several studies, it has been shown that there is a significant learning curve associated with the safe performance of CVS (23, 24). Consequently, the pregnancy loss data described previously is only valid in experienced centers.

Although there have been reports of associations between CVS and limb reduction and oromandibular defects, the risk for these anomalies is unclear (25). In an analysis by the World Health Organization, an incidence of limb-reduction defects of 6 per 10,000 was reported, which is not significantly different from the incidence in the general population (26). However, a workshop on CVS and limb reduction defects sponsored by the U.S. National Center for Environmental Health and the Centers for Disease Control and Prevention concluded that transverse limb deficiencies appeared to be more common after CVS. The frequency of limb reduction defects is highest when CVS is performed before 9 weeks of gestation (27, 28). In addition, a panel convened by the National Institute of Child Health and Development and the American College of Obstetricians and Gynecologists concluded that oromandibular–limb hypogenesis appeared to be more common among infants who were exposed to CVS and appeared to correlate with, but may not be limited to, CVS performed earlier than 7 weeks of gestation (25). Women considering CVS who are concerned about the possible association of CVS with limb defects can be reassured that when the procedure is performed after 9 weeks of gestation, the risk is low and probably not greater than the general population risk of limb defects.

Other complications after CVS include vaginal spotting or bleeding, which may occur in up to 32.2% of patients after transcervical CVS is performed. The incidence after transabdominal CVS is performed is less (29). The incidence of culture failure, amniotic fluid leakage, or infection after CVS is performed is less than 0.5% (29).

Cordocentesis

Cordocentesis, also known as percutaneous umbilical blood sampling, involves puncturing the umbilical vein under direct ultrasound guidance. Karyotype analysis of fetal blood usually can be accomplished within 24–48 hours. The procedure-related pregnancy loss rate has been reported to be less than 2% (30). Cordocentesis is rarely needed but may be useful to further evaluate chromosomal mosaicism discovered after CVS or amniocentesis is performed.

Clinical Considerations and Recommendations

▶ *Who should have the option of prenatal diagnosis for fetal chromosomal abnormalities?*

Invasive diagnostic testing for aneuploidy should be available to all women, regardless of maternal age. Pretest counseling should include a discussion of the risks and benefits of invasive testing compared with

screening tests; how many women will have a positive result (screen-positive rate) and, of those, how many will have a true positive result (detection rate); the detection rate of aneuploidies other than Down syndrome; and the type and prognosis of the aneuploidies likely to be missed by serum screening. Counseling should be provided by a practitioner familiar with these details. The differences between screening and diagnostic testing should be discussed with all women. A woman's decision of whether to have screening, an amniocentesis, or CVS is based on many factors, including the risk that the fetus will have a chromosomal abnormality, the risk of pregnancy loss from an invasive procedure, and the consequences of having an affected child. Studies that have evaluated women's preferences have shown that women weigh these potential outcomes differently. The decision to perform invasive testing should take into account these preferences and should not be based solely on age. Maternal age of 35 years alone should no longer be used as a threshold to determine who is offered screening versus who is offered invasive testing.

▶ *How is the risk of aneuploidy assessed?*

The risk for fetal aneuploidy can be determined by referring to maternal age-specific aneuploidy risk tables or using age-adjusted risks after screening. It may be helpful to compare the patient's individual risks with risk cutoffs used to indicate a positive screening test result. These cutoffs are based on the specific detection rate and screen-positive rate of the screening approach that is used.

▶ *Who is at increased risk for aneuploidy?*

Patients with an increased risk of fetal aneuploidy include the following categories:

- Previous fetus or child with autosomal trisomy— Recently, a large collaborative study reported that the risk of trisomy recurrence is 1.6–8.2 times the maternal age risk depending on the type of trisomy, whether the index pregnancy was a spontaneous abortion, maternal age at initial occurrence, and the maternal age at subsequent prenatal diagnosis (31).

- Structural anomalies identified by ultrasonography—The presence of one major or at least two minor fetal structural abnormalities increases the likelihood of aneuploidy (6, 7). However, there are some isolated malformations that are not usually associated with aneuploidy and that may not require further testing (Table 2).

- Previous fetus or child with sex chromosome abnormality—Not all sex chromosome abnormalities have maternal origin, and not all have a risk of recurrence. As with autosomal trisomies, the recurrence risk is 1.6–2.5 times the maternal age risk. A woman whose previous offspring had a 47,XYY karyotype is not at increased risk of recurrence because the extra chromosome is paternal in origin. Turner syndrome (45,X) has a nominal risk of recurrence. Parents of children with 47,XYY or 45,X karyotypes may still request prenatal diagnosis in future pregnancies for reassurance.

- Parental carrier of chromosome translocation— Women or men carrying balanced translocations, although phenotypically normal themselves, are at risk of producing unbalanced gametes, resulting in abnormal offspring. For most translocations, the observed risk of abnormal liveborn children is less than the theoretic risk because some of these gametes result in nonviable conceptions. In general, carriers of chromosome translocations that are identified after the birth of an abnormal child have a 5–30% risk of having unbalanced offspring in the future, whereas those identified for other reasons (eg, during an infertility workup) have a 0–5% risk (1). Genetic counseling may be helpful in such situations.

- Parental carrier of chromosome inversion—An inversion occurs when two breaks occur in the same chromosome and the intervening genetic material is inverted before the breaks are repaired. Although no genetic material is lost or duplicated, the rearrangement may alter gene function. Each carrier's risk of having a liveborn abnormal child is related to the method of ascertainment, the chromosome involved, and the size of the inversion; thus, risks should be determined individually. The observed risk is approximately 5–10% if the inversion is identified after the birth of an abnormal child and 1–3% if ascertainment occurs at some other time (1). One exception is a pericentric inversion of chromosome 9, which is a common variant in the general population and of no clinical consequence.

- Parental aneuploidy or mosaicism for aneuploidy— Women with trisomy 21, although subfertile, have approximately a 50% risk of having trisomic offspring. Women with 47,XXX and men with 47,XYY usually are fertile and have no discernible increase in risk of having trisomic offspring. In men with a normal karyotype who have oligospermia or whose partners conceive from intracytoplasmic sperm injection, there is an increased incidence of abnormal karyotype in the sperm (32).

▶ What type of laboratory test should be performed to diagnose aneuploidy?

Metaphase analysis of cultured amniocytes or chorionic villus cells is the preferred method for karyotype analysis. This approach is highly accurate, with results typically available 1–2 weeks after the procedure. Fluorescence in situ hybridization (FISH) analysis provides a more rapid result for specific chromosomes, most commonly chromosomes 13, 18, 21, X, and Y. Whereas FISH analysis has been shown to be accurate, false-positive and false-negative results have been reported. Therefore, clinical decision making should be based on information from FISH and at least one of the following results: confirmatory traditional metaphase chromosome analysis or consistent clinical information, such as an abnormal ultrasound finding or a positive screening test result for Down syndrome or trisomy 18 (33).

Comparative genomic hybridization (CGH) is an evolving method that identifies submicroscopic chromosomal deletions and duplications. This approach has proved useful in identifying abnormalities in individuals with developmental delay and physical abnormalities when results of traditional chromosomal analysis have been normal (34). The use of CGH in prenatal diagnosis, at present, is limited because of the difficulty in interpreting which DNA alterations revealed through CGH may be normal population variants. Until there are more data available, use of CGH for routine prenatal diagnosis is not recommended.

▶ How often does chromosomal mosaicism occur in amniocentesis or chorionic villus sampling results?

Chromosomal mosaicism, the presence of more than one cell line identified during cytogenetic analysis, occurs in approximately 0.25% of amniocentesis specimens and 1% of chorionic villus specimens. After mosaicism is found by CVS, amniocentesis typically is performed to assess whether mosaicism is present in amniocytes. In most cases, the amniocentesis result is normal, and the mosaicism is assumed to be confined to the trophoblast. Although this is unlikely to cause defects in the fetus, it may result in third-trimester growth restriction. Clinical manifestations depend on the specific mosaic cell line(s) and may range from completely normal to findings consistent with the abnormal chromosome result. Counseling following the finding of chromosomal mosaicism is complex, and referral for genetic counseling may be useful in these cases. In some instances, cordocentesis may be recommended.

A special case of mosaicism is maternal cell contamination of the fetal specimen. This can be minimized by discarding the first 1–2 milliliters of the amniocentesis specimen and by careful dissection of chorionic villi from maternal decidua.

▶ *How should you counsel women who have chronic infections, such as hepatitis B, hepatitis C or human immunodeficiency virus, about invasive prenatal testing?*

The risk of neonatal infection through amniocentesis in women who are chronically infected with hepatitis B or hepatitis C appears to be low, although the number of exposed cases in the literature is small (35). Of 115 women reported to be positive for the hepatitis B surface antigen who underwent second-trimester amniocentesis, the rate of neonatal infection was no different than in women who did not have an amniocentesis. All of the infants received hepatitis B vaccination and immunoprophylaxis beginning at birth (36–39). There is only one series reported in the literature in which 22 women who were positive for hepatitis C underwent second-trimester amniocentesis. No infants in this series were found to be hepatitis C RNA positive on postnatal testing. This group included one woman with amniotic fluid that was hepatitis C RNA positive (40). There are insufficient data in the literature to assess the risk of CVS in these women or to estimate the risk of fetal infection among women with anterior placentas, those who are hepatitis B e antigen positive or those with high hepatitis B or hepatitis C viral loads.

Amniocentesis in women with human immunodeficiency virus (HIV) has been shown to increase the vertical transmission rate in women who do not receive retroviral therapy (41). In a recent report of a small number of cases, it is suggested that amniocentesis or CVS does not increase the neonatal infection rate in newborns of women infected with HIV who are receiving retroviral therapy (42).

Because of the limited information regarding the risk of invasive procedures in women chronically infected with hepatitis B, hepatitis C, or HIV, it would be prudent to discuss noninvasive screening options with these women.

▶ *How does prenatal diagnosis differ for women with multiple gestations?*

Diagnostic options are more limited in high-order gestations (43). In women with twins, the risk of aneuploidy should be calculated by considering the maternal age-related risk of aneuploidy, population risk of dizygosity, and the probability that either one or both fetuses could be affected. Formulas and tables are available in the literature to help with these calculations (44). Counseling in this situation should include a discussion of options for pregnancy management if only one fetus is found to be

affected. These options include terminating the entire pregnancy, selective second-trimester termination of the affected fetus, and continuing the pregnancy.

Scant data exist concerning fetal loss in women with twin gestation when amniocentesis or CVS is performed. According to some small series, the fetal loss rate is approximately 3.5% when amniocentesis is performed in women with multiple gestations; this was not higher than the background loss rate for twins in the second trimester in one series with a control group (30, 45, 46). There are no data concerning loss rates after amniocentesis is performed in women with high-order multiple gestations. Similar information for twin gestations from small, non-randomized series exists for CVS (46–48).

A complex counseling issue arises in the presence of a monochorionic twin gestation, in which case the likelihood of discordance in the karyotype is low, and patients may opt for having a karyotype analysis performed on a single fetus. In this situation, it is important to discuss the accuracy of determining chorionicity by ultrasonography. The determination of chorionicity is most accurate if ultrasonography is performed at or before 14 weeks of gestation. The positive predictive value of monochorionicity is 97.8% at this stage of pregnancy. This decreases to 88% if the ultrasound examination is performed after 14 weeks of gestation (49).

▶ *What information should be provided after the diagnosis of fetal aneuploidy?*

After the diagnosis of a chromosomal abnormality, the patient should receive detailed information, if known, about the natural history of individuals with the specific chromosomal finding. In many cases, it may be very helpful to refer the patient to a genetic counselor or clinical geneticist and national groups such as The National Down Syndrome Society (www.ndss.org) or National Down Syndrome Congress (www.ndsccenter.org) to help the patient make an informed decision. The option of pregnancy termination also should be discussed. Patients may benefit from additional ultrasonography or fetal echocardiography and referral to appropriate obstetric and pediatric specialists or neonatologists to discuss pregnancy and neonatal management issues. Referral to parent support groups, counselors, social workers, or clergy may provide additional information and support.

▶ *Is there value in prenatal diagnosis for the patient who would decline pregnancy termination?*

Prenatal diagnosis is not performed solely for assistance in the decision of pregnancy termination. It can provide useful information for the physician and the patient. Nondirective counseling before prenatal diagnostic testing does not require a patient to commit to pregnancy termination if the result is abnormal. If it is determined that the fetus has a chromosomal abnormality, the physicians and family can plan ahead and develop a management plan for the remainder of the pregnancy, labor, and delivery (50).

Summary of Recommendations and Conclusions

The following recommendation is based on good and consistent scientific evidence (Level A):

▶ Early amniocentesis (at less than 15 weeks of gestation) should not be performed because of the higher risk of pregnancy loss and complications compared with traditional amniocentesis (15 weeks of gestation or later)

The following conclusions are based on limited or inconsistent scientific evidence (Level B):

▶ Amniocentesis at 15 weeks of gestation or later is a safe procedure. The procedure-related loss rate after midtrimester amniocentesis is less than 1 in 300–500.

▶ In experienced individuals and centers, CVS procedure-related loss rates may be the same as those for amniocentesis.

The following recommendation and conclusions are based primarily on consensus and expert opinion (Level C):

▶ Invasive diagnostic testing for aneuploidy should be available to all women, regardless of maternal age.

▶ Patients with an increased risk of fetal aneuploidy include women with a previous fetus or child with an autosomal trisomy or sex chromosome abnormality, one major or at least two minor fetal structural defects identified by ultrasonography, either parent with a chromosomal translocation or chromosomal inversion, or parental aneuploidy.

▶ Nondirective counseling before prenatal diagnostic testing does not require a patient to commit to pregnancy termination if the result is abnormal.

Proposed Performance Measure

The percentage of pregnant women undergoing invasive testing who were counseled about the risks of the procedure

References

1. Gardner RJ, Sutherland GR. Chromosome abnormalities and genetic counseling. 3rd ed. New York (NY): Oxford University Press; 2004. (Level III)

2. Alberman ED, Creasy MR. Frequency of chromosomal abnormalities in miscarriages and perinatal deaths. J Med Genet 1977;14:313–5. (Level III)

3. Milunsky A, Milunsky JM. Genetic counseling: preconception, prenatal, and perinatal. In: Milunsky A, editor. Genetic disorders and the fetus: diagnosis, prevention, and treatment. 5th ed. Baltimore (MD): Johns Hopkins University Press; 2004. p. 1–65. (Level III)

4. Screening for fetal chromosomal abnormalities. ACOG Practice Bulletin No. 77. American College of Obstetricians and Gynecologists. Obstet Gynecol 2007;109:217–27. (Level III)

5. Kuppermann M, Nease RF, Learman LA, Gates E, Blumberg B, Washington AE. Procedure-related miscarriages and Down syndrome-affected births: implications for prenatal testing based on women's preferences. Obstet Gynecol 2000;96:511–6. (Level II-3)

6. Williamson RA, Weiner CP, Patil S, Benda J, Varner MW, Abu-Yousef MM. Abnormal pregnancy sonogram: selective indication for fetal karyotype. Obstet Gynecol 1987;69:15–20. (Level III)

7. Wladimiroff JW, Sachs ES, Reuss A, Stewart PA, Pijpers L, Niermeijer MF. Prenatal diagnosis of chromosome abnormalities in the presence of fetal structural defects. Am J Med Genet 1988;29:289–91. (Level III)

8. Jackson LG, Zachary JM, Fowler SE, Desnick RJ, Golbus MS, Ledbetter DH, et al. A randomized comparison of transcervical and transabdominal chorionic-villus sampling. The U.S. National Institute of Child Health and Human Development Chorionic-Villus Sampling and Amniocentesis Study Group. N Engl J Med 1992;327:594–8. (Level I)

9. Mazza V, Pati M, Bertucci E, Re C, Ranzi A, Percesepe A, et al. Age-specific risk of fetal loss post second trimester amniocentesis: analysis of 5,043 cases. Prenat Diagn 2007;27:180–3. (Level II-3)

10. Eddleman KA, Malone FD, Sullivan L, Dukes K, Berkowitz RL, Kharbutli Y, et al. Pregnancy loss rates after midtrimester amniocentesis. Obstet Gynecol 2006;108:1067–72. (Level II-2)

11. Borgida AF, Mills AA, Feldman DM, Rodis JF, Egan JF. Outcome of pregnancies complicated by ruptured membranes after genetic amniocentesis. Am J Obstet Gynecol 2000;183:937–9. (Level II-2)

12. Mennuti MT, DiGaetano A, McDonnell A, Cohen AW, Liston RM. Fetal-maternal bleeding associated with genetic amniocentesis: real-time versus static ultrasound. Obstet Gynecol 1983;62:26–30. (Level II-2)

13. Romero R, Jeanty P, Reece EA, Grannum P, Bracken M, Berkowitz R, et al. Sonographically monitored amniocentesis to decrease intraoperative complications. Obstet Gynecol 1985;65:426–30. (Level II-2)

14. Leschot NJ, Verjaal M, Treffers PE. Risks of midtrimester amniocentesis; assessment in 3,000 pregnancies. Br J Obstet Gynaecol 1985 Aug;92(8):804–7. (Level III)

15. Nicolaides K, Brizot Mde L, Patel F, Snijders R. Comparison of chorionic villus sampling and amniocentesis for fetal karyotyping at 10–13 weeks' gestation [published erratum appears in: Lancet 1994;344:830]. Lancet 1994;344:435–9. (Level II-2)

16. Johnson JM, Wilson RD, Winsor EJ, Singer J, Dansereau J, Kalousek DK. The early amniocentesis study: a randomized clinical trial of early amniocentesis versus midtrimester amniocentesis. Fetal Diagn Ther 1996; 11: 85–93. (Level I)

17. Sundberg K, Bang J, Smidt-Jensen S, Brocks V, Lundsteen C, Parner J, et al. Randomised study of risk of fetal loss related to early amniocentesis versus chorionic villus sampling. Lancet 1997;350:697–703. (Level I)

18. Randomised trial to assess safety and fetal outcome of early and midtrimester amniocentesis. The Canadian Early and Mid-trimester Amniocentesis Trial (CEMAT) Group. Lancet 1998;351:242–7. (Level I)

19. Multicentre randomised clinical trial of chorion villus sampling and amniocentesis. First report. Canadian Collaborative CVS-Amniocentesis Clinical Trial Group. Lancet 1989;1:1–6. (Level I)

20. Rhoads GG, Jackson LG, Schlesselman SE, de la Cruz FF, Desnick RJ, Golbus MS, et al. The safety and efficacy of chorionic villus sampling for early prenatal diagnosis of cytogenetic abnormalities. N Engl J Med 1989;320: 609–17. (Level II-3)

21. Caughey AB, Hopkins LM, Norton ME. Chorionic villus sampling compared with amniocentesis and the difference in the rate of pregnancy loss. Obstet Gynecol 2006;108: 612–6. (Level II-2)

22. Mujezinovic F, Alfirevic Z. Procedure-related complications of amniocentesis and chorionic villous sampling: a systematic review. Obstet Gynecol 2007;110:687–94.

23. Silver RK, MacGregor SN, Sholl JS, Hobart ED, Waldee JK. An evaluation of the chorionic villus sampling learning curve. Am J Obstet Gynecol 1990;163:917–22. (Level III)

24. Wijnberger LD, van der Schouw YT, Christiaens GC. Learning in medicine: chorionic villus sampling. Prenat Diagn 2000;20:241–6. (Level II-3)

25. Holmes LB. Report of National Institute of Child Health and Human Development Workshop on Chorionic Villus Sampling and Limb and Other Defects, October 20, 1992. Teratology 1993;48:7–13. (Level III)

26. Kuliev A, Jackson L, Froster U, Brambati B, Simpson JL, Verlinsky Y, et al. Chorionic villus sampling safety. Report of World Health Organization/EURO meeting in association with the Seventh International Conference on Early Prenatal Diagnosis of Genetic Diseases, Tel-Aviv, Israel, May 21, 1994. Am J Obstet Gynecol 1996;174: 807–11. (Level III)

27. Botto LD, Olney RS, Mastroiacovo P, Khoury MJ, Moore CA, Alo CJ, et al. Chorionic villus sampling and transverse digital deficiencies: evidence for anatomic and gestational-age specificity of the digital deficiencies in two studies. Am J Med Genet 1996;62:173–8. (Level II-2)

28. Chorionic villus sampling and amniocentesis: recommendations for prenatal counseling. Centers for Disease Control and Prevention. MMWR Recomm Rep 1995;44 (RR-9):1–12. (Level III)

29. Brambati B, Tului L. Prenatal genetic diagnosis through chorionic villus sampling. In: Milunsky A. Genetic disorders and the fetus: diagnosis, prevention, and treatment. 5th ed. Baltimore (MD): Johns Hopkins University Press; 2004. p. 179–213. (Level III)

30. Ghidini A, Sepulveda W, Lockwood CJ, Romero R. Complications of fetal blood sampling. Am J Obstet Gynecol 1993;168:1339–44. (Level II-3)

31. Warburton D, Dallaire L, Thangavelu M, Ross L, Levin B, Kline J. Trisomy recurrence: a reconsideration based on North American data. Am J Hum Genet 2004;75:376–85. (Level III)

32. Burrello N, Vicari E, Calogero AE. Chromosome abnormalities in spermatozoa of patients with azoospermia and normal somatic karyotype. Cytogenet Genome Res 2005;111:363–5. (Level III)

33. Technical and clinical assessment of fluorescence in situ hybridization: an ACMG/ASHG position statement. I. Technical considerations. American College of Medical Genetics. Genet Med 2000;2:356–61. (Level III)

34. Kirchhoff M, Rose H, Lundsteen C. High resolution comparative genomic hybridisation in clinical cytogenetics. J Med Genet 2001;38:740–4. (Level III)

35. Amniocentesis and women with hepatitis B, hepatitis C, or human immunodeficiency virus. SOGC Clinical Practice Guidelines. Society of Obstetricians and Gynaecologists of Canada. J Obstet Gynaecol Can 2003;25:145–48, 149–52. (Level III)

36. Towers CV, Asra T, Rumney P. The presence of hepatitis B surface antigen and deoxyribonucleic acid in amniotic fluid and cord blood. Am J Obstet Gynecol 1999;184: 1514–8. (Level II-2)

37. Alexander JM, Ramus R, Jackson G, Sercely B, Wendel GD Jr. Risk of hepatitis B transmission after amniocentesis in chronic hepatitis B carriers. Infect Dis Obstet Gynecol 1999;7:283–6. (Level III)

38. Grosheide PM, Quartero HW, Schalm SW, Heijtink RA, Christiaens GC. Early invasive prenatal diagnosis in HBsAg-positive women. Prenat Diagn 1994;14:553–8. (Level III)

39. Ko TM, Tseng LH, Chang MH, Chen DS, Hsieh FJ, Chuang SM, et al. Amniocentesis in mothers who are hep-

atitis B virus carriers does not expose the infant to an increased risk of hepatitis B virus infection. Arch Gynecol Obstet 1994;255:25–30. (Level II-2)

40. Delamare C, Carbonne B, Heim N, Berkane N, Petit JC, Uzan S, et al. Detection of hepatitis C virus RNA (HCV RNA) in amniotic fluid: a prospective study. J Hepatol 1999;31:416–20. (Level II-2)

41. Shapiro DE, Sperling RS, Mandelbrot L, Britto P, Cunningham BE. Risk factors for perinatal human immunodeficiency virus transmission in patients receiving zidovudine prophylaxis. Pediatric AIDS Clinical Trials Group protocol 076 Study Group. Obstet Gynecol 1999;94:897–908. (Level I)

42. Somigliana E, Bucceri AM, Tibaldi C, Alberico S, Ravizza M, Savasi V, et al. Early invasive diagnostic techniques in pregnant women who are infected with the HIV: a multicenter case series. Italian Collaborative Study on HIV Infection in Pregnancy. Am J Obstet Gynecol 2005; 193:437–42. (Level III)

43. Jenkins TM, Wapner RJ. The challenge of prenatal diagnosis in twin pregnancies. Curr Opin Obstet Gynecol 2000;12:87–92. (Level III)

44. Rodis JF, Egan JF, Craffey A, Ciarleglio L, Greenstein RM, Scorza WE. Calculated risk of chromosomal abnormalities in twin gestations. Obstet Gynecol 1990;76: 1037–41. (Level III)

45. Librach CL, Doran TA, Benzie RJ, Jones JM. Genetic amniocentesis in seventy twin pregnancies. Am J Obstet Gynecol 1984;148:585–91. (Level III)

46. Wapner RJ, Johnson A, Davis G, Urban A, Morgan P, Jackson L. Prenatal diagnosis in twin gestations: a comparison between second-trimester amniocentesis and first-trimester chorionic villus sampling. Obstet Gynecol 1993;82:49–56. (Level II-2)

47. De Catte L, Liebaers I, Foulon W, Bonduelle M, Van Assche E. First trimester chorionic villus sampling in twin gestations. Am J Perinatol 1996;13:413–7. (Level II-3)

48. van den Berg C, Braat AP, Van Opstal D, Halley DJ, Kleijer WJ, den Hollander NS, et al. Amniocentesis or chorionic villus sampling in multiple gestations? Experience with 500 cases. Prenat Diagn 1999;19: 234–244. (Level II-3)

49. Lee YM, Cleary-Goldman J, Thaker HM, Simpson LL. Antenatal sonographic prediction of twin chorionicity. Am J Obstet Gynecol 2006;195:863–7. (Level II-3)

50. Clark SL, DeVore GR. Prenatal diagnosis for couples who would not consider abortion. Prenat Diagn 1989;73: 1035–7. (Level III)

The MEDLINE database, the Cochrane Library, and ACOG's own internal resources and documents were used to conduct a literature search to locate relevant articles published between January 1985 and June 2007. The search was restricted to articles published in the English language. Priority was given to articles reporting results of original research, although review articles and commentaries also were consulted. Abstracts of research presented at symposia and scientific conferences were not considered adequate for inclusion in this document. Guidelines published by organizations or institutions such as the National Institutes of Health and the American College of Obstetricians and Gynecologists were reviewed, and additional studies were located by reviewing bibliographies of identified articles. When reliable research was not available, expert opinions from obstetrician–gynecologists were used.

Studies were reviewed and evaluated for quality according to the method outlined by the U.S. Preventive Services Task Force:

I   Evidence obtained from at least one properly designed randomized controlled trial.

II-1   Evidence obtained from well-designed controlled trials without randomization.

II-2   Evidence obtained from well-designed cohort or case–control analytic studies, preferably from more than one center or research group.

II-3   Evidence obtained from multiple time series with or without the intervention. Dramatic results in uncontrolled experiments also could be regarded as this type of evidence.

III   Opinions of respected authorities, based on clinical experience, descriptive studies, or reports of expert committees.

Based on the highest level of evidence found in the data, recommendations are provided and graded according to the following categories:

Level A—Recommendations are based on good and consistent scientific evidence.

Level B—Recommendations are based on limited or inconsistent scientific evidence.

Level C—Recommendations are based primarily on consensus and expert opinion.

ISSN 1099-3630

The American College of Obstetricians and Gynecologists
409 12th Street, SW, PO Box 96920, Washington, DC 20090-6920

Invasive prenatal testing for aneuploidy. ACOG Practice Bulletin No. 88. American College of Obstetricians and Gynecologists. Obstet Gynecol 2007;110:1459–67.

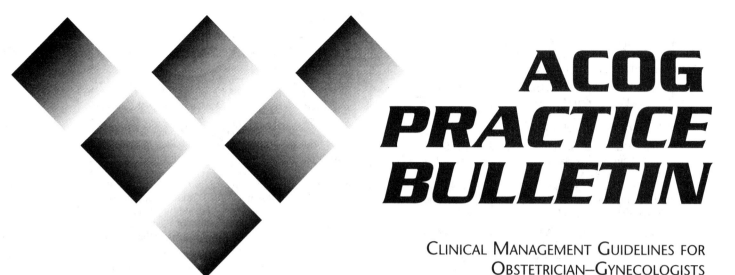

CLINICAL MANAGEMENT GUIDELINES FOR
OBSTETRICIAN–GYNECOLOGISTS
NUMBER 90, FEBRUARY 2008

Asthma in Pregnancy

Asthma is a common, potentially serious medical condition that complicates approximately 4–8% of pregnancies (1, 2). In general, the prevalence of and morbidity from asthma are increasing, although asthma mortality rates have decreased in recent years. The purpose of this document is to review the best available evidence about the management of asthma during pregnancy.

This Practice Bulletin was developed by the ACOG Committee on Practice Bulletins—Obstetrics with the assistance of Mitchell P. Dombrowski, MD and Michael Schatz, MD, MS. The information is designed to aid practitioners in making decisions about appropriate obstetric and gynecologic care. These guidelines should not be construed as dictating an exclusive course of treatment or procedure. Variations in practice may be warranted based on the needs of the individual patient, resources, and limitations unique to the institution or type of practice.

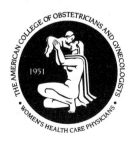

Background

Asthma is characterized by chronic airway inflammation, with increased airway responsiveness to a variety of stimuli, and airway obstruction that is partially or completely reversible (3). The pathogenesis of asthma involves airway inflammation in nearly all cases. Current medical management for asthma emphasizes treatment of airway inflammation in order to decrease airway responsiveness and prevent asthma symptoms.

The National Asthma Education and Prevention Program has found that "it is safer for pregnant women with asthma to be treated with asthma medications than it is for them to have asthma symptoms and exacerbations" (4). Mild and well-controlled moderate asthma can be associated with excellent maternal and perinatal pregnancy outcomes (5–7). Severe and poorly controlled asthma may be associated with increased prematurity, need for cesarean delivery, preeclampsia, growth restriction, other perinatal complications, and maternal morbidity and mortality (8–12). The ultimate goal of asthma therapy in pregnancy is maintaining adequate oxygenation of the fetus by preventing hypoxic episodes in the mother. Optimal management of asthma during pregnancy includes objective monitoring of lung function, avoiding or controlling asthma triggers, educating patients, and individualizing pharmacologic therapy to maintain normal pulmonary function. The step-care therapeutic approach uses the lowest amount of drug intervention necessary to control a patient's severity of asthma.

Medications

Asthma medications generally are divided into long-term control medications and rescue therapy. Long-term control medications are used for maintenance therapy to prevent asthma manifestations and include inhaled corticosteroids, cromolyn, long-acting β-agonists, and theophylline. Rescue therapy, most commonly inhaled short-acting β-agonists, provides immediate relief of symptoms. Oral corticosteroids can either be used as a form of rescue therapy to treat an asthma exacerbation or as long-term control therapy for patients with severe persistent asthma.

Certain medications, possibly used during labor and delivery, have the potential to worsen asthma. Nonselective β-blockers, carboprost (15-methyl prostaglandin $F_{2\alpha}$) and ergonovine may trigger bronchospasm. Magnesium sulfate is a bronchodilator, but indomethacin can induce bronchospasm in patients who are sensitive to aspirin. Prostaglandin E_2 or prostaglandin E_1 can be used for cervical ripening, the management of spontaneous or induced abortions, or the management of postpartum hemorrhage (13).

Asthma Severity Classification

In 2004, the National Asthma Education and Prevention Program Working Group on Asthma and Pregnancy defined mild intermittent, mild persistent, moderate persistent, and severe persistent asthma according to daytime and nighttime symptoms (wheezing, coughing, or dyspnea) and objective tests of pulmonary function (4). The most commonly used pulmonary function parameters are the peak expiratory flow rate (PEFR) and forced expiratory volume in the first second of expiration (FEV_1). Current National Asthma Education and Prevention Program guidelines suggest classifying the degree of asthma severity in patients who are not taking controller medication and the degree of asthma control in patients who are taking controller medication (Table 1).

Effects of Pregnancy on Asthma

In a large prospective study, pregnant patients with mild asthma had exacerbation rates of 12.6% and hospitalization rates of 2.3%, those with moderate asthma had exacerbation rates of 25.7% and hospitalization rates of 6.8%, and those with severe asthma had exacerbation rates of 51.9% and hospitalization rates of 26.9% (14). The effects of pregnancy on the course of asthma are variable—the symptoms of 23% of women studied improved and the symptoms of 30% became worse during pregnancy (14). Because many pregnant women have increased symptoms, pregnant patients who have asthma, even those with mild or well-controlled disease, need to be monitored with PEFR and FEV_1 testing as well as by observing their symptoms during pregnancy.

Effects of Asthma on Pregnant Women and Fetuses

There has been considerable consistency among results of prospective studies of the effects of asthma during pregnancy. Eight prospective studies, reporting maternal and infant outcomes with at least 100 participants in locations at or near sea level, have been published (5–7, 15–20). These studies show that the gravid patient with mild or moderate asthma can have excellent maternal and infant outcomes. However, suboptimal control of asthma during pregnancy may be associated with increased maternal or fetal risk (7). In fact, a significant relationship has been reported between decreased FEV_1 during pregnancy and increased risk of low birth weight and prematurity (21). Results of the two largest studies

Table 1. Classification of Asthma Severity and Control in Pregnant Patients

Asthma Severity* (Control†)	Symptom Frequency	Nighttime Awakening	Interference With Normal Activity	FEV_1 or Peak Flow (Predicted Percentage of Personal Best)
Intermittent (well controlled)	2 days per week or less	Twice per month or less	None	More than 80%
Mild persistent (not well controlled)	More than 2 days per week, but not daily	More than twice per month	Minor limitation	More than 80%
Moderate persistent (not well controlled)	Daily symptoms	More than once per week	Some limitation	60–80%
Severe persistent (very poorly controlled)	Throughout the day	Four times per week or more	Extremely limited	Less than 60%

Abbreviation: FEV_1, forced expiratory volume in the first second of expiration

*Assess severity for patients who are not taking long-term-control medications.

†Assess control in patients taking long-term-control medications to determine whether step-up therapy, step-down therapy, or no change in therapy is indicated.

indicate that classification of asthma severity and therapy tailored according to asthma severity can result in excellent infant and maternal outcomes (6, 7).

There are important caveats when interpreting the study results of asthma in pregnancy. Fewer considerable adverse associations have been found in the results of prospective studies, possibly because of better asthma surveillance and treatment. The excellent maternal and infant outcomes were achieved at centers that tended to manage asthma in pregnancy actively. In addition, women who enroll in research studies tend to be more motivated and adhere to therapeutic regimens more than the general public. The lack of more adverse outcomes among women with severe asthma also may be a function of the relatively small number of participants in this cohort and the resulting lack of power to find adverse outcomes that were statistically significant. Although the results of these prospective studies are reassuring in their consensus of good pregnancy outcomes, they do not indicate that asthma should be considered a benign condition because active asthma management was a part of these studies and may have had a positive impact on the outcomes.

Clinical Considerations and Recommendations

▶ *How is asthma diagnosed during pregnancy?*

Diagnosis of asthma in a pregnant patient is the same as that for a nonpregnant patient. Asthma typically includes characteristic symptoms (wheezing, chest cough, shortness of breath, chest tightness), temporal relationships (fluctuating intensity, worse at night), and triggers (eg, allergens, exercise, infections). Wheezing on auscultation would support the diagnosis, but its absence does not exclude the diagnosis. Ideally, the diagnosis of asthma would be confirmed by demonstrating airway obstruction on spirometry that is at least partially reversible (greater than a 12% increase in FEV_1 after bronchodilator). However, reversible airway obstruction may not be demonstrable in some patients with asthma. In patients with a clinical picture consistent with asthma, in whom reversible airway obstruction cannot be demonstrated, a trial of asthma therapy is reasonable. In such patients, a positive response to asthma therapy can be used to diagnose asthma during pregnancy.

In patients presenting with new respiratory symptoms during pregnancy, the most common differential diagnosis would be dyspnea of pregnancy. Dyspnea of pregnancy usually can be differentiated from asthma by its lack of cough, wheezing, chest tightness, or airway obstruction. Other differential diagnoses include gastroe-

sophageal reflux, chronic cough from postnasal drip, and bronchitis.

▶ *How should patients with asthma be assessed during pregnancy?*

Clinical evaluation includes subjective assessments and pulmonary function tests. Because pulmonary function and asthma severity may change during the course of pregnancy, routine evaluation of pulmonary function in pregnant women with persistent asthma is recommended. For pulmonary function assessment during outpatient visits, spirometry is preferable, but peak expiratory flow measurement with a peak flow meter also is sufficient. Patients with worsening symptoms should be evaluated with peak flow measurement and lung auscultation. Severity and control of asthma should be assessed in terms of symptom exacerbation and pulmonary impairment. It is important to identify a history of prior hospitalization (especially hospital stays that required intensive care unit admission or intubation), emergency department or other unscheduled visits for asthma treatment, or oral corticosteroid requirements. In patients who are not taking controllers, it is useful to assess pulmonary impairment based on severity classification (Table 1). Patients with two or more episodes of symptom exacerbation requiring the use of oral corticosteroids in the prior 12 months also should be considered to have persistent asthma. In patients who are taking controllers, it is useful to assess control (Table 1). Assessing the impairment domain of control consists of determining the frequency of daytime symptoms, nocturnal symptoms, activity limitation, frequency of rescue therapy, and FEV_1. The assessment in a pregnant patient with asthma also should include the effect of any prior pregnancies on asthma severity or control because this may predict the course of the asthma during subsequent pregnancies.

▶ *Can allergy shots be started or continued during pregnancy?*

The use of allergen immunotherapy, or "allergy shots," has been shown to be effective in improving asthma in patients with allergies (4). In two studies, no adverse effects of immunotherapy during pregnancy have been found (22, 23). However, anaphylaxis is a risk of allergen injections, especially early in the course of immunotherapy when the dose is being escalated, and anaphylaxis during pregnancy has been associated with maternal death, fetal death, or both. In a patient who is receiving a maintenance or near-maintenance dose, not experiencing adverse reactions to the injections and apparently deriving clinical benefit, continuation of immunotherapy is recommended. In such patients, a dose reduction may be considered to further decrease the chance of anaphylaxis. Risk–benefit considerations do not usually favor beginning allergen immunotherapy during pregnancy.

▶ *What is appropriate rescue therapy for asthma during pregnancy?*

Inhaled short-acting β_2-agonists are the rescue therapy of choice for asthma during pregnancy. Inhaled albuterol is the first-choice, short-acting β_2-agonist for pregnant women, although other agents also may be appropriate. In general, patients should use up to two treatments of inhaled albuterol (two to six puffs) or nebulized albuterol at 20-minute intervals for most mild to moderate symptoms; higher doses can be used for severe symptom exacerbation. To avoid maternal and fetal hypoxia, patients should be counseled to start rescue therapy at home when they have an exacerbation of symptoms, such as coughing, chest tightness, dyspnea, wheezing, or a 20% decrease in the PEFR. With a good response (ie, symptoms reduce or resolve, and the PEFR reaches 80% of personal best) the patient can continue normal activity. If the patient does not have a good response or if she notices a decrease in fetal activity, she should seek medical attention quickly.

▶ *What is first-line controller therapy for asthma during pregnancy?*

For those with mild, intermittent asthma, no controller therapy is indicated. Use of inhaled corticosteroids is first-line controller therapy for persistent asthma during pregnancy. For patients with mild, persistent asthma, the use of low-dose inhaled corticosteroids is recommended (see the box). For patients with moderate persistent asthma or whose symptoms are not controlled with the use of low-dose inhaled corticosteroids, the use of medium-dose inhaled corticosteroids or low-dose inhaled corticosteroids and long-acting β-agonists are indicated. See Table 2 for typical inhaled corticosteroid regimens. Budesonide is the preferred inhaled corticosteroid for use during pregnancy (4). However, there are no data indicating that the other inhaled corticosteroid preparations are unsafe during pregnancy. Therefore, the use of any inhaled corticosteroids may be continued in patients whose asthma was well controlled by these agents before pregnancy (4).

▶ *What is appropriate add-on controller therapy for asthma during pregnancy?*

Use of long-acting β_2-agonists is the preferred add-on controller therapy for asthma during pregnancy. This therapy should be added when patients' symptoms are

---

Step Therapy Medical Management of Asthma During Pregnancy

Mild Intermittent Asthma

- No daily medications, albuterol as needed

Mild Persistent Asthma

- Preferred—Low-dose inhaled corticosteroid
- Alternative—Cromolyn, leukotriene receptor antagonist, or theophylline (serum level 5–12 mcg/mL)

Moderate Persistent Asthma

- Preferred—Low-dose inhaled corticosteroid and salmeterol or medium-dose inhaled corticosteroid or (if needed) medium-dose inhaled corticosteroid and salmeterol
- Alternative—Low-dose or (if needed) medium-dose inhaled corticosteroid and either leukotriene receptor antagonist or theophylline (serum level 5–12 mcg/mL)

Severe Persistent Asthma

- Preferred—High-dose inhaled corticosteroid and salmeterol and (if needed) oral corticosteroid
- Alternative—High-dose inhaled corticosteroid and theophylline (serum level 5–12 mcg/mL) and oral corticosteroid if needed

---

not controlled with the use of medium-dose inhaled corticosteroids. Alternative add-on therapies are theophylline or leukotriene receptor antagonists (montelukast, zafirlukast). However, the use of long-acting inhaled β_2-agonists is preferred because it has been shown to be a more effective add-on therapy in nonpregnant patients than leukotriene receptor antagonists or theophylline. Long-acting inhaled β_2-agonists have fewer side effects than theophylline, which has a narrow therapeutic index and requires serum monitoring, and there are few data on the use of leukotriene receptor antagonists in humans during pregnancy. See Table 2 for typical medication dosages. Because long-acting and short-acting inhaled β_2-agonists have similar pharmacology and toxicology, long-acting inhaled β_2-agonists are expected to have a safety profile similar to that of albuterol. Two long-acting inhaled β_2-agonists are available: 1) salmeterol and 2) formoterol. Limited observational data exist on their use during pregnancy. A step-wise approach to management is advised in order to achieve control. See the box for specific therapy.

For patients whose symptoms are not well controlled (Table 1) with the use of medium-dose inhaled corticosteroids and long-acting inhaled β_2-agonists, treatment should be advanced to high-dose inhaled corticosteroids

Table 2. Comparative Daily Doses for Inhaled Corticosteroids*

Corticosteroid	Amount	Low Dose	Medium Dose	High Dose
Beclomethasone HFA	40 mcg per puff	2–6 puffs	More than 6–12 puffs	More than 12 puffs
	80 mcg per puff	1–3 puffs	More than 3–6 puffs	More than 6 puffs
Budesonide	200 mcg per inhalation	1–3 puffs	More than 3–6 puffs	More than 6 puffs
Flunisolide	250 mcg per puff	2–4 puffs	4–8 puffs	More than 8 puffs
Fluticasone HFA	44 mcg per puff	2–6 puffs		
	110 mcg per puff	2 puffs	2–4 puffs	More than 4 puffs
	220 mcg per puff		1–2 puffs	More than 2 puffs
Fluticasone DPI	50 mcg per inhalation	2–6 puffs		
	100 mcg per inhalation	1–3 puffs	3–5 puffs	More than 5 puffs
	250 mcg per inhalation	1 puff	2 puffs	More than 2 puffs
Mometasone	200 mcg per inhalation	1 puff	2 puffs	More than 2 puffs
Triamcinolone	75 mcg per puff	4–10 puffs	10–20 puffs	More than 20 puffs

*Total daily puffs is usually divided into a twice-per-day regimen.

Abbreviations: DPI, dry powder inhaler; HFA, hydrofluoroalkane

Adapted from National Heart, Lung, and Blood Institute, National Asthma Education and Prevention Program. Expert panel report 3: guidelines for the diagnosis and management of asthma. NIH Publication No. 07-4051. Bethesda (MD): NHLBI; 2007. Available at: http://www.nhlbi.nih.gov/guidelines/asthma/asthgdln.htm. Retrieved September 10, 2007.

(Table 2) and long-acting inhaled β_2-agonists (salmeterol, one puff twice daily). Some patients with severe asthma may require regular oral corticosteroid use to achieve adequate asthma control. For patients whose symptoms are very poorly controlled (Table 1), a course of oral corticosteroids may be necessary to attain control, along with a step up in therapy, as described previously and in the box.

▶ *What nonpharmacologic approaches should be used for asthma during pregnancy?*

Identifying and controlling or avoiding factors, such as allergens and irritants, that contribute to asthma severity, particularly tobacco smoke, can lead to improved maternal well-being with less need for medication (4). If gastroesophageal reflux is exacerbating the patient's asthma, nonpharmacologic measures, such as elevating the head of the bed, eating smaller meals, not eating within 2–3 hours of bedtime, and avoiding triggering foods, may help. Asthma control is enhanced by ensuring access to education about asthma, the interrelationships between asthma and pregnancy, and the skills necessary to manage asthma. These skills include self-monitoring, correct use of inhalers, following a plan for long-term management of asthma, and promptly handling signs of worsening asthma (4). Specific measures to reduce mold, dust mite exposure, animal dander, cockroaches, and other environmental triggers may be important. Animal dander control entails removing the animal from the home or, at a minimum, keeping the animal out of the patient's bedroom. Cockroaches can be controlled by poison or bait traps and eliminating exposed food or garbage.

▶ *How should asthma therapy be adjusted during pregnancy?*

The step-care therapeutic approach increases the number and dosage of medications with increasing asthma severity (see the box). At each step of therapy, medications are considered to be "preferred" or "alternative" based on efficacy and safety considerations. Patients whose symptoms are not optimally responding to treatment should receive a step up in treatment to more intensive medical therapy. Once control is achieved and sustained for several months, a step-down approach can be considered, but a change in therapy should be undertaken cautiously and administered gradually to avoid compromising the stability of the asthma control. For some patients, it may be prudent to postpone, until after birth, a reduction of therapy that is effectively controlling the patient's asthma (4).

▶ *How should acute asthma be assessed during pregnancy?*

Initial assessment of a pregnant patient presenting with acute asthma includes obtaining a brief medical history, performing a physical examination, and examining physiologic measures of airway function and fetal well-being. Pulmonary physiologic assessment includes measuring FEV_1 or PEFR and oxygen saturation. Fetal assessment depends on the stage of pregnancy, but continuous electronic fetal monitoring or biophysical profile or both should be considered if the pregnancy has reached the stage of fetal viability.

After initial treatment, repeat assessments of the patient and fetus will determine the need for continuing care. Patients with FEV_1 or PEFR measurements greater than or equal to 70% sustained for 60 minutes after last treatment, no distress, and reassuring fetal status may be discharged. For an incomplete response (FEV_1 or PEFR measurements greater than or equal to 50% but less than 70%, mild or moderate symptoms), the disposition (continued treatment in the emergency department, discharge home, or hospitalization) will need to be individualized. For patients with a poor response (FEV_1 or PEFR measurements less than 50%), hospitalization is indicated. For patients with a poor response and severe symptoms, drowsiness, confusion, or Pco_2 level greater than 42 mm Hg, intensive care unit admission is indicated and intubation should be strongly considered.

▶ *What should be the discharge regimen after an acute asthma episode?*

Patients discharged after an acute asthmatic episode should continue treatment with short-acting β_2-agonists, two to four puffs every 3–4 hours as needed. Oral corticosteroids should be continued at a dose of 40–60 mg in a single dose or two divided doses for 3–10 days. Inhaled corticosteroids should be initiated or continued until review at medical follow-up. Outpatient follow-up should be arranged within 5 days of the acute visit.

▶ *What are considerations for fetal surveillance in pregnancies complicated by asthma?*

Ultrasound examinations and antenatal fetal testing should be considered for women who have moderate or severe asthma during pregnancy. First-trimester ultrasound dating should be performed, if possible, to facilitate subsequent evaluations of fetal growth restriction and the risk of preterm birth. Serial ultrasound examinations to monitor fetal activity and growth should be considered (starting at 32 weeks of gestation) for women who have poorly controlled asthma or moderate-to-severe asthma and for women recovering from a severe asthma exacerbation. All patients should be instructed to be attentive to fetal activity.

▶ *What intrapartum concerns are unique to pregnant women with asthma?*

Asthma medication use should not be discontinued during labor and delivery. The patient should be kept hydrated

and should receive adequate analgesia in order to decrease the risk of bronchospasm. Women who are currently receiving or recently have taken systemic corticosteroids should receive intravenous administration of corticosteroids (eg, hydrocortisone 100 mg every 8 hours) during labor and for 24 hours after delivery to prevent adrenal crisis (4).

Cesarean delivery for acute exacerbation of asthma is rarely needed. Maternal and fetal compromise usually will respond to aggressive medical management. However, delivery may benefit the respiratory status of a patient with unstable asthma who has a mature fetus. Lumbar anesthesia can reduce oxygen consumption and minute ventilation during labor (24). Regional anesthesia was reported to incur a 2% incidence of bronchospasm (25). Obstetric, anesthetic, and pediatric staff should communicate to coordinate intrapartum and postpartum care.

▶ *How should women with asthma be counseled about breastfeeding?*

In general, only small amounts of asthma medications enter breast milk. The National Asthma Education and Prevention Program found that the use of prednisone, theophylline, antihistamines, inhaled corticosteroids, β_2-agonists, and cromolyn is not contraindicated for breastfeeding (4, 26).

Summary of Recommendations and Conclusions

The following recommendations and conclusions are based on limited or inconsistent scientific evidence (Level B):

▶ It is safer for pregnant women with asthma to be treated with asthma medications than it is for them to have asthma symptoms and exacerbations.

▶ Clinical evaluation of asthma includes subjective assessments and pulmonary function tests.

▶ The ultimate goal of asthma therapy in pregnancy is maintaining adequate oxygenation of the fetus by preventing hypoxic episodes in the mother.

▶ The step-care therapeutic approach increases the number and dosage of medications with increasing asthma severity.

▶ Inhaled corticosteroids are first-line controller therapy for persistent asthma during pregnancy.

▶ Budesonide is the preferred inhaled corticosteroid for use during pregnancy.

▶ Inhaled albuterol is recommended rescue therapy for pregnant women with asthma.

▶ Identifying and controlling or avoiding factors such as allergens and irritants, particularly tobacco smoke, can lead to improved maternal well-being with less need for medication.

▶ Continuation of immunotherapy is recommended in patients who are at or near a maintenance dose, not experiencing adverse reactions to the injections, and apparently deriving clinical benefit.

▶ Use of prednisone, theophylline, antihistamines, inhaled corticosteroids, β_2-agonists, and cromolyn is not contraindicated for breastfeeding.

The following recommendations and conclusions are based primarily on consensus and expert opinion (Level C):

▶ Asthma self-management skills, including self-monitoring, correct use of inhalers, and following a plan for long-term management of asthma and promptly handling signs of worsening asthma, enhance asthma control.

▶ For pulmonary function assessment of patients during outpatient visits, spirometry is preferable, but peak expiratory flow measurement with a peak flow meter also is sufficient.

▶ Ultrasound examinations and antenatal fetal testing should be considered for women who have moderate or severe asthma during pregnancy.

▶ Pregnant patients with asthma, even those with mild or well-controlled disease, need to be monitored with PEFR and FEV_1 testing as well as by observing their symptoms during pregnancy.

▶ Routine evaluation of pulmonary function in pregnant women with persistent asthma is recommended.

▶ Because pulmonary function and asthma severity may change during the course of pregnancy, routine evaluation of pulmonary function in pregnant women with persistent asthma is recommended.

Proposed Performance Measure

The percentage of pregnant patients with persistent asthma who have undergone pulmonary function testing

References

1. Alexander S, Dodds L, Armson BA. Perinatal outcomes in women with asthma during pregnancy. Obstet Gynecol 1998;92:435–40. (Level II-2)

2. Kwon HL, Belanger K, Bracken MB. Asthma prevalence among pregnant and childbearing-aged women in the United States: estimates from national health surveys. Ann Epidemiol 2003;13:317–24. (Level III)

3. Schatz M, Zeiger RS, Hoffman CP. Intrauterine growth is related to gestational pulmonary function in pregnant asthmatic women. Kaiser-Permanente Asthma and Pregnancy Study Group. Chest 1990;98:389–92. (Level II-2)

4. National Heart, Lung, and Blood Institute, National Asthma Education and Prevention Program. Working group report on managing asthma during pregnancy: recommendations for pharmacologic treatment—update 2004. NIH Publication No. 05-5236. Bethesda (MD): NHLBI; 2005. Available at: http://www.nhlbi.nih.gov/health/prof/lung/asthma/astpreg/astpreg_full.pdf. Retrieved September 10, 2007. (Level III)

5. Schatz M, Zeiger RS, Hoffman CP, Harden K, Forsythe A, Chilingar L, et al. Perinatal outcomes in the pregnancies of asthmatic women: a prospective controlled analysis. Am J Respir Crit Care Med 1995;151:1170–4. (Level II-2)

6. Bracken MB, Triche EW, Belanger K, Saftlas A, Beckett WS, Leaderer BP. Asthma symptoms, severity, and drug therapy: a prospective study of effects on 2205 pregnancies. Obstet Gynecol 2003;102:739–52. (Level II-2)

7. Dombrowski MP, Schatz M, Wise R, Momirova V, Landon M, Mabie W, et al. Asthma during pregnancy. National Institute of Child Health and Human Development Maternal–Fetal Medicine Units Network and the National Heart, Lung, and Blood Institute. Obstet Gynecol 2004;103:5–12. (Level II-2)

8. Demissie K, Breckenridge MB, Rhoads GG. Infant and maternal outcomes in the pregnancies of asthmatic women. Am J Respir Crit Care Med 1998;158:1091–5. (Level II-2)

9. Perlow JH, Montgomery D, Morgan MA, Towers CV, Porto M. Severity of asthma and perinatal outcome. Am J Obstet Gynecol 1992;167:963–7. (Level II-2)

10. Kallen B, Rydhstroem H, Aberg A. Asthma during pregnancy—a population based study. Eur J Epidemiol 2000;16:167–71. (Level II-2)

11. Greenberger PA, Patterson R. The outcome of pregnancy complicated by severe asthma. Allergy Proc 1988;9:539–43. (Level II-3)

12. Bakhireva LN, Schatz M, Chambers CD. Effect of maternal asthma and gestational asthma therapy on fetal growth. J Asthma 2007;44:71–76. (Level III)

13. Towers CV, Briggs GG, Rojas JA. The use of prostaglandin E2 in pregnant patients with asthma. Am J Obstet Gynecol 2004;190:1777–80; discussion 1780. (Level II-2)

14. Schatz M, Dombrowski MP, Wise R, Thom EA, Landon M, Mabie W, et al. Asthma morbidity during pregnancy can be predicted by severity classification. J Allergy Clin Immunol 2003;112:283–8. (Level II-2)

15. Stenius-Aarniala B, Piirila P, Teramo K. Asthma and pregnancy: a prospective study of 198 pregnancies. Thorax 1988;43:12–8. (Level II-2)

16. Mihrshahi S, Belousova E, Marks GB, Peat JK. Pregnancy and birth outcomes in families with asthma. Childhood Asthma Prevention Team. J Asthma 2003; 40:181–7. (Level II-2)

17. Minerbi-Codish I, Fraser D, Avnun L, Glezerman M, Heimer D. Influence of asthma in pregnancy on labor and the newborn. Respiration 1998;65:130–5. (Level II-2)

18. Stenius-Aarniala BS, Hedman J, Teramo KA. Acute asthma during pregnancy. Thorax 1996;51:411–4. (Level II-2)

19. Jana N, Vasishta K, Saha SC, Khunnu B. Effect of bronchial asthma on the course of pregnancy, labour and perinatal outcome. J Obstet Gynaecol 1995;21:227–32. (Level II-2)

20. Triche EW, Saftlas AF, Belanger K, Leaderer BP, Bracken MB. Association of asthma diagnosis, severity, symptoms, and treatment with risk of preeclampsia. Obstet Gynecol 2004;104:585–93. (Level II-2)

21. Schatz M, Dombrowski MP, Wise R, Momirova V, Landon M, Mabie W, et al. Spirometry is related to perinatal outcomes in pregnant women with asthma. National Institute of Child Health and Human Development Maternal–Fetal Medicine Units Network; National Heart, Lung, and Blood Institute. Am J Obstet Gynecol 2006; 194:120–6. (Level II-2)

22. Metzger WJ, Turner E, Patterson R. The safety of immunotherapy during pregnancy. J Allergy Clin Immunol 1978;61:268–72. (Level II-3)

23. Shaikh WA. A retrospective study on the safety of immunotherapy in pregnancy. Clin Exp Allergy 1993;23: 857–60. (Level II-2)

24. Hagerdal M, Morgan CW, Sumner AE, Gutsche BB. Minute ventilation and oxygen consumption during labor with epidural analgesia. Anesthesiology 1983;59:425–7. (Level II-2)

25. Fung DL. Emergency anesthesia for asthma patients. Clin Rev Allergy 1985;3:127–41. (Level III)

26. Transfer of drugs and other chemicals into human milk. American Academy of Pediatrics. Pediatrics 2001;108: 776–89. (Level III)

The MEDLINE database, the Cochrane Library, and ACOG's own internal resources and documents were used to conduct a literature search to locate relevant articles published between January 1985 and March 2007. The search was restricted to articles published in the English language. Priority was given to articles reporting results of original research, although review articles and commentaries also were consulted. Abstracts of research presented at symposia and scientific conferences were not considered adequate for inclusion in this document. Guidelines published by organizations or institutions such as the National Institutes of Health and the American College of Obstetricians and Gynecologists were reviewed, and additional studies were located by reviewing bibliographies of identified articles. When reliable research was not available, expert opinions from obstetrician–gynecologists were used.

Studies were reviewed and evaluated for quality according to the method outlined by the U.S. Preventive Services Task Force:

I   Evidence obtained from at least one properly designed randomized controlled trial.

II-1   Evidence obtained from well-designed controlled trials without randomization.

II-2   Evidence obtained from well-designed cohort or case–control analytic studies, preferably from more than one center or research group.

II-3   Evidence obtained from multiple time series with or without the intervention. Dramatic results in uncontrolled experiments also could be regarded as this type of evidence.

III   Opinions of respected authorities, based on clinical experience, descriptive studies, or reports of expert committees.

Based on the highest level of evidence found in the data, recommendations are provided and graded according to the following categories:

Level A—Recommendations are based on good and consistent scientific evidence.

Level B—Recommendations are based on limited or inconsistent scientific evidence.

Level C—Recommendations are based primarily on consensus and expert opinion.

ISSN 1099-3630

The American College of Obstetricians and Gynecologists
409 12th Street, SW, PO Box 96920, Washington, DC 20090-6920

Asthma in pregnancy. ACOG Practice Bulletin No. 90. American College of Obstetricians and Gynecologists. Obstet Gynecol 2008; 111:457–64.

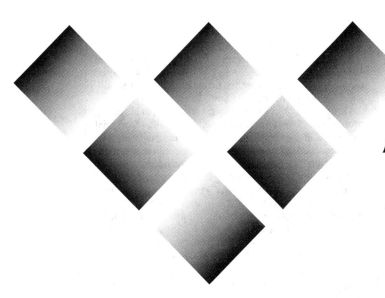

ACOG PRACTICE BULLETIN

CLINICAL MANAGEMENT GUIDELINES FOR
OBSTETRICIAN–GYNECOLOGISTS

NUMBER 92, APRIL 2008

(Replaces Practice Bulletin Number 87, November 2007)

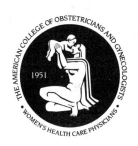

This Practice Bulletin was developed by the ACOG Committee on Practice Bulletins— Obstetrics with the assistance of Zachary N. Stowe, MD and Kimberly Ragan, MSW. The information is designed to aid practitioners in making decisions about appropriate obstetric and gynecologic care. These guidelines should not be construed as dictating an exclusive course of treatment or procedure. Variations in practice may be warranted based on the needs of the individual patient, resources, and limitations unique to the institution or type of practice.

Use of Psychiatric Medications During Pregnancy and Lactation

It is estimated that more than 500,000 pregnancies in the United States each year involve women who have psychiatric illnesses that either predate or emerge during pregnancy, and an estimated one third of all pregnant women are exposed to a psychotropic medication at some point during pregnancy (1). The use of psychotropic medications is a cause of concern for physicians and their patients because of the potential teratogenic risk, the risk of perinatal syndromes or neonatal toxicity, and the risk for abnormal postnatal behavioral development. With the limited information available on the risks of the psychotropic medications, clinical management must incorporate an appraisal of the clinical consequences of offspring exposure, the potential effect of untreated maternal psychiatric illness, and the available alternative therapies. The purpose of this document is to present current evidence on the risks and benefits of treatment for certain psychiatric illnesses during pregnancy.

Background

Advising a pregnant or breastfeeding woman to discontinue medication exchanges the fetal or neonatal risks of medication exposure for the risks of untreated maternal illness. Maternal psychiatric illness, if inadequately treated or untreated, may result in poor compliance with prenatal care, inadequate nutrition, exposure to additional medication or herbal remedies, increased alcohol and tobacco use, deficits in mother–infant bonding, and disruptions within the family environment (see Table 1). All psychotropic medications studied to date cross the placenta (1), are present in amniotic fluid (2), and can enter human breast milk (3). For known teratogens, knowledge of gestational age is helpful in the decision about drug therapy because the major risk of teratogenesis is during embryogenesis (ie, during the third through the eighth week of gestation). The U.S. Food and Drug Administration (FDA) has provided a system for categorizing individual medications (see Table 2), although this system has considerable limitations. Categories of risk for neonates from drugs used while breastfeeding also are shown in Table 2. Electronic resources for information related to the fetal and neonatal effects of psychotropic drug therapy in pregnancy and with breastfeeding include Reprotox (www.reprotox.org) and TERIS (http://depts.washington.edu/terisweb). Providing women with patient resources for online information that are well referenced is a reasonable option.

Table 1. Impact of Psychiatric Illness on Pregnancy Outcome

| Illness | Teratogenic Effects | Impact on Outcome | | Treatment Options |
		Obstetric	Neonatal	
Anxiety disorders	N/A	Increased incidence of forceps deliveries, prolonged labor, precipitate labor, fetal distress, preterm delivery, and spontaneous abortion	Decreased developmental scores and inadaptability; slowed mental development at 2 years of age	Benzodiazepines Antidepressants Psychotherapy
Major depression	N/A	Increased incidence of low birth weight, decreased fetal growth, and postnatal complications	Increased newborn cortisol and catecholamine levels, infant crying, rates of admission to neonatal intensive care units	Antidepressants Psychotherapy ECT
Bipolar disorder	N/A	See major depression	See major depression	Lithium Anticonvulsants Antipsychotics ECT
Schizophrenia	Congenital malformations, especially of cardiovascular system	Increased incidence of preterm delivery, low birth weight, small for gestational age, placental abnormalities, and antenatal hemorrhage	Increased rates of postnatal death	Antipsychotics

Abbreviations: ECT, electroconvulsive therapy; N/A, not available (eg, no studies identified)

Table 2. Psychiatric Medications in Pregnancy and Lactation*

Generic Name	Trade Name	Pregnancy Risk Category[†]	American Academy of Pediatrics Rating[‡]	Lactation Risk Category[§]
		Anxiolytic Medications		
Benzodiazepines				
Alprazolam	Xanax	D_m	Unknown, of concern	L3
Chlordiazepoxide	Librium	D	N/A	L3
Clonazepam	Klonopin	D_m	N/A	L3
Clorazepate	Tranxene	D	N/A	L3
Diazepam	Valium	D	Unknown, of concern	L3, L4 if used chronically
Lorazepam	Ativan	D_m	Unknown, of concern	L3
Oxazepam	Serax	D	N/A	L3
Benzodiazepines for Insomnia				
Estazolam	ProSom	X_m	N/A	L3
Flurazepam	Dalmane	X_m	N/A	L3
Quazepam	Doral	X_m	Unknown, of concern	L2

(continued)

Table 2. Psychiatric Medications in Pregnancy and Lactation* *(continued)*

Generic Name	Trade Name	Pregnancy Risk Category†	American Academy of Pediatrics Rating‡	Lactation Risk Category§
Anxiolytic Medications *(continued)*

Benzodiazepines for Insomnia (continued)				
Temazepam	Restoril	X_m	Unknown, of concern	L3
Triazolam	Halcion	X_m	N/A	L3
Nonbenzodiazepine Anxiolytics and Hypnotics				
Buspirone	BuSpar	B_m	N/A	L3
Chloral hydrate	Noctec	C_m	Compatible	L3
Eszoplicone	Lunesta	C_m	N/A	N/A
Zaleplon	Sonata	C_m	Unknown, of concern	L2
Zolpidem	Ambien	B_m	N/A	L3
Antiepileptic and Mood Stabilizing Medications
Lithium carbonate	Eskalith, Lithobid, Lithonate	D	Contraindicated	L4
Valproic acid	Depakote (divalproex sodium)	D_m	Compatible	L2
Carbamazepine	Tegretol	D_m	Compatible	L2
Lamotrigine	Lamictal	C_m	Unknown	L3
Antidepressants
Tricyclic and Heterocyclic Antidepressants				
Amitriptyline	Elavil, Endep	C_m	Unknown, of concern	L2
Amoxapine	Asendin	C_m	Unknown, of concern	L2
Clomipramine	Anafranil	C_m	Unknown, of concern‖	L2
Desipramine	Norpramin	C	Unknown, of concern	L2
Doxepin	Sinequan, Adapin	C	Unknown, of concern	L5
Imipramine	Tofranil	C	Unknown, of concern	L2
Maprotiline	Ludiomil	B_m	N/A	L3
Nortriptyline	Pamelor, Aventyl	C	Unknown, of concern‖	L2
Protriptyline	Vivactil	C	N/A	N/A
Selective Serotonin Reuptake Inhibitors				
Citalopram	Celexa	C_m	N/A	L3
Escitalopram	Lexapro	C_m	N/A	L3 in older infants
Fluoxetine	Prozac	C_m	Unknown, of concern	L2 in older infants, L3 if used in neonatal period
Fluvoxamine	Luvox	C_m	Unknown, of concern	L2
Paroxetine	Paxil	D_m	Unknown, of concern	L2
Sertraline	Zoloft	C_m	Unknown, of concern	L2
Other Antidepressants				
Bupropion	Wellbutrin	B_m	Unknown, of concern	L3
Duloxetine	Cymbalta	C_m	N/A	N/A
Mirtazapine	Remeron	C_m	N/A	L3
Nefazodone	Serzone	C_m	N/A	L4

(continued)

Table 2. Psychiatric Medications in Pregnancy and Lactation* *(continued)*

Generic Name	Trade Name	Pregnancy Risk Category†	American Academy of Pediatrics Rating‡	Lactation Risk Category§
Antidepressants *(continued)*				
Other Antidepressants (continued)				
Trazodone	Desyrel	C_m	Unknown, of concern	L2
Venlafaxine	Effexor	C_m	N/A	L3
Antipsychotic Medications				
Typical Antipsychotics				
Chlorpromazine	Thorazine	C	Unknown, of concern	L3
Fluphenazine	Prolixin	C	N/A	L3
Haloperidol	Haldol	C_m	Unknown, of concern	L2
Loxapine	Loxitane	C	N/A	L4
Perphenazine	Trilafon	C	Unknown, of concern	N/A
Pimozide	Orap	C_m	N/A	L4
Thioridazine	Mellaril	C	N/A	L4
Thiothixene	Navane	C	N/A	L4
Trifluoperazine	Stelazine	C	Unknown, of concern	N/A
Atypical Antipsychotics				
Aripiprazole	Abilify	C_m	N/A	L3
Clozapine	Clozaril	B_m	Unknown, of concern	L3
Olanzapine	Zyprexa	C_m	N/A	L2
Quetiapine	Seroquel	C_m	Unknown, of concern	L4
Risperidone	Risperdal	C_m	N/A	L3
Ziprasidone¶	Geodon	C	Unknown, of concern	L4

Abbreviation: N/A, not available

*The average half-life of elimination is listed for major metabolites.

†The U.S. Food and Drug Administration classifies drug safety using the following categories: A, controlled studies show no risk; B, no evidence of risk in humans; C, risk cannot be ruled out; D, positive evidence of risk; X, contraindicated in pregnancy. Risk category adapted from Briggs GG, Freeman RK, Yaffe SJ. Drugs in pregnancy and lactation. 7th ed. Philadelphia (PA): Lippincott Williams & Wilkins; 2005. The "m" subscript is for data taken from the manufacturer's package insert.

‡American Academy of Pediatrics 2001

§Lactation risk categories are listed as follows: L1, safest; L2, safer; L3, moderately safe; L4, possibly hazardous; L5, contraindicated. For more information, see Hale TW. Medications in Mother's Milk. Amaraillo (TX): Pharmasoft Publishing, 2004.

‖Original committee report 1994 listed as "compatible," and a correction was later published.

¶Not listed in Briggs. Risk category taken from Physicians' Desk Reference 1992, 1993, 1994, 1996, and 2004.

General Treatment Concepts

Optimally, shared decision making among obstetric and mental health clinicians and the patient should occur before pregnancy. Whenever possible, multidisciplinary management involving the obstetrician, mental health clinician, primary health care provider, and pediatrician is recommended to facilitate care.

A single medication at a higher dose is favored over multiple medications for treatment of psychiatric illness during pregnancy. Changing medications increases the exposure to the offspring. The selection of medication to minimize the risk of illness should be based on history of efficacy, prior exposure during pregnancy, and available reproductive safety information (see Table 3). Medications with fewer metabolites, higher protein binding (decreases placental passage), and fewer interactions with other medications are preferred.

Major Depression

Prevalence rates for depression are estimated at 17% for adults in the United States (4); women twice as often as men experience depression (5). The highest rates for

Table 3. Management Issues Associated With Medication Use During Pregnancy and Lactation

Medication Class	Management Issues					Treatment Options
	Birth Defects	Pregnancy	Delivery	Neonatal	Lactation	
Benzodiazepines	Possible increased incidence of cleft lip or palate	Ultrasonography for facial morphology	Floppy infant syndrome	Withdrawal syndrome	Infant sedation reported	Clonazepam Lorazepam Alprazolam
Selective serotonin reuptake inhibitors, selective norepinephrine reuptake inhibitors, and tricyclic antidepressants	None confirmed	Decreased serum concentrations across pregnancy	None	Neonatal, withdrawal syndrome	None	Fluoxetine Sertraline Paroxetine Citalopram Nortriptyline
Lithium	Increased incidence of heart defects	Ultrasonography or fetal echocardiography for heart development or both Decreased serum concentrations across pregnancy	Intravenous fluids Increased risk for lithium toxicity in mother	Increased risk for lithium toxicity in infant	Monitor infant complete blood count, thyroid-stimulating hormone levels, and lithium levels	Sustained release lithium
Antiepileptic Drugs	Increased incidence of birth defects	Decreased serum concentrations across pregnancy Folate supplementation, Vitamin K for some antiepileptic drugs	None	Neonatal symptoms, Vitamin K for some anti-epileptic drugs	Monitor infant complete blood count, liver enzyme levels, antiepileptic drug levels	Lamotrigine Carbemazepine
Antipsychotic Medications	None Confirmed	Avoid anticholinergic medications for side effects	None	Possible risk for neuroleptic malignant syndrome and intestinal obstruction	None	Haloperidol

depression occur in women between the ages of 25 years and 44 years (6). Symptoms include depressed or irritable mood, anhedonia, weight loss or gain, appetite and sleep changes, loss of energy, feelings of excessive guilt or worthlessness, psychomotor agitation or retardation and, in more severe cases, suicidal ideation (7). Approximately 10–16% of pregnant women fulfill diagnostic criteria for depression, and up to 70% of pregnant women report symptoms of depression (6, 8–10). Many symptoms of depression overlap with the symptoms of pregnancy and often are overlooked (6, 11). Of women taking antidepressants at conception, more than 60% experienced symptoms of depression during the pregnancy (12). In a study of pregnant women taking antidepressants before conception, a 68% relapse of depression was documented in those who discontinued medications during pregnancy (13) compared with only a 25% relapse in those who continued antidepressant medications.

Postpartum depression is classified as a major episode of depression that occurs within the first 4 weeks postpartum (7) or within the first 6 weeks postpartum

(14). Many women in whom postpartum depression was diagnosed reported having symptoms of depression during pregnancy (9, 15–17). These symptoms may be difficult to differentiate from normal postpartum adaptation. Survey tools (eg, Edinburgh Postnatal Depression Scale, Beck Depression Inventory, and the Postpartum Depression Screening Scale), are widely used to identify depression during the perinatal period (18). The detection rate is in the range of 68–100% (better for severe depression) with specificities in the range of 78–96% (19).

Untreated maternal depression is associated with an increase in adverse pregnancy outcomes, including premature birth, low birthweight infants, fetal growth restriction, and postnatal complications. This association is stronger when depression occurs in the late second to early third trimester (20). Newborns of women with untreated depression during pregnancy cry more and are more difficult to console (20–22). Maternal depression also is associated with increased life stress, decreased social support, poor maternal weight gain, smoking, and alcohol and drug use (23), all of which can adversely affect infant outcome (24–26). Later in life, children of untreated depressed mothers are more prone to suicidal behavior, conduct problems, and emotional instability and more often require psychiatric care (27, 28).

Bipolar Disorder

Bipolar disorder, historically called manic–depressive disorder, affects between 3.9% and 6.4% of Americans and affects men and women equally (4, 29–31). It commonly is characterized by distinct periods of abnormally and persistently elevated, expansive, or irritable mood and separate distinct periods of depressed mood or anhedonia (7). Women are more likely than men to experience depressive episodes of bipolar disorder (32), rapid cycling (33), and mixed episodes (34, 35). Typical onset of bipolar disorder for women is in the teens or early twenties.

Rates of postpartum relapse range from 32% (36) to 67% (37). In one study, it was reported that pregnancy had a protective effect for women with bipolar disorder (38), but the participants may have had milder illness. Perinatal episodes of bipolar disorder tend to be depressive (37, 39) and, when experienced with one pregnancy, are more likely to recur with subsequent pregnancies (37). There also is an increased risk of postpartum psychosis as high as 46% (40, 41).

Anxiety Disorders

Anxiety disorders include panic disorder, obsessive–compulsive disorder (OCD), generalized anxiety disorder (GAD), posttraumatic stress disorder (PTSD), social anxiety disorder, and specific phobias. Collectively, anxiety disorders are the most commonly occurring psychiatric disorders, with a prevalence of 18.1% among adults 18 years and older in the United States (42). Panic disorder, GAD, PTSD, agoraphobia, and specific phobias are two times more likely to be diagnosed in women than men. Anxiety and stress during pregnancy are documented as factors associated with poor obstetric outcomes, including spontaneous abortions (43), preterm delivery (44, 45), and delivery complications (46), such as prolonged labor, precipitate labor, clinical fetal distress, and forceps deliveries (47). A direct causal relationship has not been established.

Panic disorder is characterized by recurrent panic attacks that arise spontaneously in situations that are not expected to cause anxiety. Most investigators agree that women are at greatest risk for exacerbation of panic disorder during the postpartum period (48, 49). In a recent study PTSD was reported to be the third most common psychiatric diagnosis among economically disadvantaged pregnant women, with a prevalence of 7.7% (50). Women

with PTSD were significantly more likely to have a comorbid condition, principally major depression or GAD. Many reports have documented traumatic obstetric experiences (eg, emergency delivery, miscarriage, and fetal demise) as precipitants to PTSD-related symptomatology. The incidence of OCD during pregnancy is unknown. Despite limited formal investigation, most clinicians and researchers agree that pregnancy seems to be a potential trigger of OCD symptom onset, with 39% of the women in a specialized OCD clinic experiencing symptom onset during pregnancy (51). It generally is accepted that OCD worsens during the postpartum period.

Schizophrenia-Spectrum Disorders

Schizophrenia is a severe and persistent mental illness characterized by psychotic symptoms, negative symptoms, such as flat affect and lack of volition, and significant occupational and social dysfunction (7). Schizophrenia occurs in approximately 1–2% of women, with the most common age of onset during the childbearing years (52).

A variety of adverse pregnancy outcomes in women with schizophrenia have been reported, including preterm delivery, low birth weight infants, small for gestational age fetuses (53, 54), placental abnormalities and antenatal hemorrhage, increased rates of congenital malformations, especially of the cardiovascular system (55), and a higher incidence of postnatal death (53). However, in one study it was found that schizophrenic women were not at higher risk for specific obstetric complications but were at greater risk of requiring interventions during delivery, including labor induction and assisted or cesarean delivery (56). If left untreated during pregnancy, schizophrenia-spectrum disorders can have devastating effects on both mother and child, with rare reports of maternal self-mutilation (57, 58), denial of pregnancy resulting in refusal of prenatal care (59), and infanticide (60, 61).

Clinical Considerations and Recommendations

▶ *What is the evidence regarding the safety and efficacy of treatment for depression during pregnancy?*

Most data related to antidepressants in pregnancy are derived from the use of selective serotonin reuptake inhibitors (SSRIs) (fluoxetine, sertraline, citalopram, and paroxetine). Overall, there is limited evidence of teratogenic effects from the use of antidepressants in pregnancy or adverse effects from exposure during breastfeeding (62–64). There are two reports from GlaxoSmithKline based on a Swedish national registry and a U.S. insurance claims database that have raised concerns about a 1.5–2-fold increased risk of congenital cardiac malformations (atrial and ventricular septal defects) associated with first-trimester paroxetine exposure (www.gskus.com/news/paroxetine/paxil_letter_e3.pdf). The manufacturer subsequently changed paroxetine's pregnancy FDA category from C to D (www.fda.gov/cder/drug/advisory/paroxetine200512.htm).

More recently, the teratogenic effect of SSRI use during the first trimester of pregnancy was examined in two large case–control studies from multisite surveillance programs (65, 66). In the National Birth Defects Prevention Study, no significant associations were found between SSRI use overall and congenital heart defects (66). However, an association was found between SSRI use (particularly paroxetine) during early pregnancy and anencephaly, craniosynostosis, and omphalocele. Importantly, these risks were found only after more than 40 statistical tests were performed. Even if findings were not the result of chance, the absolute risks associated with SSRI use identified in this study were small. For example, a twofold to threefold increase in birth defects would occur for omphalocele (1 in 5,000 births), craniosynostosis (1 in 1,800 births) and anencephaly (1 in 1,000 births). In contrast, in the Slone Epidemiology Center Birth Defects Study no increased risk of craniosynostosis, omphalocele, or heart defects associated with SSRI use overall during early pregnancy was found (65). An association was seen between paroxetine and right ventricular outflow defects. Additionally, sertraline use was associated with omphalocele and atrial and ventricular septum defects. A limitation of this study is that the authors conducted 42 comparisons in their analyses for their main hypotheses. Both of these case–control studies were limited by the small number of exposed infants for each individual malformation. The current data on SSRI exposure during early pregnancy provide conflicting data on the risk for both overall and specific malformations. Some investigators have found a small increased risk of cardiac defects, specifically with paroxetine exposure. The absolute risk is small and generally not greater than two per 1,000 births; hence, these agents are not considered major teratogens.

Exposure to SSRIs late in pregnancy has been associated with transient neonatal complications, including jitteriness, mild respiratory distress, transient tachypnea of the newborn, weak cry, poor tone, and neonatal intensive care unit admission (67–71). A more recent FDA public health advisory highlighted concerns about the risk of an unconfirmed association of newborn persistent pulmonary hypertension with SSRI use (72) (www.fda.gov/cder/drug/advisory/SSRI_PPHN 200607. htm).

The potential risk of SSRI use in pregnancy must be considered in the context of the risk of relapse of depression if treatment is discontinued. Factors associated with relapse during pregnancy include a long history of depressive illness (more than 5 years) and a history of recurrent relapses (more than four episodes) (13). Therefore, treatment with all SSRIs or selective norepinephrine reuptake inhibitors or both during pregnancy should be individualized. At this time, paroxetine use in pregnant women and women planning pregnancy should be avoided, if possible. Fetal echocardiography should be considered for women exposed to paroxetine in early pregnancy. Because abrupt discontinuation of paroxetine has been associated with withdrawal symptoms, discontinuation of this agent should occur according to the product's prescribing information.

Tricyclic antidepressants (TCAs) have been available in the United States since 1963 and were widely used by women during pregnancy and lactation before the introduction of SSRIs. Results from initial studies, which suggested that TCA exposure might be associated with limb anomalies (73–75), have not been confirmed with subsequent studies (76, 77). Neonatal neurobehavioral effects from fetal exposure have not been reported (78).

Acute effects associated with TCA exposure include case reports of fetal tachycardia (79), neonatal symptoms such as tachypnea, tachycardia, cyanosis, irritability, hypertonia, clonus, and spasm (72–82), and transient withdrawal symptoms (83). In more recent studies, a significant link between prenatal exposure to TCAs and perinatal problems has not been documented (64, 84–86).

Atypical antidepressants are non-SSRI and non-TCA antidepressants that work by distinct pharmacodynamic mechanisms. The atypical antidepressants include bupropion, duloxetine, mirtazapine, nefazodone, and venlafaxine. The limited data of fetal exposure to these antidepressants (70, 85–89), do not suggest an increased risk of fetal anomalies or adverse pregnancy events. In the one published study of bupropion exposure in 136 patients, a significantly increased risk of spontaneous abortion, but not an increased risk of major malformations, was identified (90). In contrast, the bupropion registry maintained at GlaxoSmithKline has not identified any increased risk of spontaneous abortion, although these data have not undergone peer review.

Antidepressant medication is the mainstay of treatment for depression, although considerable data show that structured psychotherapy, such as interpersonal psychotherapy or cognitive behavioral therapy, are effective treatments for mild to moderate depression and are beneficial adjuncts to medication. In addition, electroconvulsive therapy is an effective treatment for major depression and is safe to use during pregnancy (91, 92).

What is the evidence regarding the safety and efficacy of lithium for the treatment of bipolar disorders during pregnancy?

Use of lithium in pregnancy may be associated with a small increase in congenital cardiac malformations. The initial retrospective data suggested that fetal exposure to lithium was associated with a 400-fold increase in congenital heart disease, particularly Ebstein's anomaly (93, 94). A subsequent meta-analysis of the available data calculated the risk ratio for cardiac malformations to be 1.2–7.7 and the risk ratio for overall congenital malformations to be 1.5–3 (95). In more recent small studies, limited in their statistical power, the magnitude of early estimates of teratogenic potential of lithium could not be confirmed (96–98).

Fetal exposure to lithium later in gestation has been associated with fetal and neonatal cardiac arrhythmias (99), hypoglycemia, nephrogenic diabetes insipidus (100), polyhydramnios, reversible changes in thyroid function (101), premature delivery, and floppy infant syndrome similar to that seen with benzodiazepine exposure (102). Symptoms of neonatal lithium toxicity include flaccidity, lethargy, and poor suck reflexes, which may persist for more than 7 days (103). Neurobehavioral sequelae were not documented in a 5-year follow-up of 60 school-aged children exposed to lithium during gestation (104).

The physiologic alterations of pregnancy may affect the absorption, distribution, metabolism and elimination of lithium, and close monitoring of lithium levels during pregnancy and postpartum is recommended. The decision to discontinue lithium therapy in pregnancy because of fetal risks should be balanced against the maternal risks of exacerbation of illness. In a recent study, it was reported that abrupt discontinuation of lithium was associated with a high rate of bipolar relapse among pregnant women (39). The following treatment guidelines have been suggested for women with bipolar illness who are treated with lithium and plan to conceive: 1) in women who experience mild and infrequent episodes of illness, treatment with lithium should be gradually tapered before conception; 2) in women who have more severe episodes but are only at moderate risk for relapse in the short term, treatment with lithium should be tapered before conception but reinstituted after organogenesis; 3) in women who have especially severe and frequent episodes of illness, treatment with lithium should be continued throughout gestation and the patient counseled regarding reproductive risks (95). Fetal assessment with fetal echocardiography should be considered in pregnant women exposed to lithium in the first trimester. For women in whom an unplanned conception occurs while receiving lithium therapy, the decision to continue or discontinue the use of lithium should be in part based on disease severity, course of the patient's illness, and the point of gestation at the time of exposure.

What is the evidence regarding the safety and efficacy of the antiepileptic drugs valproate and carbamazepine for the treatment of bipolar disorders during pregnancy?

Several anticonvulsants, including valproate, carbamazepine, and lamotrigine, currently are used in the treatment of bipolar disorder. Data regarding fetal effects of these drugs are derived primarily from studies of women with seizures. Whether the underlying pathology of epilepsy contributes to the teratogenic effect on the fetus is unclear. Epilepsy may not contribute to the teratogenic effects of antiepileptic drugs based on the results of a recent study that demonstrated similar rates of anomalies between infants of women without epilepsy and infants of women with epilepsy but who had not taken antiepileptic drugs during pregnancy (105).

Prenatal exposure to valproate is associated with a 1–3.8% risk of neural tube defects, with a corresponding dose–response relationship (106–113). Other congenital malformations associated with valproate use include craniofacial anomalies (114), limb abnormalities (115), and cardiovascular anomalies (116–118). A "fetal valproate syndrome" has been described with features of fetal growth restriction, facial dysmorphology, and limb and heart defects (119–121). Varying degrees of cognitive impairment, including mental development delay (122), autism (123–126), and Asperger's syndrome (124), have been reported with fetal valproate syndrome (124, 127, 128). Acute neonatal risks include hepatotoxicity (129), coagulopathies (130), neonatal hypoglycemia (131), and withdrawal symptoms (132).

Carbamazepine exposure in pregnancy is associated with a fetal carbamazepine syndrome manifest by facial dysmorphism and fingernail hypoplasia (124, 133–136). It is unclear whether carbamazepine use increases the risk of fetal neural tube defects or developmental delay (124, 127, 133–139). Fetal exposure to lamotrigine has not been documented to increase the risk of major fetal anomalies (140–145), although there may be an increased risk of midline facial clefts (0.89% of 564 exposures) as reported by one pregnancy registry (143), possibly related to higher daily maternal doses (greater than 200 mg/day) (145). The reproductive safety of lamotrigine appears to compare favorably with alternative treatments, but lacking are studies of the effectiveness of this antiepileptic drug as a mood stabilizer in pregnancy.

In managing bipolar disorders, the use of valproate and carbamazepine are superior to that of lithium for patients who experience mixed episodes or rapid cycling but exhibit limited efficacy in the treatment of bipolar depression. In contrast, lamotrigine is efficacious in the prevention of the depressed phase of illness (146, 147). Lamotrigine is a potential maintenance therapy option for pregnant women with bipolar disorder because of its protective effects against bipolar depression, general tolerability, and growing reproductive safety profile relative to alternative mood stabilizers. Because both valproate and carbamazepine are associated with adverse effects when used during pregnancy, their use, if possible should be avoided especially during the first trimester. The effectiveness of folate supplementation in the prevention of drug-associated neural tube defects has not been documented; however, folate supplementation of 4 mg/day should be offered preconceptionally and for the first trimester of pregnancy. Prenatal surveillance for congenital anomalies by maternal serum alpha-fetoprotein level testing, fetal echocardiography, or a detailed ultrasound examination of the fetal anatomy or a combination of these procedures should be considered. Whether the use of antiepileptic drugs such as carbamazepine increase the risk of neonatal hemorrhage and whether maternal vitamin K supplementation is effective remains unclear (148).

▶ *What is the evidence regarding the safety and efficacy of treatment for anxiety disorders during pregnancy?*

Use of benzodiazepines does not appear to carry a significant risk of somatic teratogenesis. In early studies of in utero exposure to diazepam, a benzodiazepine, an increased risk of oral clefts was reported (149–151). In a subsequent meta-analysis, it was demonstrated that prenatal benzodiazepine exposure increased the risk of oral cleft, although the absolute risk increased by 0.01%, from 6 in 10,000 to 7 in 10,000 (76). In a recent case–control study of 22,865 infants with congenital anomalies and 38,151 infants without congenital anomalies, an association of congenital anomalies, including oral clefts with exposure to five different benzodiazepines, was not found (152). Similar findings were documented in a case–control study of clonazepam (153). If discontinuation of benzodiazepine use is considered during pregnancy, benzodiazepines should not be abruptly withdrawn.

The data regarding neonatal toxicity and withdrawal syndromes are well documented, and neonates should be observed closely in the postpartum period. Floppy infant syndrome, characterized by hypothermia, lethargy, poor respiratory effort, and feeding difficulties, is associated with maternal use of benzodiazepines shortly before delivery (154–162). Neonatal withdrawal syndromes, characterized by restlessness, hypertonia, hyperreflexia, tremulousness, apnea, diarrhea, and vomiting, have been described in infants whose mothers were taking alprazolam (163), chlordiazepoxide (164–166), or diazepam (167, 168). These symptoms have been reported to persist for as long as 3 months postpartum (81).

The long-term neurobehavioral impact of prenatal benzodiazepine exposure is unclear. The existence of a "benzodiazepine-exposure syndrome," including growth restriction, dysmorphism, and both mental and psychomotor retardation, in infants exposed prenatally to benzodiazepines is disputed (169–171). In one study, no differences in the incidence of behavioral abnormalities at age 8 months or IQ scores at age 4 years were found among children exposed to chlordiazepoxide during gestation (172).

▶ *What is the evidence regarding the safety and efficacy of treatment for schizophrenia during pregnancy?*

The atypical antipsychotics (eg, clozapine, olanzapine, quetiapine, risperidone, ziprasidone, and aripiprazole) have replaced the typical agents as first-line medications for psychotic disorders (Table 2). The atypical antipsychotics generally are better tolerated and possibly are more effective in managing the negative symptoms of schizophrenia. They also are used increasingly for bipolar disorder, obsessive–compulsive disorder, and treatment-resistant depression. The reproductive safety data regarding the use of atypical antipsychotics remains extremely limited. In a prospective comparative study of pregnancy outcomes between groups exposed and unexposed to atypical antipsychotics, outcomes of 151 pregnancies with exposure to olanzapine, risperidone, quetiapine, and clozapine demonstrated a higher rate of low birth weight (10% in the exposed versus 2% in the nonexposed group) and therapeutic abortions (173).

The typical antipsychotic drugs have a larger reproductive safety profile and include haloperidol, thioridazine, fluphenazine, perphenazine, chlorpromazine, and trifluoperazine. No significant teratogenic effect has been documented with chlorpromazine, haloperidol, and perphenazine (174–176). In a study of 100 women treated with haloperidol (mean dose of 1.2 mg/day) for hyperemesis gravidarum, no differences in gestational duration, fetal viability, or birth weight were noted (177). In a large prospective study encompassing approximately 20,000 women treated primarily with phenothiazines for emesis (178), investigators found no significant association with neonatal survival rates or severe anomalies. Similar results have been obtained in several retrospective studies of women treated with trifluoperazine for repeated abortions and emesis (179, 180). In contrast, other investigators reported a significant association of major anomalies with prenatal exposure to phenothiazines with an aliphatic side chain but not with piperazine or piperidine class agents (181). Reanalysis of previously reported data obtained also identified a significant risk of malformations associated with phenothiazine exposure in weeks 4–10 of gestation (182). In clinical neurobehavioral outcome studies encompassing 203 children exposed to typical antipsychotics during gestation, no considerable differences have been detected in IQ scores at 4 years of age (183, 184), although relatively low antipsychotic doses were used by many women in these studies.

Fetal and neonatal toxicity reported with exposure to the typical antipsychotics includes neuroleptic malignant syndrome (185), dyskinesia (186), extrapyramidal side effects manifested by heightened muscle tone and increased rooting and tendon reflexes persisting for several months (187), neonatal jaundice (188), and postnatal intestinal obstruction (189).

Fetuses and infants also may be exposed to drugs used to manage the extrapyramidal side effects (eg, diphenhydramine, benztropine, and amantadine). In a case–control study, oral clefts were associated with a significantly higher rate of prenatal exposure to diphenhydramine than controls (149). In contrast, in several other studies diphenhydramine use has not been found to be a significant risk factor for fetal malformations (190, 191). Clinical studies of the teratogenic potential of benztropine and amantadine use are lacking.

In summary, typical antipsychotics have been widely used for more than 40 years, and the available data suggest the risks of use of these agents are minimal with respect to teratogenic or toxic effects on the fetus. In particular, use of piperazine phenothiazines (eg, trifluoperazine and perphenazine) may have especially limited teratogenic potential (181). Doses of typical antipsychotics during the peripartum should be kept to a minimum to limit the necessity of utilizing medications to manage extrapyramidal side effects. There is likewise little evidence to suggest that the currently available atypical antipsychotics are associated with elevated risks for neonatal toxicity or somatic teratogenesis. No long-term neurobehavioral studies of exposed children have yet been conducted. Therefore, the routine use of atypical antipsychotics during pregnancy and lactation cannot be recommended. In a woman who is taking an atypical antipsychotic and inadvertently conceives, a comprehensive risk–benefit assessment may indicate that continuing therapy with the atypical antipsychotic (to which the fetus has already been exposed) during gestation is preferable to switching to therapy with a typical antipsychotic (to which the fetus has not yet been exposed).

▶ *What is the risk of using psychiatric drugs while breastfeeding?*

Breastfeeding has clear benefits for both mother and infant and, in making the decision to recommend breastfeeding, these benefits should be weighed against the risks to the neonate of medication exposure while breastfeeding (Table 2). Most medications are transferred through breast milk, although most are found at very low levels and likely are not clinically relevant for the neonate. For women who breastfeed, measuring serum levels in the neonate is not recommended. Most clinical laboratory tests lack the sensitivity to detect and measure the low levels present. However, breastfeeding should be stopped immediately if a nursing infant develops abnormal symptoms most likely associated with exposure to the medication. Evaluation of the literature on drug levels in breast milk can facilitate the decision to breastfeed (192).

In the treatment of depression, published reports regarding SSRI use and lactation now consist of 173 mother–infant nursing pairs with exposure to sertraline, fluoxetine, paroxetine, fluvoxamine, and citalopram (193, 194–215). In results from studies, it has been shown that, quantitatively, medication exposure during lactation is considerably lower than transplacental exposure to these same SSRIs during gestation (193, 201, 208, 216). Generally, very low levels of SSRIs are detected in breast milk. Only a few isolated cases of adverse effects have been reported, although infant follow-up data are limited. The package insert for citalopram does report a case of an infant who experienced a transient apneic episode. Long-term neurobehavioral studies of infants exposed to SSRI antidepressants during lactation have not been conducted.

The TCAs also have been widely used during lactation. The only adverse event reported to date is respiratory depression in a nursing infant exposed to doxepin, which led to the conclusion that doxepin use should be avoided but that most TCAs are safe for use during breastfeeding (217). Data regarding the use of atypical antidepressants during lactation are limited to the use of venlafaxine (218) and bupropion (219, 220).

The existing data regarding lithium use and lactation encompass 10 mother–infant nursing dyads (103, 221–225). Adverse events, including lethargy, hypotonia, hypothermia, cyanosis, and electrocardiogram changes, were reported in two of the children in these studies (103, 223). The American Academy of Pediatrics consequently discourages the use of lithium during lactation (226). Because dehydration can increase the vulnerability to lithium toxicity, the hydration status of nursing infants of mothers taking lithium should be carefully monitored (102). There are no available reports regarding the long-term neurobehavioral sequelae of lithium exposure during lactation.

Only one adverse event, an infant with thrombocytopenia and anemia (227), has been reported in studies regarding valproate use and lactation, which includes 41 mother–infant nursing dyads (227–235). Studies of the neurobehavioral impact of valproate exposure during lactation have not been conducted. The American Academy of Pediatrics and the World Health Organization (WHO) Working Group on Drugs and Human Lactation have concluded that use of valproate is compatible with breast-feeding (226, 236). Reported adverse effects of carbamazepine in breast milk include transient cholestatic hepatitis (237, 238) and hyperbilirubinemia (239). The WHO Working Group on Drugs and Human Lactation has concluded that use of carbamazepine with breast-feeding is "probably safe" (236).

In the management of anxiety disorders, benzodiazepine use exhibits lower milk/plasma ratios than other classes of psychotropics (240, 241). Some investigators concluded that benzodiazepine use at relatively low doses does not present a contraindication to nursing (242). However, infants with an impaired capacity to metabolize benzodiazepines may exhibit sedation and poor feeding even with low maternal doses (243).

Of typical antipsychotic medications, chlorpromazine has been studied in seven breastfeeding infants, none of whom exhibited developmental deficits at 16-month and 5-year follow-up evaluations (244). However, three breastfeeding infants in another study, whose mothers were prescribed both chlorpromazine and haloperidol, exhibited evidence of developmental delay at 12–18 months of age (245).

Resources

American Academy of Pediatrics
Web: www.aap.org

American Psychiatric Association
Web: www.psych.org

National Institutes of Health
Daily medication:
http://dailymed.nlm.nih.gov/dailymed/about.cfm
Lactation medication:
toxnet.nlm.nih.gov/cgi-bin/sis/htmlgen?LACT

Summary of Recommendations and Conclusions

The following recommendations and conclusions are based on good and consistent scientific evidence (Level A):

▶ Lithium exposure in pregnancy may be associated with a small increase in congenital cardiac malformations, with a risk ratio of 1.2–7.7.

▶ Valproate exposure in pregnancy is associated with an increased risk of fetal anomalies, including neural tube defects, fetal valproate syndrome, and long-term adverse neurocognitive effects. It should be avoided in pregnancy, if possible, especially during the first trimester.

▶ Carbamazepine exposure in pregnancy is associated with fetal carbamazepine syndrome. It should be avoided in pregnancy, if possible, especially during the first trimester.

▶ Maternal benzodiazepine use shortly before delivery is associated with floppy infant syndrome.

The following recommendations and conclusions are based on limited or inconsistent scientific evidence (Level B):

▶ Paroxetine use in pregnant women and women planning pregnancy should be avoided, if possible. Fetal echocardiography should be considered for women who are exposed to paroxetine in early pregnancy.

▶ Prenatal benzodiazepine exposure increased the risk of oral cleft, although the absolute risk increased by 0.01%.

▶ Lamotrigine is a potential maintenance therapy option for pregnant women with bipolar disorder because of its protective effects against bipolar depression, general tolerability, and a growing reproductive safety profile relative to alternative mood stabilizers.

▶ Maternal psychiatric illness, if inadequately treated or untreated, may result in poor compliance with prenatal care, inadequate nutrition, exposure to additional medication or herbal remedies, increased alcohol and tobacco use, deficits in mother–infant bonding, and disruptions within the family environment.

The following recommendations and conclusions are based primarily on consensus and expert opinion (Level C):

▶ Whenever possible, multidisciplinary management involving the patient's obstetrician, mental health clinician, primary health care provider, and pediatrician is recommended to facilitate care.

▶ Use of a single medication at a higher dose is favored over the use of multiple medications for the treatment of psychiatric illness during pregnancy.

▶ The physiologic alterations of pregnancy may affect the absorption, distribution, metabolism, and elimination of lithium, and close monitoring of lithium levels during pregnancy and postpartum is recommended.

▶ For women who breastfeed, measuring serum levels in the neonate is not recommended.

▶ Treatment with all SSRIs or selective norepinephrine reuptake inhibitors or both during pregnancy should be individualized.

▶ Fetal assessment with fetal echocardiogram should be considered in pregnant women exposed to lithium in the first trimester.

References

1. Doering PL, Stewart RB. The extent and character of drug consumption during pregnancy. JAMA 1978;239:843–6. (Level III)

2. Hostetter A, Ritchie JC, Stowe ZN. Amniotic fluid and umbilical cord blood concentrations of antidepressants in three women. Biol Psychiatry 2000;48(10):1032–4. (Level III)

3. Newport DJ, Hostetter A, Arnold A, Stowe ZN. The treatment of postpartum depression: minimizing infant exposures. J Clin Psychiatry. 2002;63 (Suppl 7):31–44. (Level III)

4. Kessler RC, McGonagle KA, Zhao S, Nelson CB, Hughes M, Eshleman S, et al. Lifetime and 12-month prevalence of DSM-III-R psychiatric disorders in the United States. Results from the National Comorbidity Survey. Arch Gen Psychiatry 1994;51:8–19. (Level II-3)

5. National Institute of Mental Health (US). The numbers count: mental disorders in America. NIH Publication No. 06-4584. Bethesda (MD): NIMH; 2006. Available at: http://www.nimh.nih.gov/publicat/numbers.cfm. Retrieved December 12, 2006. (Level II-3)

6. Weissman M, Olfson M. Depression in women: implications for health care research. Science 1995;269:799–801. (Level III)

7. American Psychiatric Association. Diagnostic and statistical manual of mental disorders: DSM-IV-TR 4th ed. text version. Washington, DC: APA; 2000. (Level III)

8. O'Hara MW, Neunaber DJ, Zekoski EM. Prospective study of postpartum depression: prevalence, course and predictive factors. J Abnorm Psychol 1984;93:158–71. (Level II-3)

9. Gotlib IH, Whiffen VE, Mount JH, Milne K, Cordy NI. Prevalence rates and demographic characteristics associated with depression in pregnancy and the postpartum. J Consult Clin Psychol 1989;57:269–74. (Level III)

10. Affonso DD, Lovett S, Paul SM, Sheptak S. A standardized interview that differentiates pregnancy and postpartum symptoms from perinatal clinical depression. Birth 1990;17:121–30. (Level II-3)

11. Kumar R, Robson K. A prospective study of emotional disorders in childbearing women. Br J Psychiatry 1984;144:35–47. (Level II-3)

12. Hostetter A, Stowe ZN, Strader JR Jr, McLaughlin E, Llewellyn A. Dose of selective serotonin uptake inhibitors across pregnancy: clinical implications. Depress Anxiety 2000;11:51–7. (Level III-3)

13. Cohen LS, Altshuler LL, Harlow BL, Nonacs R, Newport DJ, Viguera AC, et al. Relapse of major depression during pregnancy in women who maintain or discontinue antidepressant treatment [published erratum appears in JAMA 2006;296:170]. JAMA 2006;295:499–507. (Level II-2)

14. Cox J. Postnatal mental disorder: towards ICD-11. World Psychiatry 2004;3:96–7. (Level III)

15. Stowe ZN, Hostetter AL, Newport DJ. The onset of postpartum depression: implications for clinical screening in obstetrical and primary care. Am J Obstet Gynecol 2005;192:522–6. (Level II-3)

16. Watson JP, Elliott SA, Rugg AJ, Brough DI. Psychiatric disorder in pregnancy and the first postnatal year. Br J Psychiatry 1984;144:453–62. (Level II-3)

17. Evans J, Heron J, Francomb H, Oke S, Golding J. Cohort study of depressed mood during pregnancy and after childbirth. BMJ 2001;323:257–60. (Level II-2)

18. Cox JL, Holden JM, Sagovsky R. Detection of postnatal depression. Development of the 10-item Edinburgh Postnatal Depression Scale. Br J Psychiatry 1987;150:782–6. (Level III)

19. Murray L, Carothers AD. The validation of the Edinburgh Post-natal Depression Scale on a community sample. Br J Psychiatry 1990;157:288–90. (Level III)

20. Hoffman S, Hatch MC. Depressive symptomatology during pregnancy: evidence for an association with decreased fetal growth in pregnancies of lower social class women. Health Psychol 2000;19:535–43. (Level II-2)

21. Field T, Diego MA, Dieter J, Hernandez-Reif M, Schanberg S, Kuhn C, et al. Depressed withdrawn and intrusive mothers' effects on their fetuses and neonates. Infant Behav Dev 2001;24:27–39. (Level II-2)

22. Zuckerman B, Bauchner H, Parker S, Cabral H. Maternal depressive symptoms during pregnancy, and newborn irritability. J Dev Behav Pediatr 1990;11:190–4. (Level II-3)

23. Zuckerman B, Amaro H, Bauchner H, Cabral H. Depressive symptoms during pregnancy: relationship to poor health behaviors. Am J Obstet Gynecol 1989;160: 1107–11. (Level II-2)

24. Zuckerman B, Frank DA, Hingson R, Amaro H, Levenson SM, Kayne H, et al. Effects of maternal marijuana and cocaine use on fetal growth. N Engl J Med 1989;320:762–8. (Level II-3)

25. Rosett HL, Weiner L, Lee A, Zuckerman B, Dooling E, Oppenheimer E. Patterns of alcohol consumption and fetal development. Obstet Gynecol 1983;61:539–46. (Level II-2)

26. Sexton M, Hebel JR. A clinical trial of change in maternal smoking and its effect on birth weight. JAMA 1984; 251:911–5. (Level I)

27. Weissman MM, Prusoff BA, Gammon GD, Merikangas KR, Leckman JF, Kidd KK. Psychopathology in the children (ages 6–18) of depressed and normal parents. J Am Acad Child Psychiatry 1984;23:78–84. (Level II-2)

28. Lyons-Ruth K, Wolfe R, Lyubchik A. Depression and the parenting of young children: making the case for early preventive mental health services. Harv Rev Psychiatry 2000;8:148–53. (Level III)

29. Judd LL, Akiskal HS. The prevalence and disability of bipolar spectrum disorders in the US population: re-analysis of the ECA database taking into account subthreshold cases. J Affect Disord 2003;73:123–31. (Level II-3)

30. Kessler RC, Chiu WT, Demler O, Merikangas KR, Walters EE. Prevalence, severity, and comorbidity of 12-month DSM-IV disorders in the National Comorbidity Survey Replication [published erratum appears in Arch Gen Psychiatry 2005;62:709]. Arch Gen Psychiatry 2005;62:617–627. (Level II-3)

31. Robins LN, Helzer JE, Weissman MM, Orvaschel H, Gruenberg E, Burke JD Jr, et al. Lifetime prevalence of specific psychiatric disorders in three sites. Arch Gen Psychiatry 1984;41:949–58. (Level II-3)

32. Angst J. The course of affective disorders. II. Typology of bipolar manic-depressive illness. Arch Psychiatr Nervenkr 1978;226:65–73. (Level III)

33. Yildiz A, Sachs GS. Characteristics of rapid cycling bipolar-I patients in a bipolar specialty clinic. J Affect Disord 2004;79:247–51. (Level II-3)

34. McElroy SL, Keck PE Jr, Pope HG Jr, Hudson JI, Faedda GL, Swan AC. Clinical and research implications of the diagnosis of dysphoric or mixed mania or hypomania. Am J Psychiatry 1992;149:1633–44. (Level III)

35. Arnold LM, McElroy SL, Keck PE Jr. The role of gender in mixed mania. Compr Psychiatry 2000;41:83–7. (Level III)

36. Akdeniz F, Vahip S, Pirildar S, Vahip I, Doganer I, Bulut I. Risk factors associated with childbearing-related episodes in women with bipolar disorder. Psychopathology 2003;36:234–8. (Level II-3)

37. Freeman MP, Smith KW, Freeman SA, McElroy SL, Kmetz GE, Wright R, et al. The impact of reproductive

events on the course of bipolar disorder in women. J Clin Psychiatry 2002;63:284–7. (Level III)

38. Grof P, Robbins W, Alda M, Berghoefer A, Vojtechovsky M, Nilsson A, et al. Protective effect of pregnancy in women with lithium-responsive bipolar disorder. J Affect Disord 2000;61:31–9. (Level III)

39. Viguera AC, Nonacs R, Cohen LS, Tondo L, Murray A, Baldessarini RJ. Risk of recurrence of bipolar disorder in pregnant and nonpregnant women after discontinuing lithium maintenance. Am J Psychiatry 2000;157:179–84. (Level II-2)

40. Kendall RE, Chalmers JC, Platz C. Epidemiology of puerperal psychosis [published erratum appears in Br J Psychiatry 1987;151:135]. Br J Psychiatry 1987;150: 662–673. (Level II-2)

41. Marks MN, Wieck A, Checkley SA, Kumar R. Contribution of psychological and social factors to psychotic and non-psychotic relapse after childbirth in women with previous histories of affective disorder. J Affect Disord 1992;24:253–63. (Level II-2)

42. Kessler RC, Berglund P, Demler O, Jin R, Merikangas KR, Walters EE. Lifetime prevalence and age-of-onset distributions of DSM-IV disorders in the National Comorbidity Survey Replication [published erratum appears in Arch Gen Psychiatry 2005;62:768]. Arch Gen Psychiatry 2005;62:593–602. (Level II-3)

43. Boyles SH, Ness RB, Grisso JA, Markovic N, Bromberger J, CiFelli D. Life event stress and the association with spontaneous abortion in gravid women at an urban emergency department. Health Psychol 2000;19: 510–4. (Level II-2)

44. Berkowitz GS, Kasl SV. The role of psychosocial factors in spontaneous preterm delivery. J Psychosom Res 1983;27:283–90. (Level II-2)

45. Perkin MR, Bland JM, Peacock JL, Anderson HR. The effect of anxiety and depression during pregnancy on obstetric complications. Br J Obstet Gynaecol 1993;100: 629–34. (Level II-2)

46. Pagel MD, Smilkstein G, Regen H, Montano D. Psychosocial influences on new born outcomes: a controlled prospective study. Soc Sci Med 1990;30:597–604. (Level II-2)

47. Taylor A, Fisk NM, Glover V. Mode of delivery and subsequent stress response. Lancet 2000;355:120. (Level II-2)

48. Northcott CJ, Stein MB. Panic disorder in pregnancy. J Clin Psychiatry 1994;55:539–42. (Level III)

49. Cohen LS, Sichel DA, Dimmock JA, Rosenbaum JF. Postpartum course in women with preexisting panic disorder. J Clin Psychiatry 1994;55:289–92. (Level III)

50. Loveland Cook CA, Flick LH, Homan SM, Campbell C, McSweeney M, Gallagher ME. Posttraumatic stress disorder during pregnancy: prevalence, risk factors, and treatment. Obstet Gynecol 2004;103:710–7. (Level II-3)

51. Neziroglu F, Anemone R, Yaryura-Tobias JA. Onset of obsessive-compulsive disorder in pregnancy. Am J Psychiatry 1992;149:947–50. (Level III)

52. Goldstein DJ, Corbin LA, Fung MC. Olanzapine-exposed pregnancies and lactation: early experience. J Clin Psychopharmacol. 2000;20:399–403. (Level III)

53. Bennedsen BE, Mortensen PB, Olesen AV, Henriksen TB. Preterm birth and intra-uterine growth retardation among children of women with schizophrenia. Br J Psychiatry 1999;175:239–45. (Level II-2)

54. Nilsson E, Lichtenstein P, Cnattingius S, Murray RM, Hultman CM. Women with schizophrenia: pregnancy outcome and infant death among their offspring. Schizophr Res 2002;58:221–9. (Level II-2)

55. Jablensky AV, Morgan V, Zubrick SR, Bower C, Yellachich LA. Pregnancy, delivery, and neonatal complications in a population cohort of women with schizophrenia and major affective disorders. Am J Psychiatry 2005;162(1):79–91. (Level II-2)

56. Bennedsen BE, Mortensen PB, Olesen AV, Henriksen TB, Frydenberg M. Obstetric complications in women with schizophrenia. Schizophr Res 2001;47:167–75. (Level II-2)

57. Coons PM, Ascher-Svanum H, Bellis K. Self-amputation of the female breast. Psychosomatics 1986;27:667–8. (Level III)

58. Yoldas Z, Iscan A, Yoldas T, Ermete L, Akyurek C. A woman who did her own caesarean section. Lancet 1996;348:135. (Level III)

59. Slayton RI, Soloff PH. Psychotic denial of third-trimester pregnancy. J Clin Psychiatry 1981;42:471–3. (Level III)

60. Bucove AD. A case of prepartum psychosis and infanticide. Psychiatr Q 1968;42:263–70. (Level III)

61. Mendlowicz MV, da Silva Filho JF, Gekker M, de Moraes TM, Rapaport MH, Jean-Louis F. Mothers murdering their newborns in the hospital. Gen Hosp Psychiatry 2000;22:53–5. (Level III)

62. Wen SW, Yang Q, Garner P, Fraser W, Olatunbosun O, Nimrod C, et al. Selective serotonin reuptake inhibitors and adverse pregnancy outcomes. Am J Obstet Gynecol 2006;194:961–6. (Level II-2)

63. Malm H, Klaukka T, Neuvonen PJ. Risks associated with selective serotonin reuptake inhibitors in pregnancy. Obstet Gynecol 2005;106:1289–96. (Level II-2)

64. Einarson TR, Einarson A. Newer antidepressants in pregnancy and rates of major malformations: a meta-analysis of prospective comparative studies. Pharmacoepidemiol Drug Saf 2005;14:823–7. (Meta-analysis)

65. Louik C, Lin AE, Werler MM, Hernandez-Diaz S, Mitchell AA. First-trimester use of selective serotonin-reuptake inhibitors and the risk of birth defects. NEJM 2007;356:2675–83. (Level II-2)

66. Alwan S, Reefhuis J, Rasmussen SA, Olney RS, Friedman JM. Use of selective serotonin-reuptake inhibitors in pregnancy and the risk of birth defects. National Birth Defects Prevention Study. NEJM 2007;356:2684–92. (Level II-2)

67. Moses-Kolko EL, Bogen D, Perel J, Bregar A, Uhl K, Levin B, et al. Neonatal signs after late in utero exposure to serotonin reuptake inhibitors: literature review and implications for clinical applications. JAMA 2005; 293:2372–83. (Level III)

68. Chambers CD, Johnson KA, Dick LM, Felix RJ, Jones KL. Birth outcomes in pregnant women taking fluoxetine. N Engl J Med 1996;335:1010–15. (Level II-2)

69. Costei AM, Kozer E, Ho T, Ito S, Koren G. Perinatal outcome following third trimester exposure to paroxetine. Arch Pediatr Adolesc Med 2002;156:1129–32. (Level II-2)

70. Kallen B. Neonate characteristics after maternal use of antidepressants in late pregnancy. Arch Pediatr Adolesc Med 2004;158:312–316. (Level II-2)

71. Zeskind PS, Stephens LE. Maternal selective serotonin reuptake inhibitor use during pregnancy and newborn neurobehavior. Pediatrics 2004;113:368–75. (Level II-2)

72. Chambers CD, Hernandez-Diaz S, Van Marter LJ, Werler MM, Louik C, Jones KL, et al. Selective serotonin-reuptake inhibitors and risk of persistent pulmonary hypertension of the newborn. N Engl J Med 2006;354:579–87. (Level II-2)

73. Barson AJ. Malformed infant. Br Med J 1972;2:45. (Level III)

74. Elia J, Katz IR, Simpson GM. Teratogenicity of psychotherapeutic medications. Psychopharmacol Bull 1987;23: 531–86. (Level III)

75. McBride WG. Limb deformities associated with iminodibenzyl hydrochloride. Med J Austr 1972;1:492. (Level III)

76. Altshuler LL, Cohen L, Szuba MP, Burt VK, Gitlin M, Mintz J. Pharmacologic management of psychiatric illness during pregnancy: dilemmas and guidelines. Am J Psychiatry 1996;153:592–606. (Level III)

77. McElhatton PR, Garbis HM, Elefant E, Vial T, Bellemin B, Mastroiacovo P, et al. The outcome of pregnancy in 689 women exposed to therapeutic doses of antidepressants. A collaborative study of the European Network of Teratology Information Services (ENTIS). Reprod Toxicol 1996;10:285–94. (Level III)

78. Nulman I, Rovet J, Stewart DE, Wolpin J, Gardner HA, Theis JA et al. Neurodevelopment of children exposed in utero to antidepressant drugs. N Engl J Med 1997;336: 258–62. (Level II-2)

79. Prentice A, Brown R. Fetal tachyarrhythmia and maternal antidepressant treatment. BMJ 1989;298:190. (Level III)

80. Eggermont E. Withdrawal symptoms in neonates associated with maternal imipramine therapy. Lancet 1973;2: 680. (Level III)

81. Miller LJ. Clinical strategies for the use of psychotropic drugs during pregnancy. Psychiatr Med 1991;9:275–98. (Level III)

82. Webster PA. Withdrawal symptoms in neonates associated with maternal antidepressant therapy. Lancet 1973; 2:318–9. (Level III)

83. Misri S, Sivertz K. Tricyclic drugs in pregnancy and lactation: a preliminary report. Int J Psychiatry Med 1991; 21:157–71. (Level II-3)

84. Simon GE, Cunningham ML, Davis RL. Outcomes of prenatal antidepressant exposure. Am J Psychiatry 2002; 159:2055–61. (Level II-2)

85. Yaris F, Kadioglu M, Kesim M, Ulku C, Yaris E, Kalyoncu NI, et al. Newer antidepressants in pregnancy: prospective outcome of a case series. Reprod Toxicol 2004;19:235–8. (Level II-3)

86. Yaris F, Ulku C, Kesim M, Kadioglu M, Unsal M, Dikici MF, et al. Psychotropic drugs in pregnancy: a case-control study. Prog Neuropsychopharmacol Biol Psychiatry 2005;29:333–8. (Level II-2)

87. Kesim M, Yaris F, Kadioglu M, Yaris E, Kalyoncu NI, Ulku C. Mirtazapine use in two pregnant women: is it safe? Teratology 2002;66:204. (Level III)

88. Rohde A, Dembinski J, Dorn C. Mirtazapine (Remergil) for treatment resistant hyperemesis gravidarum: rescue of a twin pregnancy. Arch Gynecol Obstet 2003;268: 219–21. (Level III)

89. Einarson A, Bonari L, Voyer-Lavigne S, Addis A, Matsui D, Johnson Y, et al. A multicentre prospective controlled study to determine the safety of trazodone and nefazodone use during pregnancy. Can J Psychiatry 2003;48: 106–10. (Level II-2)

90. Chun-Fai-Chan B, Koren G, Fayez I, Kalra S, Voyer-Lavigne S, Boshier A, et al. Pregnancy outcome of women exposed to bupropion during pregnancy: a prospective comparative study. Am J Obstet Gynecol 2005;192:932–6. (Level II-2)

91. Miller LJ. Use of electroconvulsive therapy during pregnancy. Hosp Community Psychiatry 1994;45:444–50. (Level III)

92. Rabheru K. The use of electroconvulsive therapy in special patient populations. Can J Psychiatry 2001;46: 710–9. (Level III)

93. Nora JJ, Nora AH, Toews WH. Lithium, Ebstein's anomaly, and other congenital heart defects [letter]. Lancet 1974;2:594–5. (Level III)

94. Weinstein MR, Goldfield M. Cardiovascular malformations with lithium use during pregnancy. Am J Psychiatry 1975;132:529–31. (Level III)

95. Cohen LS, Friedman JM, Jefferson JW, Johnson EM, Weiner ML. A reevaluation of risk of in utero exposure to lithium [published erratum appears in JAMA 1994;271: 1485]. JAMA 1994;271:146–50. (Level III)

96. Kallen B, Tandberg A. Lithium and pregnancy. A cohort of manic-depressive women. Acta Psychiatr Scand 1983;68:134–9. (Level II-2)

97. Jacobson SJ, Jones K, Johnson K, Ceolin L, Kaur P, Sahn D, et al. Prospective multicentre study of pregnancy outcome after lithium exposure during first trimester. Lancet 1992;339:530–3. (Level II-2)

98. Friedman JM, Polifka JE. Teratogenic effects of drugs: a resource for clinicians (TERIS). 2nd ed. Baltimore (MD): Johns Hopkins University Press; 2000. (Level III)

99. Wilson N, Forfar JC, Godman MJ. Atrial flutter in the newborn resulting from maternal lithium ingestion. Arch Dis Child 1983;58:538–9. (Level III)

100. Mizrahi EM, Hobbs JF, Goldsmith DI. Nephrogenic diabetes insipidus in transplacental lithium intoxication. J Pediatr 1979;94:493–5. (Level III)

101. Karlsson K, Lindstedt G, Lundberg PA, Selstam U. Transplacental lithium poisoning: reversible inhibition of fetal thyroid [letter]. Lancet 1975;1:1295. (Level III)

102. Llewellyn A, Stowe ZN, Strader JR Jr. The use of lithium and management of women with bipolar disorder during pregnancy and lactation. J Clin Psychiatry 1998;59(suppl 6):57–64;discussion 65. (Level III)

103. Woody JN, London WL, Wilbanks GD Jr. Lithium toxicity in a newborn. Pediatrics 1971;47:94–6. (Level III)

104. Schou M. What happened later to the lithium babies? A follow-up study of children born without malformations. Acta Psychiatr Scand 1976;54:193–7. (Level II-2)

105. Holmes LB, Harvey EA, Coull BA, Huntington KB, Khoshbin S, Hayes AM. The teratogenicity of anticonvulsant drugs. N Engl J Med 2001;344:1132–8. (Level 11-2)

106. Jager-Roman E, Deichl A, Jakob S, Hartmann AM, Koch S, Rating D, et al. Fetal growth, major malformations, and minor anomalies in infants born to women receiving valproic acid. J Pediatr 1986;108:997–1004. (Level II-2)

107. Lindhout D, Schmidt D. In-utero exposure to valproate and neural tube defects. Lancet 1986;1:1392–3. (Level III-3)

108. Spina bifida incidence at birth—United States, 1983–1990. Centers for Disease Control (CDC). MMWR Morb Mortal Wkly Rep 1992;41:497–500. (Level II-3)

109. Samren E, van Duijn CM, Koch S, Hiilesmaa VK, Klepel H, Bardy AH, et al. Maternal use of antiepileptic drugs and the risk of major congenital malformations: a joint European prospective study of human teratogenesis associated with maternal epilepsy. Epilepsia 1997;38:981–90. (Level II-2)

110. Omtzigt JG, Los FJ, Meiger JW, Lindhout D. The 10, 11-epoxide-10, 11-diol pathway of carbamazepine in early pregnancy in maternal serum, urine, and amniotic fluid: effect of dose, comedication, and relation to outcome of pregnancy. Ther Drug Monit 1993;15:1–10. (Level II-3)

111. Samren E, van Duijn CM, Christiaens GC, Hofman A, Lindhout D. Antiepileptic drug regimens and major congenital abnormalities in the offspring. Ann Neurol 1999; 46:739–46. (Level II-2)

112. Canger R, Battino D, Canevini MP, Fumarola C, Guidolin L, Vignoli A, et al. Malformations in offspring of women with epilepsy: a prospective study. Epilepsia 1999;40:1231–6. (Level II-2)

113. Kaneko S, Battino D, Andermann E, Wada K, Kan R, Takeda A, et al. Congenital malformations due to antiepileptic drugs. Epilepsy Res 1999;33:145–58. (Level II-2)

114. Paulson GW, Paulson RB. Teratogenic effects of anticonvulsants. Arch Neurol 1981;38:140–3. (Level III)

115. Rodriguez-Pinilla E, Arroyo I, Fondevilla J, Garcia MJ, Martinez-Frias ML. Prenatal exposure to valproic acid during pregnancy and limb deficiencies: a case-control study. Am J Med Genet 2000;90:376–81. (Level II-2)

116. Dalens B, Raynaud EJ, Gaulme J. Teratogenicity of valproic acid. J Pediatr 1980:97:332–3. (Level III)

117. Koch S, Jager-Roman E, Rating D, Helge H. Possible teratogenic effect of valproate during pregnancy. J Pediatr 1983;103:1007–8. (Level III)

118. Sodhi P, Poddar B, Parmar V. Fatal cardiac malformation in fetal valproate syndrome. Indian J Pediatr 2001;68: 989–90. (Level III)

119. Winter RM, Donnai D, Burn J, Tucker SM. Fetal valproate syndrome: is there a recognisable phenotype? J Med Genet 1987;24:692–5. (Level III)

120. Ardinger HH, Atkin JF, Blackston RD, Elsas LJ, Clarren SK, Livingstone S, et al. Verification of the fetal valproate syndrome phenotype. Am J Med Genet 1988;29: 171–85. (Level III)

121. Martinez-Frias ML. Clinical manifestation of prenatal exposure to valproic acid using case reports and epidemiologic information. Am J Med Genet 1990;37: 277–82. (Level III)

122. Kozma C. Valproic acid embryopathy: report of two siblings with further expansion of the phenotypic abnormalities and a review of the literature. Am J Med Genet 2001;98:168–75. (Level III)

123. Williams PG, Hersh JH. A male with fetal valproate syndrome and autism. Dev Med Child Neurol 1997;39: 632–4. (Level III)

124. Moore SJ, Turnpenny P, Quinn A, Glover S, Lloyd DJ, Montgomery T, et al. A clinical study of 57 children with fetal anticonvulsant syndromes. J Med Genet 2000;37: 489–97. (Level III)

125. Bescoby-Chambers N, Forster P, Bates G. Foetal valproate syndrome and autism: additional evidence of an association [letter]. Dev Med Child Neurol 2001;43:847. (Level III)

126. Williams G, King J, Cunningham M, Stephan M, Kerr B, Hersh JH. Fetal valproate syndrome and autism: additional evidence of an association. Dev Med Child Neurol 2001;43:202–6. (Level III)

127. Gaily E, Kantola-Sorsa E, Granstrom ML. Specific cognitive dysfunction in children with epileptic mothers. Dev Med Child Neurol 1990;32:403–14. (Level II-2)

128. Adab N, Jacoby A, Smith D, Chadwick D. Additional educational needs in children born to mothers with epilepsy. J Neurol Neurosurg Psychiatry 2001;70:15–21. (Level II-2)

129. Kennedy D, Koren G. Valproic acid use in psychiatry: issues in treating women of reproductive age. J Psychiatry Neurosci 1998;23:223–8. (Level III)

130. Mountain KR, Hirsch J, Gallus AS. Neonatal coagulation defect due to anticonvulsant drug treatment in pregnancy. Lancet 1970;1:265–8. (Level II-3)

131. Thisted E, Ebbesen F. Malformations, withdrawal manifestations, and hypoglycaemia after exposure to valproate in utero. Arch Dis Child 1993;69:288–91. (Level III)

132. Ebbesen F, Joergensen A, Hoseth E, Kaad PH, Moeller M, Holsteen V, et al. Neonatal hypoglycaemia and withdrawal symptoms after exposure in utero to valproate. Arch Dis Child Fetal Neonatal Ed 2000;83:F124–9. (Level II-2)

133. Jones KL, Lacro RV, Johnson KA, Adams J. Pattern of malformations in the children of women treated with carbamazepine during pregnancy. N Engl J Med 1989; 320:1661–6. (Level II-3)

134. Scolnik D, Nulman I, Rovet J, Gladstone D, Czuchta D, Gardner HA, et al. Neurodevelopment of children exposed in utero to phenytoin and carbamazepine monotherapy [published erratum appears in JAMA 1994; 271:1745]. JAMA 1994;271:767–70. (Level II-2)

135. Wide K, Winbladh B, Tomson T, Sars-Zimmer K, Berggren E. Psychomotor development and minor anomalies in children exposed to antiepileptic drugs in utero: a prospective population-based study [published erratum appears in Dev Med Child Neurol 2000;42:356]. Dev Med Child Neurol 2000;42:87–92. (Level II-2)

136. Ornoy A, Cohen E. Outcome of children born to epileptic mothers treated with carbamazepine during pregnancy. Arch Dis Child 1996;75:517–20. (Level II-2)

137. Gaily E, Granstrom ML, Liukkonen E. Oxcarbazepine in the treatment of epilepsy in children and adolescents with intellectual disability. J Intellect Disabil Res. 1998;42 (suppl 1):41–5. (Level III)

138. Van der Pol MC, Hadders-Algra M, Huisjes MJ, Touwen BC. Antiepileptic medication in pregnancy: late effects on the children's central nervous system development. Am J Obstet Gynecol 1991;164:121–8. (Level II-2)

139. Matalon S, Schechtman S, Goldzweig G, Ornoy A. The teratogenic effect of carbamazepine: a meta-analysis of 1255 exposures. Reprod Toxicol 2002;16:9–17. (Meta-analysis)

140. Vajda FJ, O'Brien TJ, Hitchcock A, Graham J, Lander C. The Australian registry of anti-epileptic drugs in pregnancy: experience after 30 months. J Clin Neurosci 2003; 10:543–9. (Level II-2)

141. Sabers A, Dam M, A-Rogvi-Hansen B, Boas J, Sidenius P, Laue Friis M, et al. Epilepsy and pregnancy: lamotrigine as main drug used. Acta Neurol Scand 2004;109: 9–13. (Level III)

142. Cunnington M, Tennis P. Lamotrigine and the risk of malformations in pregnancy. International Lamotrigine Pregnancy Registry Scientific Advisory Committee. Neurology 2005;64:955–60. (Level III)

143. Holmes LB, Wyszynski DF. North American antiepileptic drug pregnancy registry. Epilepsia 2004;45:1465. (Level III)

144. Meador KJ, Baker GA, Finnell RH, Kalayjian LA, Liporace JD, Loring DW, et al. In utero antiepileptic drug exposure: fetal death and malformations. NEAD Study Group. Neurology 2006;67:407–12. (Level II-2)

145. Morrow J, Russell A, Guthrie E, Parsons L, Robertson I, Waddell R, et al. Malformation risks of antiepileptic drugs in pregnancy: a prospective study from the UK Epilepsy and Pregnancy Register. J Neurol Neurosurg Psychiatry 2006;77:193–8. (Level II-2)

146. Baldessarini RJ, Faedda GL, Hennen J. Risk of mania with antidepressants. Arch Pediatr Adolesc Med 2005; 159:298. (Level III)

147. Newport DJ, Viguera AC, Beach AJ, Ritchie JC, Cohen LS, Stowe ZN. Lithium placental passage and obstetrical outcome: implications for clinical management during late pregnancy. Am J Psychiatry 2005;162:2162–70. (Level III)

148. Choulika S, Grabowski E, Holmes LB. Is antenatal vitamin K prophylaxis needed for pregnant women taking anticonvulsants? Am J Obstet Gynecol 2004;190:882–3. (Level II-2)

149. Saxen I. Cleft palate and maternal diphenhydramine intake [letter]. Lancet 1974;1:407–8. (Level III)

150. Aarkog D. Association between maternal intake of diazepam and oral clefts [letter]. The Lancet 1975;2:921. (Level II-2)

151. Saxen I. Associations between oral clefts and drugs taken during pregnancy. Int J Epidemiol 1975;4:37–44. (Level II-2)

152. Eros E, Czeizel AE, Rockenbauer M, Sorensen HT, Olsen J. A population-based case-control teratologic study of nitrazepam, medazepam, tofisopam, alprazolum and clonazepam treatment during pregnancy. Euro J Obstet, Gynecol Reprod Biol 2002;101:147–54. (Level II-2)

153. Lin AE, Peller AJ, Westgate MN, Houde K, Franz A, Holmes LB. Clonazepam use in pregnancy and the risk of malformations. Birth Defects Res A Clin Mol Teratol 2004;70:534–6. (Level III-3)

154. Haram K. "Floppy infant syndrome" and maternal diazepam. Lancet 1977;2:612–3. (Level III)

155. Speight AN. Floppy-infant syndrome and maternal diazepam and/or nitrazepam. Lancet 1977;2:878. (Level III)

156. Woods DL, Malan AF. Side-effects of maternal diazepam on the newborn infant. S Afr Med J 1978;54:636. (Level III)

157. Kriel RL, Cloyd J. Clonazepam and pregnancy. Ann Neurol 1982;11:544. (Level III)

158. McAuley DM, O'Neill MP, Moore J, Dundee JW. Lorazepam premedication for labour. Br J Obstet Gynaecol 1982;89:149–54. (Level I)

159. Erkkola R, Kero P, Kanto J, Aaltonen L. Severe abuse of psychotropic drugs during pregnancy with good perinatal outcome. Ann Clin Res 1983;15:88–91. (Level III)

160. Fisher JB, Edgren BE, Mammel MC, Coleman JM. Neonatal apnea associated with maternal clonazepam therapy: a case report. Obstet Gynecol. 1985;66(suppl): 34s–35s. (Level III)

161. Sanchis A, Rosique D, Catala J. Adverse effects of maternal lorazepam on neonates. DICP 1991;25:1137–8. (Level III)

162. Whitelaw AG, Cummings AJ, McFadyen IR. Effect of maternal lorazepam on the neonate. Br Med J (Clin Res Ed) 1981;282:1106–8. (Level II-2)

163. Barry WS, St Clair S. Exposure to benzodiazepines in utero. Lancet 1987;1:1436–7. (Level III)

164. Bitnun S. Possible effect of chlordiazepoxide on the fetus. Can Med Assoc J 1969;100:351. (Level III)

165. Stirrat GM, Edington PT, Berry DJ. Transplacental passage of chlordiazepoxide [letter]. Br Med J 1974;2:729. (Level III)

166. Athinarayanan P, Pierog SH, Nigam SK, Glass L. Chloriazepoxide withdrawal in the neonate. Am J Obstet Gynecol 1976;124:212–3. (Level III)

167. Mazzi E. Possible neonatal diazepam withdrawal: a case report. Am J Obstet Gynecol 1977;129:586–7. (Level III)

168. Backes CR, Cordero L. Withdrawal symptoms in the neonate from presumptive intrauterine exposure to diazepam: report of case. J Am Osteopath Assoc 1980; 79:584–5. (Level III)

169. Laegreid L, Olegard R, Wahlstrom J, Conradi N. Abnormalities in children exposed to benzodiazepines in utero. Lancet 1987;1:108–109. (Level III)

170. Gerhardsson M, Alfredsson L. In utero exposure to benzodiazepines [letter]. Lancet 1987:628. (Level III)

171. Winter RM. In-utero exposure to benzodiazepines [letter]. Lancet 1987;1:627. (Level III)

172. Hartz SC, Heinonen OP, Shapiro S, Siskind V, Slone D. Antenatal exposure to meprobamate and chlordiazepoxide in relation to malformations, mental development, and childhood mortality. N Engl J Med 1975;292:726–8. (Level II-2)

173. McKenna K, Koren G, Tetelbaum M, Wilton L, Shakir S, Diav-Citrin O, et al. Pregnancy outcome of women using atypical antipsychotic drugs: a prospective comparative study. J Clin Psychiatry 2005;66:444–9;quiz 546. (Level III-3)

174. Goldberg HL, DiMascio A. Psychotropic drugs in pregnancy. In: Lipton MA, DiMascio A, Killam KF, editors. Psychopharmacology: a generation of progress. New York (NY): Raven Press; 1978. p.1047–55. (Level III)

175. Hill RM, Stern L. Drugs in pregnancy: effects on the fetus and newborn. Drugs 1979;17:182–97. (Level III)

176. Nurnberg HG, Prudic J. Guidelines for treatment of psychosis during pregnancy. Hosp Community Psychiatry 1984;35:67–71. (Level III)

177. Van Waes A, Van de Velde E. Safety evaluation of haloperidol in the treatment of hyperemesis gravidarum. J Clin Pharmacol 1969;9:224–7. (Level II-2)

178. Miklovich L, van den Berg BJ. An evaluation of the teratogenicity of certain antinauseant drugs. Am J Obstet Gynecol 1976;125:244–8. (Level II-2)

179. Moriarty AJ, Nance NR. Trifluoperazine and pregnancy [letter]. Can Med Assoc J 1963;88:375–6. (Level III)

180. Rawlings WJ. Use of medroxyprogesterone in the treatment of recurrent abortion. Med J Aust 1963;50:183–4. (Level III)

181. Rumeau-Rouquette C, Goujard J, Huel G. Possible teratogenic effect of phenothiazines in human beings. Teratology 1977;15:57–64. (Level II-2)

182. Edlund MJ, Craig TJ. Antipsychotic drug use and birth defects: an epidemiologic reassessment. Compr Psychiatry 1984;25:32–7. (Level II-2)

183. Kris EB. Children of mothers maintained on pharmacotherapy during pregnancy and postpartum. Curr Ther Res Clin Exp 1965;7:785–9. (Level III)

184. Slone D, Siskind V, Heinonen OP, Monson RR, Kaufman DW, Shapiro S. Antenatal exposure to the phenothiazines in relation to congenital malformations, perinatal mortality rate, birth weight, and intelligence quotient score. Am J Obstet Gynecol. 1977;128:486–8. (Level II-2)

185. James ME. Neuroleptic malignant syndrome in pregnancy. Psychosomatics 1988;29:119–22. (Level III)

186. Collins KO, Comer JB. Maternal haloperidol therapy associated with dyskinesia in a newborn. Am J Health Syst Pharm 2003;60:2253–5. (Level III)

187. Hill RM, Desmond MM, Kay JL. Extrapyramidal dysfunction in an infant of a schizophrenic mother. J Pediatr 1966;69:589–95. (Level III)

188. Scokel PW 3rd, Jones WN. Infant jaundice after phenothiazine drugs for labor: an enigma. Obstet Gynecol 1962;20:124–7. (Level II-2)

189. Falterman CG, Richardson CJ. Small left colon syndrome associated with maternal ingestion of psychotropic drugs. J Pediatr 1980;97:308–10. (Level III)

190. Heinonen OP, Shapiro S, Slone D. Birth defects and drugs in pregnancy. Littleton (MA): Publishing Sciences Group; 1977. (Level III)

191. Nelson MM, Forfar JO. Associations between drugs administered during pregnancy and congenital abnormalities of the fetus. Br Med J 1971;1:523–7. (Level III)

192. Hale TW. Medications in Mother's Milk. Amaraillo (TX): Pharmasoft Publishing, 2004. (Level III)

193. Stowe ZN, Owens MJ, Landry JC, Kilts CD, Ely T, Llewellyn A, et al. Sertraline and desmethylsertraline in human breast milk and nursing infants. Am J Psychiatry 1997;154:1255–60. (Level II-3)

194. Altshuler LL, Burt VK, McMullen M, Hendrick V. Breastfeeding and sertraline: a 24-hour analysis. J Clin Psychiatry 1995;56:243–5. (Level III)

195. Epperson CN, Anderson GM, McDougle CJ. Sertraline and breast-feeding. N Engl J Med 1997;336:1189–90. (Level III)

196. Kristensen JH, Ilett KF, Dusci LJ, Hackett LP, Yapp P, Wojnar-Horton RE, et al. Distribution and excretion of sertraline and N-desmethylsertraline in human milk. Br J Clin Pharmacol 1998;45:453–7. (Level III)

197. Mammen O, Perel JM, Wheeler S. Antidepressants and breast-feeding. Am J Psychiatry 1997;154:1174–5. (Level III)

198. Wisner KL, Perel JM, Blumer J. Serum sertraline and N-desmethylsertraline levels in breast-feeding mother-infant pairs. Am J Psychiatry 1998;155:690–2. (Level III)

199. Birnbaum CS, Cohen LS, Bailey JW, Grush LR, Robertson LM, Stowe ZN. Serum concentrations of antidepressants and benzodiazepines in nursing infants: a case series. Pediatrics 1999;104(1):e11. (Level III)

200. Dodd S, Buist A, Norman TR. Antidepressants and breast-feeding: a review of the literature. Paediatr Drugs 2000;2:183–92. (Level III)

201. Stowe ZN, Cohen LS, Hostetter A, Ritchie JC, Owens MJ, Nemeroff CB. Paroxetine in human breast milk and nursing infants. Am J Psychiatry 2000;157:185–9. (Level II-3)

202. Epperson N, Czarkowski KA, Ward-O'Brien D, Weiss E, Gueorguieva R, Jatlow P, et al. Maternal sertraline treatment and serotonin transport in breast-feeding mother-infant pairs. Am J Psychiatry 2001;158:1631–7. (Level II-3)

203. Hendrick V, Fukuchi A, Altshuler L, Widawski M, Wertheimer A, Brunhuber MV. Use of sertraline, paroxetine and fluvoxamine by nursing women. Br J Psychiatr 2001;179:163–6. (Level II-3)

204. Burch KJ, Wells BG. Fluoxetine/norfluoxetine concentrations in human milk. Pediatrics 1992;89:676–7. (Level III)

205. Lester BM, Cucca J, Andreozzi L, Flanagan P, Oh W. Possible association between fluoxetine hydrochloride and colic in an infant. J Am Acad Child Adolesc Psychiatry 1993;32:1253–5. (Level III)

206. Taddio A, Ito S, Koren G. Excretion of fluoxetine and its metabolite, norfluoxetine, in human breast milk. J Clin Pharmacol 1996;36:42–7. (Level II-3)

207. Yoshida K, Kumar RC, Smith B, Craggs M. Psychotropic drugs in breast milk: no evidence for adverse effects on prepulse modulation of startle reflex or on cognitive level in infants. Dev Psychobiol 1998;32:249–56. (Level II-2)

208. Cohen LS, Heller V, Bailey JW, Grush L, Ablon JS, Bouffard SM. Birth outcomes following prenatal exposure to fluoxetine. Biol Psychiatry 2000;48:996–1000. (Level II-2)

209. Spigset O, Carleborg L, Norstrom A, Sandlund M. Paroxetine level in breast milk. J Clin Psychiatry 1996; 57:39. (Level III)

210. Ohman R, Hagg S, Carleborg L, Spigset O. Excretion of paroxetine into breast milk. J Clin Psychiatry 1999;60: 519–23. (Level III)

211. Wright S, Dawling S, Ashford JJ. Excretion of fluvoxamine in breast milk. British Journal of Clinical Pharmacology 1991;31(2):209. (Level III)

212. Piontek CM, Wisner KL, Perel JM, Peindl KS. Serum fluvoxamine levels in breastfed infants. J Clin Psychiatry 2001;62:111–3. (Level III)

213. Jensen PN, Olesen OV, Bertelsen A, Linnet K. Citalopram and desmethylcitalopram concentrations in breast milk and in serum of mother and infant. Ther Drug Monit 1997;19:236–9. (Level III)

214. Spigset O, Carieborg L, Ohman R, Norstrom A. Excretion of citalopram in breast milk. Br J Clin Pharmacol 1997;44:295–8. (Level III)

215. Schmidt K, Olesen OV, Jensen PN. Citalopram and breast-feeding: serum concentration and side effects in the infant. Biol Psychiatry 2000;47:164–5. (Level III)

216. Stowe ZN, Hostetter AL, Owens MJ, Ritchie JC, Sternberg K, Cohen LS, et al. The pharmacokinetics of sertraline excretion into human breast milk: determinants of infant serum concentrations. J Clin Psychiatry 2003; 64:73–80. (Level III)

217. Matheson I, Pande H, Alertsen AR. Respiratory depression caused by N-desmethyldoxepin in breast milk. Lancet 1985;2:1124. (Level III)

218. Ilett KF, Hackett LP, Dusci LJ, Roberts MJ, Kristensen JH, Paech M, et al. Distribution and excretion of venlafaxine and O-desmethylvenlafaxine in human milk. Br J Clin Pharmacol 1998;45:459–62. (Level III)

219. Briggs GG, Samson JH, Ambrose PJ, Schroeder DH. Excretion of bupropion in breast milk. Ann Pharmacother 1993;27:431–3. (Level III)

220. Baab SW, Peindl KS, Piontek CM, Wisner KL. Serum bupropion levels in 2 breastfeeding mother-infant pairs. J Clin Psychiatry 2002;63:910–1. (Level III)

221. Weinstein MR, Goldfield M. Lithium carbonate treatment during pregnancy; report of a case. Dis Nerv Syst 1969;30:828–32. (Level III)

222. Fries H. Lithium in pregnancy. Lancet 1970;1:1233. (Level III)

223. Tunnessen WW Jr, Hertz CG. Toxic effects of lithium in newborn infants: a commentary. J Pediatr 1972;81: 804–7. (Level III)

224. Schou M, Amdisen A. Lithium and pregnancy. 3.: lithium ingestion by children breast-fed by women on lithium treatment. BMJ 1973;2:138. (Level III)

225. Sykes PA, Quarrie J, Alexander FW. Lithium carbonate and breast-feeding [letter]. BMJ 1976;2:1299. (Level III)

226. Transfer of drugs and other chemicals into human milk. American Academy of Pediatrics Committee on Drugs. Pediatrics 2001;108:776–89. (Level III)

227. Stahl MM, Neiderud J, Vinge E. Thrombocytopenic purpura and anemia in a breast-fed infant whose mother was treated with valproic acid. J Pediatr 1997;130:1001–3. (Level III)

228. Alexander FW. Sodium valproate and pregnancy. Arch Dis Child 1979;54:240–1. (Level III)

229. Dickinson RG, Harland RC, Lynn RK, Smith WB, Gerber N. Transmission of valproic acid (Depakene) across the placenta: half-life of the drug in mother and baby. J Pediatr 1979;94:832–5. (Level III)

230. Nau H, Rating D, Koch S, Hauser I, Helge H. Valproic acid and its metabolites: placental transfer, neonatal pharmacokinetics, transfer via mother's milk and clinical status in neonates of epileptic mothers. J Pharmacol Exp Ther 1981;219:768–77. (Level II-3)

231. Bardy AH, Teramo K, Hiilesmaa VK. Apparent plasma clearances of phenytoin, phenobarbitone, primidone, and carbamazepine during pregnancy: results of the Prospective Helsinki Study. In: Janz D, Dam M, Richens A, Bossi L, Helge H, Schmidt D, editors. Epilepsy, pregnancy, and the child. New York (NY): Raven Press; 1982. p.141–5. (Level III-3)

232. von Unruh GE, Froescher W, Hoffmann F, Niesen M. Valproic acid in breast milk: how much is really there? Ther Drug Monit 1984;6:272–6. (Level III)

233. Tsuru N, Maeda T, Tsuruoka M. Three cases of delivery under sodium valproate—placental transfer, milk transfer and probable teratogenicity of sodium valproate. Jpn J Psychiatry Neurol 1988;42:89–96. (Level III)

234. Wisner KL, Perel JM. Serum levels of valproate and carbamazepine in breastfeeding mother-infant pairs. J Clin Psychopharmacol 1998;18:167–9. (Level III)

235. Piontek CM, Baab S, Peindl KS, Wisner KL. Serum valproate levels in 6 breastfeeding mother-infant pairs. J Clin Psychiatry 2000;61:170–2. (Level III)

236. Bennett PN, editor. Drugs and human lactation. 2nd ed. New York (NY): Elsevier; 1996. (Level III)

237. Frey B, Braegger CP, Ghelfi D. Neonatal cholestatic hepatitis from carbamazepine exposure during pregnancy and breast feeding. Ann Pharmacother 2002;36:644–7. (Level III)

238. Frey B, Schubiger G, Musy JP. Transient cholestatic hepatitis in a neonate associated with carbamazepine exposure during pregnancy and breast-feeding. Eur J Pediatr 1990;150:136–8. (Level III)

239. Merlob P, Mor N, Litwin A. Transient hepatic dysfunction in an infant of an epileptic mother treated with carbamazepine during pregnancy and breastfeeding. Ann Pharmacother 1992;26:1563–5. (Level III)

240. Wretlind M. Excretion of oxazepam in breast milk. Eur J Clin Pharmacol 1987;33:209–10. (Level III)

241. Summerfield RJ, Nielsen MS. Excretion of lorazepam into breast milk. Br J Anaesth 1985;57:1042–3. (Level III)

242. Buist A, Norman TR, Dennerstein L. Breastfeeding and the use of psychotropic medication: a review. J Affect Disord 1990;19:197–206. (Level III)

243. Wesson DR, Camber S, Harkey M, Smith DE. Diazepam and desmethyldiazepam in breast milk. J Psychoactive Drugs 1985;17(1):55–56. (Level III)

244. Kris EB, Carmichael DM. Chlorpromazine maintenance therapy during pregnancy and confinement. Psychiatr Q 1957;31:690–5. (Level III)

245. Yoshida K, Smith B, Craggs M, Kumar R. Neuroleptic drugs in breast-milk: a study of pharmacokinetics and of possible adverse effects in breast-fed infants. Psychol Med 1998;28:81–91. (Level II-2)

The MEDLINE database, the Cochrane Library, and ACOG's own internal resources and documents were used to conduct a literature search to locate relevant articles published between January 1985 and June 2007. The search was restricted to articles published in the English language. Priority was given to articles reporting results of original research, although review articles and commentaries also were consulted. Abstracts of research presented at symposia and scientific conferences were not considered adequate for inclusion in this document. Guidelines published by organizations or institutions such as the National Institutes of Health and the American College of Obstetricians and Gynecologists were reviewed, and additional studies were located by reviewing bibliographies of identified articles. When reliable research was not available, expert opinions from obstetrician–gynecologists were used.

Studies were reviewed and evaluated for quality according to the method outlined by the U.S. Preventive Services Task Force:

I   Evidence obtained from at least one properly designed randomized controlled trial.

II-1   Evidence obtained from well-designed controlled trials without randomization.

II-2   Evidence obtained from well-designed cohort or case–control analytic studies, preferably from more than one center or research group.

II-3   Evidence obtained from multiple time series with or without the intervention. Dramatic results in uncontrolled experiments also could be regarded as this type of evidence.

III   Opinions of respected authorities, based on clinical experience, descriptive studies, or reports of expert committees.

Based on the highest level of evidence found in the data, recommendations are provided and graded according to the following categories:

Level A—Recommendations are based on good and consistent scientific evidence.

Level B—Recommendations are based on limited or inconsistent scientific evidence.

Level C—Recommendations are based primarily on consensus and expert opinion.

ISSN 1099-3630

The American College of Obstetricians and Gynecologists
409 12th Street, SW, PO Box 96920, Washington, DC 20090-6920

Use of psychiatric medications during pregnancy and lactation. ACOG Practice Bulletin No. 92. American College of Obstetricians and Gynecologists. Obstet Gynecol 2008;111:1001–20.

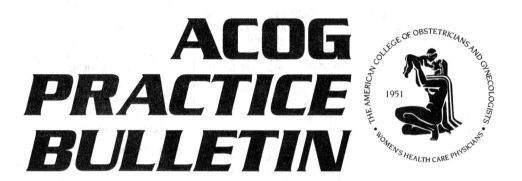

ACOG PRACTICE BULLETIN

CLINICAL MANAGEMENT GUIDELINES FOR OBSTETRICIAN–GYNECOLOGISTS

NUMBER 95, JULY 2008

Anemia in Pregnancy

This Practice Bulletin was developed by the ACOG Committee on Practice Bulletins—Obstetrics with the assistance of Maureen Malee, PhD, MD. The information is designed to aid practitioners in making decisions about appropriate obstetric and gynecologic care. These guidelines should not be construed as dictating an exclusive course of treatment or procedure. Variations in practice may be warranted based on the needs of the individual patient, resources, and limitations unique to the institution or type of practice.

Anemia, the most common hematologic abnormality, is a reduction in the concentration of erythrocytes or hemoglobin in blood. The two most common causes of anemia in pregnancy and the puerperium are iron deficiency and acute blood loss. Iron requirements increase during pregnancy, and a failure to maintain sufficient levels of iron may result in adverse maternal–fetal consequences. The purpose of this document is to provide a brief overview of the causes of anemia in pregnancy, review iron requirements, and provide recommendations for screening and clinical management of anemia during pregnancy.

Background

Classification

The definition of *anemia* recommended by the Centers for Disease Control and Prevention is a hemoglobin (Hgb) or hematocrit (Hct) value less than the fifth percentile of the distribution of Hgb or Hct in a healthy reference population based on the stage of pregnancy. Classification derived from an iron-supplemented population lists the following levels as anemic: Hgb (g/dL) and Hct (percentage) levels below 11 g/dL and 33%, respectively, in the first trimester; 10.5 g/dL and 32%, respectively, in the second trimester; and 11 g/dL and 33%, respectively, in the third trimester (1).

Anemias may be categorized by the underlying causative mechanism, red blood cell morphology, or by whether they are inherited or acquired (see the boxes). A mechanistic approach categorizes anemias caused by decreased red blood cell production, increased red blood cell destruction, and blood loss. Decreased production may result from a lack of nutrients, such as iron, vitamin B_{12}, or folate. This lack may be a result of dietary deficiency, malabsorption, or bleeding. Bone marrow disorders or suppression, hormone deficiencies, and chronic disease or infection also may lead to decreased production. Hemolytic anemias are associated with increased destruction.

THE AMERICAN COLLEGE OF OBSTETRICIANS AND GYNECOLOGISTS
WOMEN'S HEALTH CARE PHYSICIANS

Anemia Classification

Acquired

- Deficiency anemia (eg, iron, vitamin B$_{12}$, folate)
- Hemorrhagic anemia
- Anemia of chronic disease
- Acquired hemolytic anemia
- Aplastic anemia

Inherited

- Thalassemias
- Sickle cell anemia
- Hemoglobinopathies (other than sickle cell anemia)
- Inherited hemolytic anemias

Anemias Characterized by Mechanism

Decreased red blood cell production

- Iron deficiency anemia
- Anemia associated with vitamin B$_{12}$ deficiency
- Folic acid deficiency anemia
- Anemia associated with bone marrow disorders
- Anemia associated with bone marrow suppression
- Anemia associated with low levels of erythropoietin
- Anemia associated with hypothyroidism

Increased red blood cell destruction

- Inherited hemolytic anemias
  - Sickle cell anemia
  - Thalassemia major
  - Hereditary spherocytosis
- Acquired hemolytic anemias
  - Autoimmune hemolytic anemia
  - Hemolytic anemia associated with thrombotic thrombocytopenic purpura
  - Hemolytic anemia associated with hemolytic uremic syndrome
  - Hemolytic anemia associated with malaria
- Hemorrhagic anemia

Anemias Classified by Mean Corpuscular Volume

Microcytic (MCV less than 80 fL)

- Iron deficiency anemia
- Thalassemias
- Anemia of chronic disease
- Sideroblastic anemia
- Anemia associated with copper deficiency
- Anemia associated with lead poisoning

Normocytic (MCV 80–100 fL)

- Hemorrhagic anemia
- Early iron deficiency anemia
- Anemia of chronic disease
- Anemia associated with bone marrow suppression
- Anemia associated with chronic renal insufficiency
- Anemia associated with endocrine dysfunction
- Autoimmune hemolytic anemia
- Anemia associated with hypothyroidism or hypopituitarism
- Hereditary spherocytosis
- Hemolytic anemia associated with paroxysmal nocturnal hemoglobinuria

Macrocytic (MCV greater than 100 fL)

- Folic acid deficiency anemia
- Anemia associated with vitamin B$_{12}$ deficiency
- Drug-induced hemolytic anemia (eg, zidovudine)
- Anemia associated with reticulocytosis
- Anemia associated with liver disease
- Anemia associated with ethanol abuse
- Anemia associated with acute myelodysplastic syndrome

Abbreviation: MCV, mean corpuscular volume

Anemias also may be classified by cell size. In contemporary practice, this typically is done by an automated cell counter. Macrocytic anemias are associated with a mean corpuscular volume (MCV) greater than 100 fL. Reticulocytosis also may cause an increased MCV. A common cause of macrocytic anemia is folate deficiency. Microcytic anemias are associated with an MCV less than 80 fL. The most common cause of microcytic anemia is iron deficiency. Another common cause of microcytic anemia in certain ethnic groups is hemoglobinopathy (2).

Anemia in Pregnancy

Pregnancy is associated with physiologic changes that may complicate the diagnosis of hematologic disorders. There is an increased iron requirement during pregnancy because blood volume expands by approximately 50%

(1,000 mL), and total red blood cell mass expands by approximately 25% (300 mL) during a singleton gestation (3). The greater expansion in plasma typically is reflected by decreases in Hgb and Hct levels.

The total amount of iron in the body is determined by intake, loss, and storage (4). There are approximately 2.3 g of total body iron in women. Additional iron stores during pregnancy (approximately 1 g) support this increased red blood cell mass, the fetus and placenta, and the anticipated blood loss accompanying a vaginal delivery. When there is adequate iron to meet needs, more than 70% is classified as functional iron, and the remainder as storage iron. Of the functional iron, more than 80% is found in the red blood cell mass as hemoglobin, with the remainder in myoglobin and in respiratory enzymes (5).

Iron Deficiency Anemia

Iron deficiency can be defined as abnormal values on biochemical test results, increases in hemoglobin concentrations of more than 1 g/dL after iron treatment, or absent bone marrow iron stores as determined by a bone marrow iron smear (1). The spectrum of iron deficiency ranges from iron depletion, when stored iron is low, to iron deficient erythropoiesis, when both stored and transport iron are low, to iron deficiency anemia, when stored, transport, and functional iron are low (6).

Measurements of serum Hgb concentration or Hct are the primary screening tests for identifying anemia but are nonspecific for identifying iron deficiency. Normal iron indices are listed in Table 1. Laboratory test results characteristic of iron deficiency anemia are a microcytic, hypochromic anemia with evidence of depleted iron stores, low plasma iron levels, high total iron-binding capacity, low serum ferritin levels, and increased levels of free erythrocyte protoporphyrin.

Measurement of ferritin levels has the highest sensitivity and specificity for diagnosing iron deficiency in anemic patients (7). Levels of less than 10–15 micrograms/L confirm iron-deficiency anemia. The Centers for Disease Control and Prevention recommends screening for iron deficiency anemia in pregnant women and universal iron supplementation to meet the iron requirements

of pregnancy except in the presence of certain genetic disorders, such as hemochromatosis (1, 8). The rationale is that treatment maintains maternal iron stores and may be beneficial for neonatal iron stores. The typical diet confers 15 mg of elemental iron per day. The recommended daily dietary allowance of ferrous iron during pregnancy is 27 mg, which is present in most prenatal vitamins (8). Available iron supplements are listed in Table 2. Perinatal iron supplementation is important because the typical American diet and endogenous stores are insufficient sources for the increased iron requirements during pregnancy. Sustained-release or enteric-coated preparations dissolve poorly and may be less effective.

Prevalence, Etiologies, and Risk Factors

A national study of anemia in pregnancy in the United States found a prevalence of 21.55 per 1,000 women when anemia was defined as a hemoglobin concentration less than 10 g/dL (9). The prevalence of anemia in pregnancy in non-Hispanic black women (35.38 per 1,000 women) was two times higher than that of non-Hispanic white women (18.02 per 1,000 women) (9). Teenaged mothers had the highest prevalence of anemia in pregnancy of all races (9). Prevalence data specific to iron deficiency anemia in pregnancy are limited (10). A recent report estimates that in a low income, mostly minority population, rates of iron deficiency anemia are 1.8% in the first trimester, 8.2% in the second trimester, and 27.4% in the third trimester (11).

In reproductive-aged women of all races, risk factors for iron deficiency anemia include a diet poor in iron-rich foods, such as clams, oysters, liver, beef, shrimp, turkey, enriched breakfast cereals, beans, and lentils; a diet poor in iron absorption enhancers, such as orange juice, grapefruit, strawberries, broccoli, and peppers; a diet rich in foods that diminish iron absorption, such as dairy products, soy products, spinach, coffee, and tea; pica (eating nonfood substances such as clay or laundry starch); gastrointestinal disease affecting

Table 1. Normal Iron Indices in Pregnancy

Test	Normal Value
Plasma iron level	40–175 micrograms/dL
Plasma total iron-binding capacity	216–400 micrograms/dL
Transferrin saturation	16–60%
Serum ferritin level	More than 10 micrograms/dL
Free erythrocyte protoporphyrin level	Less than 3 micrograms/g

Table 2. Iron Supplements

Preparation	Dose
Ferrous fumarate	106 mg elemental iron per 325 mg tablet
Ferrous sulfate	65 mg elemental iron per 325 mg tablet
Ferrous gluconate	34 mg elemental iron per 300 mg tablet
Iron dextran	50 mg elemental iron per milliliter, intramuscularly or intravenously
Ferric gluconate	12.5 mg iron per milliliter, intravenously only
Iron sucrose	20 mg iron per milliliter, intravenously only

absorption; heavy menses; short interpregnancy interval; and blood loss at delivery exceeding that of an uncomplicated vaginal delivery.

Iron deficiency anemia during pregnancy has been associated with an increased risk of low birth weight, preterm delivery, and perinatal mortality (11, 12). In addition, there may be an association between maternal iron deficiency anemia and postpartum depression, with poor results in mental and psychomotor performance testing in offspring (13–15).

Macrocytic Anemia

Macrocytic anemia may be megaloblastic or nonmegaloblastic. Causes of megaloblastic anemia include folate and vitamin B_{12} deficiency and pernicious anemia. Causes of nonmegaloblastic anemia include alcoholism, liver disease, myelodysplasia, aplastic anemia, hypothyroidism, and an increased reticulocyte count. Macrocytic anemia is characterized by an MCV greater than 100 fL. Levels greater than 115 fL are almost exclusively seen in patients with folic acid or vitamin B_{12} deficiencies. The diagnosis may be confirmed by measurement of serum folic acid or vitamin B_{12} levels. Measurement of red cell folate also has been proposed (16). In the United States, macrocytic anemia beginning during pregnancy is overwhelmingly caused by folic acid deficiency. It is associated with diets lacking fresh leafy vegetables, legumes, or animal proteins. During pregnancy, folic acid requirements increase from 50 micrograms to 400 micrograms per day. Treatment of pregnancy-induced folic acid deficiency should include a nutritious diet and folic acid and iron supplementation. Treatment with 1 mg of folic acid, administered orally, each day typically produces an appropriate response. Macrocytic anemia in pregnancy caused by vitamin B_{12} (cyanocobalamin) deficiency may be encountered in women who have had a partial or total gastric resection or in women with Crohn disease. Women who have had a total gastrectomy require 1,000 micrograms of vitamin B_{12}, intramuscularly, at monthly intervals.

Clinical Considerations and Recommendations

▶ *Who should be screened for anemia during pregnancy?*

All pregnant women should be screened for anemia during pregnancy. Those with iron deficiency anemia should be treated with supplemental iron, in addition to prenatal vitamins. Patients with anemia other than iron deficiency anemia should be further evaluated.

▶ *When should evaluation of an asymptomatic patient with mild anemia be considered?*

Asymptomatic women who meet the criteria for anemia (Hct levels less than 33% in the first and third trimesters and less than 32% in the second trimester) should be evaluated. Living at a high altitude and tobacco abuse cause a generalized upward shift in Hgb and Hct levels, and adjustments for these potential confounders may be appropriate (17–19). Hemoglobin and Hct levels are lower in African-American women compared with white women, even after correction for income (20, 21). Thus, applying the same criteria to all women could inappropriately classify almost 30% of African-American women as iron deficient. For African-American adults, the Institute of Medicine recommends lowering the cut-off levels for Hgb and Hct by 0.8 g/dL and 2%, respectively (21, 22).

▶ *How should asymptomatic pregnant women with mild to moderate anemia be evaluated?*

The initial evaluation of pregnant women with mild to moderate anemia may include a medical history, physical examination, and measurements of the complete blood count, red blood cell indices, serum iron levels, and ferritin levels. Examination of a peripheral smear is helpful for the diagnosis of hemolytic or parasitic disease. In certain ethnic groups, an Hgb electrophoresis is indicated (2). Using biochemical tests, iron deficiency anemia is defined by results of abnormal values for levels of serum ferritin, transferrin saturation, and levels of free erythrocyte protoporphyrin, along with low Hgb or Hct levels (see Table 1 and Table 3). In practice, the diagnosis of mild to moderate iron deficiency anemia is often presumptive. In patients without evidence of causes of anemia other than iron deficiency, it may be reasonable to empirically initiate iron therapy without first obtaining iron test results. When pregnant women with moderate iron deficiency anemia are given adequate iron therapy, reticulocytosis may be observed 7–10 days after iron therapy, followed by an increase in Hgb and Hct levels in subsequent weeks. Failure to respond to iron therapy should prompt further investigation and may suggest an incorrect diagnosis, coexisting disease, malabsorption (sometimes caused by the use of enteric-coated tablets or concomitant use of antacids), noncompliance, or blood loss.

▶ *Are there benefits of iron supplementation for patients who are not anemic?*

Iron supplementation decreases the prevalence of maternal anemia at delivery (23). However, it is unclear

Table 3. Biochemical Tests for Diagnosis of Anemia

Test	Results Indicating Iron Deficiency Anemia	Results Indicating Thalassemia	Results Indicating Anemia of Chronic Disease
Iron level	Decreased level	Normal	Decreased level
Total iron-binding capacity	Increased capacity	Normal	Decreased capacity
Ferritin level	Decreased level	Normal	Increased level
Iron/total iron-binding capacity	Less than 18%	Normal	More than 18%

whether iron supplementation in well-nourished pregnant women who are not anemic affects perinatal outcomes. There is little evidence that iron supplementation results in morbidity beyond gastrointestinal symptoms, except in patients with hemochromatosis or certain other genetic disorders.

▶ *When should transfusion be considered in the antepartum or preoperative patient?*

Transfusions of red cells seldom are indicated unless hypovolemia from blood loss coexists or an operative delivery must be performed on a patient with anemia. The need for transfusion in women with antepartum complications can be predicted in only 24% of those who ultimately require blood products (24). The most common diagnoses associated with transfusion include trauma caused by instrumented delivery, uterine atony, placenta previa, retained products of conception, placental abruption, and coagulopathy (eg, the syndrome of hemolysis, elevated liver enzymes, and low platelet count [HELLP]). The presence of these diagnoses in a patient with anemia should prompt consideration of transfusion, particularly in the presence of unstable vital signs (24).

Severe anemia with maternal Hgb levels less than 6 g/dL has been associated with abnormal fetal oxygenation, resulting in nonreassuring fetal heart rate patterns, reduced amniotic fluid volume, fetal cerebral vasodilatation, and fetal death (25, 26). Thus, maternal transfusion should be considered for fetal indications in cases of severe anemia.

▶ *When should parenteral iron be used in pregnant patients? Is there a role for erythropoietin?*

Parenteral iron is used in the rare patient who cannot tolerate or will not take modest doses of oral iron. Patients with a malabsorption syndrome and severe iron deficiency anemia may benefit from parenteral therapy. Anaphylactic reactions have been reported in 1% of patients receiving parenteral iron dextran. In comparison with patients who take iron dextran, patients who take ferrous sucrose have fewer allergic reactions (8.7 versus 3.3 allergic events per 1,000,000 doses) and a significantly lower fatality rate (31 versus 0, $P < .001$) (27). In a recent randomized trial of the use of oral versus intravenous iron sucrose for postpartum anemia, women treated with intravenous iron had significantly higher Hgb levels on days 5 and 14 than women treated with an oral supplement. However, by day 40, there was no significant difference between the Hgb levels of the two groups (28). Thus, in most clinical circumstances, oral preparations are appropriate and sufficient.

Few studies have examined the role of erythropoietin in pregnant patients with anemia. In a randomized, controlled trial that examined the time to reach the targeted Hgb value and changes in efficacy measurements, including reticulocyte count and Hct levels, the use of both parenteral iron and parenteral iron plus erythropoietin improved measured parameters. However, the use of adjuvant erythropoietin alone was associated with a significantly shorter time to the targeted hemoglobin level and improved indices (reticulocyte count, Hct levels) in less than 2 weeks after treatment was initiated. No differences in maternal–fetal safety parameters were reported (29). In contrast, a randomized trial of women with postpartum anemia showed no additional benefit of the use of erythropoietin and iron versus iron alone (30).

▶ *Is there a role for autologous transfusion?*

Case reports suggest a role for autologous transfusion in patients with diagnoses placing them at high risk of symptomatic blood loss, such as placenta previa. Suggested criteria for consideration of autologous donation include an Hct level greater than 32% at 32 weeks of gestation (31). However, autologous transfusions rarely are performed, and the inability to predict the eventual need for transfusion has led to the conclusion that they are not cost-effective (32).

Summary of Recommendations and Conclusions

The following conclusion is based on good and consistent scientific evidence (Level A):

▶ Iron supplementation decreases the prevalence of maternal anemia at delivery.

The following recommendation and conclusions are based on limited or inconsistent scientific data (Level B):

▶ Iron deficiency anemia during pregnancy has been associated with an increased risk of low birth weight, preterm delivery, and perinatal mortality.

▶ Severe anemia with maternal Hgb levels less than 6 g/dL has been associated with abnormal fetal oxygenation resulting in nonreassuring fetal heart rate patterns, reduced amniotic fluid volume, fetal cerebral vasodilatation, and fetal death. Thus, maternal transfusion should be considered for fetal indications.

The following recommendations are based primarily on consensus and expert opinion (Level C):

▶ All pregnant women should be screened for anemia, and those with iron deficiency anemia should be treated with supplemental iron, in addition to prenatal vitamins.

▶ Patients with anemia other than iron deficiency anemia should be further evaluated.

▶ Failure to respond to iron therapy should prompt further investigation and may suggest an incorrect diagnosis, coexisting disease, malabsorption (sometimes caused by the use of enteric-coated tablets or concomitant use of antacids), noncompliance, or blood loss.

Proposed Performance Measure

Percentage of pregnant patients with iron deficiency anemia treated with supplemental iron in addition to prenatal vitamins

References

1. Recommendations to prevent and control iron deficiency in the United States. Centers for Disease Control and Prevention. MMWR Recomm Rep 1998;47(RR-3):1–29. (Level III)

2. Angastiniotis M, Modell B. Global epidemiology of hemoglobin disorders. Ann N Y Acad Sci 1998;850: 251–69. (Level II-3)

3. Pitkin RM. Nutritional influences during pregnancy. Med Clin North Am 1977;61:3–15. (Level III)

4. Bothwell TH. Overview and mechanisms of iron regulation. Nutr Rev 1995;53:237–45. (Level III)

5. Bothwell TH, Charlton RW. Iron deficiency in women. Washington, DC: The Nutrition Foundation; 1981. (Level III)

6. Baynes RD. Iron deficiency. In: Brock JH, Halliday JW, Pippard MJ, Powell LW, editors. Iron metabolism in health and disease. Philadelphia (PA): W.B. Saunders; 1994. p.189–225. (Level III)

7. Ontario Association of Medical Laboratories. Guidelines for the use of serum tests for iron deficiency. Guidelines for Clinical Laboratory Practice CLP 002. North York (ON): OAML; 1995. Available at: http://www.oaml.com/PDF/CLP002.pdf. Retrieved April 4, 2008. (Level III)

8. Institute of Medicine (US). Dietary reference intakes for vitamin A, vitamin K, arsenic, boron, chromium, copper, iodine, iron, manganese, molybdenum, nickel, silicon, vanadium, and zinc. Washington, DC: National Academy Press 2002. (Level III)

9. Adebisi OY, Strayhorn G. Anemia in pregnancy and race in the United States: blacks at risk. Fam Med 2005;37: 655–62. (Level III)

10. Agency for Healthcare Research and Quality. Screening for iron deficiency anemia in childhood and pregnancy: update of the 1996 U.S. Preventive Task Force review. AHRQ Publication No. 06-0590-EF-1. Rockville (MD): AHRQ; 2006. (Level III)

11. Scholl TO. Iron status during pregnancy: setting the stage for mother and infant. Am J Clin Nutr 2005;81: 1218S–22S. (Level III)

12. Rasmussen K. Is there a causal relationship between iron deficiency or iron-deficiency anemia and weight at birth, length of gestation and perinatal mortality? J Nutr 2001;131:590S,601S; discussion 601S–603S. (Level III)

13. Tamura T, Goldenberg RL, Hou J, Johnston KE, Cliver SP, Ramey SL et al. Cord serum ferritin concentrations and mental and psychomotor development of children at five years of age. J Pediatr 2002;140:165–70. (Level II-2)

14. Corwin EJ, Murray-Kolb LE, Beard JL. Low hemoglobin level is a risk factor for postpartum depression. J Nutr 2003;133:4139–42. (Level II-3)

15. Perez EM, Hendricks MK, Beard JL, Murray-Kolb LE, Berg A, Tomlinson M, et al. Mother-infant interactions and infant development are altered by maternal iron deficiency anemia. J Nutr 2005;135:850–5. (Level I)

16. Snow CF. Laboratory diagnosis of vitamin B12 and folate deficiency: a guide for the primary care physician. Arch Intern Med 1999;159:1289–98. (Level III)

17. CDC criteria for anemia in children and childbearing-aged women. Centers for Disease Control (CDC). MMWR Morb Mortal Wkly Rep 1989;38:400–4. (Level III)

18. Dirren H, Logman MH, Barclay DV, Freire WB. Altitude correction for hemoglobin. Eur J Clin Nutr 1994;48: 625–32. (Level II-3)

19. Nordenberg D, Yip R, Binkin NJ. The effect of cigarette smoking on hemoglobin levels and anemia screening. JAMA 1990;264:1556–9. (Level II-2)

20. Johnson-Spear MA, Yip R. Hemoglobin difference between black and white women with comparable iron status: justification for race-specific anemia criteria. Am J Clin Nutr 1994;60:117–21. (Level III)

21. Perry GS, Byers T, Yip R, Margen S. Iron nutrition does not account for the hemoglobin differences between blacks and whites. J Nutr 1992;122:1417–24. (Level II-3)

22. Institute of Medicine (US). Iron deficiency anemia: recommended guidelines for the prevention, detection, and management among U.S. children and women of childbearing age. Washington, DC: National Academy Press; 1993. (Level III)

23. Pena-Rosas JP, Viteri FE. Effects of routine oral iron supplementation with or without folic acid for women during pregnancy. Cochrane Database of Systematic Reviews 2006, Issue 3. Art. No.: CD004736. DOI: 10.1002/14651858.CD004736.pub2. (Level III)

24. Sherman SJ, Greenspoon JS, Nelson JM, Paul RH. Obstetric hemorrhage and blood utilization. J Reprod Med 1993;38:929–34. (Level II-2)

25. Carles G, Tobal N, Raynal P, Herault S, Beucher G, Marret H, et al. Doppler assessment of the fetal cerebral hemodynamic response to moderate or severe maternal anemia. Am J Obstet Gynecol 2003;188:794–9. (Level II-3)

26. Sifakis S, Pharmakides G. Anemia in pregnancy. Ann N Y Acad Sci 2000;900:125–36. (Level III)

27. Faich G, Strobos J. Sodium ferric gluconate complex in sucrose: safer intravenous iron therapy than iron dextrans. Am J Kidney Dis 1999;33:464–70. (Level III)

28. Bhandal N, Russell R. Intravenous versus oral iron therapy for postpartum anaemia. BJOG 2006;113:1248–52. (Level I)

29. Breymann C, Visca E, Huch R, Huch A. Efficacy and safety of intravenously administered iron sucrose with and without adjuvant recombinant human erythropoietin for the treatment of resistant iron-deficiency anemia during pregnancy. Am J Obstet Gynecol 2001;184:662–7. (Level I)

30. Wagstrom E, Akesson A, Van Rooijen M, Larson B, Bremme K. Erythropoietin and intravenous iron therapy in postpartum anaemia. Acta Obstet Gynecol Scand 2007;86: 957–62. (Level I)

31. Toedt ME. Feasibility of autologous blood donation in patients with placenta previa. J Fam Pract 1999;48: 219–21. (Level II-3)

32. Etchason J, Petz L, Keeler E, Calhoun L, Kleinman S, Snider C, et al. The cost effectiveness of preoperative autologous blood donations. N Engl J Med 1995;332: 719–24. (Level III)

The MEDLINE database, the Cochrane Library, and ACOG's own internal resources and documents were used to conduct a literature search to locate relevant articles published between January 1985 and September 2007. The search was restricted to articles published in the English language. Priority was given to articles reporting results of original research, although review articles and commentaries also were consulted. Abstracts of research presented at symposia and scientific conferences were not considered adequate for inclusion in this document. Guidelines published by organizations or institutions such as the National Institutes of Health and the American College of Obstetricians and Gynecologists were reviewed, and additional studies were located by reviewing bibliographies of identified articles. When reliable research was not available, expert opinions from obstetrician–gynecologists were used.

Studies were reviewed and evaluated for quality according to the method outlined by the U.S. Preventive Services Task Force:

I   Evidence obtained from at least one properly designed randomized controlled trial.

II-1 Evidence obtained from well-designed controlled trials without randomization.

II-2 Evidence obtained from well-designed cohort or case–control analytic studies, preferably from more than one center or research group.

II-3 Evidence obtained from multiple time series with or without the intervention. Dramatic results in uncontrolled experiments also could be regarded as this type of evidence.

III   Opinions of respected authorities, based on clinical experience, descriptive studies, or reports of expert committees.

Based on the highest level of evidence found in the data, recommendations are provided and graded according to the following categories:

Level A—Recommendations are based on good and consistent scientific evidence.

Level B—Recommendations are based on limited or inconsistent scientific evidence.

Level C—Recommendations are based primarily on consensus and expert opinion.

ISSN 1099-3630

The American College of Obstetricians and Gynecologists
409 12th Street, SW, PO Box 96920, Washington, DC 20090-6920

Anemia in pregnancy. ACOG Practice Bulletin No. 95. American College of Obstetricians and Gynecologists. Obstet Gynecol 2008;112: 201–7.

ACOG PRACTICE BULLETIN

CLINICAL MANAGEMENT GUIDELINES FOR OBSTETRICIAN–GYNECOLOGISTS

NUMBER 97, SEPTEMBER 2008

Replaces Educational Bulletin Number 230, November 1996

This Practice Bulletin was developed by the ACOG Committee on Practice Bulletins—Obstetrics with the assistance of William N.P. Herbert, MD, and Thomas Peng, MD. The information is designed to aid practitioners in making decisions about appropriate obstetric and gynecologic care. These guidelines should not be construed as dictating an exclusive course of treatment or procedure. Variations in practice may be warranted based on the needs of the individual patient, resources, and limitations unique to the institution or type of practice.

THE AMERICAN COLLEGE OF OBSTETRICIANS AND GYNECOLOGISTS
WOMEN'S HEALTH CARE PHYSICIANS

Fetal Lung Maturity

Respiratory difficulties are common in neonates born with immature lung development. Assessment of fetal lung maturity is an important component in determining the timing of delivery in certain patients who experience complications during pregnancy. Enhancement of fetal pulmonary function with the use of antenatal steroids and the administration of surfactant lessens the prevalence and severity of neonatal respiratory distress syndrome (RDS) and its sequelae. However, RDS remains a major clinical issue. Commonly used tests to determine fetal lung maturity are reviewed in this Practice Bulletin.

Background

The status of fetal lung maturation can assist the clinician in determining when delivery should occur. Testing for fetal lung maturity should not be performed, and is contraindicated, when delivery is mandated for fetal or maternal indications. Conversely, a mature fetal lung maturity test result before 39 weeks of gestation, in the absence of appropriate clinical circumstances, is not an indication for delivery. Respiratory distress syndrome, intraventricular hemorrhage, necrotizing enterocolitis, and other complications have been reported in premature newborns delivered with mature lecithin (phosphatidylcholine)/sphingomyelin ratios or the presence of phosphatidylglycerol (1, 2).

Indications for Assessing Fetal Maturity

To prevent iatrogenic prematurity, fetal pulmonary maturity should be confirmed before scheduled delivery at less than 39 weeks of gestation unless fetal maturity can be inferred from any of the following historic criteria:

- Ultrasound measurement at less than 20 weeks of gestation supports gestational age of 39 weeks or greater.
- Fetal heart tones have been documented as present for 30 weeks by Doppler ultrasonography.

- It has been 36 weeks since a positive serum or urine human chorionic gonadotropin pregnancy test result.

If any of these criteria confirms a gestational age of 39 weeks or more, it is appropriate to schedule delivery at that time. Ultrasonography may be considered to confirm menstrual dates if there is a gestational age agreement within 1 week by crown–rump measurements obtained in the first trimester or within 10 days by an average of multiple fetal biometric measurements (eg, crown–rump length, biparietal diameter, head and abdominal circumference, and femur length) obtained in the second trimester (up to 20 weeks of gestation).

The risk of RDS is increased significantly in infants born by electively scheduled cesarean delivery between 37 6/7 weeks and 38 6/7 weeks of gestation (3). In a retrospective study of 1,284 elective cesarean deliveries, RDS was diagnosed at a rate of 25 per 1,000 live births when cesarean delivery occurred between 37 6/7 weeks and 38 6/7 weeks of gestation, versus a significantly lower rate of RDS, 7 per 1,000 with cesarean delivery after 39 6/7 weeks of gestation. Neonatal RDS with vaginal deliveries did not vary (3–4/1000) across these gestational ages.

Physiology and Pathophysiology

Fetal Lung Development

The development of the pulmonary system begins approximately 3 weeks after conception and continues well into childhood. From approximately 16–24 weeks of gestation, early bronchioles develop, and the epithelium vascularizes and differentiates. It is in the alveolar phase of pulmonary development, which begins at approximately 22–23 weeks of gestation, that subsequent bronchiolar division occurs such that thin spherical saccules known as alveoli develop. The concomitant proliferation of capillaries around these alveoli makes effective gas exchange possible after delivery.

The alveoli are lined by type II pneumocytes, which produce phospholipids that are "packaged" into lamellar bodies. Surfactant is the name given to a group of "surface-active" phospholipid compounds that can be released from these lamellar bodies and reduce the surface tension within the alveolar spaces. Maintaining a low surface tension within the alveoli allows the sacs to remain expanded, which permits continuous and maximal effective gas exchange. During the latter portion of pregnancy, fetal respiratory activity permits the passage of surfactant into the amniotic fluid where its quantity or function can be evaluated. The most prominent of these surfactant compounds is lecithin, which generally appears earlier in gestation than another component of surfactant, phosphatidylglycerol.

Respiratory Distress Syndrome

A deficiency in the quantity of surfactant in premature infants leads to higher surface tension within the alveoli, causing alveolar collapse and difficult gas exchange. The result is neonatal hypoxia, with further worsening of pulmonary status manifested by acidosis and increased shunting within the lungs. Signs of RDS include neonatal tachypnea, grunting, inspiratory thoracic retractions, and cyanosis, often occurring within several hours of birth.

Other complications associated with RDS include necrotizing enterocolitis, patent ductus arteriosus, intraventricular hemorrhage, and infection. Some survivors will experience bronchopulmonary dysplasia, or chronic lung disease.

Fetal Lung Maturity Tests

Laboratory tests measure either the concentration of particular components of pulmonary surfactant (biochemical tests) or the surface-active effects of these phospholipids (biophysical tests). Common biochemical tests include measuring the lecithin/sphingomyelin ratio and determining the presence of phosphatidylglycerol. Biophysical tests include fluorescence polarization. Lamellar body counts also are generally available. Less frequently used tests include foam stability index and optical density of amniotic fluid at 650 nm.

Commonly used fetal lung maturity tests include fluorescence polarization (TDx-FLM II), lecithin/sphingomyelin ratio, phosphatidylglycerol presence, and lamellar body counts. No test has been conclusively shown to be superior, and each requires its own standard to define the risk of neonatal RDS. Comparisons between the different tests have shown varying results. A comparison of lecithin/sphingomyelin ratio to lamellar body counts in 833 neonates born within 72 hours of fetal lung maturity testing (prevalence of RDS was 12%) noted that both tests had similar sensitivity (proportion of immature test result in neonates with RDS) of 81.8% and 88.9%, respectively, and negative predictive values (probability of no RDS with a mature fetal lung maturity test result) 96.8% and 97.7%, respectively (4). Comparisons of lamellar body counts (cutoff greater than 50,000) and TDx-FLM II assay results (greater than 55 mg/g) also demonstrated similar test characteristics in sensitivity (92% and 83%, respectively) and negative predictive values (99% and 98%, respectively) (5). Studies comparing lecithin/sphingomyelin ratios with TDx-FLM II assay results demonstrate that both tests yield high sensitivity for RDS and high negative predictive values. Neonates of 109 pregnant women were delivered within 72 hours of the fetal lung maturity test, and RDS was diagnosed in 9 (8%) (6). In this study, using cutoff values of 45 mg/g for TDx-FLM II assay results and 2 for lecithin/sphingomyelin ratios, the sensitivity and negative predictive values were 100% for both tests (6).

A multiinstitutional study compared test characteristics of lecithin/sphingomyelin ratio, phosphatidylglycerol presence, lamellar body counts, and TDx-FLM II assays. The investigators found that characteristics were similar in a population of 220 neonates delivered within 48 hours of testing (7). Cutoff values were lecithin/sphingomyelin ratios of 2.5, phosphatidylglycerol presence greater than 0.5, TDx-FLM II assay results greater than 40 mg/g, and lamellar body counts greater than 30,000. Of the 13 (6%) neonates diagnosed with RDS, the lecithin/sphingomyelin ratios were falsely reassuring (greater than 2.5) in five, as were the TDx-FLM II assay results, phosphatidylglycerol presence measurements, and lamellar body counts in one amniotic fluid sample. As noted by the authors, a probability risk of RDS that takes into account the fetal gestation may be more helpful than a cutoff value to define mature versus immature neonatal lung function.

Ideally, laboratories should develop their own reference standards for fetal lung maturity testing, but few have a sufficient number of amniotic fluid samples and outcomes for such internal evaluations. The predictive values of fetal lung maturity tests will vary with the prevalence of RDS in the population sampled. In addition, it should be noted that there is a risk of RDS even with a positive mature fetal lung maturity test result and that this risk varies by gestational age (7–9).

Fluorescence Polarization

Fetal lung maturity testing using fluorescence polarization is based on competitive binding of a fluorescent probe to albumin and surfactant. When the probe is bound to albumin, net polarization values are high; when bound to surfactant, polarization values are low. In amniotic fluid samples, the fluorescence polarization measured by an automated analyzer reflects the ratio of surfactant to albumin, a value that correlates with lung maturity. Recent modifications of this concept provide a simple, automated, rapid test that is widely available, varies minimally between laboratories, and requires only a small volume of amniotic fluid (typically 1 mL). In the recently modified commercial version of this assay (TDx-FLM II), values above 55 mg surfactant per 1 g albumin are considered mature (10); values below 40 mg surfactant per 1 g albumin are considered immature; and values between 40 mg surfactant per 1 g albumin and 54 mg surfactant per 1 g albumin are considered indeterminate. In a retrospective analysis of 185 samples (15 with

RDS and 170 without RDS), a cutoff value of greater than or equal to 45 mg/g yielded a sensitivity of 100% (95% confidence interval [CI], 82–100%), specificity (proportion of mature result in a neonate without RDS) of 84% (95% CI, 78–89%) (11). The assay compares favorably with other direct tests, but blood and meconium contamination interfere with its interpretation (Table 1).

Lecithin/Sphingomyelin Ratio

The lecithin/sphingomyelin ratio measures the ratio of lecithin to sphingomyelin in amniotic fluid. As gestational age advances, the concentration of lecithin increases, whereas the concentration of sphingomyelin remains relatively constant. Reporting results in a ratio takes into account the increasing amniotic fluid volume as gestational age progresses.

Determination of the lecithin/sphingomyelin ratio involves thin-layer chromatography after organic solvent extraction. A value of 2 is the commonly accepted standard indicating pulmonary maturity in the fetus, although laboratories may define a different ratio to indicate fetal lung maturity.

Compared with newer tests, popularity of the lecithin/sphingomyelin ratio has diminished substantially in recent years. The technique is more costly, has a longer turnaround time (average of 5–6 hours), and requires highly trained personnel. Blood and meconium contamination can interfere with test interpretation (Table 1).

Phosphatidylglycerol Presence

Phosphatidylglycerol is a minor constituent of surfactant. Because phosphatidylglycerol enhances the spread of phospholipids on the alveolar surface, its presence indicates a more advanced state of fetal pulmonary maturity. Phosphatidylglycerol can be determined using thin-layer chromatography as an extension of the lecithin/sphingomyelin ratio. In addition, a slide-agglutination test has been developed using antisera specific for phosphatidylglycerol. This test can be performed quickly and generally is not affected by the presence of blood, meconium, or other contaminants. Its relatively late appearance in pregnancy means that its false-postive rate (proportion of neonates without RDS with an immature FLM test result) for RDS is high. Older studies noted that when phosphatidylglycerol was present, the risk of RDS was very low (less than 1%). When phosphatidylglycerol was absent, the risk of RDS was in the range of 25%, which is poorly predictive of occurrence of RDS (12).

Lamellar Body Counts

Surfactant is stored within type II pneumocytes in the form of lamellar bodies. These bodies are actively

Table 1. Commonly Used Direct Tests of Fetal Lung Maturity

Test*	Technique	Time and Ease of Testing†	Threshold	Typical Predictive Value (%)		Blood Contamination Affects Results	Meconium Contamination Affects Results	Vaginal Pool Sample
				Mature Negative Predictive Value	Immature Positive‡ Predictive Value			
Fluorescence polarization	Fluorescence polarization with TDx-FLM II	1+	55 mg/g or greater of albumin§	96–100	47–61	Yes	Yes	Yes
Lecithin/sphingomyelin ratio	Thin-layer chromatography	4+	2–3.5	95–100	33–50	Yes	Yes	No
Phosphatidyl-glycerol	Thin-layer chromatography	4+	Present (usually greater than 3% of total phospholipids)	95–100	23–53	No	No	Yes
	Antisera with AminoStat-FLM	1+	0.5 = low positive 2 = high positive	95–100	23–53	No	No	Yes
Lamellar body counts	Counts using commercial hematology counter	2+	30,000–40,000 (still investigational)	97–98	29–35	Yes	No	Not available
Optical density at 650 nm	Spectrophotometric reading	1+	Optical density of 0.15 or greater	98	13	Not available	Not available	Not available
Foam stability index	Ethanol added to amniotic fluid, solution shaken, presence of stable bubbles at meniscus noted	2+	47–48 or greater	95	51	Yes	Yes	No

*Commercial versions are available for all tests except optical density and lamellar body counts.

†Range in complexity: 1+ indicates procedure is simple, procedure is available all the time, procedure time is short, and personnel effort is not intensive; 4+ indicates procedure is complex or difficult, time consuming, and, therefore, frequently not available at all times.

‡Positive predictive value is the probability of neonatal respiratory distress syndrome when the fetal lung maturity test result is immature.

§The manufacturer has reformulated the product and revised the testing procedure. Currently, the threshold for maturity is 55; with the original assay, it was 70.

secreted into the alveoli space and hence into the amniotic fluid. The similarity of lamellar body size to that of platelets permits the use of a standard hematologic counter to determine lamellar body concentrations. Such counting is simple, rapid, inexpensive, and reliably predictive of pulmonary maturity. However, there are no clearly established protocols, consistent instrumentation, guidelines, or consensus on cutoff values for a lamellar body count that predicts absence of RDS.

Neonatal RDS may be reduced by acceptance of a higher threshold, a higher lamellar body count. In a cohort study of 527 neonates, two cutoff values, a lamellar body count of greater than 30,000 and a count of greater than 50,000, were defined as indicating pulmonary maturity (13). Neonatal intensive care unit admissions, neonatal respiratory assistance, and overall neonatal complications were less frequent with a cutoff value of greater than 50,000. A similar study of 80 pregnancies documented a negative predictive value of 93% when a cutoff value for maturity of lamellar body counts of greater than 50,000 was used (14). Meconium contamination may marginally increase the lamellar body count, and blood contamination can lead to falsely increased lamellar body counts because of platelet contamination (Table 1) (4, 15). If testing is not performed rapidly, coagulation will reduce the lamellar body count.

Interpretation of Tests and Testing Strategies

As shown in Table 1, the negative predictive value for mature neonatal lung function is high, and if one of these test results for fetal lung maturity is positive, RDS is

Table 2. Fetal Lung Maturity Testing in Twin Gestations

Gestational Age	Amniocentesis to Test Fetal Lung Maturity
30 %–32 % weeks of gestation	Both twins
33 %–35 % weeks of gestation	
Concordant gender	Either twin
Discordant gender and discordant weight less than 10% or greater than 20%	Either twin
Discordant gender and discordant weight 10–20%	One twin (prefer nonpresenting or male)
Greater than 35 % weeks of gestation	Either twin

Data from Mackenzie MW. Predicting concordance of biochemical lung maturity in the preterm twin gestation. J Matern Fetal Neonat Med 2002;12:50–8.

unlikely. The main value for fetal lung maturity testing is predicting the absence of RDS. An immature test result for fetal lung maturity is less reliable in predicting the presence of RDS.

Fetal lung maturity testing traditionally has been based on the result alone, not taking into account the gestational age of the fetus. More recently, it has been recognized that the probability of neonatal RDS is dependent on both the fetal lung maturity test result and the gestational age at which the fetal lung maturity test was performed (7, 8, 16, 17). The prevalence of RDS within a population will alter the positive predictive value of the fetal lung maturity test results. Nonetheless, combining test results and gestational age improves the clinician's ability to counsel patients about perinatal management and the neonatal risks, including the risk of RDS, with elective delivery. Another factor in choosing which amniotic fluid test to perform is the effect of various contaminants on test results (Table 1).

Clinical Considerations and Recommendations

▶ *What are the complications of third-trimester amniocentesis?*

Complications from third-trimester amniocentesis for fetal lung maturity are uncommon when performed with ultrasound guidance (18, 19). One study of 562 amniocenteses documented a 0.7% rate of complications, which included one each of preterm labor, premature rupture of membranes, placental abruption, and fetal–maternal hemorrhage (18). None of the complications required urgent delivery. One study documented complications requiring urgent delivery on the day of amniocentesis in 6 patients (0.7%) from 913 amniocenteses for fetal lung maturity.

Complications were isolated events but included three fetal heart rate abnormalities and one each of placental bleeding, placental abruption, and uterine rupture.

▶ *Is there a gestational age below which there is no utility of fetal lung maturity testing?*

Before 32 weeks of gestation, fetal lung maturity testing generally is not indicated because most test results will indicate immaturity. Thus, delivery is indicated at this gestational age only for specific maternal or fetal indications.

▶ *What is the impact of corticosteroid administration on fetal lung maturity test results?*

Corticosteroid administration significantly reduces the incidence of RDS but may not have an impact on the results of fetal lung maturity testing (20, 21). In a cohort study of pregnant patients with hypertension and similar gestational ages at the time of amniocenteses for fetal lung maturity, 34 patients were treated with betamethasone before amniocentesis and 34 were not treated. Amniocentesis for fetal lung maturity occurred within 5 days of the corticosteroid administration. Compared with no corticosteroid exposure, patients with hypertension who were treated with corticosteroids had significantly higher values for lecithin/sphingomyelin ratios and lamellar body counts, but no difference in phosphatidylglycerol presence. (21). No such increases in lecithin/sphingomyelin ratios were noted in a subset of patients enrolled in a study of dexamethasone versus placebo for fetal lung maturation. No difference in the lecithin/sphingomyelin ratio was found in the amniotic fluid obtained a week after dexamethasone administration in 25 women compared with the placebo group of 20 women (20).

▶ *In a patient with a twin pregnancy, should fetal lung maturity testing be performed for each fetus?*

Information concerning pulmonary maturation and testing in twin pregnancies is mixed. Studies have reported that values of fetal maturity test results in twin pregnancies are higher compared with those in singleton pregnancies at similar gestations (22, 23). In a study of 27 twin pregnancies and 143 singleton pregnancies, the higher values of TDx FLM assay results were noted in the twin pregnancies after 31 weeks of gestation (23). Other studies have found no difference (24).

In twin pregnancies, data are not clear as to whether assessing fetal lung maturity in one twin is sufficient or whether assessing both twins is necessary to predict the risk of neonatal RDS. Several studies suggest good correlation of fetal lung maturity assay values between both twins with correlation coefficients of 0.83–0.86 (25, 26). The correlation was not affected by the presenting versus nonpresenting twin, by gender discordance, or by birth-weight discordance (26). Discordant values (one twin with a fetal lung maturity value in the mature range and the other twin with a fetal lung maturity value in the immature range) appear to occur more frequently at earlier gestational ages (26, 27). Many of these reports used the lecithin/sphingomyelin ratio for fetal lung maturity testing, which, because of larger differences in interlaboratory and intralaboratory variation, may have contributed to the varying results in concordance. These data suggest that amniocentesis of both twins be performed when the gestation is between 30 6/7 weeks and 32 6/7 weeks of gestation. Amniocentesis of one twin appears to be sufficient when gestation is greater than 32 6/7 weeks (27) (Table 2).

Before elective delivery, fetal lung maturity testing in twins with well defined gestational ages of 38 6/7 weeks or greater may not be necessary. A descriptive study of 126 twins electively delivered without fetal lung testing noted five pregnancies in which one or both twins were diagnosed with RDS (28). For all five, delivery occurred at less than 38 6/7 weeks of gestation. Of the 47 twin pregnancies delivered at 38 6/7 weeks or greater, one infant was affected by transient tachypnea of the newborn.

▶ *How do abnormal amniotic fluid volumes (hydramnios, oligohydramnios) affect fetal lung maturity test results?*

Very few studies have addressed this question. Based on the results of one clinical study, the effect of amniotic fluid volume on the results of fetal lung maturity testing appears to be minimal. In a study of patients with oligohydramnios (an amniotic fluid index of 5 cm or less), the lecithin/sphingomyelin ratios, phosphatidylglycerol presence, and lamellar body counts were similar to controls of similar gestation but with a normal amniotic fluid index. However, in patients with polyhydramnios (an amniotic fluid index greater than 25), the lecithin/sphingomyelin ratios, lamellar body counts, and phosphatidylglycerol presence were lower compared with the control group (29).

▶ *Are results of fetal lung maturity tests performed on samples collected vaginally reliable?*

Studies comparing results of fetal lung maturity tests of amniotic fluid collected vaginally with those collected by transabdominal amniocentesis demonstrated that when results from fluid collected vaginally are mature, the results are reliable (30, 31). In a study of 16 patients with preterm premature rupture of membranes, amniotic fluid was collected both vaginally and by transabdominal amniocentesis within twelve hours of each other. Twelve samples collected by transabdominal amniocentesis indicated mature lung development compared with four samples collected vaginally. Results of a TDx-FLM assay were lower in the fluid collected vaginally then fluid collected by transabdominal amniocentesis, but when the assay of the fluid collected vaginally was mature, it was always confirmed by results of the fluid collected by transabdominal amniocentesis (31). Compared with transabdominal amniocentesis, fluid collected vaginally for fetal lung maturity testing yields higher specificity (100%) and positive predictive value (100%) but had lower sensitivity (42%) and negative predictive value (36%) for neonatal RDS.

▶ *How does blood and meconium contamination affect fetal lung maturity test results?*

Contamination of amniotic fluid with blood appears to increase the number of falsely immature fetal lung maturity test results. With an in vitro system, increasing aliquots of blood added to samples of amniotic fluid produced fetal lung maturity test results that were less mature (32). Table 1 lists the effects of various substances on the reliability of interpretation of tests of fetal lung maturity.

▶ *How are results interpreted in the presence of diabetes mellitus? Are there additional tests that may be helpful?*

In general, the same threshold values for fetal lung maturity tests that predict low risk of neonatal RDS in pregnancies of women who are not diabetic apply to pregnancies of women who are diabetic, whether the woman has gestational diabetes mellitus or pregestational diabetes mellitus. Most studies have evaluated the performance of lecithin/sphingomyelin ratios, tests for the presence of phosphatidylglycerol, and TDx-FLM and TDx-FLM II assays. The manufacturer of TDx-FLM II assays recommends a value of 55 mg/g or higher as compatible with a mature lung profile. In a series of 45 pregnant women with diabetes mellitus who gave birth within 72 hours of the performance of a fetal lung maturity test, 40 had fetuses with a mature profile (TDx-FLM II value was equal to 55 mg/g or greater), and no neonatal RDS occurred (17). The remaining five had fetuses with an indeterminate profile (TDx-FLM II value between 40 mg/g and 55 mg/g), and one had RDS. Therefore, testing with fluorescence polarization (TDx-FLM II), using a defined mature profile of a value of 55 mg/g or greater, is appropriate for the determination of risk of neonatal RDS in pregnant women with diabetes mellitus.

Similar findings were noted with the older version of the fluorescence polarization test, TDx-FLM, in which values greater than 70 mg/g in amniotic fluid obtained by amniocentesis were associated with a very low risk of neonatal RDS (33, 34). In one series of 182 pregnant women with diabetes mellitus, five neonates born within 4 days of the amniocentesis experienced severe RDS. The TDx-FLM values of these five neonates ranged from 18–59 mg/g. Mild RDS, requiring hood oxygenation, occurred in three neonates with fetal lung maturity values of 47, 74, and 81 mg/g (33). In another series of 121 pregnant women with diabetes mellitus who gave birth within 72 hours of fetal lung maturity testing, one neonate had RDS with a TDx-FLM value of 7.2 mg/g. No RDS was noted when the value was 70 mg/g or greater (108 patients) (34).

Evaluation of lecithin/sphingomyelin ratios and tests for the presence of phosphatidylglycerol in an older study of pregnant women with and without diabetes mellitus confirmed that a mature lecithin/sphingomyelin ratio predicted very low risk of neonatal RDS in both populations (1.6% and 1.8%, respectively), and when phosphatidylglycerol was present, no RDS was identified in either group (35).

The effect of diabetes mellitus or glucose control on the development of a mature phospholipid profile in amniotic fluid is unclear (36). Some reports indicate a delay in production of phosphatidylglycerol in fetuses of pregnant women with diabetes mellitus (37, 38) and a higher proportion of immature profiles in women with poorly controlled compared with well controlled diabetes mellitus (39). Others report no difference in phospholipid profiles between patients with diabetes mellitus and patients without diabetes mellitus (40, 41). There is more of a consensus that the extent of glycemic control is related to the timing of pulmonary maturation and fetal lung maturity testing.

In pregnant women with diabetes mellitus and good glycemic control, amniocentesis for fetal lung maturity testing is not indicated before scheduled delivery at or beyond 39 weeks of gestation. It has been suggested that with the rare risk of RDS in pregnant women with well-controlled diabetes mellitus, amniocentesis for fetal lung maturity may be eliminated in women with a well-dated pregnancy at or beyond 38 weeks of gestation (42). In patients with diabetes mellitus and poor glucose control, fetal lung maturity testing is recommended if delivery is contemplated at less than 39 weeks of gestation.

▶ *How is an immature or indeterminate test result managed? What is the interval for repeat testing?*

If the test results following the first amniocentesis are immature, individual circumstances can guide decision making. The risks of untoward fetal or maternal outcome if the pregnancy continues and the results of the testing (very immature or indeterminate) can be helpful in such situations. With an indeterminate test result, the practitioner should consider incorporation of the gestational age of the fetus into the interpretation of the fetal lung maturity value and risk of neonatal RDS.

For borderline lecithin/sphingomyelin ratios (1.8–1.9), the risk of neonatal morbidity and mortality if delivered within 72 hours of the test appear significant. In a group of 63 pregnancies at a gestation of 27–36 weeks delivered within 72 hours of the fetal lung maturity test, there was a 13% neonatal morbidity rate and 3% neonatal mortality rate when the lecithin/sphingomyelin ratio was 1.8 compared with a 3% morbidity rate and no mortality when the lecithin/sphingomyelin ratio was 1.9. All the major neonatal morbidity occurred in gestations less than 32–34 weeks (43). Increased risk of RDS was noted with TDx-FLM II results in the indeterminate zone (40–55 mg/g), with proportional increases in the risk of RDS as fetal gestation decreased (16).

No consensus exists as to whether repeat testing is required or when to perform a repeat test when the fetal lung maturity test is either immature or indeterminate. TDx-FLM II results derived from two sequential amniocenteses in a group of 85 pregnant women documented that as fetal gestation progresses, the increase in the value of TDx-FLM II results appear to be constant, increasing approximately 14.4 plus or minus 9.9 mg/g (95% CI, 12.3–16.5) per week over a broad range of gestations (31–38 weeks of gestation) (44). This may provide guidance on whether repeat testing is necessary and when to consider repeat testing.

Summary of Recommendations and Conclusions

The following recommendations and conclusions are based on limited or inconsistent scientific evidence (Level B:)

▶ Testing for fetal lung maturity should not be performed, and is contraindicated, when delivery is mandated for fetal or maternal indications.

▶ Fetal pulmonary maturity should be confirmed before scheduled delivery at less than 39 weeks of gestation unless fetal maturity can be inferred from historic criteria.

▶ The probability of neonatal RDS is dependent on both the fetal lung maturity test result and the gestational age at which the fetal lung maturity test was performed.

▶ Fluorescence polarization assays (TDx FLM II) using a defined mature profile of 55 mg/g or greater is appropriate for the determination of risk of neonatal RDS in pregnancies of women with diabetes mellitus.

▶ Fetal lung maturity test results from amniotic fluid collected vaginally compared with those from fluid collected by transabdominal amniocentesis demonstrate that when results from fluid collected vaginally are mature, the results are reliable.

▶ Complications from third-trimester amniocentesis for fetal lung maturity are uncommon when performed with ultrasound guidance.

The following conclusions are based primarily on consensus and expert opinion (Level C):

▶ In general, the same threshold values for fetal lung maturity tests that predict low risk of neonatal RDS in pregnancies of women who do not have diabetes mellitus apply to pregnancies of women who have diabetes mellitus, whether it is gestational diabetes mellitus or pregestational diabetes mellitus.

▶ Data suggest that amniocentesis of both twins be performed when the gestation is between 30 % weeks and 32 % weeks of gestation. Amniocentesis of one twin appears to be sufficient when gestation is greater than 32 % weeks.

▶ Prior to elective delivery, fetal lung maturity testing in twins with well defined gestational ages at 38 % weeks or greater may not be necessary.

Proposed Performance Measure

Documentation of discussion or performance of fetal lung maturity testing in elective cesarean deliveries at a gestation less than 39 % weeks

References

1. Wigton TR, Tamura RK, Wickstrom E, Atkins V, Deddish R, Socol ML. Neonatal morbidity after preterm delivery in the presence of documented lung maturity. Am J Obstet Gynecol 1993;169:951–5. (Level III)

2. Ghidini A, Hicks C, Lapinski RH, Lockwood CJ. Morbidity in the preterm infant with mature lung indices. Am J Perinatol 1997;14:75–8. (Level II-3)

3. Zanardo V, Simbi AK, Franzoi M, Solda G, Salvadori A, Trevisanuto D. Neonatal respiratory morbidity risk and mode of delivery at term: influence of timing of elective caesarean delivery. Acta Paediatr 2004;93:643–7. (Level II-2)

4. Neerhof MG, Haney EI, Silver RK, Ashwood ER, Lee IS, Piazze JJ. Lamellar body counts compared with traditional phospholipid analysis as an assay for evaluating fetal lung maturity. Obstet Gynecol 2001;97:305–9. (Level II-3)

5. Haymond S, Luzzi VI, Parvin CA, Gronowski AM. A direct comparison between lamellar body counts and fluorescent polarization methods for predicting respiratory distress syndrome. Am J Clin Pathol 2006;126:894–9. (Level II-3)

6. Winn-McMillan T, Karon BS. Comparison of the TDx-FLM II and lecithin to sphingomyelin ratio assays in predicting fetal lung maturity. Am J Obstet Gynecol 2005; 193:778–82. (Level II-3)

7. Karcher R, Sykes E, Batton D, Uddin Z, Ross G, Hockman E, et al. Gestational age-specific predicted risk of neonatal respiratory distress syndrome using lamellar body count and surfactant-to-albumin ratio in amniotic fluid. Am J Obstet Gynecol 2005;193:1680–4. (Level II-3)

8. Parvin CA, Kaplan LA, Chapman JF, McManamon TG, Gronowski AM. Predicting respiratory distress syndrome using gestational age and fetal lung maturity by fluorescent polarization. Am J Obstet Gynecol 2005;192: 199–207. (Level III)

9. Pinette MG, Blackstone J, Wax JR, Cartin A. Fetal lung maturity indices—a plea for gestational age-specific interpretation: a case report and discussion. Am J Obstet Gynecol 2002;187:1721–2. (Level III)

10. Kesselman EJ, Figueroa R, Garry D, Maulik D. The usefulness of the TDx/TDxFLx fetal lung maturity II assay in the initial evaluation of fetal lung maturity. Am J Obstet Gynecol 2003;188:1220–2. (Level II-3)

11. Fantz CR, Powell C, Karon B, Parvin CA, Hankins K, Dayal M, et al. Assessment of the diagnostic accuracy of the TDx-FLM II to predict fetal lung maturity. Clin Chem 2002;48:761–5. (Level II-3)

12. Field NT, Gilbert WM. Current status of amniotic fluid tests of fetal maturity. Clin Obstet Gynecol 1997;40: 366–86. (Level III)

13. Ventolini G, Neiger R, Hood DL, Belcastro MR. Changes in the threshold of fetal lung maturity testing and neonatal outcome of infants delivered electively before 39 weeks gestation: implications and cost-effectiveness. J Perinatol 2006;26:264–7. (Level II-3)

14. Khazardoost S, Yahyazadeh H, Borna S, Sohrabvand F, Yahyazadeh N, Amini E. Amniotic fluid lamellar body count and its sensitivity and specificity in evaluating of fetal lung maturity. J Obstet Gynaecol 2005;25:257–9. (Level II-3)

15. Torday JS, Rehan VK. Testing for fetal lung maturation: a biochemical "window" to the developing fetus. Clin Lab Med 2003;23:361–83. (Level III)

16. Kaplan LA, Chapman JF, Bock JL, Santa Maria E, Clejan S, Huddleston DJ, et al. Prediction of respiratory distress

syndrome using the Abbott FLM-II amniotic fluid assay. Clin Chim Acta 2002;326:61–8. (Level III)

17. Melanson SE, Jarolim P, McElrath TF, Berg A, Tanasijevic MJ. Fetal lung maturity testing in diabetic mothers. Lab Med 2007;38:553–5. (Level III)

18. Gordon MC, Narula K, O'Shaughnessy R, Barth WH Jr. Complications of third-trimester amniocentesis using continuous ultrasound guidance. Obstet Gynecol 2002;99: 255–9. (Level II-3)

19. Stark CM, Smith RS, Lagrandeur RM, Batton DG, Lorenz RP. Need for urgent delivery after third-trimester amniocentesis. Obstet Gynecol 2000;95:48–50. (Level II-3)

20. Farrell PM, Engle MJ, Zachman RD, Curet LB, Morrison JC, Rao AV, et al. Amniotic fluid phospholipids after maternal administration of dexamethasone. Am J Obstet Gynecol 1983;145:484–90. (Level II-2)

21. Piazze JJ, Maranghi L, Nigro G, Rizzo G, Cosmi EV, Anceschi MM. The effect of glucocorticoid therapy on fetal lung maturity indices in hypertensive pregnancies. Obstet Gynecol 1998;92:220–5. (Level II-2)

22. Leveno KJ, Quirk JG, Whalley PJ, Herbert WN, Trubey R. Fetal lung maturation in twin gestation. Am J Obstet Gynecol 1984;148:405–11. (Level III)

23. McElrath TF, Norwitz ER, Robinson JN, Tanasijevic MJ, Lieberman ES. Differences in TDx fetal lung maturity assay values between twin and singleton gestations. Am J Obstet Gynecol 2000;182:1110–2. (Level II-3)

24. Winn HN, Romero R, Roberts A, Liu H, Hobbins JC. Comparison of fetal lung maturation in preterm singleton and twin pregnancies. Am J Perinatol 1992;9:326–8. (Level II-3)

25. Spellacy WN, Cruz AC, Buhi WC, Birk SA. Amniotic fluid L/S ratio in twin gestation. Obstet Gynecol 1977;50:68–70. (Level II-3)

26. Whitworth NS, Magann EF, Morrison JC. Evaluation of fetal lung maturity in diamniotic twins. Am J Obstet Gynecol 1999;180:1438–41. (Level II-3)

27. Mackenzie MW. Predicting concordance of biochemical lung maturity in the preterm twin gestation. J Matern Fetal Neonatal Med 2002;12:50–8. (Level II-3)

28. Chasen ST, Madden A, Chervenak FA. Cesarean delivery of twins and neonatal respiratory disorders. Am J Obstet Gynecol 1999;181:1052–6. (Level II-3)

29. Piazze JJ, Maranghi L, Cosmi EV, Anceschi MM. The effect of polyhydramnios and oligohydramnios on fetal lung maturity indexes. Am J Perinatol 1998;15:249–52. (Level II-2)

30. Edwards RK, Duff P, Ross KC. Amniotic fluid indices of fetal pulmonary maturity with preterm premature rupture of membranes. Obstet Gynecol 2000;96:102–5. (Level II-3)

31. Cleary-Goldman J, Connolly T, Chelmow D, Malone F. Accuracy of the TDx-FLM assay of amniotic fluid: a comparison of vaginal pool samples with amniocentesis. J Matern Fetal Neonatal Med 2002;11:374–7. (Level II-3)

32. Carlan SJ, Gearity D, O'Brien WF. The effect of maternal blood contamination on the TDx-FLM II assay. Am J Perinatol 1997;14:491–4. (Level III)

33. Livingston EG, Herbert WN, Hage ML, Chapman JF, Stubbs TM. Use of the TDx-FLM assay in evaluating fetal lung maturity in an insulin-dependent diabetic population. The Diabetes and Fetal Maturity Study Group. Obstet Gynecol 1995;86:826–9. (Level II-3)

34. Del Valle GO, Adair CD, Ramos EE, Gaudier FL, Sanchez-Ramos L, Morales R. Interpretation of the TDx-FLM fluorescence polarization assay in pregnancies complicated by diabetes mellitus. Am J Perinatol 1997;14:241–4. (Level II-3)

35. Curet LB, Tsao FH, Zachman RD, Olson RW, Henderson PA. Phosphatidylglycerol, lecithin/sphingomyelin ratio and respiratory distress syndrome in diabetic and non-diabetic pregnancies. Int J Gynaecol Obstet 1989;30: 105–8. (Level II-2)

36. Langer O. The controversy surrounding fetal lung maturity in diabetes in pregnancy: a re-evaluation. J Matern Fetal Neonatal Med 2002;12:428–32. (Level III)

37. Piper JM, Xenakis EM, Langer O. Delayed appearance of pulmonary maturation markers is associated with poor glucose control in diabetic pregnancies. J Matern Fetal Med 1998;7:148–53. (Level II-2)

38. Moore TR. A comparison of amniotic fluid fetal pulmonary phospholipids in normal and diabetic pregnancy. Am J Obstet Gynecol 2002;186:641–50. (Level II-2)

39. Piper JM, Langer O. Does maternal diabetes delay fetal pulmonary maturity? Am J Obstet Gynecol 1993;168: 783–6. (Level II-2)

40. Berkowitz K, Reyes C, Saadat P, Kjos SL. Fetal lung maturation. Comparison of biochemical indices in gestational diabetic and nondiabetic pregnancies. J Reprod Med 1997;42:793–800. (Level II-2)

41. Piazze JJ, Anceschi MM, Maranghi L, Brancato V, Marchiani E, Cosmi EV. Fetal lung maturity in pregnancies complicated by insulin-dependent and gestational diabetes: a matched cohort study. Eur J Obstet Gynecol Reprod Biol 1999;83:145–50. (Level II-2)

42. Piper JM. Lung maturation in diabetes in pregnancy: if and when to test. Semin Perinatol 2002;26:206–9. (Level III)

43. Burkhart AE, Towers CV, Rumney PJ, Lewis DF. Neonatal outcome when delivery follows a borderline immature lecithin to sphingomyelin ratio. J Perinatol 2000;20:157–60. (Level III)

44. Bildirici I, Moga CN, Gronowski AM, Sadovsky Y. The mean weekly increment of amniotic fluid TDx-FLM II ratio is constant during the latter part of pregnancy. Am J Obstet Gynecol 2005;193:1685–90. (Level III)

The MEDLINE database, the Cochrane Library, and ACOG's own internal resources and documents were used to conduct a literature search to locate relevant articles published between January 1985 and October 2007. The search was restricted to articles published in the English language. Priority was given to articles reporting results of original research, although review articles and commentaries also were consulted. Abstracts of research presented at symposia and scientific conferences were not considered adequate for inclusion in this document. Guidelines published by organizations or institutions such as the National Institutes of Health and the American College of Obstetricians and Gynecologists were reviewed, and additional studies were located by reviewing bibliographies of identified articles. When reliable research was not available, expert opinions from obstetrician–gynecologists were used.

Studies were reviewed and evaluated for quality according to the method outlined by the U.S. Preventive Services Task Force:

I   Evidence obtained from at least one properly designed randomized controlled trial.

II-1 Evidence obtained from well-designed controlled trials without randomization.

II-2 Evidence obtained from well-designed cohort or case–control analytic studies, preferably from more than one center or research group.

II-3 Evidence obtained from multiple time series with or without the intervention. Dramatic results in uncontrolled experiments also could be regarded as this type of evidence.

III   Opinions of respected authorities, based on clinical experience, descriptive studies, or reports of expert committees.

Based on the highest level of evidence found in the data, recommendations are provided and graded according to the following categories:

Level A—Recommendations are based on good and consistent scientific evidence.

Level B—Recommendations are based on limited or inconsistent scientific evidence.

Level C—Recommendations are based primarily on consensus and expert opinion.

ISSN 1099-3630

The American College of Obstetricians and Gynecologists
409 12th Street, SW, PO Box 96920, Washington, DC 20090-6920

Fetal lung maturity. ACOG Practice Bulletin No. 97. American College of Obstetricians and Gynecologists. Obstet Gynecol 2008;112: 717–26.

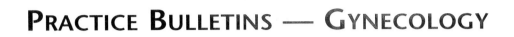

PRACTICE BULLETINS — GYNECOLOGY

PRACTICE BULLETINS — GYNECOLOGY

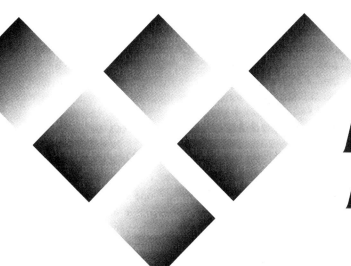

ACOG PRACTICE BULLETIN

CLINICAL MANAGEMENT GUIDELINES FOR
OBSTETRICIAN–GYNECOLOGISTS

NUMBER 81, MAY 2007

This Practice Bulletin was developed by the ACOG Committee on Practice Bulletins— Gynecology with the assistance of Malcolm G. Munro, MD. The information is designed to aid practitioners in making decisions about appropriate obstetric and gynecologic care. These guidelines should not be construed as dictating an exclusive course of treatment or procedure. Variations in practice may be warranted based on the needs of the individual patient, resources, and limitations unique to the institution or type of practice.

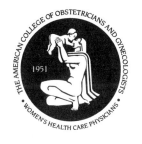

Endometrial Ablation

Endometrial ablation refers to a number of minimally invasive surgical procedures designed to treat abnormal uterine bleeding in selected women who have no desire for future fertility. In this document, standard resectoscopic endometrial ablation will be compared with the newer nonresectoscopic endometrial ablation devices and techniques. Evidence comparing endometrial ablation with other techniques for treating abnormal uterine bleeding also will be reviewed. The purpose of this document is to review the efficacy, safety, indications, and limitations of techniques for endometrial ablation.

Background

History

The technique of targeted endometrial destruction, using a radiofrequency electrosurgical probe passed through the cervical canal into the endometrial cavity without endoscopic guidance, was originally developed in 1937. Another blind technique, called cryoendometrial ablation, using a probe that supercooled the endometrial lining, was introduced in 1967 (1). Despite these early introductions, endometrial ablation did not become more widely adopted until the advent of hysteroscopically directed techniques. The first of these was laser endometrial ablation, introduced in 1981, using the neodymium:yttrium–aluminum–garnet (Nd:YAG) laser through the instrument channel of an operating hysteroscope (2). Subsequently, a number of investigators described case series using a urological resectoscope to resect (3), electrodesiccate (4), or vaporize (5) the endometrium. For most gynecologic surgeons, these techniques replaced the generally more cumbersome and expensive laser-based approach to endometrial destruction.

The rediscovery of nonresectoscopic endometrial ablation techniques led to the development of a number of systems that use different energy sources to achieve destruction of the endometrium, including tissue freezing, radiofrequency electricity, microwaves, and heated fluid, either freely circulating in the endometrial cavity or contained within a balloon. The first of these devices was approved by the U.S. Food and Drug Administration (FDA) in 1997, and others were released over the next few years. Currently, five systems are now approved for use in the United States.

Indications

Endometrial ablation is indicated for the treatment of menorrhagia or patient-perceived heavy menstrual bleeding in premenopausal women with normal endometrial cavities who have no desire for future fertility. In general, such patients will have experienced failure of or will be intolerant of medical therapy. When menorrhagia or excessive menstrual bleeding occurs in the context of submucosal myomata, endometrial ablation may be effective, depending on the location and diameter of the myomata as well as the system used for performing endometrial ablation. Patients who choose endometrial ablation should be willing to accept normalization of menstrual flow, not necessarily amenorrhea, as an outcome. The presence of anemia or failure or intolerance of medical therapy are important considerations but should not be construed as prerequisites for the procedure. The use of endometrial ablation in postmenopausal women or in women with disorders of hemostasis has not been rigorously evaluated.

The process of informed consent for endometrial ablation should include device- or system-appropriate information regarding risk and a realistic discussion of the potential outcomes of surgery because amenorrhea is not achieved in a substantial number of cases. Furthermore, given the persistence of endometrial tissue, premenopausal patients undergoing endometrial ablation should be counseled to use appropriate contraception.

Preoperative Evaluation

The structure and histology of the endometrial cavity should be thoroughly evaluated, both to assess for malignancy or endometrial hyperplasia and to ensure that the length and configuration is suitable for endometrial ablation. These parameters will vary depending on the technique or system used. Endometrial sampling, typically with an outpatient technique, can be used to evaluate all women for hyperplasia or malignancy, and results should be reviewed before ablation is scheduled. Women with endometrial hyperplasia or uterine cancer should not undergo endometrial ablation. Sounding and the use of transvaginal ultrasonography, saline infusion sonohysterography, hysteroscopy, or a combination of these procedures should be performed to measure the length of the cavity and to evaluate the internal architecture for structural anomalies and, in particular, for intracavitary or sub-

mucosal myomata. If such myomata are identified, it is important to characterize them by quantifying their diameter and determining the proportion of the lesion(s) that extend into the endometrial cavity.

Devices and Mechanisms of Action

Laser and Resectoscopic Endometrial Ablation

The modified urological resectoscope that uses radio-frequency-alternating current has become the most commonly used instrument, initially described using a resection technique by way of a loop electrode (6) and subsequently the combination of electrosurgical tissue desiccation and coagulation with a ball or barrel-shaped electrode (4). Another modification was introduced using grooved or spiked electrodes and higher wattage that allowed the surgeon to electrosurgically vaporize the endometrium (5, 7). This technique results in an endomyometrial furrow similar to that made by a loop electrode, without the creation of tissue "chips," and a slightly greater degree of coagulation in the adjacent tissue, a feature that has been shown, in the context of a comparative trial, to be associated with markedly reduced systemic absorption of distention media (8).

Nonresectoscopic Systems

Nonresectoscopic endometrial ablation refers to destruction of the endometrium using any of a number of techniques or devices, placed within the endometrial cavity, that do not require a uterine resectoscope. These systems appear to require less training and experience than for resectoscopic endometrial ablation, and they seem to result in clinical outcomes similar to those achieved by experienced resectoscopic surgeons. Performance of endometrial ablation with each of these systems comprises manual positioning of a device through the cervical canal to the endometrial cavity. The device controller unit is then activated and energy is applied, usually with microprocessor-based monitoring that aids in the determination of the treatment endpoint or that actually terminates the process when that endpoint is reached.

Cryotherapy. The FDA-approved cryotherapy system, Her Option, comprises a disposable 4.5-mm outside-diameter (OD) probe attached to a handle and cable that is connected to a dedicated controller unit. The cervix is exposed, and cervical dilation, if necessary, is performed. The device is passed into the endometrial cavity and then directed to one cornual area where a progressively expanding elliptical freeze zone, involving the surrounding endomyometrium, is created. This is repeated on the contralateral cornu. In some instances, an additional application may be made lower in the endometrial cavity. The typical treatment time is approximately 10 minutes.

Heated Free Fluid. The Hydro ThermAblator heated free fluid system also is FDA approved and achieves endometrial ablation with heated normal saline. It is the only system with integrated hysteroscopic monitoring. The device comprises a single use 7.8-mm OD sheath that adapts to any of a number of 2.7–3-mm OD hysteroscopes. The controller unit automates the processes of distending the uterus, creating a closed circuit, heating fluid, and monitoring of temperature and circuit volume. The distending media is normal saline drawn from a bag mounted on an attached, modified intravenous fluid pole. The process takes approximately 3 minutes to heat the fluid to 90°C, 10 minutes to maintain that temperature to ablate the endometrium, and approximately 1 minute for the fluid to cool down, allowing the device to be removed. If there is egress of more than 10 mL of distending media, either via the cervix or fallopian tubes, the system shuts off automatically. The depth of necrosis attained is 3–4 mm (9).

Microwave. Microwaves occupy the part of the electromagnetic spectrum between radio and infrared waves and exert their effect both directly and, in adjacent deeper layers, by thermal propagation. There currently are two FDA-approved versions of the microwave endometrial ablation device, one reusable and one disposable, each of which comprises an 8-mm OD probe attached by a reusable cable to a dedicated control module. The probe also contains an integrated thermal coupling device that transmits information about adjacent tissue temperature back to the control module for display on a screen. The surgeon controls activation and manipulation of the device.

The microwave probe is inserted to the uterine fundus and, when the measured temperature of the tissue around the probe reaches 30°C, the machine is activated. The operator moves the probe across the entire endometrial surface from the fundus down as the device gradually is withdrawn. Treatment time depends, in part, on cavity size but is usually 2–4 minutes.

Radiofrequency Electricity. The NovaSure system is an FDA-approved nonresectoscopic endometrial ablation device that uses radiofrequency electricity to perform automated endometrial ablation. The system is based around a dedicated microprocessor-based control unit and a single-use 7.2-mm OD probe with a bipolar gold mesh electrode array located at the distal end. To detect inadvertent perforation of the myometrium, the probe contains a system for determining the integrity of the endometrial cavity based on injection of a fixed volume of CO_2.

The electrode assembly is inserted transcervically and the mesh electrode is deployed by retraction of the outer sleeve. The unit is used to apply radiofrequency energy to the bipolar mesh while simultaneously applying suction, thereby evacuating steam and carbonized debris. This process allows for electrosurgical vaporization and underlying desiccation in a relatively rapid fashion (approximately 80–90 seconds).

Thermal Balloon. A balloon-tipped catheter probe is positioned in the endometrial cavity and then distended with fluid that is subsequently heated to a temperature that is high enough to destroy the endometrium. Although there are a number of such devices available worldwide, the ThermaChoice system currently is the only one approved by the FDA.

This system comprises a single-use balloon catheter, a connecting cable, and a dedicated controller unit. The OD of the catheter is 5.5 mm, and the heating element is contained within the balloon itself. The microprocessor-determined duration of treatment is 8 minutes (10).

After exposure of the cervix and any required dilation, the balloon tipped catheter is passed through the cervical canal into the endometrial cavity. The surgeon uses a syringe to inflate the balloon with 5% dextrose and water to a predetermined pressure of 160–180 mm Hg. The dedicated controller unit is then activated, thereby heating the element and the fluid. The microprocessor in the controller then monitors the parameters of balloon pressure and fluid temperature and automates treatment duration.

Clinical Considerations and Recommendations

▶ *How do endometrial ablation outcomes compare with medical therapy?*

Oral medical therapy has been compared with endometrial ablation in a high-quality randomized trial (11). By 5 years, only 10% of those patients randomized to medical therapy continued receiving medical treatment, whereas 77% had undergone surgery. Of the group allocated to resectoscopic endometrial ablation, 27% had further surgery, including 18% with hysterectomy. Patients randomized to oral medical therapy were significantly less likely to be satisfied than those undergoing resectoscopic endometrial ablation.

A different picture emerges when intrauterine medical therapy is compared with endometrial ablation. The Cochrane meta-analyses showed that quality of life and satisfaction measures were similar for patients undergoing endometrial ablation and receiving the intrauterine levonorgestrel-releasing system at 1 year (12, 13). In addition, whereas endometrial ablation was more effective at controlling uterine bleeding at 1 year, by years 2 and 3 there was no difference between the interventions.

▶ *Is pretreatment needed with these devices?*

Resectoscopic Endometrial Ablation

Mechanically thinning the endometrium with curettage or by direct suppression or inhibition of ovarian steroidogenesis has been used a presurgical adjuvant to resectoscopic endometrial ablation. A meta-analysis demonstrated that either preoperative danazol or gonadotropin-releasing hormone (Gn-RH) agonists result in shorter procedures, greater ease of surgery, a lower rate of postoperative dysmenorrhea, and a higher rate of post-surgical amenorrhea (14). Whether the short-term increase in amenorrhea rates associated with adjuvant medical suppression is sustained for multiple years is not known.

At this time, there are no high-quality data that allow for objective evaluation of similar outcomes associated with other preoperative approaches such as systemic progestins or mechanical preparation of the endometrium with curettage.

Nonresectoscopic Endometrial Ablation

Because single-layer thickness of the endometrium is typically up to 6 mm in the luteal phase (even thicker for women who are anovulatory) and most of the nonresectoscopic endometrial ablation systems typically treat to a depth of 4–6 mm, preoperative endometrial thinning seems to be logical. Endometrial thinning may not be necessary with the NovaSure system, which appears to vaporize and remove tissue, thereby, at least theoretically, increasing the thickness of endometrium that could be treated. With the exception of the NovaSure system (15), most of the randomized trials involving nonresectoscopic endometrial ablation devices have been performed on women who have had pretreatment to thin the endometrium. The ThermaChoice balloon ablation system was evaluated after suction curettage (16). For other devices, medical therapy, usually with Gn-RH agonists, was used (17–19).

▶ *What is the efficacy of resectoscope endometrial ablation?*

There are six randomized controlled trials (RCT) comparing endometrial ablation (almost exclusively resectoscopic endometrial ablation) with hysterectomy; four are from the United Kingdom (20–23), one is from Italy (24), and one is from North America (25, 26). Each of these tri-

als has resulted in a number of important additional publications comparing hysterectomy with endometrial ablation, including the Cochrane meta-analyses (27, 28).

These studies conclude that total hysterectomy is superior in attaining amenorrhea and, although satisfaction with resectoscopic endometrial ablation is high, there usually are somewhat greater patient satisfaction rates when the uterus is removed (21–23). Women who received resectoscopic endometrial ablation had shorter hospital stays and fewer postoperative complications, and they resumed activities earlier than those undergoing hysterectomy (20–23).

In clinical trials with long follow-up intervals, reoperation rates for women assigned to endometrial ablation increased steadily over time. Up to 36% of women at 4 years had either repeat ablation or hysterectomy, and treatment with hysterectomy was at least 24% (26, 29).

There is a relative paucity of randomized trials comparing the different techniques of resectoscopic endometrial ablation; those that are available are reviewed in the Cochrane systematic review (28). In the RCT conducted by the Aberdeen group, patients assigned to endometrial ablation were subsequently randomized to either laser ablation or endometrial resection (30). Whereas both procedures were associated with similar patient satisfaction and clinical outcomes at 12 months, laser ablation was associated with longer procedure time. Compared with loop resection, resectoscopic endometrial ablation with a vaporizing electrode was associated with significantly reduced systemic absorption of distending media during surgery and similar 1-year clinical outcomes (8). Resectoscopic endometrial ablation with rollerball electrodesiccation was compared with loop resection in an RCT in which 120 patients were recruited, with a 5-year follow-up involving 94% of the original sample. There were no differences in complications, bleeding outcomes, or the incidence of repeat surgery, which included a hysterectomy rate of 15% (31).

▶ *What is the efficacy of nonresectoscopic endometrial ablation therapy?*

Table 1 summarizes amenorrhea rates and patient satisfaction rates based on pivotal RCTs for nonresectoscopic endometrial ablation devices.

Thermal Balloon

The original ThermaChoice system underwent a multicenter RCT comparing it to resectoscopic endometrial ablation with rollerball electrosurgical coagulation and desiccation. Primary outcomes were reported at 1 year (16) with subsequent reports at 2 (32), 3 (33), and 5 years (34). Patient satisfaction with the therapeutic results was

Table 1. Patient Satisfaction and Amenorrhea Rates Associated With Nonresectoscope Endometrial Ablation Compared With Resectoscopic Ablation at 12 Months*

Device	Nonresectoscopic/Resectoscopic Ablation (%)		
	Satisfaction Rate	Amenorrhea Rate[†]	Diary Success (Score: 75 or Less)
ThermaChoice (thermal balloon)	96/99[‡]	13.2/27.2	80.2/84.3
Hydro ThermAblator (heated free fluid)	—[§]	35.3/47.1	68.4/76.4
Her Option (cryotherapy)	86/88[¶]	22.2/46.5	67.4/73.3
NovaSure (radiofrequency electricity)	92/93[‡]	36/32.2	77.7/74.4
Microwave Endometrial Ablation System (microwave energy)	92/93[‡]	55.3/45.8	87/83.2

*Based on U.S. Food and Drug Administration pivotal trials.

[†]Based on intent to treat.

[‡]Patients reported being satisfied or very satisfied.

[§]Quality-of-life scores compared with baseline only.

[¶]Patients reported being very or extremely satisfied.

Adapted from Sharp HT. Assessment of new technology in the treatment of idiopathic menorrhagia and uterine leiomyomata. Obstet Gynecol 2006;108:990–1003.

equal at 1 year (balloon ablation 95.9%, resectoscopic endometrial ablation 99.1%) and the success rates defined by the FDA (Pictorial Blood Loss Assessment Chart score less than 75) were equivalent. At 5 years, 122 (48%) of the original 255 patients treated were available for evaluation, an equal number from each group. By this time, 21 of the women available for evaluation in each of the groups had undergone hysterectomy; three and two underwent repeat ablation, respectively. However, with a high attrition rate and reporting based on the patients available for evaluation, it is possible that repeat surgery rates could be higher in the subset of women not available for evaluation.

Another single-institution RCT from the Netherlands also compared the original ThermaChoice balloon ablation system with resectoscopic endometrial ablation in 137 patients (35, 36). Perioperatively, complications with resectoscopic endometrial ablation included uterine perforation and electrolyte imbalance related to excess absorption of distention media; no such complications were seen in the balloon ablation group. At 24 months, the reduction in bleeding (measured by the same Pictorial Blood Loss Assessment Chart system used in the U.S. trial) was greater with balloon ablation, but success rates (Pictorial Blood Loss Assessment Chart score less than 185) and satisfaction rates (resectoscopic endometrial ablation 75%, ThermaChoice balloon ablation system 80%) were equivalent.

Although not randomized, a large multicenter, multinational cohort study described results of ThermaChoice balloon ablation for 260 women with dysfunctional uterine bleeding (37). Of the 260 original patients, 188 (72%) were available for 5 years of follow-up. Of these, 75% had avoided subsequent surgery altogether, whereas 21 had repeat ablation and 25 had undergone hysterectomy.

Cryotherapy

Published data regarding the FDA-approved Her Option cryotherapy system has been limited to endometrial cavities without submucosal myomata and that sound to 10 cm or less. The clinical outcomes from the pivotal trial designed for the FDA approval process have been published at 12 months (17) and 24 months (38). The total enrollment was 279 participants with a 2:1 randomization ratio (193 patients assigned to cryotherapy system and 86 assigned to resectoscopic endometrial electrodesiccation). At 12 months, 156 of the patients assigned to the cryotherapy system were available for evaluation, whereas 94 took part in the 24-month follow-up. For the resectoscopic ablation group at 12 months and 24 months, 72 and 43 patients were available for evaluation, respectively. Success rates, defined by reduction of the Pictorial Blood Loss Assessment Chart scores to less than 75, were equivalent in the two groups at 12 months (cryotherapy system 84.6%, resectoscopic endometrial ablation 88.9%). Amenorrhea rates are not reported at 2 years postablation. However, the investigators report that 7% of the patients assigned to the cryotherapy system and 8.1% of the patients assigned to resectoscopic endometrial ablation underwent hysterectomy in the follow-up period, whereas repeat ablations were performed on 8.1% and 1.2% of the patients, respectively (38). These 2-year outcomes also must be considered in the context of a relatively high attrition rate, with less than 50% of the original cohort available for follow-up at 2 years.

Heated Free Fluid

The only published clinical trial for the heated free fluid system was a comparison of 276 patients with dysfunctional uterine bleeding or heavy menstrual bleeding (no intracavitary or submucosal leiomyomata or endometrial polyps) treated with either the Hydro ThermAblator or with resectoscopic rollerball ablation in a 2:1 randomization scheme (18). A report in which the 3-year results were described also has been published (39). Of the 177 patients treated with the Hydro ThermAblator according to protocol, 167 were available for evaluation at 12 months and 135 were available for data collection at 3 years. At 1 year, bleeding was reduced to normal or less in 127 (94%) of these patients, with 72 (53%) experiencing amenorrhea. Each of these results was similar to those for resectoscopic electrodesiccation and coagulation (91% and 46%, respectively). At 3 years, satisfaction was high for the patients in both groups (98% for those treated with the Hydro ThermAblator, 97% for those treated with resectoscopic endometrial electrodesiccation), and hysterectomy was performed in 16 (9%) of the group treated with the Hydro ThermAblator and five (6%) of the patients treated with resectoscopic endometrial ablation. There were three repeat ablations in each group—2% of the patients treated with the Hydro ThermAblator and 4% of the patients treated with resectoscopic endometrial ablation.

Two retrospective studies have indicated that women with intracavitary myomata may have outcomes similar to women with normal cavities (40, 41), but prospective trials will be necessary to confirm such an impression.

Microwave

The Microwave Endometrial Ablation System has been the subject of a number of high-quality randomized trials. The first published RCT involved 263 women and compared the Microwave Endometrial Ablation System with resectoscopic endometrial ablation by expert surgeons, with outcomes published at 1 (42), 2 (43), and 5 years (44). Surgical time was shorter for those treated with the Microwave Endometrial Ablation System. At 1 year of follow-up, 116 (90%) of the 129 assigned to the Microwave Endometrial Ablation System and 124 (93%) of the 134 assigned to resectoscopic endometrial ablation were available for evaluation, with three fourths of each group satisfied with their outcome at 12 months following treatment. At 5 years, 236 (90%) of the original 263 women were available for follow-up. Bleeding and pain scores both were significantly reduced, and amenorrhea rates were similar (65% for those treated with the Microwave Endometrial Ablation System, 69% for those treated with resectoscopic endometrial ablation); however, those assigned to the Microwave Endometrial Ablation System were more likely to be satisfied with therapy than those who underwent resectoscopic endometrial ablation (86% compared with 74%).

Another RCT compared the Microwave Endometrial Ablation System to resectoscopic endometrial ablation performed by expert surgeons using rollerball electrosurgical desiccation and coagulation (19). In this trial, 322 participants were randomized to either the Microwave Endometrial Ablation System or resectoscopic endometrial ablation in a 2:1 allocation scheme. Of the 215 patients allocated to the Microwave Endometrial Ablation System, 209 were treated with the Microwave Endometrial Ablation System, with 194 available for evaluation at 1 year; of the 107 designated for resectoscopic endometrial ablation, 106 were treated, with 96 available for evaluation at 12 months. The Microwave Endometrial Ablation System treatment time was 3.45 minutes, whereas that for rollerball electrodesiccation was 20.22 minutes. At 12 months, and using intention-to-treat analysis, 87% of the patients treated with the Microwave Endometrial Ablation System and 83.2% of the patients treated with resectoscopic endometrial ablation had successful outcomes (Pictorial Blood Loss Assessment Chart scores less than 75). If only cases available for evaluation were considered (ie, only those treated according to assignment and available for evaluation at 12 months), the rate increased to 96.4% and 92.7%, respectively. The rate of amenorrhea in patients available for evaluation was 61.3% for those treated with the Microwave Endometrial Ablation System and 51% for those treated with resectoscopic endometrial ablation. At 1 year, 98.5% of the women undergoing treatment with the Microwave Endometrial Ablation System and 99% of those treated with resectoscopic endometrial ablation were either satisfied or highly satisfied with their treatment.

This trial was unique in that it included participants with submucosal myomata of up to 3 cm in diameter, provided that the myomata did not interfere with the positioning of the probe; such patients were available for subgroup evaluation. This is a similar diameter and configuration to those reported in the study on Therma-

Choice balloon ablation (45). In the subgroup analysis of the patients treated by the Microwave Endometrial Ablation System, success, amenorrhea, and patient satisfaction rates for women with submucosal myomata did not differ from those of women with normally configured endometrial cavities without submucosal leiomyomata.

Radiofrequency Electricity

In the RCT performed in North America (15), 265 participants were enrolled at nine clinical centers in a 2:1 randomization scheme. The resectoscopic endometrial ablation procedure was different from all of the other U.S. nonresectoscopic endometrial ablation trials to date because resection was used with subsequent electrosurgical desiccation with a rollerball electrode. At 1 year, success (Pictorial Blood Assessment Chart scores less than or equal to 75) was experienced by 88.3% of the patients treated with the NovaSure system and 81.7% of those treated with endometrial resection and ablation. The amenorrhea rates at 1 year were 41% for patients treated with the NovaSure system and 35% for those treated with resectoscopic endometrial ablation. In the first year, there were three hysterectomies in the group treated with the NovaSure system (1.3%) and two in the resectoscopic endometrial ablation cohort (2.2%). The 1-year patient satisfaction rates also were similar, with 92.8% of the patients treated with the NovaSure system and 93.9% of the patients treated with resectoscopic endometrial ablation reporting that they were satisfied or very satisfied with the outcome. Trials comparing the NovaSure system with other nonresectoscopic endometrial ablation methods will be discussed later.

The NovaSure system also has been subjected to prospective observational studies with follow-up data up to 3 (46) or 4 (47) years. Data from these studies suggest that repeat surgery rates may stay low and satisfaction rates high beyond the 12-month follow-up interval reported in the single North American RCT.

In the North American RCT, participants with polyps or submucosal leiomyomata smaller than 2 cm in diameter were allowed, but there was no subgroup analysis of patients with such lesions (15). Consequently, the efficacy of the NovaSure system in the presence of submucosal myomata, even smaller than 2 cm in diameter, remains unknown.

▶ *How do clinical outcomes of nonresectoscopic endometrial ablation devices compare with each other?*

Although there are abundant trials comparing resectoscopic endometrial ablation with nonresectoscopic endometrial ablation techniques, there has been a rela-

tive paucity of comparative studies involving two or more nonresectoscopic endometrial ablation devices. In a review of the literature via MEDLINE and the Cochrane Database, no comparative trials were found involving the Hydro ThermAblator device or the cryotherapy system called Her Option. However, there have been trials involving the Microwave Endometrial Ablation System, the NovaSure system, and the ThermaChoice balloon ablation system.

Two double-blinded RCTs have been published comparing the radiofrequency electrosurgical endometrial ablation system, NovaSure, with thermal balloon ablation systems; however, one involved the Cavaterm system, which is not currently available in the United States (48). The RCT comparing the NovaSure system with the original ThermaChoice system (49) followed a 2:1 randomization scheme, with 83 of the 126 participants assigned to the NovaSure system and 43 to the thermal balloon ablation system. Patients assigned to the ThermaChoice system underwent preprocedural mechanical thinning of the endometrium with suction curettage. There also was a generator problem encountered with the NovaSure system controller unit that was not discovered until 44 participants had been treated. The generator was replaced and enrollment into the trial continued with clinical outcomes reported by considering both the entire treatment cohort (intent to treat analysis) and including only the patients who were randomized following replacement of the generator. The patients were monitored to 12 months postprocedure using a validated semiquantitative Pictorial Blood Loss Assessment Chart as the primary outcome. The rate of amenorrhea in the entire cohort in the group assigned to the NovaSure system was 43% (34:83) and 8% (3:43) for those assigned to the ThermaChoice system. When the patients who were treated before changing the generator were excluded, 56% of those treated with the NovaSure system experienced amenorrhea, a proportion that is consistent with the results obtained in other RCTs. For both treatment groups, therapy was generally successful, as the mean Pictorial Blood Loss Assessment Chart scores decreased to the normal range, but the magnitude of the decrease was significantly greater for the group assigned to the NovaSure system. There were four hysterectomies in each group in the 12-month follow-up interval.

▶ *What are the reported complications associated with ablation devices?*

Both resectoscopic endometrial ablation and nonresectoscopic endometrial ablation have been associated with a number of adverse events (Table 2). Unique to resectoscopic endometrial ablation are complications related to

Table 2. Percentages of Postoperative Adverse Events Occurring Within Two Weeks of Nonresectoscopic Endometrial Ablation Surgery*

Complication	ThermaChoice (Thermal Balloon)	Hydro ThermAblator (Heated Free Fluid)	Her Option (Cryotherapy)	NovaSure (Radiofrequency Electricity)	Microwave Ablation System (Microwave Energy)
Urinary tract infection	0.8	2	3	0.6	0.5
Vaginal infection	0.8	0	1	0.6	2.3
Fever	0	0	0	0	1.4
Endometritis	2.1	1	0	0	2.8
Thermal injury†	0	1	0	0	0
Abdominal pain	0	2	4	0.6	3.2
Hematometra	0	0	0	0.6	0
Bacteremia	0	0	0	0	0.5

*Reported During U.S. Food and Drug Administration pivotal trials.
†Involving an extremity.
Sharp HT. Assessment of new technology in the treatment of idiopathic menorrhagia and uterine leiomyomata. Obstet Gynecol 2006;108:990–1003.

fluid overload and electrolyte disturbances, but both approaches have been associated with bleeding, injury of the cervix and vagina, and uterine perforation with potential damage to surrounding structures. Postprocedural infection as well as pregnancy, malignancy, and a painful syndrome associated with prior or concomitant tubal ligation have all been described.

Distention Media Fluid Overload

Distention media are required for hysteroscopic and resectoscopic surgery and, on occasion, substantial volumes of such media can be absorbed into the systemic circulation. Such complications do not occur in association with nonresectoscopic endometrial ablation.

Standard radiofrequency electrosurgical operative hysteroscopy or resectoscopy with monopolar instrumentation requires the use of electrolyte-free, low-viscosity solutions, such as 3% sorbitol, 1.5% glycine, 5% mannitol, and combined solutions of sorbitol and mannitol, each of which, if sufficiently absorbed into the systemic circulation, will result in dilutional hyponatremia and, with the possible exception of mannitol, hypoosmolality (50, 51). These electrolyte-free fluids can result in hyponatremia, hyposmolality, subsequent brain edema, and, in some instances, permanent neurologic damage or death. Such outcomes may be more common in premenopausal women because of the inhibitory impact of estrogen and progesterone on the brain's sodium pump, making such women more vulnerable to cerebral edema (52). As a result, appropriate fluid management is critical to the safety of resectoscopic and operative hysteroscopic surgery. The development of hysteroscopic electrosurgical systems that can operate in electrolyte-rich media, such as normal saline, has provided an opportu-

nity to eliminate the risk of hyponatremia (53, 54), but risks of fluid overload remain.

The volume of systemically absorbed distention media may be reduced with the preoperative use of Gn-RH analogues (52, 55) or the immediate preoperative administration of dilute intracervical vasopressin (56) or both. There are a number of other measures that should reduce the extent of systemic intravasation, including operating at the lowest effective intrauterine pressure and avoidance of preoperative overhydration. Early detection of intravasation is enhanced by adherence to a strict fluid measurement and management protocol that is recommended to include an automated system that measures fluid inflow and captures fluid from three sources: 1) the resectoscope, 2) the perineal collection drape, and 3) the floor. Such systems allow for real-time measurement of systemic intravasation of distention media. The management of intraoperatively recognized excessive intravasation varies according to the patient's baseline medical condition, her intraoperative assessment, the status of the procedure, and the amount of measured fluid intravasation.

Uterine Trauma

The uterus may be injured at the time of endometrial ablation, either with lacerations of the cervix or secondary to perforation of the corpus, an event that may be associated with damage to surrounding structures, such as blood vessels or viscera. The largest published evaluation of resectoscopic complications reflects the experience in the United Kingdom and suggests that techniques involving endometrial resection are most often associated with serious complications secondary to hemorrhage or perforation (57). This study also documents that experience is an important variable because these complications were most commonly encountered in the first 100 cases of a given surgeon.

The Cochrane systematic review showed that both cervical lacerations and perforation of the corpus were more commonly associated with resectoscopic endometrial ablation when compared with the various published nonresectoscopic endometrial ablation systems, despite the fact that, in most instances, those performing resectoscopic endometrial ablation in these trials were highly experienced. Given this information, the reported incidence of complications found in the literature from series and trials may not reflect the risk in the population at large because of the expertise and the experience of most published investigators.

The risk of cervical laceration can be reduced with the preoperative use of mechanical dilators, such as laminaria, or the use of vaginal misoprostol to soften the cervix (58). Alternatively, the injection of a low volume of a diluted vasopressin solution has been demonstrated to reduce the force required for dilation (59).

Although it is not possible to completely avoid the complication of perforation of the uterine corpus, serious complications should be minimized if the surgeon avoids advancing an activated electrode at all times. Should perforation with an activated electrode occur or if the activation status of the electrode at perforation is unknown, exploration of the peritoneal cavity is mandatory. Although laparotomy generally is the best method for evaluation of the bowel, laparoscopy may be selected in certain instances, provided there is adequate training and expertise of the surgeon.

Lower Tract Thermal Injury

A number of instances of burns to the vagina and vulva associated with the use of monopolar instrumentation for resectoscopic endometrial ablation have been reported (60). These lesions appear to be the result of shorting or capacitative coupling of current to the external sheath of the resectoscope (61–64). Careful attention to technique or the use of bipolar resectoscopes should minimize the incidence of these uncommon complications (64).

Postablation Tubal Ligation Syndrome

Shortly after the introduction of resectoscopic endometrial ablation, postablation tubal ligation syndrome was first described as a complication of endometrial ablation performed in women with previous tubal occlusion for purposes of contraception (65). Patients experienced cyclical pelvic pain presumably related to residual and trapped endometrium in one or both cornua. Women undergoing endometrial ablation with previous or con-

comitant laparoscopic sterilization are at low risk for the development of cyclic or intermittent pelvic pain subsequent to the procedure. The incidence of this syndrome is unclear but has been reported to be as high as 10% (66). Hysteroscopic decompression and laparoscopic salpingectomy are frequently not effective, and hysterectomy has been described as the most effective treatment (66).

Pregnancy

Pregnancy following endometrial ablation can occur and has been reported (67, 68). Although a limited number of women elect to carry the pregnancy, those that do so appear to experience high rates of malpresentation, prematurity, placenta accreta, and perinatal mortality. As a result, premenopausal women undergoing endometrial ablation should be counseled that pregnancy is possible and that an appropriate contraception method should be used.

Endometrial Malignancy

An early concern about endometrial ablation was the potential for delaying the diagnosis of a subsequent endometrial carcinoma. However, it appears that in most instances, an intrauterine cavity remains, allowing egress of bleeding from retained endometrium. Consequently, delay in the diagnosis of endometrial carcinoma is unlikely because of the absence of uterine bleeding.

Infection Rates

The incidence of infection following the performance of endometrial ablation is low. In the randomized trials comparing treatments of nonresectoscopic endometrial ablation and resectoscopic endometrial ablation performed in North America, endometritis was diagnosed in approximately 1% of the patients in each treatment group. Such patients seemed to respond to antibiotic therapy (15–19).

Nonresectoscopic Endometrial Ablation Complications

High-quality evidence from the RCTs involving nonresectoscopic endometrial ablation devices suggest that there are fewer complications with these devices, particularly with respect to distention fluid overload, cervical lacerations, perforation of the corpus and postprocedural hematometra (28).

Nonetheless, as is the case for any surgical device, complications can occur with nonresectoscopic endometrial ablation systems, and the incidence may be greater than that suggested by published clinical trials. In a review of the FDA's Manufacturer and User Facility Device Experience database, a number of complications were reported with the use of all nonresectoscopic endometrial ablation devices on the market at that time. These complications, not previously noted in the published literature, included uterine perforation, with at least one bowel injury in three of the four reports, and one death (69). This review was published shortly after introduction of three of the devices and before the introduction of one, and, consequently, underrepresents the incidence and extent of these complications. One example is the uncommon, but occasional, thermal injury to the vagina and vulva from spilled heated fluid while using the Hydro ThermAblator system. In addition, uterine perforation and thermal injury to the bowel have now been associated with all of five nonresectoscopic endometrial ablation devices approved by the FDA for distribution in the United States.

▶ *What forms of anesthesia are indicated?*

To date, most trials describing the use of nonresectoscopic endometrial ablation devices with local anesthesia include the use of parenteral conscious sedation, which precludes these procedures in most office environments. The NovaSure and ThermaChoice devices have been compared in a prospective study that suggested less pain for a shorter duration in the group assigned to the NovaSure system (70). In an RCT, treatment with the Microwave Endometrial Ablation System was performed with local anesthesia and, frequently, parenteral conscious sedation or general anesthesia (71). There was no particular advantage to the local or intravenous sedation group. Some investigators have described the successful performance of treatment with the ThermaChoice system without anesthesia (10) or with only local paracervical anesthetics and a rectal suppository containing a nonsteroidal analgesic (72, 73). Use of the Hydro ThermAblator system has been reported to be feasible with similar analgesics and intracervical or paracervical block (74).

To date, ideal regimens for using local anesthetic agents have not been determined. The fact that the cervix is innervated via the sacral S-2–S-3 nerve roots, whereas the corpus receives its nerve supply from the thoracic T-8–T-10 nerves, should be considered when designing such regimens. Paracervical and intracervical anesthesia will address only the S-2–S-3 nerve region, whereas intracavitary anesthesia with topical agents may have to be considered to address pain from the corpus (75–77). Clinicians also should consider the time required for local anesthetics to reach maximum action before performing uterine manipulations in the office setting.

▶ *Can nonresectoscopic endometrial ablation be performed in the presence of uterine leiomyomata?*

Data derived from RCTs involving the Microwave Endometrial Ablation System device (19, 42, 44) and one involving the ThermaChoice device (45) support the hypothesis that these systems can be used to treat women with abnormal uterine bleeding and selected submucosal leiomyomata up to 3 cm in diameter. With these devices, bleeding and satisfaction outcomes were similar to those achieved in women with normal endometrial cavities. Lesser quality evidence is available regarding the use of both the Hydro ThermAblator (40, 41) and NovaSure devices (78).

There is a relative paucity of information regarding the use of the ThermaChoice device in women with abnormal endometrial cavities, particularly those distorted by leiomyomata. However, a randomized trial involving 93 participants compared treatment results of the use of the ThermaChoice device (under local anesthesia with conscious sedation) with resectoscopic endometrial ablation in patients with type II myomata (with less than 50% of the diameter within the endometrial cavity) that were up to 3 cm in diameter. At 1 year, bleeding outcomes were significantly and equally reduced in the two treatment groups (45). At the time of this publication, there are no available studies or trials evaluating the currently distributed ThermaChoice III system.

▶ *What are the relative and absolute contraindications to endometrial ablation?*

All of the currently available nonresectoscopic endometrial ablation devices have limitations with respect to the size of the endometrial cavity and the nature and extent of anatomic distortion of the endometrial surface. Consequently, they are not recommended for use in women with endometrial cavities that exceed device limitations. Similar circumstances apply for resectoscopic endometrial ablation as well, but the manual nature of the technique may allow it to be applied to a wider spectrum of endometrial cavity sizes and configurations. Indeed, there is evidence that, at least in experienced and able hands, success rates in uteri greater than 12 gestational weeks in size may be equivalent to that of women with smaller sized uteri (79).

Table 3 demonstrates parameters such as the current limitations in both minimum- and maximum-sounded length and for the type and diameter of submucosal leiomyomata for the nonresectoscopic endometrial ablation devices currently available in the United States.

Table 3. Nonresectoscopic Endometrial Ablation Device Comparisons

Method	Pretreatment	Outside Diameter (mm)	Approximate Treatment Time (min)	*Sounded Uterine Length (cm) Minimum	Maximum	Treatment in the Presence of Submucosal Leiomyomata Published Evidence	Type	Diameter (cm)	U.S. Food and Drug Administration Approval
ThermaChoice (thermal balloon)	Mechanical (suction aspiration)	5.5	8	4	10	Yes (Level I)	II	Smaller than or equal to 3	No
Her Option (cryotherapy)	Gonadotropin-releasing hormone agonist	4.5	10–18	Not specified	10	None	Not applicable	Not applicable	No
Hydro ThermAblator (heated free fluid)	Gonadotropin-releasing hormone agonist	7.8	14	4	10.5	Yes (Level II-3)	I†, II	Not specified	No
Microwave Endometrial Ablation System (microwave energy)	Gonadotropin-releasing hormone agonist	8.5	2.5–4.5	6	14	Yes (Level I)	I†, II	Smaller than or equal to 3†	Yes
NovaSure (radiofrequency electricity)	None	7.2	1–2	6	10	Yes (Level II-2)	I, II	Smaller than or equal to 3	No

*From device activation to withdrawal

†Selected

Women who have abnormal uterine bleeding and a sounded cavity length or submucosal myomata outside the parameters of the devices available to the surgeon should consider either resectoscopic endometrial ablation or alternative approaches to the clinical problem. The impact of preoperative administration of Gn-RH agonists on the sounded length of the uterus or of submucosal myoma characteristics has not been specifically evaluated.

The presence of disorders of müllerian fusion or absorption also presents obstacles to the performance of endometrial ablation, and there are no data that specifically evaluate the performance of any system in the presence of such anomalies. The impact of müllerian fusion anomalies likely differs based in part on the anomaly itself and in part on the specific device or system. For example, it would seem that septate uteri may be successfully treated using heated free fluid or resectoscopic endometrial ablation, but other devices are less likely to be successful. Given that there are no existing data regarding this issue, clinicians are encouraged to individualize the therapy of such patients.

There are a number of circumstances in which endometrial ablation should probably be avoided. Certainly, the procedure should not be performed with recent pregnancy or in the presence of active or recent uterine infection, endometrial malignancy, or hyperplasia. Selected disorders or distortions of uterine structure may unduly enhance the risks associated with the procedure or make success unlikely. For example, extreme uterine version or flexion may make it impossible to position a device safely within the endometrial cavity. Another concern exists when areas of the myometrium are extremely thin, which may be the case in the presence of previous uterine surgery, such as abdominal or laparoscopic myomectomy, cesarean delivery (in particular classic cesarean delivery), and even with previous endometrial ablation. In such instances, there may be an increased risk of transmural thermal injury that could involve the adjacent bowel or bladder. Preoperative ultrasound evaluation of myometrial thickness is a prerequisite for the Microwave Endometrial Ablation System, with patients excluded from the procedure if any part of the myometrium is less than 10 mm in thickness. However, there is no available evidence evaluating the ability of such ultrasound myometrial evaluation to identify a group of patients with previous transmural uterine surgery who are at low risk for the use of nonresectoscopic endometrial ablation techniques.

Summary of Recommendations and Conclusions

The following recommendations and conclusions are based on good and consistent scientific evidence (Level A):

▶ For women with normal endometrial cavities, resectoscopic endometrial ablation and nonresectoscopic endometrial ablation systems appear to be equivalent with respect to successful reduction in menstrual flow and patient satisfaction at 1 year following index surgery.

▶ Resectoscopic endometrial ablation is associated with a high degree of patient satisfaction but not as high as hysterectomy.

The following recommendations and conclusions are based on limited or inconsistent scientific evidence (Level B):

▶ Hysterectomy rates associated with both resectoscopic endometrial ablation and nonresectoscopic endometrial ablation are at least 24% within 4 years following the procedure.

▶ Women undergoing endometrial ablation with previous or concomitant laparoscopic sterilization are at low risk for the development of cyclic or intermittent pelvic pain subsequent to the procedure.

▶ Patient satisfaction and reduction in menstrual blood flow after endometrial ablation in women with normal endometrial cavities is similar to that experienced by women using the levonorgestrel-secreting intrauterine system.

The following recommendations and conclusions are based primarily on consensus and expert opinion (Level C):

▶ Patients who choose endometrial ablation should be willing to accept normalization of menstrual flow, not necessarily amenorrhea, as an outcome.

▶ Premenopausal patients undergoing endometrial ablation should be counseled to use appropriate contraception.

▶ Nonresectoscope endometrial ablation is not recommended in women with endometrial cavities that exceed device limitations.

▶ The endometrium of all candidates for endometrial ablation should be sampled, and histopathologic results should be reviewed before the procedure.

▶ Women with endometrial hyperplasia or uterine cancer should not undergo endometrial ablation.

▶ Performance of nonresectoscopic endometrial ablation in patients with prior classic cesarean delivery or transmural myomectomy may increase the risk of damage to surrounding structures. If endometrial ablation is to be performed in such patients, it may be best to perform resectoscopic endometrial ablation with laparoscopic monitoring. Safety of nonresectoscopic endometrial ablation in women with low transverse cesarean delivery has not been adequately studied.

▶ For resectoscopic endometrial ablation, it is recommended that a fluid management and monitoring system that provides "real-time" output of fluid balance be used.

Proposed Performance Measure

The percentage of patients who have endometrial sampling performed and results of histopathology reviewed before endometrial ablation

References

1. Cahan WG, Brockunier A Jr. Cryosurgery of the uterine cavity. Am J Obstet Gynecol 1967;99:138–53. (Level III)

2. Goldrath MH, Fuller TA, Segal S. Laser photovaporization of endometrium for the treatment of menorrhagia. Am J Obstet Gynecol 1981;140:14–9. (Level II-3)

3. DeCherney AH, Diamond MP, Lavy G, Polan ML. Endometrial ablation for intractable uterine bleeding: hysteroscopic resection. Obstet Gynecol 1987;70:668–70. (Level III)

4. Vancaillie TG. Electrocoagulation of the endometrium with the ball-end resectoscope. Obstet Gynecol 1989; 74:425–7. (Level II-3)

5. Vercellini P, Oldani S, De Giorgi O, Milesi M, Merlo D, Crosignani PG. Endometrial ablation with a vaporizing electrode. II. Clinical outcome of a pilot study. Acta Obstet Gynecol Scand. 1998;77:688–93. (Level II-2)

6. DeCherney A, Polan ML. Hysteroscopic management of intrauterine lesions and intractable uterine bleeding. Obstet Gynecol 1983;61:392–7. (Level II-3)

7. Glasser MH. Endometrial ablation and hysteroscopic myomectomy by electrosurgical vaporization. J Am Assoc Gynecol Laparosc 1997;4:369–74. (Level II-3)

8. Vercellini P, Oldani S, Yaylayan L, Zaina B, De Giorgi O, Crosignani PG. Randomized comparison of vaporizing electrode and cutting loop for endometrial ablation. Obstet Gynecol 1999;94:521–7. (Level I)

9. Richart RM, das Dores GB, Nicolau SM, Focchi GR, Cordeiro VC. Histologic studies of the effects of circulating hot saline on the uterus before hysterectomy. J Am Assoc Gynecol Laparosc 1999;6:269–73. (Level II-1)

10. Marsh F, Thewlis J, Duffy S. Thermachoice endometrial ablation in the outpatient setting, without local anesthesia or intravenous sedation: a prospective cohort study. Fertil Steril 2005;83:715–20. (Level II-1)

11. Cooper KG, Jack SA, Parkin DE, Grant AM. Five-year follow up of women randomised to medical management or transcervical resection of the endometrium for heavy menstrual loss: clinical and quality of life outcomes. BJOG 2001;108:1222–8. (Level I)

12. Lethaby AE, Cooke I, Rees M. Progesterone or progestogen-releasing intrauterine systems for heavy menstrual bleeding. Cochrane Database Systematic Reviews 2005, Issue 4. Art No.: CD002126. DOI: 10.1002/14651858. CD002126.pub2. (Meta-Analysis)

13. Marjoribanks J, Lethaby A, Farquhar C. Surgery versus medical therapy for heavy menstrual bleeding. Cochrane Database Systematic Reviews 2006, Issue 2. Art No.: CD003855. DOI: 10.1002/14651858.CD003855.pub2. (Meta-Analysis)

14. Sowter MC, Lethaby A, Singla AA. Pre-operative endometrial thinning agents before endometrial destruction for heavy menstrual bleeding. Cochrane Database of Systematic Reviews 2002, Issue 3. Art No.:CD001124. DOI:10.1002/14651858.CD001124. (Meta-Analysis)

15. Cooper J, Gimpelson R, Laberge P, Galen D, Garza-Leal JG, Scott J, et al. A randomized, multicenter trial of safety and efficacy of the NovaSure system in the treatment of menorrhagia. J Am Assoc Gynecol Laparosc 2002; 9:418–28. (Level I)

16. Meyer WR, Walsh BW, Grainger DA, Peacock LM, Loffer FD, Steege JF. Thermal balloon and rollerball ablation to treat menorrhagia: a multicenter comparison. Obstet Gynecol 1998;92:98–103. (Level I)

17. Duleba AJ, Heppard MC, Soderstrom RM, Townsend DE. Randomized study comparing endometrial cryoablation and rollerball electroablation for treatment of dysfunctional uterine bleeding. J Am Assoc Gyencol Laparosc 2003;10:17–26. (Level I)

18. Corson SL. A multicenter evaluation of endometrial ablation by Hydro ThermAblator and rollerball for treatment of menorrhagia. J Am Assoc Gynecol Laparosc 2001; 8:359–67. (Level 1)

19. Cooper JM, Anderson TL, Fortin CA, Jack SA, Plentl MB. Microwave endometrial ablation vs. rollerball electroablation for menorrhagia: a multicenter randomized trial. J Am Assoc Gynecol Laparosc 2004;11:394–403. (Level I)

20. Gannon MJ, Holt EM, Fairbank J, Fitzgerald M, Molne MA, Crystal AM, et al. A randomised trial comparing endometrial resection and abdominal hysterectomy for the treatment of menorrhagia. BMJ 1991;303(6814):1362–4. (Level I)

21. Dwyer N, Hutton J, Stirrat GM. Randomised controlled trial comparing endometrial resection with abdominal hysterectomy for the surgical treatment of menorrhagia. Br J Obstet Gynaecol 1993;100:237–43. (Level I)

22. Pinion SB, Parkin DE, Abramovich DR, Naji A, Alexander DA, Russell IT, et al. Randomised trial of hysterectomy, endometrial laser ablation, and transcervical endometrial resection for dysfunctional uterine bleeding. BMJ 1994;309:979–83. (Level I)

23. O'Connor H, Broadbent JA, Magos AL, McPherson K. Medical Research Council randomised trial of endometrial resection versus hysterectomy in management of menorrhagia. Lancet 1997;349:897–901. (Level I)

24. Crosignani PG, Vercellini P, Apolone G, De Giorgi O, Cortesi I, Meschia M. Endometrial resection versus vaginal hysterectomy for menorrhagia: long-term clinical and quality-of-life outcomes. Am J Obstet Gynecol 1997; 177:95–101. (Level I)

25. Weber AM, Munro MG. Endometrial ablation versus hysterectomy: STOP-DUB. Medscape Womens Health 1998; 3:3. (Level III)

26. Dickersin K, Munro MG, Langenberg P, Scherer R, Frick KD, Weber AM, et al. Surgical Treatments Outcomes Project for Dysfunctional Uterine Bleeding (STOP-DUB): design and methods. Surgical Treatments Outcomes Project for Dysfunctional Uterine Bleeding Research Group. Control Clin Trials 2003;24:591–609. (Level III)

27. Lethaby A, Shepperd S, Cooke I, Farquhar C. Endometrial resection and ablation versus hysterectomy for heavy menstrual bleeding. Cochrane Database Systematic Reviews 1999, Issue 2. Art. No.:CD000329. DOI: 10.1002/14651858.CD000329. (Meta-Analysis)

28. Lethaby A, Hickey M, Garry R. Endometrial destruction techniques for heavy menstrual bleeding. Cochrane Database of Systematic Reviews 2005, Issue 4. Art. No.: CD001501. DOI: 10.1002/14651858.CD001501.pub2. (Meta-Analysis)

29. A randomised trial of endometrial ablation versus hysterectomy for the treatment of dysfunctional uterine bleeding: outcome at four years. Aberdeen Endometrial Ablation Trials Group [published erratum appears in Br J Obstet Gynaecol 1999;106:360–6]. Br J Obstet Gynaecol 1999;106:360–6. (Level II-2)

30. Bhattacharya S, Cameron IM, Parkin DE, Abramovich DR, Mollison J, Pinion SB, et al. A pragmatic randomised comparison of transcervical resection of the endometrium with endometrial laser ablation for the treatment of menorrhagia. Br J Obstet Gynaecol 1997;104(5):601–7. (Level I)

31. Boujida VH, Philipsen T, Pelle J, Joergensen JC. Five-year follow-up of endometrial ablation: endometrial coagulation versus endometrial resection. Obstet Gynecol 2002;99:988–92. (Level I)

32. Grainger DA, Tjaden BL, Rowland C, Meyer WR. Thermal balloon and rollerball ablation to treat menorrha-

gia: two-year results of a multicenter, prospective, randomized, clinical trial. J Am Assoc Gynecol Laparosc 2000;7:175–9. (Level I)

33. Loffer FD. Three-year comparison of thermal balloon and rollerball ablation in treatment of menorrhagia [published erratum appears in J Am Assoc Gynecol Laparosc 2001;8:330]. J Am Assoc Gynecol Laparosc 2001;8: 48–54. (Level I)

34. Loffer FD, Grainger D. Five-year follow-up of patients participating in a randomized trial of uterine balloon therapy versus rollerball ablation for treatment of menorrhagia. J Am Assoc Gynecol Laparosc 2002;9:429–35. (Level I)

35. Van Zon-Rabelink IA, Vleugels MP, Merkus HM, de Graaf R. Endometrial ablation by rollerball electrocoagulation compared to uterine balloon thermal ablation. Technical and safety aspects. Eur J Obstet Gynecol Reprod Biol 2003;110:220–3. (Level I)

36. van Zon-Rabelink IA, Vleugels MP, Merkus HM, De Graaf R. Efficacy and satisfaction rate comparing endometrial ablation by rollerball electrocoagulation to uterine balloon thermal ablation in a randomised controlled trial. Eur J Obstet Gynecol Reprod Biol 2004; 114:97–103. (Level I)

37. Amso NN, Stabinsky SA, McFaul P, Blanc B, Pendley L, Neuwirth R. Uterine thermal balloon therapy for the treatment of menorrhagia: the first 300 patients from a multicentre study. International Collaborative Uterine Thermal Balloon Working Group. Br J Obstet Gynaecol 1998;105: 517–23. (Level II-2)

38. Townsend DE, Duleba AJ, Wilkes MM. Durability of treatment effects after endometrial cryoablation versus rollerball electroablation for abnormal uterine bleeding: two-year results of a multicenter randomized trial. Am J Obstet Gynecol 2003;188:699–701. (Level I)

39. Goldrath MH. Evaluation of HydroThermAblator and rollerball endometrial ablation for menorrhagia 3 years after treatment. J Am Assoc Gynecol Laparosc 2003;10: 505–11. (Level II-3)

40. Glasser MH, Zimmerman JD. The HydroThermAblator system for management of menorrhagia in women with submucous myomas: 12- to 20-month follow-up. J Am Assoc Gynecol Laparosc 2003;10:521–7. (Level II-3)

41. Rosenbaum SP, Fried M, Munro MG. Endometrial hydrothermablation: a comparison of short-term clinical effectiveness in patients with normal endometrial cavities and those with intracavitary pathology. J Minim Invasive Gynecol 2005;12:144–9. (Level II-2)

42. Cooper KG, Bain C, Parkin DE. Comparison of microwave endometrial ablation and transcervical resection of the endometrium for treatment of heavy menstrual loss: a randomised trial. Lancet 1999;354(9193):1859–63. (Level I)

43. Bain C, Cooper KG, Parkin DE. Microwave endometrial ablation versus endometrial resection: a randomized controlled trial. Obstet Gynecol 2002;99:983–7. (Level I)

44. Cooper KG, Bain C, Lawrie L, Parkin DE. A randomised comparison of microwave endometrial ablation with transcervical resection of the endometrium; follow up at a minimum of five years. BJOG 2005;112:470–5. (Level I)

45. Soysal ME, Soysal SK, Vicdan K. Thermal balloon ablation in myoma-induced menorrhagia under local anesthesia. Gynecol Obstet Invest 2001;51:128–33. (Level I)

46. Gallinat A, Nugent W. NovaSure impedance-controlled system for endometrial ablation. J Am Assoc Gynecol Laparosc 2002;9:283–9. (Level II-3)

47. Baskett TF, Clough H, Scott TA. NovaSure bipolar radiofrequency endometrial ablation: report of 200 cases. J Obstet Gynaecol Can 2005;27:473–6. (Level II-2)

48. Abbott J, Hawe J, Hunter D, Garry R. A double-blind randomized trial comparing the Cavaterm and the NovaSure endometrial ablation systems for the treatment of dysfunctional uterine bleeding. Fertil Steril 2003;80:203–8. (Level I)

49. Bongers MY, Bourdrez P, Mol BW, Heintz AP, Brolmann HA. Randomised controlled trial of bipolar radio-frequency endometrial ablation and balloon endometrial ablation. BJOG 2004;111:1095–102. (Level I)

50. Istre O, Skajaa K, Schjoensby AP, Forman A. Changes in serum electrolytes after transcervical resection of endometrium and submucous fibroids with use of glycine 1.5% for uterine irrigation. Obstet Gynecol 1992;80: 218–22. (Level II-2)

51. Kim AH, Keltz MD, Arici A, Rosenberg M, Olive DL. Dilutional hyponatremia during hysteroscopic myomectomy with sorbitol-mannitol distention medium. J Am Assoc Gynecol Laparosc 1995;2(2):237–42. (Level II-2)

52. Taskin O, Buhur A, Birincioglu M, Burak F, Atmaca R, Yilmay I, et al. Endometrial Na+, K+-ATPase pump function and vasopressin levels during hysteroscopic surgery in patients pretreated with GnRH agonist. J Am Assoc Gynecol Laparosc 1998;5:119–24. (Level I)

53. Isaacson K, Nardella P. Development and use of a bipolar resectoscope in endometrial electrosurgery. J Am Assoc Gynecol Laparosc 1997;4:385–91. (Level III)

54. Vilos GA. Intrauterine surgery using a new coaxial bipolar electrode in normal saline solution (Versapoint): a pilot study. Fertil Steril 1999;72(4):740–3. (Level III)

55. Donnez J, Vilos G, Gannon MJ, Stampe-Sorensen S, Klinte I, Miller RM. Goserelin acetate (Zoladex) plus endometrial ablation for dysfunctional uterine bleeding: a large randomized, double-blind study. Fertil Steril 1997;68:29–36. (Level I)

56. Goldenberg M, Zolti M, Bider D, Etchin A, Sela BA, Seidman DS. The effect of intracervical vasopressin on the systemic absorption of glycine during hysteroscopic endometrial ablation. Obstet Gynecol 1996;87:1025–9. (Level I)

57. Overton C, Hargreaves J, Maresh M. A national survey of the complications of endometrial destruction for menstrual disorders: the MISTLETOE study. Minimally Invasive Surgical Techniques—Laser, EndoThermal or Endoresection. Br J Obstet Gynaecol 1997;104:1351–9. (Level II-2)

58. Preutthipan S, Herabutya Y. Vaginal misoprostol for cervical priming before operative hysteroscopy: a randomized controlled trial. Obstet Gynecol 2000;96:890–4. (Level I)

59. Phillips DR, Nathanson HG, Milim SJ, Haselkorn JS. The effect of dilute vasopressin solution on the force needed for cervical dilatation: a randomized controlled trial. Obstet Gynecol 1997;89:507–11. (Level I)

60. Vilos GA, Brown S, Graham G, McCulloch S, Borg P. Genital tract electrical burns during hysteroscopic endometrial ablation: report of 13 cases in the United States and Canada. J Am Assoc Gynecol Laparosc 2000;7:141–7. (Level III)

61. Vilos GA, McCulloch S, Borg P, Zheng W, Denstedt J. Intended and stray radiofrequency electrical currents during resectoscopic surgery. J Am Assoc Gynecol Laparosc 2000;7:55–63. (Level III)

62. Vilos GA, Newton DW, Odell RC, Abu-Rafea B, Vilos AG. Characterization and mitigation of stray radiofrequency currents during monopolar resectoscopic electrosurgery. J Minim Invasive Gynecol 2006;13:134–40. (Level III)

63. Munro MG. Capacitive coupling: a comparison of measurements in four uterine resectoscopes. J Am Assoc Gynecol Laparosc 2004;11:379–87. (Level III)

64. Munro MG. Mechanisms of thermal injury to the lower genital tract with radiofrequency resectoscopic surgery. J Minim Invasive Gynecol 2006;13:36–42. (Level III)

65. Townsend DE, McCausland V, McCausland A, Fields G, Kauffman K. Post-ablation-tubal sterilization syndrome. Obstet Gynecol 1993;82:422–4. (Level III)

66. McCausland AM, McCausland VM. Frequency of symptomatic cornual hematometra and postablation tubal sterilization syndrome after total rollerball endometrial ablation: a 10-year follow-up. Am J Obstet Gynecol 2002;186:1274–80; discussion 1280–3. (Level II-3)

67. Hare AA, Olah KS. Pregnancy following endometrial ablation: a review article. J Obstet Gynaecol 2005;25:108–14. (Level III)

68. Lo JS, Pickersgill A. Pregnancy after endometrial ablation: English literature review and case report. J Minim Invasive Gynecol 2006;13:88–91. (Level III)

69. Gurtcheff SE, Sharp HT. Complications associated with global endometrial ablation: the utility of the MAUDE database. Obstet Gynecol 2003;102:1278–82. (Level III)

70. Laberge PY, Sabbah R, Fortin C, Gallinat A. Assessment and comparison of intraoperative and postoperative pain associated with NovaSure and ThermaChoice endometrial ablation systems. J Am Assoc Gynecol Laparosc 2003;10:223–32. (Level II-1)

71. Wallage S, Cooper KG, Graham WJ, Parkin DE. A randomised trial comparing local versus general anaesthesia for microwave endometrial ablation. BJOG 2003;110 (9):799–807. (Level I)

72. McAllister KF, Bigrigg A. Uterine balloon therapy for menorrhagia: a feasibility study of its use in the community setting. J Fam Plann Reprod Health Care 2002; 28:133–4. (Level II-3)

73. Fernandez H, Capella S, Audibert F. Uterine thermal balloon therapy under local anaesthesia for the treatment of menorrhagia: a pilot study. Hum Reprod 1997;12: 2511–4. (Level II-3)

74. Farrugia M, Hussain SY. Hysteroscopic endometrial ablation using the Hydro ThermAblator in an outpatient hysteroscopy clinic: feasibility and acceptability. J Minim Invasive Gynecol 2006;13(3):178–82. (Level II-3)

75. Zupi E, Luciano AA, Marconi D, Valli E, Patrizi G, Romanini C. The use of topical anesthesia in diagnostic hysteroscopy and endometrial biopsy. J Am Assoc Gynecol Laparosc 1994;1:249–52. (Level I)

76. Cicinelli E, Didonna T, Fiore G, Parisi C, Matteo MG, Castrovilli G. Topical anesthesia for hysteroscopy in postmenopausal women. J Am Assoc Gynecol Laparosc 1996;4:9–12. (Level I)

77. Rattanachaiyanont M, Leerasiri P, Indhavivadhana S. Effectiveness of intrauterine anesthesia for pain relief during fractional curettage. Obstet Gynecol 2005;106: 533–9. (Level I)

78. Sabbah R, Desaulniers G. Use of the NovaSure Impedance Controlled Endometrial Ablation System in patients with intracavitary disease: 12-month follow-up results of a prospective, single-arm clinical study. J Minim Invasive Gynecol 2006;13:467–71. (Level II-3)

79. Eskandar MA, Vilos GA, Aletebi FA, Tummon IS. Hysteroscopic endometrial ablation is an effective alternative to hysterectomy in women with menorrhagia and large uteri. J Am Assoc Gynecol Laparosc 2000;7: 339–45. (Level II-2)

The MEDLINE database, the Cochrane Library, and ACOG's own internal resources and documents were used to conduct a literature search to locate relevant articles published between January 1985 and October 2006. The search was restricted to articles published in the English language. Priority was given to articles reporting results of original research, although review articles and commentaries also were consulted. Abstracts of research presented at symposia and scientific conferences were not considered adequate for inclusion in this document. Guidelines published by organizations or institutions such as the National Institutes of Health and the American College of Obstetricians and Gynecologists were reviewed, and additional studies were located by reviewing bibliographies of identified articles. When reliable research was not available, expert opinions from obstetrician–gynecologists were used.

Studies were reviewed and evaluated for quality according to the method outlined by the U.S. Preventive Services Task Force:

I   Evidence obtained from at least one properly designed randomized controlled trial.

II-1   Evidence obtained from well-designed controlled trials without randomization.

II-2   Evidence obtained from well-designed cohort or case–control analytic studies, preferably from more than one center or research group.

II-3   Evidence obtained from multiple time series with or without the intervention. Dramatic results in uncontrolled experiments also could be regarded as this type of evidence.

III   Opinions of respected authorities, based on clinical experience, descriptive studies, or reports of expert committees.

Based on the highest level of evidence found in the data, recommendations are provided and graded according to the following categories:

Level A—Recommendations are based on good and consistent scientific evidence.

Level B—Recommendations are based on limited or inconsistent scientific evidence.

Level C—Recommendations are based primarily on consensus and expert opinion.

ISSN 1099-3630

The American College of Obstetricians and Gynecologists
409 12th Street, SW, PO Box 96920, Washington, DC 20090-6920

Endometrial ablation. ACOG Practice Bulletin No. 81. American College of Obstetricians and Gynecologists. Obstet Gynecol 2007; 109:1233–48.

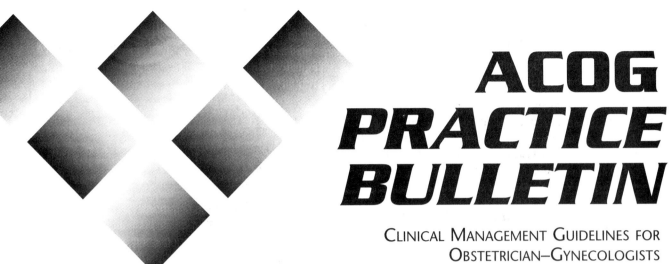

ACOG PRACTICE BULLETIN

CLINICAL MANAGEMENT GUIDELINES FOR
OBSTETRICIAN–GYNECOLOGISTS

NUMBER 83, JULY 2007

This Practice Bulletin was developed by the ACOG Committee on Practice Bulletins—Gynecology with the assistance of Michael Berman, MD, and Leslie Randall-Whitis, MD. The information is designed to aid practitioners in making decisions about appropriate obstetric and gynecologic care. These guidelines should not be construed as dictating an exclusive course of treatment or procedure. Variations in practice may be warranted based on the needs of the individual patient, resources, and limitations unique to the institution or type of practice.

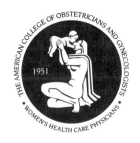

Management of Adnexal Masses

A suspected ovarian neoplasm is a common clinical problem that affects women of all ages. In the United States, a woman has a 5–10% lifetime risk of undergoing surgery for a suspected ovarian neoplasm and, within that group, an estimated 13–21% chance of receiving a diagnosis of ovarian cancer (1). Although most adnexal masses are benign, the goal of the diagnostic evaluation is to exclude malignancy. Management decisions often are influenced by the age and family history of the patient. The purpose of this document is to review the most recent data on imaging modalities, operative assessment of the adnexal mass, and preoperative models to predict the probability of ovarian malignancy.

Background

Adnexal masses are commonly encountered in gynecologic practice and often present both diagnostic and management dilemmas. Whereas some women present with acute torsion or rupture of a mass requiring immediate surgical intervention, most masses are detected incidentally. In these situations, the physician must try to differentiate masses likely to be benign from those likely to be malignant. Masses with a low likelihood of malignancy often can be managed conservatively. Conversely, those that are more likely to be malignant are best managed with prompt surgery by a physician with advanced training and expertise in the management of ovarian cancer, such as a gynecologic oncologist. Masses that are less clearly benign or malignant usually require surgery; however, many can be managed laparoscopically, with ovarian preservation. This document includes a review of the patient factors, physical findings, imaging results, and serum markers that help separate masses into the categories of probably benign, uncertain, and likely malignant, helping to guide appropriate management.

The differential diagnosis of the adnexal mass includes both gynecologic and nongynecologic sources and, when arising from the ovary, may be benign, malignant, or of low malignant potential (Box 1). The most important factor in narrowing the possibilities is the stage of the woman's reproductive life. For example, masses in menstruating women are almost always gynecologic, and most are functional cysts. In contrast, the most common masses in postmenopausal women are benign neoplasms, such as cystadenomas, but the risk of malignancy is much greater than in premenopausal women (2). Even metastatic cancers, especially those from the breast, colon, or stomach, may first present as adnexal masses.

Ovarian Cancer Incidence, Morbidity, and Mortality

A woman's lifetime risk of developing ovarian cancer is approximately 1 in 70 (3). It is estimated that in the United States 22,430 new ovarian cancer cases will be diagnosed, and 15,280 women will die of disease annually (4). The 5-year survival rate in women in whom Stage I ovarian cancer has been diagnosed exceeds 90%; however, only 20% of cancers are detected at this stage (5). Indeed, 65–70% are diagnosed at an advanced stage, when the 5-year survival rate is 30–55% (6). Despite the poor prognosis for women with advanced cancers, the figures reflect modest survival improvements achieved over the past two decades, attributable to advances in cytoreductive surgery and more effective first- and second-line chemotherapeutic agents.

Risk Factors

Age is the most important independent risk factor for ovarian cancer in the general population, with the incidence increasing sharply after the onset of menopause (4). According to data reported by the Surveillance, Epidemiology, and End Results program, from 2000 to 2003, the median age at ovarian cancer diagnosis was 63 years, and ovarian cancer was diagnosed in 68.6% of patients after the age of 55 years (3). Thus, adnexal masses in postmenopausal women are more likely to be malignant than those in premenopausal women.

A family history of breast or ovarian cancer increases the lifetime risk for ovarian cancer, but the magnitude of that increase in women without identifiable genetic risk factors is unknown. The Hereditary Ovarian Cancer Clinical Study Group reported that *BRCA1* carriers have a 60-fold increased risk and *BRCA2* carriers have a 30-fold increased risk of developing ovarian cancer by the age of 60 years compared with the general population (7). Additionally, women affected with hereditary nonpolyposis colorectal cancer or Lynch II syndrome have approximately a 13-fold greater risk of developing ovarian cancer than the general population (8). Additional

---

Box 1. Differential Diagnosis of Adnexal Mass

Gynecologic
- Benign
  - Functional cyst
  - Leiomyomata
  - Endometrioma
  - Tuboovarian abscess
  - Ectopic pregnancy
  - Mature teratoma
  - Serous cystadenoma
  - Mucinous cystadenoma
  - Breast cancer
  - Hydrosalpinx
- Malignant
  - Germ cell tumor
  - Sex-cord or stromal tumor
  - Epithelial carcinoma

Nongynecologic
- Benign
  - Diverticular abscess
  - Appendiceal abscess or mucocele
  - Nerve sheath tumors
  - Ureteral diverticulum
  - Pelvic kidney
  - Paratubal cysts
  - Bladder diverticulum
- Malignant
  - Gastrointestinal cancers
  - Retroperitoneal sarcomas
  - Metastases

---

factors that increase ovarian cancer risk include nulliparity, primary infertility, and endometriosis (9).

Aside from prophylactic oophorectomy, use of combined oral contraceptives is the only strategy consistently shown to decrease the risk of epithelial ovarian cancer. The magnitude of protection is a function of duration of use. A large cohort study following 103,551 women for up to 9 years reported a 40% reduction in ovarian cancer risk in women who have ever used oral contraceptives (relative risk [RR], 0.6; 95% confidence interval [CI], 0.5–0.7) and a 90% reduction for women who were long-term users (15 years or longer) of oral contraceptives (RR, 0.1; 95% CI, 0.01–0.6) (10). Protection was observed to a lesser degree in patients with a known *BRCA1* or *BRCA2* mutation (11).

Clinical Tests

Physical Examinations

Pelvic examinations, including a rectal exam, even under anesthesia, have shown limited ability to identify an adnexal mass, especially with increasing patient body mass index (BMI) greater than 30 (12). Even so, features most consistently associated with an adnexal malignancy include a mass that is irregular; has a solid consistency; is fixed, nodular, or bilateral; or is associated with ascites. Benign conditions that can produce many of these findings, especially in premenopausal women, include endometriosis, chronic pelvic infections, hemorrhagic corpus luteum, and uterine leiomyoma.

Ultrasonography

High-frequency, gray-scale transvaginal ultrasonography can produce high-resolution images of an adnexal mass that approximate its gross anatomic appearance. Advantages of transvaginal ultrasonography include its widespread availability, good patient tolerability, and cost-effectiveness, making transvaginal ultrasonography the most widely used imaging modality to evaluate adnexal masses. In asymptomatic women (both premenopausal or postmenopausal) with pelvic masses, transvaginal ultrasonography is the imaging modality of choice. No alternative imaging modality has demonstrated sufficient superiority to transvaginal ultrasonography to justify its routine use (Table 1).

Although image quality is operator dependent, interobserver agreement among experienced ultrasonographers is quite high ($\kappa = 0.85$) (13). The main limitation of transvaginal ultrasonography use alone relates to its lack of specificity and low positive predictive value for cancer, especially in premenopausal women. Abdominal

Table 1. Modalities for the Evaluation of Adnexal Masses

Modality	Sensitivity	Specificity
Gray-scale transvaginal ultrasonography	0.82–0.91%	0.68–0.81%
Doppler ultrasonography	0.86%	0.91%
Computed tomography	0.90%	0.75%
Magnetic resonance imaging	0.91%	0.88%
Positron emission tomography	0.67%	0.79%
CA 125 level measurement	0.78%	0.78%

Agency for Healthcare Research and Quality. Management of adnexal mass. Evidence Based Report/Technology Assessment No. 130. AHRQ Publication No. 06-E004. Rockville (MD): AHRQ; 2006.

ultrasonography is very useful as an adjuvant to transvaginal ultrasonography because transvaginal ultrasonography may not provide an accurate image of masses that are both pelvic and abdominal.

Information provided should include the size and consistency of the mass (cystic, solid, or mixed), whether the mass was unilateral or bilateral, presence or absence of septations, mural nodules, papillary excrescences, and free fluid in the pelvis. In premenopausal or postmenopausal women, excrescences, ascites, and mural nodules raise the suspicion for cancer, whereas absence of these findings suggests a benign diagnosis. Ultrasound findings should be correlated with physical findings, and a refined differential diagnosis should be constructed.

In an effort to quantify cancer risk based on morphology, several transvaginal ultrasound scoring systems have been proposed (14–19). Whereas scoring criteria vary among these systems, most assign low risk scores to sonolucent cysts with smooth walls, thin or absent septations, and absence of solid components. In initial publications, scoring systems were able to distinguish benign from malignant masses in most instances (sensitivity, 65–100% and specificity, 67–95%); however, prospective validation studies have provided consistently lower figures for each scoring system so evaluated (17, 20–22). In a rigorous meta-analysis of these scoring systems, the pooled sensitivities and specificities ranged from 86% to 91% and from 68% to 83%, respectively (23).

One morphology index assigns a morphologic score to the ultrasound image of the adnexal mass by considering three criteria: 1) ovarian tumor volume, 2) cyst wall structure, and 3) septa structure (16) (Table 2). Volume is calculated using an ellipsoid formula: length $\times$ width $\times$ height $\times$ 0.523, and each component is assigned a score from 0 to 4 for a possible composite score of 0–12. For example, a sonolucent, smooth-walled mass measuring less than 10 cm^3 would be assigned a composite score of 0, whereas a multiseptate mass with irregular wall structure or solid component measuring 100 cm^3 would be assigned a score of 10. Although, in a study of 213 patients (24), a composite score of 5 or more was associated with an 89% sensitivity to distinguish a malignant mass from a benign mass, the positive predictive value of a score of 5 or more was only 46%. In other words, more than one half of the masses that were classified as malignant based on a score of 5 or more were actually benign. In addition, intraobserver variation in assigning scores for wall and septal structure was quite high ($\kappa = 0.41$ and 0.47, respectively).

Color Doppler Ultrasonography

Color Doppler ultrasonography permits measurement of blood flow in and around a mass. Based on the hypothe-

Table 2. Morphology Index for Ovarian Tumors

Score	0	1	2	3	4	5
Volume	Less than 10 cm³	10–50 cm³	Greater than 50–100 cm³	Greater than 100–200 cm³	Greater than 200–500 cm³	Greater than 500 cm³
Structure	Smooth wall, sonolucent	Smooth wall, diffuse echogenicity	Wall thickening, less than 3 mm fine septa	Papillary projection equal to or greater than 3 mm thick	Complex, predominantly solid	Complex, solid and cystic areas with extratumoral fluid

Liu JH, Gass M. Management of the perimenopause. New York (NY): © The McGraw-Hill Companies, Inc; 2006.

sis that hypoxic tissue in tumors will recruit low-resistance, high-flow blood vessels, the ultimate goal of color Doppler ultrasonography is to increase the specificity of gray-scale two-dimensional ultrasonography alone. Color Doppler ultrasonography performed at the time of transvaginal ultrasonography measures various blood flow indices, including resistive index, pulsatility index, and maximum systolic velocity (25–31). The current role of color Doppler ultrasonography in evaluating pelvic masses remains controversial because the ranges of values of resistive index, pulsatility index, and maximum systolic velocity between benign and malignant masses overlap considerably in most publications on this subject.

In an attempt to overcome the overlap among color Doppler ultrasonography blood flow indices, "vascular sampling" of suspicious areas (papillary projections, solid areas, and thick septations) using both three-dimensional transvaginal ultrasonography and power Doppler ultrasonography has been investigated (13, 32–35). In addition, three-dimensional ultrasound examination of vascular architecture has proved to be highly discriminatory in distinguishing benign masses from cancers in some reports (36). In particular, a "chaotic" vascular architecture correlated highly with malignancy. These newer approaches deserve prospective clinical trials to define their role in distinguishing benign from malignant masses.

Other Imaging Modalities

Computed tomography (CT), magnetic resonance imaging (MRI), and positron emission tomography (PET) are not recommended for use in the initial evaluation of adnexal masses. In addition, after a thorough transvaginal ultrasound examination is performed, additional imaging with these modalities usually is of limited value. Because of their high cost, use of these imaging modalities should be reserved for specific situations. Based on limited data, MRI might have superior ability compared with transvaginal ultrasonography in correctly classifying malignant masses at the expense of a lower overall

detection rate (37–40). Gadolinium-contrast MRI can improve sensitivity (37, 41, 42), but in addition to its expense, its inconvenience precludes its routine use over transvaginal ultrasonography. However, MRI often will be helpful in differentiating the origin of nonadnexal pelvic masses, especially leiomyomata (43).

Currently, the best use of CT imaging is not to detect and characterize pelvic masses but to evaluate the abdomen for metastasis when a cancer is suspected based on transvaginal ultrasound images, examination results, or serum markers. A CT scan can detect omental metastases, peritoneal implants, pelvic or periaortic lymph node enlargement, hepatic metastases, obstructive uropathy, and possibly an alternate primary cancer site, including pancreas or colon.

Because of the much higher cost with no clear advantage over transvaginal ultrasonography, current data do not support the use of PET scanning in the preoperative assessment of adnexal masses.

Serum Marker Screening

The most extensively studied serum marker to distinguish benign from malignant pelvic masses is CA 125. It is most useful when nonmucinous epithelial cancers are present, but it is not of value in distinguishing other categories of ovarian malignancy (44). The serum marker CA 125 level is elevated in 80% of patients with epithelial ovarian cancer but only in 50% of patients with stage I disease at the time of diagnosis, hence its lack of utility as a screening test (1). Additionally, β-hCG, L-lactate dehydrogenase (LDH), and alpha-fetoprotein (AFP) levels may be elevated in the presence of certain malignant germ cell tumors, and inhibin A and B sometimes are markers for granulosa cell tumors of the ovary. The overall sensitivity of CA 125 screening in distinguishing benign from malignant adnexal masses reportedly ranges from 61% to 90%; specificity ranges from 71% to 93%, positive predictive value ranges from 35% to 91%, and negative predictive value ranges from 67% to 90% (26–28, 45–48). Wide variations in these figures reflect differences in cancer prevalence in the study population, the proportion of patients who are postmenopausal, and the threshold of CA 125 levels considered abnormal. The low sensitivity occurs because the CA 125 level is elevated in only one half of early stage epithelial ovarian cancers and rarely in germ cell, stromal, or mucinous cancers. The low specificity occurs because the CA 125 level frequently is elevated in many commonly encountered clinical conditions, including uterine leiomyomata, endometriosis, acute or chronic pelvic inflammatory disease, ascites of any etiology, and even inflammatory conditions such as systemic lupus erythematosus and inflammatory bowel disease. Because most of these clinical conditions occur in premenopausal women and because most epithelial ovarian cancers occur in postmenopausal women, the sensitivity and specificity of an elevated CA 125 level in concert with a pelvic mass is highest after menopause.

Clinical Considerations and Recommendations

▶ What ultrasound findings are suggestive of benign disease?

Unilocular, thin-walled sonolucent cysts with smooth, regular borders are overwhelmingly benign, regardless of menopausal status or cyst size, with malignancy rates in most series of 0–1% (49–53). In the largest prospective study published to date, 2,763 postmenopausal women with unilocular cysts no larger than 10 cm were evaluated using serial ultrasonography at 6-month intervals. Spontaneous resolution occurred in more than two thirds of patients, and no cancers were detected after a mean follow-up of 6.3 years, suggesting that the risk of malignancy in such patients was virtually nonexistent (51). Therefore, simple cysts up to 10 cm in diameter as measured by ultrasonography are almost universally benign and may safely be followed without intervention, even in postmenopausal patients.

Small descriptive studies have reported ultrasound characteristics that may be specific for selected benign diagnoses. Typical findings reported for endometriomas include a round homogeneous-appearing cyst containing low-level echoes within the ovary, with sensitivity of 83% and specificity of 89% in differentiating them from other types of ovarian cysts (54, 55). Mature teratomas typically contain a hypoechoic attenuating component with multiple small homogeneous interfaces; these were determined with 98% accuracy in a series of 155 suspected dermoid cysts (56). In addition, hydrosalpinges appear as tubular-shaped sonolucent cysts, with a sensitivity of 93% and specificity of 99.6% for differentiating this diagnosis from other adnexal masses (57).

▶ When is a CA 125 test warranted?

The value of elevated CA 125 levels is in distinguishing between benign and malignant masses in postmenopausal women. Few studies evaluate the predictive value of CA 125 levels stratified by menopausal status but, of those that do, specificity and positive predictive value are consistently higher in postmenopausal patients. In a prospective study of 158 patients undergoing laparotomy for a pelvic mass, the positive predictive value of an elevated CA 125 level was 98% in postmenopausal women (cancer prevalence 63%) but was only 49% in premenopausal women (cancer prevalence 15%) (58).

Whereas CA 125 level measurement is less valuable in premenopausal than postmenopausal women in predicting cancer risk, extreme values can be helpful. For example, although premenopausal women with masses and either normal or mildly elevated CA 125 levels usually have benign diagnoses, a markedly elevated CA 125 level raises a much greater concern for malignancy, even though women with benign conditions such as endometriomas can have CA 125 level elevations of 1,000 units/mL or greater (59). A normal CA 125 level in the absence of transvaginal ultrasound findings suspicious for cancer can justify observation in the asymptomatic woman.

Typically CA 125 values will increase over time when a cancer is present, whereas this is not necessarily so for benign masses. Although this observation is intuitive, there are few studies published that specifically address this hypothesis (60).

▶ What evaluation is necessary in the premenopausal woman?

Almost all pelvic masses in premenopausal women are benign. The initial evaluation in this age group is influenced by the presence or absence of abdominal or pelvic symptomatology. Symptomatic patients typically have diagnoses that require immediate interventions, including antibiotics and possibly surgery for tuboovarian abscesses, medical management or surgical intervention for ectopic pregnancies, surgical management for torsion of an ovarian cyst, and expectant management for most ruptured ovarian cysts. Appropriate evaluation for such women includes a medical history and physical examination, quantitative β-hCG level evaluation, complete blood count, and transvaginal ultrasonography. Additional studies may be indicated, including serial hematocrit measurements and appropriate cultures.

Rarely, a patient with acute symptomatology might have a malignancy. Acute hemorrhage into a cancerous ovary or rapid growth of a malignancy can present in such a manner. Such malignant tumors often are germ cell tumors, occurring in adolescents or women in their late teens or twenties (61, 62). In such a situation, tumor markers specific for many such germ cell tumors, including β-hCG, AFP, and LDH in conjunction with transvaginal ultrasonography, might aid in the diagnosis.

▶ *What evaluation is necessary in the post-menopausal woman?*

The exclusion of many common diagnoses of premenopausal women (eg, functional cyst, endometriosis, tuboovarian abscess, and ectopic pregnancy) and the greater probability that a mass will be malignant in postmenopausal women results in a much higher index of suspicion for malignancy when a mass is present in women in this age group. The hallmark for evaluation of such women includes transvaginal ultrasonography and CA 125 level measurements. Any elevation of CA 125 levels is highly suspicious for malignancy in women in this age group (45, 63) as are transvaginal ultrasound findings of masses that contain solid areas or excrescences or that are associated with free fluid in the abdomen or pelvis or both. With the exception of simple cysts on a transvaginal ultrasound finding, most pelvic masses in postmenopausal women will require surgical intervention.

It also is important to note that the ovary is a relatively common site for metastases from uterine, breast, colorectal, or gastric cancers. All postmenopausal women with a mass should have breast and digital rectal examinations as well as mammography if it has not been performed in the past 12 months. An endometrial biopsy should be performed if transvaginal ultrasound findings show a thickened endometrial lining and abnormal uterine bleeding is present. Additionally, if the patient is found to be anemic, has a positive fecal occult blood test result, and is older than 50 years, upper and lower gastrointestinal endoscopy should be performed to rule out primary gastric or colon cancer.

▶ *Is aspiration of cyst fluid appropriate?*

Aspiration of nonunilocular cyst fluid for both diagnosis and treatment of an adnexal mass may seem quicker, less invasive, and less expensive than surgery; however, it is typically regarded as contraindicated in postmenopausal women for several reasons, especially when there is a suspicion for cancer. First, diagnostic cytology has poor sensitivity to detect malignancy, ranging from 25% to 82% (64–69). In addition, even when a benign mass is aspirated, the procedure often is not therapeutic. Approximately 25% of cysts in perimenopausal and postmenopausal women will recur within 1 year of the procedure (70). Finally, aspiration of a malignant mass may induce spillage and seeding of cancer cells into the peritoneal cavity, thereby changing the stage and prognosis. Although definitive evidence supporting this notion is lacking, there have been many cases of aspirated malignant masses recurring along the needle tract through which the aspiration was done (71, 72). Furthermore, there is strong evidence that spillage at the time of surgery decreases overall survival of stage I cancer patients compared with patients with tumors that were removed intact (73, 74).

An exception to avoiding aspiration of a mass exists for those patients who have clinical and radiographic evidence of advanced ovarian cancer and who are medically unfit to undergo surgery. In these women, malignant cytology confirmed in this fashion will establish a cancer diagnosis, thereby permitting initiation of neoadjuvant chemotherapy (75, 76).

▶ *When is observation appropriate?*

Repeat imaging is most appropriate when either the morphology of the mass on an ultrasound finding suggests benign disease (49), or when morphology is less certain but there is a compelling reason to avoid surgical intervention. Examples include functional cysts in ovulating women, suspected endometriomas in asymptomatic women with normal or elevated, but not increasing, CA 125 levels, simple cysts in any setting, and hydrosalpinges. Specific diagnostic criteria for most of these conditions were discussed previously. Thus, repeat imaging is recommended whenever there is uncertainty of a diagnosis and when cancer or a benign neoplasm is in the differential diagnosis (77). Furthermore, some women for whom the usual management of a mass would require surgical intervention are at substantial risk for perioperative morbidity and mortality. In such instances, repeat imaging often is safer than immediate operative intervention, although the frequency of repeat imaging has not been determined.

▶ *Which patients may benefit from referral to a gynecologic oncologist?*

It has been well-established that women with ovarian cancer whose care is managed by a physician who has advanced training and expertise in the treatment of women with gynecologic cancer, such as a gynecologic oncologist, have improved overall survival rates as compared with those treated without such collaboration. Improved survival rates reflect both proper staging, thereby identifying some patients with unexpected occult metastasis who require adjuvant chemotherapy and aggressive debulking of advanced disease (78–80).

The Society of Gynecologic Oncologists (SGO) performed a multi-center, retrospective validation trial of

SGO–American College of Obstetricians and Gynecologists (ACOG) guidelines (Box 2) in which referral criteria and final histology of 1,035 women undergoing surgical exploration for a pelvic mass in six referral centers were reviewed (81). The prevalence of primary ovarian cancer was 30.7%, and the prevalence of cancers metastatic to the ovary was 4.8%. When applying the referral criteria, the positive predictive value was 33.8% and 59.5% in premenopausal and postmenopausal women, respectively. The negative predictive value was 92% for premenopausal and 91.1% for postmenopausal women. A second set of SGO guidelines referenced premenarchal patients and young adults with elevated germ cell tumor marker levels who may require surgical staging and adjuvant chemotherapy for malignant germ cell tumors (82) and supported the referral criteria recommended in the guidelines.

▶ *How should adnexal masses be managed in pregnancy?*

Despite the widespread use of ultrasonography during pregnancy, creating opportunities for detection of pelvic masses, there are few studies regarding adnexal masses in pregnancy. The prevalence of adnexal masses in pregnant women is 0.05–3.2% of live births (83–87). The most commonly reported pathologic diagnoses are mature teratomas and paraovarian or corpus luteum cysts (87–89). Malignancy is diagnosed in only 3.6–6.8% of patients with persistent masses and, in this age group, most malignancies are either germ cell, stromal, or epithelial tumors of low malignant potential.

The best approach to evaluate the pregnant patient with a mass is similar to that of the premenopausal patient described earlier. Depending on gestational age, abdominal ultrasonography may be used in addition to transvaginal ultrasonography because the ovaries may be outside of the pelvis later in gestation. Magnetic resonance imaging is the modality of choice if additional imaging is needed because it poses no fetal radiation exposure. Levels of CA 125 peak in the first trimester (range, 7–251 units/mL) and decrease consistently thereafter (90). Accordingly, low-level elevations in pregnancy typically are not associated with malignancy.

Despite a lack of supporting data, surgical removal of persistent masses in the second trimester is a common practice, with the intent to prevent emergent intervention for torsion or rupture. Several investigators have examined the role of expectant management; they report that 51–70% of adnexal masses will resolve during pregnancy (86–91), with predictors of persistence being mass size greater than 5 cm and "complex" morphology on transvaginal ultrasound findings. The actual occurrence of acute complications is reportedly less than 2% (85). Therefore, because adnexal masses in pregnancy appear to have low risk for both malignancy and acute complications, they may be considered for expectant management.

▶ *When should laparotomy versus laparoscopy be used in the management of the unilateral adnexal mass?*

Advancements in the preoperative assessment of pelvic masses permit the distinction of benign from malignant masses with a relatively high degree of confidence in most cases. Given such advancements in diagnosis, coupled with advancements in minimally invasive surgical techniques, laparoscopic management of many women with benign pelvic masses is appropriate and desirable. In general, if a mass is suspicious for cancer based on transvaginal ultrasound findings, CA 125 levels, and clinical assessment, laparoscopic surgery usually is considered contraindicated, although laparoscopic staging and management of ovarian cancer have been reported (92–94).

Several retrospective studies addressing the laparoscopic management of pelvic masses have confirmed

---

Box 2. Society of Gynecologic Oncologists and American College of Obstetricians and Gynecologists Referral Guidelines for a Newly Diagnosed Pelvic Mass

Premenopausal (younger than 50 years)

• CA 125 levels greater than 200 units/mL

• Ascites

• Evidence of abdominal or distant metastasis (by results of examination or imaging study)

• Family history of breast or ovarian cancer (in a first-degree relative)

Postmenopausal (older than 50 years)

• Elevated CA 125 levels

• Ascites

• Nodular or fixed pelvic mass

• Evidence of abdominal or distant metastasis (by results of examination or imaging study)

• Family history of breast or ovarian cancer (in a first-degree relative)

Im SS, Gordon AN, Buttin BM, Leath CA 3rd, Gostout BS, Shah C, et al. Validation of referral guidelines for women with pelvic masses. Obstet Gynecol 2005;105:35–41.

low complication rates ranging from 0% to 10%. Higher complication rates occur when masses are suspicious for cancer (95–102). In these studies, the mean conversion rate from laparoscopy to laparotomy was 6.4% (range, 0–25%), and the mean rate of cancer diagnosis was 4.3% (range, 0–17%). When compared with women undergoing laparotomy, the most consistent endpoints showing statistical significance are shortened length of hospital stay, decreased pain, and decreased convalescence time for women in whom masses are managed laparoscopically (97–101).

Three published randomized trials comprising 394 patients compare the findings and outcome of laparoscopy versus laparotomy in women with clinically benign pelvic masses (102–104). Conversion to laparotomy was performed only for endoscopic suspicion of cancer with conversion rates ranging from 0% to 1.5%. Rates of intraoperative cyst rupture were equal between the two approaches. In each study, statistically significant decreases in operative time, perioperative morbidity, length of hospital stay, and postoperative pain following laparoscopy versus laparotomy were demonstrated.

▶ *When is removal of the uterus and contralateral adnexa appropriate?*

The extent of surgery typically is a function of diagnosis, age, and patient wishes for ovarian function or future fertility. In premenopausal women, the operation of choice is cystectomy, when feasible, including most if not all mature teratomas and many endometriomas and cystadenomas. When ovarian tissue cannot be preserved, a unilateral oophorectomy or salpingo-oophorectomy is indicated. Patients must be advised about the risk of bilaterality, which can be as high as 25% for benign serous tumors, approximately 15% for benign teratomas, and as low as 2–3% for benign mucinous tumors. Wedge biopsy of a normal appearing contralateral ovary is not advised because doing so might adversely affect fertility (105). Perimenopausal or postmenopausal patients also may choose to undergo cystectomy or unilateral salpingo-oophorectomy. However, hysterectomy or bilateral salpingo-oophorectomy or both are considered appropriate options following completion of childbearing to reduce the risk of requiring future pelvic surgery and to exclude the risk of developing uterine, cervical, or ovarian cancer. It is unclear whether the potential benefits of ovarian preservation outweigh the risks of leaving them in situ. One decision-analysis model performed in women at average risk demonstrated excess mortality risk largely because of coronary heart disease and hip fracture if oophorectomy is performed before age 59 years (106).

▶ *When is conservative surgery an option in ovarian cancer management?*

Regardless of menopausal status, when cancers are present, including tumors of low malignant potential, the standard management includes hysterectomy with bilateral salpingo-oophorectomy and staging procedures by a physician with advanced training and experience with gynecologic cancer. Exceptions exist for some premenopausal women who wish to preserve their childbearing capabilities. Conservative surgery to preserve future fertility, including unilateral salpingo-oophorectomy or even ovarian cystectomy, does not appear to be associated with compromised prognosis in premenopausal women when the cancer is a germ cell tumor (107–109), a stage I stromal tumor, a tumor of low malignant potential (83, 92, 110–113), and even cases of stage IA, grade 1–2 invasive cancers (114, 115). Such patients should undergo complete surgical staging even when the uterus and opposite ovary will be preserved. Rates of recurrence are relatively low, being reported as 0–18.5% in low-malignant-potential tumors (83, 110, 112, 113) and 9.6–14.7% in patients with stage IA, grade 1–2 tumors (114, 115). Long-term survival rates in these series exceeded 90% for all tumors. Reproductive outcomes generally are favorable; however, these cases remain small in number.

The surgeon often may rely on frozen-section evaluation for operative decision making. The accuracy of frozen-section diagnosis varies from 72% to 88.7% (116). In addition, diagnostic accuracy has been shown to be lower in masses greater than 10 cm (74%) because of possible sampling errors with large masses, tumors of low malignant potential (78%), and ovarian cancers (75%) (116).

Summary of Recommendations and Conclusions

The following recommendations and conclusions are based on limited or inconsistent scientific evidence (Level B):

▶ In asymptomatic women with pelvic masses, whether premenopausal or postmenopausal, transvaginal ultrasonography is the imaging modality of choice. No alternative imaging modality has demonstrated sufficient superiority to transvaginal ultrasonography to justify its routine use.

▶ Specificity and positive predictive value of CA 125 level measurements are consistently higher in postmenopausal women compared with premenopausal women. Any CA 125 elevation in a postmenopausal woman with a pelvic mass is highly suspicious for malignancy.

▶ Simple cysts up to 10 cm in diameter on ultrasound findings are almost universally benign and may safely be followed without intervention, even in postmenopausal patients.

▶ Unilateral salpingo-oophorectomy or ovarian cystectomy in patients with germ cell tumors, stage I stromal tumors, tumors of low malignant potential, and stage IA, grade 1–2 invasive cancer who undergo complete surgical staging and who wish to preserve fertility does not appear to be associated with compromised prognosis.

The following recommendations and conclusions are based primarily on consensus and expert opinion (Level C):

▶ Women with ovarian cancer whose care is managed by physicians who have advanced training and expertise in the treatment of women with ovarian cancer, such as gynecologic oncologists, have improved overall survival rates compared with those treated without such collaboration.

▶ Most masses in pregnancy appear to have a low risk for both malignancy and acute complications and, thus, may be considered for expectant management.

Proposed Performance Measure

The percentage of patients evaluated for an asymptomatic pelvic mass who receive a transvaginal ultrasound examination

References

1. National Institutes of Health Consensus Development Conference Statement. Ovarian cancer: screening, treatment, and follow-up. Gynecol Oncol 1994;55:S4–14. (Level III)

2. Koonings P, Campbell K, Mishell D, Daniel R, Grimes DA. Relative frequency of primary ovarian neoplasms: a 10-year review. Obstet Gynecol 1989;74(6):921–6. (Level II-3).

3. Reis LA, Harkins D, Krapcho M, Mariotto A, Miller BA, Feuer EJ, et al. editors. SEER cancer statistics review, 1975–2003. Bethesda (MD): National Cancer Institute; 2006. Available at: http://seer.cancer.gov/csr/1975_2003. Retrieved February 16, 2007. (Level III)

4. American Cancer Society, Cancer facts and figures 2007. Atlanta (GA): ACS; 2007. Available at: http://www.cancer.org/downloads/STT/CAFF2007PWSecured.pdf. Retrieved February 16, 2007. (Level III)

5. Heintz AP, Odicino F, Maisonneuve P, Beller U, Benedet JL, Creasman WT, et al. Carcinoma of the ovary. Int J Gynaecol Obstet 2003;83(suppl 1):135–66. (Level II-3)

6. Jemal A, Siegel R, Ward E, Murray T, Xu J, Smigal C, et al. Cancer statistics, 2006. CA Cancer J Clin 2006; 56:106–30. (Level II-3)

7. Finch A, Beiner M, Lubinski J, Lynch HT, Moller P, Rosen B, et al. Salpingo-oophorectomy and the risk of ovarian, fallopian tube, and peritoneal cancers in women with a BRCA1 or BRCA2 mutation. Hereditary Ovarian Cancer Clinical Study Group. JAMA 2006;296:185–92. (Level II-2)

8. Aarnio M, Sankila R, Pukkala E, Salovaara R, Aaltonen LA, de la Chapelle A, et al. Cancer risk in mutation carriers of DNA-mismatch-repair genes. Int J Cancer 1999;81(2):214–8. (Level II-2)

9. Brinton LA, Lamb EJ, Moghissi KS, Scoccia B, Althuis MD, Mabie JE, et al. Ovarian cancer risk associated with varying causes of infertility. Fertil Steril 2004;82: 405–14. (Level II-2)

10. Kumle M, Weiderpass E, Braaten T, Adami HO, Lund E. Risk for invasive and borderline epithelial ovarian neoplasias following use of hormonal contraceptives: the Norwegian-Swedish Women's Lifestyle and Health Cohort Study. Norwegian-Swedish Women's Lifestyle and Health Cohort Study. Br J Cancer 2004;90:1386–91. (Level II-2)

11. Whittemore AS, Balise RR, Pharoah PD, Dicioccio RA, Oakley-Girvan I, Ramus SJ, et al. Oral contraceptive use and ovarian cancer risk among carriers of BRCA1 or BRCA2 mutations. Br J Cancer 2004;91:1911–5. (Level II-2)

12. Padilla LA, Radosevich DM, Milad MP. Limitations of the pelvic examination for evaluation of the female pelvic organs. Int J Gynaecol Obstet 2005;88:84–8. (Level II-3)

13. Timmerman D, Schwarzler P, Collins WP, Claerhout F, Coenen M, Amant F, et al. Subjective assessment of adnexal masses with the use of ultrasonography: an analysis of interobserver variability and experience. Ultrasound Obstet Gynecol 1999;13:11–6. (Level III)

14. Granberg S, Norstrom A, Wikland M. Tumors in the lower pelvis as imaged by vaginal sonography. Gynecol Oncol 1990;37:224–9. (Level III)

15. Sassone AM, Timor-Tritsch IE, Artner A, Westhoff C, Warren WB. Transvaginal sonographic characterization of ovarian disease: evaluation of a new scoring system to predict ovarian malignancy. Obstet Gynecol 1991;78: 70–6. (Level II-3)

16. DePriest PD, Shenson D, Fried A, Hunter JE, Andrews SJ, Gallion HH, et al. A morphology index based on sonographic findings in ovarian cancer. Gynecol Oncol 1993;51:7–11. (Level II-2)

17. Ferrazzi E, Zanetta G, Dordoni D, Berlanda N, Mezzopane R, Lissoni AA. Transvaginal ultrasonographic characterization of ovarian masses: comparison of five scoring systems in a multicenter study [published erratum appears in Ultrasound Obstet Gynecol 1998;11:v]. Ultrasound Obstet Gynecol 1997;10:192–7. (Level II-3)

18. Lerner JP, Timor-Tritsch IE, Federman A, Abramovich G. Transvaginal ultrasonographic characterization of ovarian masses with an improved, weighted scoring system. Am J Obstet Gynecol 1994;170:81–5. (Level II-3)

19. Finkler NJ, Benacerraf B, Lavin PT, Wojciechowski C, Knapp RC. Comparison of serum CA 125, clinical impression, and ultrasound in the preoperative evaluation of ovarian masses. Obstet Gynecol 1988;72:659–64. (Level III)

20. Mol BW, Boll D, De Kanter M, Heintz AP, Sijmons EA, Oei SG, et al. Distinguishing the benign and malignant adnexal mass: an external validation of prognostic models. Gynecol Oncol 2001;80:162–7. (Level II-3)

21. Alcazar JL, Merce LT, Laparte C, Jurado M, Lopez-Garcia G. A new scoring system to differentiate benign from malignant adnexal masses. Am J Obstet Gynecol 2003;88:685–92. (Level II-2)

22. Caruso A, Caforio L, Testa AC, Ciampelli M, Panici PB, Mancuso S. Transvaginal color Doppler ultrasonography in the presurgical characterization of adnexal masses. Gynecol Oncol 1996;63:184–91. (Level II-2)

23. Agency for Healthcare Research and Quality. Management of adnexal mass. Evidence Based Report/Technology Assessment No. 130. AHRQ Publication No. 06-E004. Rockville (MD): AHRQ; 2006. (Level II-2)

24. DePriest PD, Varner E, Powell J, Fried A, Puls L, Higgins R, et al. The efficacy of a sonographic morphology index in identifying ovarian cancer: a multi-institutional investigation. Gynecol Oncol 1994;55(2):174–8. (Level III)

25. Szpurek D, Moszyniki R, Sajdak S. Clinical value of the ultrasound Doppler index in determination of ovarian tumor malignancy. Eur J Gynaecol Oncol 2004;25:442–4. (Level III)

26. Antonic J, Rakar S. Validity of colour and pulsed Doppler US and tumour marker CA 125 in differentiation between benign and malignant ovarian masses. Eur J Gynaecol Oncol 1996;17:29–35. (Level II-3)

27. Alcazar JL, Errasti T, Zornoza A, Minguez JA, Galan MJ. Transvaginal color Doppler ultrasonography and CA-125 in suspicious adnexal masses. Int J Gynaecol Obstet 1999;66:255–61. (Level III)

28. Itakura T, Kikkawa F, Kajiyama H, Mitsui T, Kawai M, Mizutani S. Doppler flow and arterial location in ovarian tumors. Int J Gynaecol Obstet 2003;83:277–83. (Level II-2)

29. Marret H, Ecochard R, Giraudeau B, Golfier F, Raudrant D, Lansac J. Color Doppler energy prediction of malignancy in adnexal masses using logistic regression models. Ultrasound Obstet Gynecol 2002;20:597–604. (Level II-3)

30. Stein SM, Laifer-Narin S, Johnson MB, Roman LD, Muderspach LI, Tyszka JM, et al. Differentiation of benign and malignant adnexal masses: relative value of gray-scale, color Doppler, and spectral Doppler sonography. AJR Am J Roentgenol 1995;164:381–6. (Level II-3)

31. Schneider VL, Schneider A, Reed KL, Hatch KD. Comparison of Doppler with two-dimensional sonography and CA 125 for prediction of malignancy of pelvic masses. Obstet Gynecol 1993;81:983–8. (Level II-3)

32. Alcazar JL, Lopez-Garcia G. Transvaginal color Doppler assessment of venous flow in adnexal masses. Ultrasound Obstet Gynecol 2001;17:434–8. (Level II-3)

33. Marret H, Sauget S, Giraudeau B, Body G, Tranquart F. Power Doppler vascularity index for predicting malignancy of adnexal masses. Ultrasound Obstet Gynecol 2005;25:508–13. (Level II-3)

34. Alcazar JL, Castillo G. Comparison of 2-dimensional and 3-dimensional power-Doppler imaging in complex adnexal masses for the prediction of ovarian cancer. Am J Obstet Gynecol 2005;192:807–12. (Level II-2)

35. Guerriero S, Alcazar JL, Coccia ME, Ajossa S, Scarselli G, Boi M, et al. Complex pelvic mass as a target of evaluation of vessel distribution by color Doppler sonography for the diagnosis of adnexal malignancies: results of a multicenter European study. J Ultrasound Med 2002; 21:1105–11. (Level II-2)

36. Kurjak A, Jukic S, Kupesic S, Babic D. A combined Doppler and morphopathological study of ovarian tumors. Eur J Obstet Gynecol Reprod Biol 1997;71:147–50. (Level II-3)

37. Komatsu T, Konishi I, Mandai M, Togashi K, Kawakami S, Konishi J, et al. Adnexal masses: transvaginal US and gadolinium-enhanced MR imaging assessment of intratumoral structure. Radiology 1996;198:109–15. (Level III)

38. Grab D, Flock F, Stohr I, Nussle K, Rieber A, Fenchel S, et al. Classification of asymptomatic adnexal masses by ultrasound, magnetic resonance imaging, and positron emission tomography. Gynecol Oncol 2000;77:454–9. (Level II-3)

39. Sohaib SA, Mills TD, Sahdev A, Webb JA, Vantrappen PO, Jacobs IJ, et al. The role of magnetic resonance imaging and ultrasound in patients with adnexal masses. Clin Radiol 2005;60:340–8. (Level II-3)

40. Buist MR, Golding RP, Burger CW, Vermorken JB, Kenemans P, Schutter EM, et al. Comparative evaluation of diagnostic methods in ovarian carcinoma with emphasis on CT and MRI. Gynecol Oncol 1994;52:191–8. (Level II-3)

41. Yamashita Y, Torashima M, Hatanaka Y, Harada M, Higashida Y, Takahashi M, et al. Adnexal masses: accuracy of characterization with transvaginal US and precontrast and postcontrast MR imaging. Radiology 1995;194: 557–65. (Level II-3)

42. Hricak H, Chen M, Coakley FV, Kinkel K, Yu KK, Sica G, et al. Complex adnexal masses: detection and characterization with MR imaging—multivariate analysis. Radiology 2000;214:39–46. (Level II-3)

43. Chang SD, Cooperberg PL, Wong AD, Llewellyn PA, Bilbey JH. Limited-sequence magnetic resonance imaging in the evaluation of the ultrasonographically indeter-

minate pelvic mass. Can Assoc Radiol J 2004;55:87–95. (Level II-3)

44. Jacobs IJ, Fay TN, Stabile I, Bridges JE, Oram DH, Grudzinskas JG. The distribution of CA 125 in the reproductive tract of pregnant and non-pregnant women. Br J Obstet Gynaecol 1988;95:1190–4. (Level III)

45. Maggino T, Gadducci A, D'Addario V, Pecorelli S, Lissoni A, Stella M, et al. Prospective multicenter study on CA 125 in postmenopausal pelvic masses. Gynecol Oncol 1994;54:117–23. (Level II-2)

46. Schutter EM, Kenemans P, Sohn C, Kristen P, Crombach G, Westermann R, et al. Diagnostic value of pelvic examination, ultrasound, and serum CA 125 in postmenopausal women with a pelvic mass. An international multicenter study. Cancer 1994;74:1398–406. (Level II-3)

47. Sehouli J, Akdogan Z, Heinze T, Konsgen D, Stengel D, Mustea A, et al. Preoperative determination of CASA (Cancer Associated Serum Antigen) and CA-125 for the discrimination between benign and malignant pelvic tumor mass: a prospective study. Anticancer Res 2003; 23:1115–8. (Level II-2)

48. Manjunath AP, Pratapkumar, Sujatha K, Vani R. Comparison of three risk of malignancy indices in evaluation of pelvic masses. Gynecol Oncol 2001;81:225–9. (Level III)

49. Alcazar JL, Castillo G, Jurado M, Garcia GL. Is expectant management of sonographically benign adnexal cysts an option in selected asymptomatic premenopausal women? Hum Reprod 2005;20:3231–4. (Level II-2)

50. Castillo G, Alcazar JL, Jurado M. Natural history of sonographically detected simple unilocular adnexal cysts in asymptomatic postmenopausal women. Gynecol Oncol 2004;92:965–9. (Level II-2)

51. Modesitt SC, Pavlik EJ, Ueland FR, DePriest PD, Kryscio RJ, van Nagell JR Jr. Risk of malignancy in unilocular ovarian cystic tumors less than 10 centimeters in diameter. Obstet Gynecol 2003;102:594–9. (Level II-1)

52. Brown DL, Doubilet PM, Miller FH, Frates MC, Laing FC, DiSalvo DN, et al. Benign and malignant ovarian masses: selection of the most discriminating gray-scale and Doppler sonographic features. Radiology 1998;208: 103–10. (Level II-3)

53. Ekerhovd E, Wienerroith H, Staudach A, Granberg S. Preoperative assessment of unilocular adnexal cysts by transvaginal ultrasonography: a comparison between ultrasonographic morphologic imaging and histopathologic diagnosis. Am J Obstet Gynecol 2001;184:48–54. (Level II-2)

54. Guerriero S, Mais V, Ajossa S, Paoletti AM, Angiolucci M, Labate F, et al. The role of endovaginal ultrasound in differentiating endometriomas from other ovarian cysts. Clin Exp Obstet Gynecol 1995;22:20–2. (Level II-2)

55. Kupfer MC, Schwimer SR, Lebovic J. Transvaginal sonographic appearance of endometriomata: spectrum of findings. J Ultrasound Med 1992;11:129–33. (Level III)

56. Ekici E, Soysal M, Kara S, Dogan M, Gokmen O. The efficiency of ultrasonography in the diagnosis of dermoid cysts. Zentralbl Gynakol 1996;118:136–41. (Level II-2)

57. Guerriero S, Ajossa S, Lai MP, Mais V, Paoletti AM, Melis GB. Transvaginal ultrasonography associated with colour Doppler energy in the diagnosis of hydrosalpinx. Hum Reprod 2000;15:1568–72. (Level II-3)

58. Malkasian GD Jr, Knapp RC, Lavin PT, Zurawski VR Jr, Podratz KC, Stanhope CR, et al. Preoperative evaluation of serum CA 125 levels in premenopausal and postmenopausal patients with pelvic masses: discrimination of benign from malignant disease. Am J Obstet Gynecol 1988;159:341–6. (Level II-1)

59. Kitawaki J, Ishihara H, Koshiba H, Kiyomizu M, Teramoto M, Kitaoka Y, et al. Usefulness and limits of CA-125 in diagnosis of endometriosis without associated ovarian endometriomas. Hum Reprod 2005;20: 1999–2003. (Level II-2)

60. Skates SJ, Menon U, MacDonald N, Rosenthal AN, Oram DH, Knapp RC, et al. Calculation of the risk of ovarian cancer from serial CA-125 values for preclinical detection in postmenopausal women. J Clin Oncol 2003; 21(suppl):206–10. (Level II-3)

61. Deligeoroglou E, Eleftheriades M, Shiadoes V, Botsis D, Hasiakos D, Kontoravdis A, et al. Ovarian masses during adolescence: clinical, ultrasonographic and pathologic findings, serum tumor markers and endocrinological profile. Gynecol Endocrinol 2004;19:1–8. (Level III)

62. van Winter JT, Simmons PS, Podratz KC. Surgically treated adnexal masses in infancy, childhood, and adolescence. Am J Obstet Gynecol 1994;170:1780–6; discussion 1786–9. (Level III)

63. Jacobs IJ, Skates S, Davies AP, Woolas RP, Jeyerajah A, Weidemann P, et al. Risk of diagnosis of ovarian cancer after raised serum CA 125 concentration: a prospective cohort study. BMJ 1996;313:1355–8. (Level II-2)

64. Moran O, Menczer J, Ben-Baruch G, Lipitz S, Goor E. Cytologic examination of ovarian cyst fluid for the distinction between benign and malignant tumors. Obstet Gynecol 1993;82:444–6. (Level II-3)

65. Higgins RV, Matkins JF, Marroum MC. Comparison of fine-needle aspiration cytologic findings of ovarian cysts with ovarian histologic findings. Am J Obstet Gynecol 1999;180:550–3. (Level II-3)

66. Martinez-Onsurbe P, Ruiz Villaespesa A, Sanz Anquela JM, Valenzuela Ruiz PL. Aspiration cytology of 147 adnexal cysts with histologic correlation. Acta Cytol 2001; 45:941–7. (Level III)

67. Gaetje R, Popp LW. Is differentiation of benign and malignant cystic adnexal masses possible by evaluation of cysts fluids with respect to color, cytology, steroid hormones, and tumor markers? Acta Obstet Gynecol Scand 1994;73:502–7. (Level III)

68. Ganjei P, Dickinson B, Harrison T, Nassiri M, Lu Y. Aspiration cytology of neoplastic and non-neoplastic ovarian cysts: is it accurate? Int J Gynecol Pathol 1996; 15:94–101. (Level II-3)

69. Vercellini P, Oldani S, Felicetta I, Bramante T, Rognoni MT, Crosignani PG. The value of cyst puncture in the differential diagnosis of benign ovarian tumours. Hum Reprod 1995;10:1465–9. (Level II-3)

70. Bonilla-Musoles F, Ballester MJ, Simon C, Serra V, Raga F. Is avoidance of surgery possible in patients with perimenopausal ovarian tumors using transvaginal ultrasound and duplex color Doppler sonography? J Ultrasound Med 1993;12:33–9. (Level II-3)

71. Perrin RG, Bernstein M. Iatrogenic seeding of anaplastic astrocytoma following stereotactic biopsy. J Neurooncol 1998 Feb;36:243–6. (Level III)

72. Kim JE, Kim CY, Kim DG, Jung HW. Implantation metastasis along the stereotactic biopsy tract in anaplastic astrocytoma: a case report. J Neurooncol 2003;61:215–8. (Level III)

73. Mizuno M, Kikkawa F, Shibata K, Kajiyama H, Suzuki T, Ino K, et al. Long-term prognosis of stage I ovarian carcinoma. Prognostic importance of intraoperative rupture. Oncology 2003;65:29–36. (Level III)

74. Sainz de la Cuesta R, Goff BA, Fuller AF Jr, Nikrui N, Eichhorn JH, Rice LW. Prognostic importance of intraoperative rupture of malignant ovarian epithelial neoplasms. Obstet Gynecol 1994;84:1–7. (Level III)

75. Vergote I, De Wever I, Tjalma W, Van Gramberen M, Decloedt J, van Dam P. Neoadjuvant chemotherapy or primary debulking surgery in advanced ovarian carcinoma: a retrospective analysis of 285 patients. Gynecol Oncol 1998;71:431–6. (Level III)

76. Chan YM, Ng TY, Ngan HY, Wong LC. Quality of life in women treated with neoadjuvant chemotherapy for advanced ovarian cancer: a prospective longitudinal study. Gynecol Oncol 2003;88:9–16. (Level II-2)

77. Kinkel K, Lu Y, Mehdizade A, Pelte MF, Hricak H. Indeterminate ovarian mass at US: incremental value of second imaging test for characterization—meta-analysis and Bayesian analysis. Radiology 2005;236:85–94. (Level II-3)

78. Wolfe CD, Tilling K, Raju KS. Management and survival of ovarian cancer patients in south east England. Eur J Cancer. 1997;33:1835–40. (Level II-2)

79. Junor EJ, Hole DJ, McNulty L, Mason M, Young J. Specialist gynaecologists and survival outcome in ovarian cancer: a Scottish national study of 1866 patients. Br J Obstet Gynaecol 1999;106:1130–6. (Level III)

80. McGowan L, Lesher LP, Norris HJ, Barnett M. Misstaging of ovarian cancer. Obstet Gynecol 1985;65:568–72. (Level III)

81. Im SS, Gordon AN, Buttin BM, Leath CA 3rd, Gostout BS, Shah C et al. Validation of referral guidelines for women with pelvic masses. Obstet Gynecol 2005;105:35–41. (Level III)

82. Guidelines for referral to a gynecologic oncologist: rationale and benefits. The Society of Gynecologic Oncologists. Gynecol Oncol 2000;78:S1–13. (Level III)

83. Zanetta G, Rota S, Chiari S, Bonazzi C, Bratina G, Mangioni C. Behavior of borderline tumors with particular interest to persistence, recurrence, and progression to invasive carcinoma: a prospective study. J Clin Oncol 2001;19:2658–64. (Level II-2)

84. Schmeler KM, Mayo-Smith WW, Peipert JF, Weitzen S, Manuel MD, Gordinier ME. Adnexal masses in pregnancy: surgery compared with observation. Obstet Gynecol 2005;105:1098–103. (Level III)

85. Whitecar MP, Turner S, Higby MK. Adnexal masses in pregnancy: a review of 130 cases undergoing surgical management. Am J Obstet Gynecol 1999;181:19–24. (Level III)

86. Bernhard LM, Klebba PK, Gray DL, Mutch DG. Predictors of persistence of adnexal masses in pregnancy. Obstet Gynecol 1999;93:585–9. (Level II-3)

87. Platek DN, Henderson CE, Goldberg GL. The management of a persistent adnexal mass in pregnancy. Am J Obstet Gynecol 1995;173:1236–40. (Level III)

88. Bromley B, Benacerraf B. Adnexal masses during pregnancy: accuracy of sonographic diagnosis and outcome. J Ultrasound Med 1997;16:447–52; quiz 453–4. (Level II-3)

89. Sunoo CS, Terada KY, Kamemoto LE, Hale RW. Adnexal masses in pregnancy: occurrence by ethnic group. Obstet Gynecol 1990;75:38–40. (Level III)

90. Spitzer M, Kaushal N, Benjamin F. Maternal CA-125 levels in pregnancy and the puerperium. J Reprod Med 1998;43:387–92. (Level II-3)

91. Zanetta G, Mariani E, Lissoni A, Ceruti P, Trio D, Strobelt N, et al. A prospective study of the role of ultrasound in the management of adnexal masses in pregnancy. BJOG 2003;110:578–83. (Level II-2)

92. Fauvet R, Boccara J, Dufournet C, Poncelet C, Darai E. Laparoscopic management of borderline ovarian tumors: results of a French multicenter study. Ann Oncol 2005;16:403–10. (Level III)

93. Lecuru F, Desfeux P, Camatte S, Bissery A, Blanc B, Querleu D. Impact of initial surgical access on staging and survival of patients with stage I ovarian cancer. Int J Gynecol Cancer 2006;16:87–94. (Level III)

94. Chi DS, Abu-Rustum NR, Sonoda Y, Ivy J, Rhee E, Moore K, et al. The safety and efficacy of laparoscopic surgical staging of apparent stage I ovarian and fallopian tube cancers. Am J Obstet Gynecol 2005;192:1614–9. (Level II-2)

95. Canis M, Mage G, Pouly JL, Wattiez A, Glowaczower E, Raiga J, et al. Laparoscopic management of suspicious adnexal masses [abstract]. J Am Assoc Gynecol Laparosc 1994;1:S6. (Level II-3)

96. Havrilesky LJ, Peterson BL, Dryden DK, Soper JT, Clarke-Pearson DL, Berchuck A. Predictors of clinical outcomes in the laparoscopic management of adnexal masses. Obstet Gynecol 2003;102:243–51. (Level III)

97. Mendilcioglu I, Zorlu CG, Trak B, Ciftci C, Akinci Z. Laparoscopic management of adnexal masses. Safety and effectiveness. J Reprod Med 2002;47:36–40. (Level II-3)

98. Serur E, Emeney PL, Byrne DW. Laparoscopic management of adnexal masses. JSLS 2001;5:143–51. (Level III)

99. Childers JM, Nasseri A, Surwit EA. Laparoscopic management of suspicious adnexal masses. Am J Obstet Gynecol 1996;175:1451–7; discussion 1457–9. (Level III)

100. Hidlebaugh DA, Vulgaropulos S, Orr RK. Treating adnexal masses. Operative laparoscopy vs. laparotomy. J Reprod Med 1997;42:551–8. (Level III)

101. Parker WH, Levine RL, Howard FM, Sansone B, Berek JS. A multicenter study of laparoscopic management of selected cystic adnexal masses in postmenopausal women. J Am Coll Surg 1994;179:733–7. (Level II-3)

102. Yuen PM, Yu KM, Yip SK, Lau WC, Rogers MS, Chang A. A randomized prospective study of laparoscopy and laparotomy in the management of benign ovarian masses. Am J Obstet Gynecol 1997;177:109–14. (Level I)

103. Fanfani F, Fagotti A, Ercoli A, Bifulco G, Longo R, Mancuso S, et al. A prospective randomized study of laparoscopy and minilaparotomy in the management of benign adnexal masses. Hum Reprod 2004;19:2367–71. (Level I)

104. Deckardt R, Saks M, Graeff H. Comparison of minimally invasive surgery and laparotomy in the treatment of adnexal masses. J Am Assoc Gynecol Laparosc 1994;1: 333–8. (Level I)

105. Comerci JT Jr, Licciardi F, Bergh PA, Gregori C, Breen JL. Mature cystic teratoma: a clinicopathologic evaluation of 517 cases and review of the literature. Obstet Gynecol 1994;84:22–8. (Level III)

106. Parker WH, Broder MS, Liu Z, Shoupe D, Farquhar C, Berek JS. Ovarian conservation at the time of hysterectomy for benign disease. Obstet Gynecol 2005;106: 219–26. (Level II-2)

107. Low JJ, Perrin LC, Crandon AJ, Hacker NF. Conservative surgery to preserve ovarian function in patients with malignant ovarian germ cell tumors. A review of 74 cases. Cancer 2000;89:391–8. (Level III)

108. Perrin LC, Low J, Nicklin JL, Ward BG, Crandon AJ. Fertility and ovarian function after conservative surgery for germ cell tumours of the ovary. Aust N Z J Obstet Gynaecol 1999;39:243–5. (Level III)

109. Kanazawa K, Suzuki T, Sakumoto K. Treatment of malignant ovarian germ cell tumors with preservation of fertility: reproductive performance after persistent remission. Am J Clin Oncol 2000;23:244–8. (Level III)

110. Rao GG, Skinner EN, Gehrig PA, Duska LR, Miller DS, Schorge JO. Fertility-sparing surgery for ovarian low malignant potential tumors. Gynecol Oncol 2005;98: 263–6. (Level III)

111. Donnez J, Munschke A, Berliere M, Pirard C, Jadoul P, Smets M, et al. Safety of conservative management and fertility outcome in women with borderline tumors of the ovary. Fertil Steril 2003;79:1216–21. (Level III)

112. Chan JK, Lin YG, Loizzi V, Ghobriel M, DiSaia PJ, Berman ML. Borderline ovarian tumors in reproductive-age women. Fertility-sparing surgery and outcome. J Reprod Med 2003;48:756–60. (Level III)

113. Boran N, Cil AP, Tulunay G, Ozturkoglu E, Koc S, Bulbul D, et al. Fertility and recurrence results of conservative surgery for borderline ovarian tumors. Gynecol Oncol 2005;97:845–51. (Level III)

114. Schilder JM, Thompson AM, DePriest PD, Ueland FR, Cibull ML, Kryscio RJ, et al. Outcome of reproductive age women with stage IA or IC invasive epithelial ovarian cancer treated with fertility-sparing therapy. Gynecol Oncol 2002;87:1–7. (Level III)

115. Morice P, Leblanc E, Rey A, Baron M, Querleu D, Blanchot J, et al. Conservative treatment in epithelial ovarian cancer: results of a multicentre study of the GCCLCC (Groupe des Chirurgiens de Centre de Lutte Contre le Cancer) and SFOG (Societe Francaise d'Oncologie Gynecologique). GCCLCC and SFOG. Hum Reprod 2005;20:1379–85. (Level III)

116. Canis M, Mashiach R, Wattiez A, Botchorishvili R, Rabischong B, Jardon K, et al. Frozen section in laparoscopic management of macroscopically suspicious ovarian masses. J Am Assoc Gynecol Laparosc 2004;11:365–9. (Level II-3)

The MEDLINE database, the Cochrane Library, and ACOG's own internal resources and documents were used to conduct a literature search to locate relevant articles published between January 1985 and January 2007. The search was restricted to articles published in the English language. Priority was given to articles reporting results of original research, although review articles and commentaries also were consulted. Abstracts of research presented at symposia and scientific conferences were not considered adequate for inclusion in this document. Guidelines published by organizations or institutions such as the National Institutes of Health and the American College of Obstetricians and Gynecologists were reviewed, and additional studies were located by reviewing bibliographies of identified articles. When reliable research was not available, expert opinions from obstetrician–gynecologists were used.

Studies were reviewed and evaluated for quality according to the method outlined by the U.S. Preventive Services Task Force:

I   Evidence obtained from at least one properly designed randomized controlled trial.

II-1   Evidence obtained from well-designed controlled trials without randomization.

II-2   Evidence obtained from well-designed cohort or case–control analytic studies, preferably from more than one center or research group.

II-3   Evidence obtained from multiple time series with or without the intervention. Dramatic results in uncontrolled experiments also could be regarded as this type of evidence.

III   Opinions of respected authorities, based on clinical experience, descriptive studies, or reports of expert committees.

Based on the highest level of evidence found in the data, recommendations are provided and graded according to the following categories:

Level A—Recommendations are based on good and consistent scientific evidence.

Level B—Recommendations are based on limited or inconsistent scientific evidence.

Level C—Recommendations are based primarily on consensus and expert opinion.

ISSN 1099-3630

The American College of Obstetricians and Gynecologists
409 12th Street, SW, PO Box 96920, Washington, DC 20090-6920

Management of adnexal masses. ACOG Practice Bulletin No. 83. American College of Obstetricians and Gynecologists. Obstet Gynecol 2007;110:201–14.

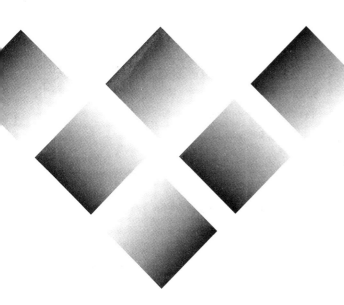

ACOG
PRACTICE
BULLETIN

CLINICAL MANAGEMENT GUIDELINES FOR
OBSTETRICIAN–GYNECOLOGISTS

NUMBER 84, AUGUST 2007

(Replaces Practice Bulletin Number 21, October 2000)

This Practice Bulletin was developed by the ACOG Committee on Practice Bulletins— Gynecology with the assistance of Daniel Clarke-Pearson, MD, and Lisa N. Abaid, MD, MPH. The information is designed to aid practitioners in making decisions about appropriate obstetric and gynecologic care. These guidelines should not be construed as dictating an exclusive course of treatment or procedure. Variations in practice may be warranted based on the needs of the individual patient, resources, and limitations unique to the institution or type of practice.

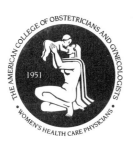

Prevention of Deep Vein Thrombosis and Pulmonary Embolism

Despite advances in prophylaxis, diagnosis, and treatment, venous thromboembolism remains a leading cause of disability and death in postoperative, hospitalized patients (1–3). Venous thromboembolism most commonly occurs in the form of a deep vein thrombosis or pulmonary embolism. Beyond the acute sequelae, venous thromboembolism may result in chronic conditions, including postthrombotic syndrome, venous insufficiency, and pulmonary hypertension. The purpose of this bulletin is to review the current literature on the use of thromboprophylaxis in gynecology patients and to provide evidence-based recommendations to guide clinical decision making.

Background

Magnitude of the Problem and Epidemiology

Deep vein thrombosis (DVT) and pulmonary embolism are collectively referred to as *venous thromboembolic* events. The prevalence of DVT in patients undergoing major gynecologic surgery ranges from 15% to 40% in the absence of thromboprophylaxis (4). The presence of an asymptomatic DVT is highly linked to the development of a clinically significant pulmonary embolism (5). Most patients who die from a pulmonary embolism succumb within 30 minutes of the event, leaving little time for therapeutic interventions. Thus, clinicians should focus on identifying at-risk patients and instituting consistent, effective thromboprophylaxis to reduce the incidence of this frequent, often preventable cause of death.

Deep vein thrombosis is diagnosed in two million Americans each year, and nearly one third of these patients will develop a pulmonary embolism, resulting in 60,000 deaths each year (6). The incidence of a first venous thromboembolism is 1–2 per 1,000 individuals per year (7, 8). Pulmonary embolism is associated with a case-fatality rate of 11–12%, although this rate is lower in young patients and higher in patients with cancer (8, 9). Additionally, patients undergoing bed rest are nearly nine times more likely to develop a venous thromboembolism (10). Hospitalization and surgery also are associated with an increased thrombosis risk, with odds ratios of 11.1 and 5.9, respectively (10).

A recent trial of more than 2,000 patients undergoing surgery for cancer showed a 2% rate of clinical venous thromboembolism formation, despite the use of in-hospital prophylaxis by more than 80% of patients (11). Overall mortality was 1.72% within 35 days of surgery, and despite prophylaxis, 46% of the deaths were attributed to venous thromboembolism. Given these increased odds, it is important to identify high-risk patients because aggressive thromboprophylaxis will decrease the risk of a potentially fatal venous thromboembolism. Risk factors are listed in the box.

Definitions of Low, Medium, High, and Highest Risk

Patients should be classified preoperatively into one of four risk categories—1) low, 2) medium, 3) high, and 4) highest risk—to determine the appropriate thromboprophylaxis regimen. The risk of venous thromboembolism is determined based on procedure type and duration, age, and presence of other risk factors (see box and Table 1). Patients have different risk factors, and some prophylactic regimens are neither appropriate nor effective in certain risk groups. Therefore, proper risk classification is important in order to prescribe the best prophylactic regimen. Recommendations for venous thromboembolism prevention are described in Table 1.

Prophylaxis in Gynecologic Surgery

Rates of venous thromboembolism after gynecologic surgery are similar to those reported in the general surgery literature and average 15–40% in an untreated population (4, 12). Graded compression stockings, intermittent pneumatic compression devices, low-dose unfractionated heparin, and low molecular weight heparin (LMWH) have each been shown to effectively reduce venous thromboembolism development. In two randomized trials and a large retrospective series, the incidence of venous thromboembolism was reported to be 1–6.5% in a gynecologic oncology patient population treated with one of the previously mentioned modalities (13–15). A combined regimen of medical and mechanical prophylaxis may improve efficacy, especially in the patients at highest risk for venous

Venous Thromboembolism Risk Factors
Surgery
Trauma (major or lower extremity)
Immobility, paresis
Malignancy
Cancer therapy (hormonal, chemotherapy, or radiotherapy)
Previous venous thromboembolism
Increasing age
Pregnancy and the postpartum period
Estrogen-containing oral contraception or hormone therapy
Selective estrogen receptor modulators
Acute medical illness
Heart or respiratory failure
Inflammatory bowel disease
Myeloproliferative disorders
Paroxysmal nocturnal hemoglobinuria
Nephrotic syndrome
Obesity
Smoking
Varicose veins
Central venous catheterization
Inherited or acquired thrombophilia

Geerts WH, Pineo GF, Heit JA, Bergqvist D, Lassen MR, Colwell CW, et al. Prevention of venous thromboembolism: the Seventh ACCP Conference on Antithrombotic and Thrombolytic Therapy. Chest 2004;126(suppl):338S–400S.

thromboembolism. Although limited data exist to support this approach in gynecology patients, studies from the general surgery and neurosurgery literature suggest significant benefit from a combined regimen (16, 17). Until more evidence is accumulated, patients undergoing laparoscopic surgery should be stratified by risk category (and provided prophylaxis) similar to patients undergoing laparotomy.

Hypercoagulable States

Numerous environmental, inherited, and acquired risk factors influence coagulability. Most inherited factors do not result in clot formation until the onset of a precipitating event, such as pregnancy, surgery, or exogenous hormone use (18). The most prevalent genetic and acquired thrombophilias are listed in Table 2. Factor V Leiden

Table 1. Risk Classification for Venous Thromboembolism in Patients Undergoing Surgery Without Prophylaxis

Level of Risk	Definition	Successful Prevention Strategies
Low	Surgery lasting less than 30 minutes in patients younger than 40 years with no additional risk factors	No specific prophylaxis; early and "aggressive" mobilization
Moderate	Surgery lasting less than 30 minutes in patients with additional risk factors; surgery lasting less than 30 minutes in patients aged 40–60 years with no additional risk factors; major surgery in patients younger than 40 years with no additional risk factors	Low-dose unfractionated heparin (5,000 units every 12 hours), low molecular weight heparin (2,500 units dalteparin or 40 mg enoxaparin daily), graduated compression stockings, or intermittent pneumatic compression device
High	Surgery lasting less than 30 minutes in patients older than 60 years or with additional risk factors; major surgery in patients older than 40 years or with additional risk factors	Low-dose unfractionated heparin (5,000 units every 8 hours), low molecular weight heparin (5,000 units dalteparin or 40 mg enoxaparin daily), or intermittent pneumatic compression device
Highest	Major surgery in patients older than 60 years plus prior venous thromboembolism, cancer, or molecular hypercoagulable state	Low-dose unfractionated heparin (5,000 units every 8 hours), low molecular weight heparin (5,000 units dalteparin or 40 mg enoxaparin daily), or intermittent pneumatic compression device/graduated compression stockings + low-dose unfractionated heparin or low molecular weight heparin
		Consider continuing prophylaxis for 2–4 weeks after discharge.

Modified from Geerts WH, Pineo GF, Heit JA, Bergqvist D, Lassen MR, Colwell CW, et al. Prevention of venous thromboembolism: the Seventh ACCP Conference on Antithrombotic and Thrombolytic Therapy. Chest 2004;126(suppl):338S–400S.

mutation and prothrombin gene mutation G20210A are the most common mutations found in patients with a venous thromboembolism. The presence of one of these conditions during pregnancy or major surgery confers an increased venous thromboembolism risk and may place a patient into the highest risk category.

Factor V Leiden, identified in 1993 as the major cause of activated protein C resistance, is the most common inherited thrombophilia, and is carried by 5% of Caucasians (19, 20). One half of patients with thrombophilia and 20% of patients with venous thromboembolism carry this mutation. Heterozygotes have a threefold to eightfold increased risk of venous thromboembolism; homozygotes are more severely affected, with a 50- to 80-fold increase in risk (21). Prothrombin G20210A mutation is found almost exclusively in Caucasians and in 6% of patients with venous thromboembolism. This mutation causes an abnormally elevated prothrombin level, which results in a venous thromboembolism rate three times higher than baseline (22). Factor V Leiden mutation and prothrombin mutation may be diagnosed by DNA analysis; factor V Leiden mutation also can be detected in an abnormal activated protein C resistance assay.

Antithrombin-III (AT-III), protein C, and protein S are natural inhibitors of coagulation, and deficiencies of these result in an increased risk of venous thromboembolism. Although these deficiencies are an uncommon cause of thrombosis, they should be considered in patients with a strong family history of clots who test negative for factor V Leiden and prothrombin mutation. Heterozygotes for these three conditions have a 10-fold increased risk of

venous thromboembolism, whereas most homozygotes have severe thrombotic events in early infancy (23). All three disorders are diagnosed using serum assays. However, activity levels are unreliable during acute thrombosis and while receiving anticoagulation.

Elevated homocysteine levels have been correlated with an increase in venous thromboembolism. Hyperhomocysteinemia can result from both genetic and acquired conditions. Homozygous carriers of the methylenetetrahydrofolate reductase variant 677T have mildly elevated homocysteine levels and modest increases in risk of thrombosis and arteriosclerosis (24). Acquired hyperhomocysteinemia is associated with dietary deficiencies in folate, vitamin B_6, and vitamin B_{12} (25). It is currently unclear whether homocysteine is a causative agent or merely a marker, and whether lowering homocysteine levels would similarly decrease venous thromboembolism risk (26).

Antiphospholipid syndrome is another acquired thrombophilia associated with arterial and venous thrombosis, and it is manifested by a wide variety of symptoms. One half of patients with systemic lupus erythematosus (SLE) test positive for antiphospholipid antibodies. Testing includes serum assays for both lupus anticoagulant and anticardiolipin antibodies. Lupus anticoagulant is the more relevant test because it detects β_2-glycoprotein-1 antibodies, which correlate highly with thromboembolic complications and pregnancy morbidity (27). Testing should be considered in patients with venous thromboembolism and other risk factors such as SLE, recurrent pregnancy loss, early or severe preeclampsia, or thrombocytopenia (28).

Table 2. Common Hypercoagulable States

Abnormality	Prevalence in the General Population	Prevalence in Patients With Thrombosis	Testing Methods	Can Patients Be Tested During Pregnancy?	Is the Test Reliable During Acute Thrombosis?	Is the Test Reliable in Patients Using Anticoagulant therapy?
Factor V Leiden						
Heterozygous	5%	20%	Activated protein C resistance assay	No	Yes	Yes
Homozygous	0.02%	—	DNA analysis	Yes	Yes	Yes
Prothrombin gene mutation G20210A	2–3%	6%	DNA analysis	Yes	Yes	Yes
Antiphospholipid antibody	1–2%	5%	Functional assay (eg, dilute Russell viper venom time)	Yes	Yes	Yes
			Anticardiolipin antibodies			
			β_2-Glycoprotein-1 antibodies			
Protein C deficiency	0.2–0.5%	3%	Protein C activity	Yes	No	No
Protein S deficiency	0.03–0.13%	3.2%	Protein S total and free antigen	Yes	No	No
Antithrombin-III deficiency	0.2–0.4%	Less than 1%	Antithrombin-III activity	Yes	No	No
Acquired hyperhomocysteinemia	—	8–25%	Fasting plasma homocystine	Yes	Unclear	Yes
Methylenetetrahydrofolate reductase 677T carriers (homozygous)	10%	25%	DNA analysis	Yes	Yes	Yes

Data from Rosendaal FR. Venous thrombosis: the role of genes, environment, and behavior. Hematology Am Soc Hematol Educ Program 2005;1–12 and Kyrle PA, Eichinger S. Deep vein thrombosis. Lancet 2005;365:1163–74.

Prophylaxis Options

A variety of prophylactic methods will effectively reduce DVT formation. Although DVT in the leg or pelvic veins precedes most fatal pulmonary emboli, most studies have not been sufficiently powered to show a reduction in mortality as a result of thromboprophylaxis. However, it seems reasonable to assume that the prevention of DVT also will result in the reduction of pulmonary embolism.

Prophylactic methods can be divided into mechanical and pharmacologic methods. Mechanical methods reduce venous stasis and may promote endogenous fibrinolysis. Pharmacologic methods prevent clot formation by effects at different points on the clotting cascade. Cost, benefit, risk, and feasibility of each method should be weighed in determining the appropriate prophylaxis for an individual patient.

Graduated Compression Stockings

Most postoperative thrombi develop within 24 hours after surgery, and these predominantly occur in the capacitance veins of the calf. In addition to early postoperative ambulation and elevating the foot of the bed, graduated compression stockings prevent pooling of blood in the calves. A Cochrane review of randomized, controlled trials reported a 50% reduction in DVT formation with graduated compression stockings, and they were more effective when combined with a second prophylactic method (29). Low cost and simplicity are the main advantages of using graduated compression stockings. Correct fit is essential because improperly fitted stockings may act as a tourniquet at the knee or mid-thigh, causing an increase in venous stasis (30). Knee-length stockings are as effective as thigh-length stockings and should be preferentially used (31).

Pneumatic Compression

Intermittent pneumatic compression devices reduce stasis by regularly compressing the calf with an inflatable pneumatic sleeve. When used during and after major gynecologic surgery, the devices are as effective as low-dose heparin and low molecular weight heparin in reducing

DVT incidence (14, 15, 32). Most studies have included a small number of patients and are underpowered to prove efficacy in lowering pulmonary embolism incidence or mortality. The benefits of using intermittent pneumatic compression devices have been postulated to include an increase in systemic fibrinolysis (33, 34). However, data reported from a larger series have failed to confirm this finding (35, 36). The devices should be used continuously until ambulation and discontinued only at the time of hospital discharge (4). In a study of patients with gynecologic malignancies undergoing surgery, the devices were placed intraoperatively and their use was continued for 5 days (37). Their use was associated with a threefold reduction in venous thromboembolism.

Low-Dose Unfractionated Heparin

Low-dose unfractionated heparin is the most extensively studied method of thromboprophylaxis. When administered subcutaneously starting 2 hours before surgery and continued every 8–12 hours postoperatively, numerous controlled trials have shown low-dose unfractionated heparin to be effective in preventing DVT (4). Two large meta-analyses of randomized clinical trials of patients who had undergone general surgery showed a two-thirds reduction in fatal pulmonary embolism with the use of low-dose unfractionated heparin every 8 hours compared with placebo or no prophylaxis (38, 39).

Patients undergoing major gynecologic surgery for benign indications also benefit from low-dose unfractionated heparin given in a preoperative dose and postoperatively at 12-hour intervals (4). This approach was found to be ineffective in patients with gynecologic cancer (40). However, the administration of 5,000 units of heparin beginning 2 hours preoperatively and continued every 8 hours postoperatively does provide effective venous thromboembolism prophylaxis in women with gynecologic malignancies (41).

Advantages of low-dose unfractionated heparin include well-studied efficacy and low cost. With perioperative low-dose unfractionated heparin use, a major concern is increased intraoperative and postoperative bleeding. Although blood loss during surgery does not seem to be increased by the preoperative use of low-dose unfractionated heparin administration, an increase in postoperative bleeding has been noted, specifically in wound hematoma formation (38, 42). Additionally, use for more than 4 days warrants monitoring of platelet counts because 6% of patients will experience heparin-induced thrombocytopenia (42).

Low Molecular Weight Heparin

Advantages of low molecular weight heparin include greater bioavailability and a once-daily dosage. These ben-

efits result from a longer half-life, more predictable pharmacokinetics, and equivalent efficacy when compared with prophylactic use of low-dose unfractionated heparin (43). Low molecular weight heparin has more antifactor Xa and less antithrombin activity than low-dose unfractionated heparin, which may decrease medical bleeding and wound hematoma formation. However, low molecular weight heparin is more expensive than low-dose unfractionated heparin. Heparin-induced thrombocytopenia is rarely observed with low molecular weight heparin, and screening for this is not recommended (44).

Since initial reports in 1985 (45), multiple well designed trials have shown low molecular weight heparin to be a reliable method of thromboprophylaxis. Effective venous thromboembolism prophylaxis also was shown in patients undergoing surgery for gynecologic malignancies. Equivalent risk reductions were seen with the use of preoperative and daily postoperative low molecular weight heparin when compared with intermittent pneumatic compression devices (15). A major prospective trial including 2,373 patients showed a 2% incidence of clinical venous thromboembolism in patients undergoing general, urologic, and gynecologic surgery for cancer who received low molecular weight heparin prophylaxis (11). A retrospective analysis of more than 3,500 patients showed a statistically significant reduction in DVT and fatal pulmonary embolism in patients receiving low molecular weight heparin prophylaxis compared with those who did not, although the investigators did not control for use of mechanical methods (46).

Duration of prophylaxis varies depending on risk factors. Major risk factors for the development of a clinical venous thromboembolism include age older than 60 years, cancer, prior venous thromboembolism, and prolonged surgery or bed rest (11, 13). Of patients with cancer who develop a venous thromboembolism, 40% will do so more than 21 days after surgery (11). A placebo-controlled trial of low molecular weight heparin administered for 1 week versus 4 weeks postoperatively showed a 60% reduction in venous thromboembolism with 4 weeks of treatment and no increase in bleeding or thrombocytopenia (47). Patients at the highest risk for venous thromboembolism may benefit from prolonged low molecular weight heparin prophylaxis.

Dual Prophylaxis

The combined use of two prophylactic methods has been examined in the general surgery literature, specifically in patients undergoing colorectal surgery. A Cochrane review of 19 studies showed that low-dose unfractionated heparin combined with graduated compression stockings was four times more effective in preventing venous thromboembolism than low-dose unfractionated heparin alone (17). A randomized trial of 307 patients undergoing neurosurgical procedures showed a significant reduction in venous thromboembolism with the use of low molecular weight heparin and graduated compression stockings combined over graduated compression stockings alone (16). A decision analysis in high-risk gynecologic oncology patients determined that combined intermittent pneumatic compression devices and low molecular weight heparin use is cost-effective (16).

No randomized trial data exist in the gynecology literature on the benefits of using a combination of mechanical and pharmacologic prophylaxis. However, having two of three identified risk factors that are associated with the ineffectiveness of intermittent pneumatic compression devices (age older than 40 years, cancer, prior venous thromboembolism) places patients in the highest-risk category for the development of venous thromboembolism (13). As a result, the use of a combined approach possesses inherent appeal because it may reduce both hypercoagulability and venous stasis in highest-risk patients undergoing surgery. Although data from randomized trials in gynecology patients are lacking, a combined approach seems appropriate in the highest-risk patients, and this practice is recommended by the Seventh American College of Chest Physicians Consensus Conference (4).

Anesthesia Concerns

Use of regional anesthesia is associated with a 50% decrease in DVT risk compared with general anesthesia (48). However, use of spinal and epidural anesthesia in patients receiving pharmacologic thromboprophylaxis is a cause for concern. The risk of spinal hematoma with low molecular weight heparin use was underscored by a 1997 public health advisory released by the U.S. Food and Drug Administration. It described 41 patients who developed epidural or spinal hematomas, with resultant long-term neurologic injury, after using enoxaparin and undergoing epidural or spinal anesthesia (49). Many of these patients had multiple risk factors, including additional antithrombotic drug use and vascular or anatomic spinal abnormalities. Additional risk factors for the development of a spinal hematoma include an underlying coagulopathy, traumatic or repeated catheter insertion, advanced age, female sex, and catheter removal while receiving prophylactic or therapeutic anticoagulation (4).

Although the previously mentioned risk factors are relatively common, development of a spinal hematoma is a rare event, and limited data exist to guide evidence-based recommendations. The American College of Chest Physicians suggests that spinal and epidural anesthesia be avoided in patients with a bleeding disorder or recent use of antithrombotic drugs, including low-dose unfractionated heparin, low molecular weight heparin, platelet inhibitors such as clopidogrel and ticlopidine, and vitamin K antagonists such as warfarin. Use of nonsteroidal antiinflammatory drugs such as aspirin and ibuprofen has not been linked to spinal hematoma formation. Before using neuraxial anesthesia, platelet inhibitors should be discontinued for 5–14 days, low-dose unfractionated heparin or twice daily low molecular weight heparin for 8–12 hours, and daily low molecular weight heparin for at least 18 hours. Additionally, anticoagulant prophylaxis should be delayed following a hemorrhagic aspirate and for 2 hours after removal of an epidural or spinal catheter. Epidural and spinal catheters should be removed during the nadir of the anticoagulant effect, just before the next scheduled dose of low-dose unfractionated heparin or low molecular weight heparin (4).

Clinical Considerations and Recommendations

▶ *Who are candidates for perioperative venous thromboembolism prophylaxis?*

Candidates for perioperative venous thromboembolism prophylaxis are those who have an increased risk of postoperative venous thromboembolism. A complete history and physical examination will identify risk factors, which may be grouped by level of risk (Table 1).

In addition, prophylaxis should be prescribed for patients who have deficiencies of protein C, protein S, or AT-III, and for heterozygous carriers of the factor V Leiden or prothrombin gene mutation G20210A without a personal history of thrombosis (15, 19, 43, 45).

▶ *Which prophylactic methods should be considered for low-, medium-, high-, and highest-risk patients undergoing surgery?*

The recommended prophylactic options for patients in each of the four risk categories are described in Table 1. Low-risk patients do not require prophylaxis beyond early and aggressive mobilization.

Most patients will require one method of thromboprophylaxis, and intermittent pneumatic compression devices have been shown to be safe, efficacious, and cost-effective in both moderate- and high-risk patients, especially in patients at risk for bleeding complications. Graduated compression stockings are not as extensively studied as intermittent pneumatic compression devices and, if used, should be limited to the knee-high length (31). In patients with multiple risk factors, such as those in the highest-risk category, consideration should be given to combination prophylaxis with or without continued anticoagulant prophylaxis for up to 28 days.

▶ *What is the optimal timing for prophylactic therapy?*

Studies of the natural history of postoperative venous thromboembolism document that nearly 50% of occurrences of venous thromboembolism will begin in the first 24 hours postoperatively and 75% will begin within 72 hours of surgery (50, 51). Because venous thromboembolism begins in the perioperative period, most clinical trials evaluating either mechanical or pharmacologic prophylaxis have initiated the prophylactic method before surgery. Both graduated compression stockings and pneumatic compression devices should be placed before initiation of surgery and continued until the patient is fully ambulatory. Concern is commonly expressed by surgeons that the preoperative administration of low-dose unfractionated heparin or low molecular weight heparin will result in increased intraoperative bleeding. Meta-analysis of many randomized trials shows that there is an increase in intraoperative and postoperative bleeding. However, most complications are minor wound hematomas, and there is no increase in serious, life-threatening bleeding.

Optimal timing of the initial low molecular weight heparin dose currently is unresolved. A prospective, randomized trial including nearly 10,000 patients undergoing elective general surgical, gynecologic, or urologic procedures showed no difference in venous thromboembolism formation or bleeding complications with administration of 20 mg of enoxaparin 2 hours before surgery, compared with administration 12 hours before surgery (52). However, the enoxaparin dose used was lower than the 30–40-mg dose currently used for thromboprophylaxis, and in most studies, low molecular weight heparin was initiated 12 hours before surgery. When initiating low molecular weight heparin postoperatively, no data exist in the gynecology literature to guide clinical decision making. Recent data from patients undergoing orthopedic surgery describe a window of optimal low molecular weight heparin initiation from 6 hours to 12 hours postoperatively. Starting low molecular weight heparin therapy less than 6 hours after surgery is associated with increased bleeding complications, but prolonging the first dose more than 12 hours after surgery may reduce protection from venous thromboembolism (53).

▶ *Should patients discontinue use of hormonal contraceptives or postmenopausal hormone therapy before surgery?*

Hormone therapy and oral contraceptive use have been associated with an increased risk of venous thromboembolism. In the Women's Health Initiative, participants using estrogen plus progestin therapy showed a doubling in risk of venous thrombosis from 1.7 to 3.5 events per 1,000 person-years (hazard ratio 2.1; 95% confidence interval [CI], 1.6–2.7) (54). When using estrogen alone, venous thromboembolism risk remains modestly elevated with a hazard ratio of 1.32 (95% CI, 0.99–1.75) (55). Although venous thromboembolism is associated with estrogen and progesterone use, the overall number of events is low. No trials exist that show a reduction in postsurgical venous thromboembolism with preoperative discontinuation of hormone therapy; thus, this practice should not be routinely recommended.

Prospectively collected data show a small increase in postoperative venous thromboembolism from 0.5% to 0.96% in users of oral contraceptives (56). Despite a large sample size of more than 17,000 women, this did not reach statistical significance. The risk of venous thromboembolism with oral contraceptive use is directly related to estrogen dose, with a decreased risk associated with low-estrogen formulations. A case–control study including more than 5,000 participants showed a 60% increase in venous thromboembolism risk with the use of 50-mcg pills, and a 40% reduction in venous thromboembolism with the use of 20-mcg products, compared with 30–40-mcg formulations (57). However, venous thromboembolism risk remains about four times higher for oral contraceptive users than for nonusers (58).

Prothrombotic clotting factor changes appear to persist for 4–6 weeks after discontinuing oral contraceptive use (59). Accordingly, the risks associated with stopping oral contraception 1 month or more before major surgery should be balanced against the risks of an unintended pregnancy (60). In current users of oral contraceptives having major surgical procedures, heparin prophylaxis should be considered (60). Because of the low perioperative risk of venous thromboembolism, it is currently not considered necessary to discontinue combination oral contraceptives before laparoscopic tubal sterilization or other brief surgical procedures.

▶ *Which patients should be tested for clotting abnormalities, and which tests should be ordered?*

Because of the high prevalence of the factor V Leiden mutation in the Caucasian population, all patients who are not Hispanic, Asian, or African American and have a history of DVT may be tested (61–69). In non-Caucasian patients, the decision to test should be individualized. Patients with histories of extensive or recurrent thrombosis or family histories of thrombosis may have the factor V Leiden mutation in combination with another congenital or acquired disorder (21). Patients with a strong family history of thrombosis who are negative for the factor V

Leiden mutation may benefit from testing for the pro-thrombin gene mutation G20210A and deficiencies in the natural inhibitors, including protein C, protein S, and AT-III. Patients with a history of thrombosis, recurrent fetal loss, early or severe preeclampsia, severe unexplained intrauterine growth restriction, or unexplained thrombocy-topenia may be tested for antiphospholipid antibodies. Fasting plasma homocystine levels may be assessed, especially in women of childbearing age who have had venous or arterial thrombosis, because elevated levels can be treated with vitamins (folic acid, vitamin B_{12}, and vitamin B_6). The specific tests and optimal timing for testing are described in Table 2.

▶ *What special considerations should be given when using low molecular weight heparin in patients undergoing regional anesthesia?*

Low molecular weight heparin has a longer half-life than heparin. Caution should be used in the timing of spinal or epidural anesthesia in patients using low molecular weight heparin to avoid the development of a spinal hematoma. Activity of low molecular weight heparin is measured by an antifactor-Xa level, which may not be widely available. In addition, normalization of the antifactor-Xa level has not been correlated with a reduction in spinal hematoma risk. Given these concerns, patients receiving twice-daily low molecular weight heparin should not receive regional anesthesia for 8–12 hours after the last dose, and for 18 hours after a once-daily low molecular weight heparin dose. Administration of low molecular weight heparin should be held for 2 hours after removal of a spinal or epidural catheter (4).

▶ *Which prophylactic methods are considered cost-effective?*

Two cost-effectiveness analyses have been performed in patients who have undergone gynecologic surgery. All methods were cost-effective, with pneumatic compression being the most cost-effective (70). Another study revealed the potential cost-effectiveness of combined prophylaxis in high-risk gynecologic cancer patients. The authors concluded that the use of intermittent pneumatic compression devices combined with low molecular weight heparin was cost-effective in a high-risk group (71).

▶ *What is the appropriate treatment for patients who are taking other medications (including botanicals) that may alter their risks?*

An estimated 38 million Americans use herbs or complementary medicines each year, with more than 20% of American women reporting some use in the preceding 12 months (72). Some of these medications can interact with commonly prescribed drugs, including anticoagulants, underscoring the importance of taking a complete medication history. A number of common herbs, in addition to nonsteroidal antiinflammatory drugs and antiplatelet medications such as clopidogrel, can potentiate the activity of low molecular weight heparin, unfractionated heparin, and vitamin K antagonists and result in excessive bleeding. A list of herbs and supplements with antiplatelet or anticoagulant activity is found in the box.

Warfarin originally was derived from the sweet clover plant, and related herbs can potentiate its action through direct vitamin K antagonism or by intrinsic antiplatelet activity (73). Conversely, ginseng and hypericum, or St. John's wort, can reduce warfarin concentrations resulting in subtherapeutic levels. Hypericum has been associated with breakthrough bleeding and unin-

---

Herbs and Supplements That May Interfere With Anticoagulant Therapy

Chinese wolfberry

Coenzyme Q_{10}

Cranberry juice

Curbicin

Danshen

Devil's claw

Dong quai

Fenugreek

Garlic

Ginger

Gingko

Ginseng

Glucosamine-chondroitin

Grapefruit juice

Green tea

Melatonin

Omega-3 fish oil

Papaya extract

Quilinggao

St. John's wort

Data from Wittkowsky AK. A systematic review and inventory of supplement effects on warfarin and other anticoagulants. Thromb Res 2005;117:81–6; discussion 113–5 and Basila D, Yuan CS. Effects of dietary supplements on coagulation and platelet function. Thromb Res 2005;117:49–53; discussion 65–7.

tended pregnancy when used with oral contraceptives. These effects likely result from decreased levels of circulating hormones due to cytochrome P-450 upregulation (74, 75). Although many of these effects are derived from case reports and clinical observations, avoidance of drugs known to interact with antithrombotic medication is advised for patients using oral or injected anticoagulants.

Summary of Conclusions and Recommendations

The following recommendations are based on good and consistent scientific evidence (Level A).

▶ Alternatives for thromboprophylaxis for moderate-risk patients include the following:

1. Graduated compression stockings placed before initiation of surgery and continued until the patient is fully ambulatory

2. Pneumatic compression devices placed before the initiation of surgery and continued until the patient is fully ambulatory

3. Unfractionated heparin (5,000 units) administered subcutaneously 2 hours before surgery and every 12 hours after surgery until discharge

4. Low molecular weight heparin (dalteparin 2,500 antifactor-Xa units, or enoxaparin 40 mg) administered subcutaneously, 12 hours before surgery and once a day postoperatively until discharge

▶ Alternatives for prophylaxis for high-risk patients undergoing gynecologic surgery include the following:

1. Pneumatic compression devices placed before surgery and continued until hospital discharge

2. Unfractionated heparin (5,000 units) administered subcutaneously 2 hours before surgery and every 8 hours postoperatively and continued until discharge

3. Low molecular weight heparin (dalteparin 5,000 antifactor-Xa units or enoxaparin 40 mg) administered subcutaneously, 12 hours before surgery and once daily postoperatively until discharge

The following recommendations are based on limited scientific evidence (Level C).

▶ Alternatives for prophylaxis for highest-risk patients include the following:

1. Combination prophylaxis (such as the combination of pneumatic compression and either low-dose unfractionated heparin or low molecular weight heparin)

2. Consideration of continuing low molecular weight heparin prophylaxis as an outpatient for up to 28 days postoperatively

▶ If administration of low molecular weight heparin 12 hours before surgery is impractical, initial dosing should commence 6–12 hours postoperatively.

▶ Low-risk patients who are undergoing gynecologic surgery do not require specific prophylaxis other than early ambulation.

▶ Until more evidence is accumulated, patients undergoing laparoscopic surgery should be stratified by risk category (and provided prophylaxis) similar to patients undergoing laparotomy.

References

1. Hoyert DL, Heron MP, Murphy SL, Kung HC. Deaths: final data for 2003. Natl Vital Stat Rep 2006;54:1–120. (Level II-3)

2. Rubinstein I, Murray D, Hoffstein V. Fatal pulmonary emboli in hospitalized patients. An autopsy study. Arch Intern Med 1988;148:1425–6. (Level III)

3. Kaunitz AM, Hughes JM, Grimes DA, Smith JC, Rochat RW, Kafrissen ME. Causes of maternal mortality in the United States. Obstet Gynecol 1985;65:605–12. (Level II-3)

4. Geerts WH, Pineo GF, Heit JA, Bergqvist D, Lassen MR, Colwell CW, et al. Prevention of venous thromboembolism: the Seventh ACCP Conference on Antithrombotic and Thrombolytic Therapy. Chest 2004;126(suppl): 338S–400S. (Level III)

5. Ibrahim EH, Iregui M, Prentice D, Sherman G, Kollef MH, Shannon W. Deep vein thrombosis during prolonged mechanical ventilation despite prophylaxis. Crit Care Med 2002;30:771–4. (Level II-3)

6. Hirsh J, Hoak J. Management of deep vein thrombosis and pulmonary embolism. A statement for healthcare professionals. Council on Thrombosis (in consultation with the Council on Cardiovascular Radiology), American Heart Association. Circulation 1996;93:2212–45. (Level III)

7. Oger E. Incidence of venous thromboembolism: a community-based study in Western France. EPI-GETBP Study Group. Groupe d'Etude de la Thrombose de Bretagne Occidentale. Thromb Haemost 2000;83:657–60. (Level II-3)

8. Cushman M, Tsai AW, White RH, Heckbert SR, Rosamond WD, Enright P, et al. Deep vein thrombosis and pulmonary embolism in two cohorts: the longitudinal investigation of thromboembolism etiology. Am J Med 2004;117:19–25. (Level I)

9. Anderson FA Jr, Wheeler HB, Goldberg RJ, Hosmer DW, Patwardhan NA, Jovanovic B, et al. A population-based perspective of the hospital incidence and case-fatality

rates of deep vein thrombosis and pulmonary embolism. The Worcester DVT Study. Arch Intern Med 1991;151: 933–8. (Level III)

10. van der Meer FJ, Koster T, Vandenbroucke JP, Briet E, Rosendaal FR. The Leiden Thrombophilia Study (LETS). Thromb Haemost 1997;78:631–5. (Level II-2)

11. Agnelli G, Bolis G, Capussotti L, Scarpa RM, Tonelli F, Bonizzoni E, et al. A clinical outcome-based prospective study on venous thromboembolism after cancer surgery: the @RISTOS project. Ann Surg 2006;243:89–95. (Level II-3)

12. Geerts WH, Heit JA, Clagett GP, Pineo GF, Colwell CW, Anderson FA Jr, et al. Prevention of venous thromboembolism. Chest 2001;119(suppl):132S–75S. (Level III)

13. Clarke-Pearson DL, Dodge RK, Synan I, McClelland RC, Maxwell GL. Venous thromboembolism prophylaxis: patients at high risk to fail intermittent pneumatic compression. Obstet Gynecol 2003;101:157–63. (Level II-2)

14. Clarke-Pearson DL, Synan IS, Dodge R, Soper JT, Berchuck A, Coleman RE. A randomized trial of low-dose heparin and intermittent pneumatic calf compression for the prevention of deep venous thrombosis after gynecologic oncology surgery. Am J Obstet Gynecol 1993;168: 1146–53; discussion 1153–4. (Level I)

15. Maxwell GL, Synan I, Dodge R, Carroll B, Clarke-Pearson DL. Pneumatic compression versus low molecular weight heparin in gynecologic oncology surgery: a randomized trial. Obstet Gynecol 2001;98:989–95. (Level I)

16. Agnelli G, Piovella F, Buoncristiani P, Severi P, Pini M, D'Angelo A, et al. Enoxaparin plus compression stockings compared with compression stockings alone in the prevention of venous thromboembolism after elective neurosurgery. N Engl J Med 1998;339:80–5. (Level I)

17. Wille-Jorgensen P, Rasmussen MS, Andersen BR, Borly L. Heparins and mechanical methods for thromboprophylaxis in colorectal surgery. Cochrane Database of Systematic Reviews 2004, Issue 1. Art. No.: CD001217. DOI: 10.1002/14651858.CD001217. (Level III)

18. Middeldorp S, Henkens CM, Koopman MM, van Pampus EC, Hamulyak K, van der Meer J, et al. The incidence of venous thromboembolism in family members of patients with factor V Leiden mutation and venous thrombosis. Ann Intern Med 1998;128:15–20. (Level II-3)

19. Dahlback B, Carlsson M, Svensson PJ. Familial thrombophilia due to a previously unrecognized mechanism characterized by poor anticoagulant response to activated protein C: prediction of a cofactor to activated protein C. Proc Natl Acad Sci U S A 1993;90:1004–8. (Level III)

20. Rees DC, Cox M, Clegg JB. World distribution of factor V Leiden. Lancet 1995;346:1133–4. (Level II-3)

21. Rosendaal FR, Koster T, Vandenbroucke JP, Reitsma PH. High risk of thrombosis in patients homozygous for factor V Leiden (activated protein C resistance). Blood 1995; 85:1504–8. (Level II-2)

22. Poort SR, Rosendaal FR, Reitsma PH, Bertina RM. A common genetic variation in the 3′-untranslated region of the prothrombin gene is associated with elevated plasma prothrombin levels and an increase in venous thrombosis. Blood 1996;88:3698–703. (Level II-2)

23. Rosendaal FR. Venous thrombosis: the role of genes, environment, and behavior. Hematology Am Soc Hematol Educ Program 2005;1–12. (Level III)

24. Kluijtmans LA, den Heijer M, Reitsma PH, Heil SG, Blom HJ, Rosendaal FR. Thermolabile methylenetetrahydrofolate reductase and factor V Leiden in the risk of deep-vein thrombosis. Thromb Haemost 1998;79:254–8. (Level II-2)

25. Oger E, Lacut K, Le Gal G, Couturaud F, Guenet D, Abalain JH, et al. Hyperhomocysteinemia and low B vitamin levels are independently associated with venous thromboembolism: results from the EDITH study: a hospital-based case-control study. EDITH Collaborative Study Group. J Thromb Haemost 2006;4:793–9. (Level II-2)

26. Lentz SR. Mechanisms of homocysteine-induced atherothrombosis. J Thromb Haemost 2005;3:1646–54. (Level III)

27. de Groot PG, Derksen RH. The antiphospholipid syndrome: clinical characteristics, laboratory features and pathogenesis. Curr Opin Infect Dis 2005;18:205–10. (Level III)

28. Bertolaccini ML, Khamashta MA, Hughes GR. Diagnosis of antiphospholipid syndrome. Nat Clin Pract Rheumatol 2005;1:40–6. (Level III)

29. Amaragiri SV, Lees TA. Elastic compression stockings for prevention of deep vein thrombosis. Cochrane Database of Systematic Reviews 2000, Issue 1. Art. No.: CD001484. DOI: 10.1002/14651858.CD001484. (Level III)

30. Byrne B. Deep vein thrombosis prophylaxis: the effectiveness and implications of using below-knee or thigh-length graduated compression stockings. Heart Lung 2001;30:277–84. (Level III)

31. Agu O, Hamilton G, Baker D. Graduated compression stockings in the prevention of venous thromboembolism. Br J Surg 1999;86:992–1004. (Level III)

32. Ginzburg E, Cohn SM, Lopez J, Jackowski J, Brown M, Hameed SM. Randomized clinical trial of intermittent pneumatic compression and low molecular weight heparin in trauma. Miami Deep Vein Thrombosis Study Group. Br J Surg 2003;90:1338–44. (Level I)

33. Kohro S, Yamakage M, Sato K, Sato JI, Namiki A. Intermittent pneumatic foot compression can activate blood fibrinolysis without changes in blood coagulability and platelet activation. Acta Anaesthesiol Scand 2005; 49:660–4. (Level II-3)

34. Tarnay TJ, Rohr PR, Davidson AG, Stevenson MM, Byars EF, Hopkins GR. Pneumatic calf compression, fibrinolysis, and the prevention of deep venous thrombosis. Surgery 1980;88:489–96. (Level II-1)

35. Killewich LA, Cahan MA, Hanna DJ, Murakami M, Uchida T, Wiley LA, et al. The effect of external pneumatic compression on regional fibrinolysis in a prospective randomized trial. J Vasc Surg 2002;36:953–8. (Level I)

36. Cahan MA, Hanna DJ, Wiley LA, Cox DK, Killewich LA. External pneumatic compression and fibrinolysis in abdominal surgery. J Vasc Surg 2000;32:537–43. (Level I)

37. Clarke-Pearson DL, Synan IS, Hinshaw WM, Coleman RE, Creasman WT. Prevention of postoperative venous thromboembolism by external pneumatic calf compres-

sion in patients with gynecologic malignancy. Obstet Gynecol 1984;63:92–8. (Level I)

38. Clagett GP, Reisch JS. Prevention of venous thromboembolism in general surgical patients. Results of meta-analysis. Ann Surg 1988;208:227–40. (Meta-analysis)

39. Collins R, Scrimgeour A, Yusuf S, Peto R. Reduction in fatal pulmonary embolism and venous thrombosis by perioperative administration of subcutaneous heparin. Overview of results of randomized trials in general, orthopedic, and urologic surgery. N Engl J Med 1988;318:1162–73. (Level III)

40. Clarke-Pearson DL, Coleman RE, Synan IS, Hinshaw W, Creasman WT. Venous thromboembolism prophylaxis in gynecologic oncology: a prospective, controlled trial of low-dose heparin. Am J Obstet Gynecol 1983;145:606–13. (Level I)

41. Clarke-Pearson DL, DeLong E, Synan IS, Soper JT, Creasman WT, Coleman RE. A controlled trial of two low-dose heparin regimens for the prevention of postoperative deep vein thrombosis. Obstet Gynecol 1990;75:684–9. (Level I)

42. Clarke-Pearson DL, DeLong ER, Synan IS, Creasman WT. Complications of low-dose heparin prophylaxis in gynecologic oncology surgery. Obstet Gynecol 1984;64:689–94. (Level II-1)

43. Holzheimer RG. Prophylaxis of thrombosis with low-molecular-weight heparin (LMWH). Eur J Med Res 2004;9:150–70. (Level III)

44. Warkentin TE, Greinacher A. Heparin-induced thrombocytopenia: recognition, treatment, and prevention: the Seventh ACCP Conference on Antithrombotic and Thrombolytic Therapy [published erratum appears in: Chest 2005;127:416]. Chest 2004;126(suppl):311S–37S. (Level III)

45. Kakkar VV, Murray WJ. Efficacy and safety of low-molecular-weight heparin (CY216) in preventing postoperative venous thrombo-embolism: a co-operative study. Br J Surg 1985;72:786–91. (Level I)

46. Cyrkowicz A. Reduction in fatal pulmonary embolism and venous thrombosis by perioperative administration of low molecular weight heparin. Gynecological ward retrospective analysis. Eur J Obstet Gynecol Reprod Biol 2002;100:223–6. (Level II-2)

47. Bergqvist D, Agnelli G, Cohen AT, Eldor A, Nilsson PE, Le Moigne-Amrani A, et al. Duration of prophylaxis against venous thromboembolism with enoxaparin after surgery for cancer. ENOXACAN II Investigators. N Engl J Med 2002;346:975–80. (Level I)

48. Roderick P, Ferris G, Wilson K, Halls H, Jackson D, Collins R, et al. Towards evidence-based guidelines for the prevention of venous thromboembolism: systematic reviews of mechanical methods, oral anticoagulation, dextran and regional anaesthesia as thromboprophylaxis. Health Technol Assess 2005 Dec;9:iii–iv, ix–x, 1–78. (Level III)

49. Food and Drug Administration (US). Subject: Reports of epidural or spinal hematomas with the concurrent use of low molecular weight heparin and spinal/epidural anesthesia or spinal puncture. FDA Public Health Advisory. Rockville (MD): FDA; 1997. Available at: http://www.fda.gov/medwatch/safety/1997/antico.htm. Retrieved April 26, 2007. (Level III)

50. Kakkar VV, Howe CT, Flanc C, Clarke MB. Natural history of postoperative deep-vein thrombosis. Lancet 1969;2:230–2. (Level II-3)

51. Clarke-Pearson DL, Synan IS, Colemen RE, Hinshaw W, Creasman WT. The natural history of postoperative venous thromboemboli in gynecologic oncology: a prospective study of 382 patients. Am J Obstet Gynecol 1984;148:1051–4. (Level II-3)

52. Haas S, Flosbach CW. Prevention of postoperative thromboembolism with Enoxaparin in general surgery: a German multicenter trial. Semin Thromb Hemost 1993;19(suppl 1):164–73. (Level I)

53. Raskob GE, Hirsh J. Controversies in timing of the first dose of anticoagulant prophylaxis against venous thromboembolism after major orthopedic surgery. Chest 2003;124(suppl):379S–85S. (Level III)

54. Cushman M, Kuller LH, Prentice R, Rodabough RJ, Psaty BM, Stafford RS, et al. Estrogen plus progestin and risk of venous thrombosis. Women's Health Initiative Investigators. JAMA 2004;292:1573–80. (Level I)

55. Curb JD, Prentice RL, Bray PF, Langer RD, Van Horn L, Barnabei VM, et al. Venous thrombosis and conjugated equine estrogen in women without a uterus. Arch Intern Med 2006;166:772–80. (Level I)

56. Vessey M, Mant D, Smith A, Yeates D. Oral contraceptives and venous thromboembolism: findings in a large prospective study. Br Med J 1986;292:526. (Level II-2)

57. Lidegaard O, Edstrom B, Kreiner S. Oral contraceptives and venous thromboembolism: a five-year national case-control study. Contraception 2002;65:187–96. (Level II-2)

58. Rosendaal FR, Helmerhorst FM, Vandenbroucke JP. Female hormones and thrombosis. Arterioscler Thromb Vasc Biol 2002;22:201–10. (Level III)

59. Robinson GE, Burren T, Mackie IJ, Bounds W, Walshe K, Faint R, et al. Changes in haemostasis after stopping the combined contraceptive pill: implications for major surgery. BMJ 1991;302:269–71. (Level III)

60. Bonnar J. Can more be done in obstetric and gynecologic practice to reduce morbidity and mortality associated with venous thromboembolism? Am J Obstet Gynecol 1999;180:784–91. (Level III)

61. Florell SR, Rodgers GM. Inherited thrombotic disorders: an update. Am J Hematol 1997;54:53–60. (Level III)

62. Bokarewa MI, Bremme K, Blomback M. Arg506-Gln mutation in factor V and risk of thrombosis during pregnancy. Br J Haematol 1996;92:473–8. (Level II-3)

63. Dahlback B. Resistance to activated protein C as risk factor for thrombosis: molecular mechanisms, laboratory investigation, and clinical management. Semin Hematol 1997;34:217–34. (Level III)

64. Dizon-Townson DS, Nelson LM, Jang H, Varner MW, Ward K. The incidence of the factor V Leiden mutation in an obstetric population and its relationship to deep vein thrombosis. Am J Obstet Gynecol 1997;176:883–6. (Level III)

65. Faioni EM, Razzari C, Martinelli I, Panzeri D, Franchi F, Mannucci PM. Resistance to activated protein C in unse-

lected patients with arterial and venous thrombosis. Am J Hematol 1997;55:59–64. (Level II-2)

66. Hellgren M, Svensson PJ, Dahlback B. Resistance to activated protein C as a basis for venous thromboembolism associated with pregnancy and oral contraceptives. Am J Obstet Gynecol 1995;173:210–3. (Level II-2)

67. Rintelen C, Mannhalter C, Ireland H, Lane DA, Knobl P, Lechner K, et al. Oral contraceptives enhance the risk of clinical manifestation of venous thrombosis at a young age in females homozygous for factor V Leiden. Br J Haematol 1996;93:487–90. (Level III)

68. Vandenbroucke JP, Koster T, Briet E, Reitsma PH, Bertina RM, Rosendaal FR. Increased risk of venous thrombosis in oral-contraceptive users who are carriers of factor V Leiden mutation. Lancet 1994;344:1453–7. (Level II-2)

69. Simioni P, Prandoni P, Lensing AW, Manfrin D, Tormene D, Gavasso S, et al. Risk for subsequent venous thromboembolic complications in carriers of the prothrombin or the factor V gene mutation with a first episode of deep-vein thrombosis. Blood 2000;96:3329–33. (Level II-2)

70. Maxwell GL, Myers ER, Clarke-Pearson DL. Cost-effectiveness of deep venous thrombosis prophylaxis in gynecologic oncology surgery. Obstet Gynecol 2000;95:206–14. (Level III)

71. Dainty L, Maxwell GL, Clarke-Pearson DL, Myers ER. Cost-effectiveness of combination thromboembolism prophylaxis in gynecologic oncology surgery. Gynecol Oncol 2004;93:366–73. (Level III)

72. Kennedy J. Herb and supplement use in the US adult population. Clin Ther 2005;27:1847–58. (Level II-3)

73. Samuels N. Herbal remedies and anticoagulant therapy. Thromb Haemost 2005;93:3–7. (Level III)

74. Schwarz UI, Buschel B, Kirch W. Unwanted pregnancy on self-medication with St John's wort despite hormonal contraception. Br J Clin Pharmacol 2003;55:112–3. (Level III)

75. Hu Z, Yang X, Ho PC, Chan SY, Heng PW, Chan E, et al. Herb-drug interactions: a literature review. Drugs 2005; 65:1239–82. (Level III)

The MEDLINE database, the Cochrane Library, and ACOG's own internal resources and documents were used to conduct a literature search to locate relevant articles published between January 1985 and November 2006. The search was restricted to articles published in the English language. Priority was given to articles reporting results of original research, although review articles and commentaries also were consulted. Abstracts of research presented at symposia and scientific conferences were not considered adequate for inclusion in this document. Guidelines published by organizations or institutions such as the National Institutes of Health and the American College of Obstetricians and Gynecologists were reviewed, and additional studies were located by reviewing bibliographies of identified articles. When reliable research was not available, expert opinions from obstetrician–gynecologists were used.

Studies were reviewed and evaluated for quality according to the method outlined by the U.S. Preventive Services Task Force:

I   Evidence obtained from at least one properly designed randomized controlled trial.

II-1   Evidence obtained from well-designed controlled trials without randomization.

II-2   Evidence obtained from well-designed cohort or case–control analytic studies, preferably from more than one center or research group.

II-3   Evidence obtained from multiple time series with or without the intervention. Dramatic results in uncontrolled experiments also could be regarded as this type of evidence.

III   Opinions of respected authorities, based on clinical experience, descriptive studies, or reports of expert committees.

Based on the highest level of evidence found in the data, recommendations are provided and graded according to the following categories:

Level A—Recommendations are based on good and consistent scientific evidence.

Level B—Recommendations are based on limited or inconsistent scientific evidence.

Level C—Recommendations are based primarily on consensus and expert opinion.

ISSN 1099-3630

The American College of Obstetricians and Gynecologists
409 12th Street, SW, PO Box 96920, Washington, DC 20090-6920

Prevention of deep vein thrombosis and pulmonary embolism. ACOG Practice Bulletin No. 84. American College of Obstetricians and Gynecologists. Obstet Gynecol 2007;110:429–40.

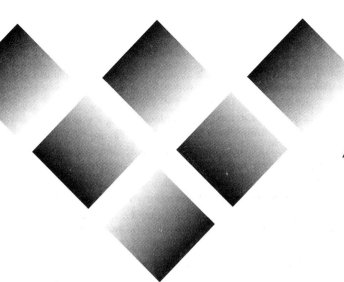

ACOG PRACTICE BULLETIN

CLINICAL MANAGEMENT GUIDELINES FOR
OBSTETRICIAN–GYNECOLOGISTS

NUMBER 85, SEPTEMBER 2007

(Replaces Practice Bulletin Number 79, February 2007)

Pelvic Organ Prolapse

This Practice Bulletin was developed by the ACOG Committee on Practice Bulletins—Gynecology with the assistance of Scott W. Smilen, MD, and Anne M. Weber, MD, MS. The information is designed to aid practitioners in making decisions about appropriate obstetric and gynecologic care. These guidelines should not be construed as dictating an exclusive course of treatment or procedure. Variations in practice may be warranted based on the needs of the individual patient, resources, and limitations unique to the institution or type of practice.

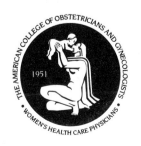

With the advancing age of the U.S. population, obstetrician–gynecologists are likely to encounter women with pelvic organ prolapse with greater frequency. The lifetime risk (to age 80 years) for undergoing surgery for prolapse or urinary incontinence has been estimated at 11% (1). Approximately 200,000 inpatient procedures for prolapse are performed annually in the United States (2). The most common indication for hysterectomy in women aged 55 years and older in the United States is prolapse (3). The purpose of this document is to review current treatment options.

Background

Pelvic organ prolapse occurs with descent of one or more pelvic structures: the uterine cervix or vaginal apex, anterior vagina (usually with bladder, cystocele), posterior vagina (usually with rectum, rectocele), or peritoneum of the cul-de-sac (usually with small intestine, enterocele). However, a specific definition of what constitutes clinically significant prolapse remains elusive. Although almost half of parous women can be identified as having prolapse by physical examination criteria, most are not clinically affected (4); the finding of prolapse on physical examination is not well correlated with specific pelvic symptoms.

Possible risk factors for pelvic organ prolapse include genetic predisposition, parity (particularly vaginal birth [5]), menopause, advancing age, prior pelvic surgery, connective tissue disorders, and factors associated with elevated intraabdominal pressure (eg, obesity, chronic constipation with excessive straining) (6, 7). Whether hysterectomy for conditions other than prolapse is a risk factor for subsequent prolapse is still controversial. Until recently, advocates of supracervical (or subtotal) hysterectomy claimed that preservation of the cervix (and, more important, the upper vagina and its pelvic attachments through the cardinal–uterosacral ligament complex) would prevent the development of subsequent prolapse. However, evidence from randomized trials comparing supracervical hysterectomy with total hysterectomy has shown no difference in vaginal support with short-term follow-up after hysterectomy, regardless of cervical preservation or removal (8, 9).

Evaluation

Each woman's condition should be thoroughly evaluated to ascertain the nature and severity of her symptoms along with the extent of prolapse. Many patients with prolapse are asymptomatic and seek only reassurance or a better understanding of their condition. Women with asymptomatic or mildly symptomatic prolapse can be counseled that treatment is appropriate only when symptoms warrant it. It cannot be assumed that nonspecific symptoms, such as pelvic pressure or back pain, will be alleviated with prolapse treatment. The most specific symptom of prolapse is when the woman can see or feel a bulge of tissue that protrudes to or past the vaginal opening. Because prolapse is a dynamic condition responsive to the effects of gravity when women are in an erect position, some women may experience little or no bulging early in the day with progressively more protrusion as the day goes on, especially after long periods of physical exertion, such as lifting or standing.

Patients with prolapse, perhaps particularly anterior vaginal prolapse, may experience difficulty voiding or incomplete bladder emptying; however, symptoms of urinary urgency or frequency or urge incontinence are not related to prolapse severity. Women with advanced prolapse may recall symptoms of stress incontinence in the past that gradually improved and even resolved as the prolapse became worse. Some women with severe prolapse discover they can void more completely when the prolapse is reduced. Similarly, some women with posterior vaginal prolapse use manual pressure applied to the perineum or posterior vagina to assist defecation. Because many women will not volunteer such information, it is critically important that clinicians ask specific questions to assess voiding and defecating.

The maximum degree of descent may be observed on physical examination with the patient supine in heel stirrups, performing a Valsalva maneuver. If the patient suggests that her prolapse is not being seen at its worst extent, she can be asked to strain while in the standing position. Efficiency of bladder emptying should be evaluated by measuring the patient's voided volume when she has a comfortably full bladder, followed by assessment of postvoid residual urine volume by catheterization or bladder ultrasonography. Valsalva and cough stress testing can be performed with the prolapse reduced to determine if a subjectively stress-continent patient has occult (or potential) stress incontinence; however, cur-

rently, there is no consensus on how to best reduce prolapse for stress testing nor on how to use information from stress testing with and without prolapse reduction in making recommendations for care.

Several systems have been developed to classify pelvic organ prolapse. The Baden–Walker system (or some modification) is in widespread clinical use (see box, "Baden–Walker System for the Evaluation of Pelvic Organ Prolapse on Physical Examination"); the Pelvic Organ Prolapse Quantification (POP-Q) system (10) was introduced for use in clinical practice and research. Some have argued that the nine points of the POP-Q system may be more detailed than necessary for clinical practice, and the full POP-Q system may be better suited for clinical research purposes. The Baden–Walker system is probably adequate for clinical practice as long as descent or protrusion affecting all pelvic compartments (anterior, apical, and posterior) is assessed. It often is useful to include an estimation or measurement of the extent of protrusion relative to the hymen, as in the POP-Q system, to better assess change over time (see box, "Stages of Pelvic Organ Prolapse").

Clinical Considerations and Recommendations

▶ *Are effective nonsurgical treatments available for women with pelvic organ prolapse?*

The option of nonsurgical management should be discussed with all women with prolapse. Although pessary use is the only specific nonsurgical treatment, pelvic floor muscle rehabilitation and symptom-directed therapy may be offered, despite the lack of data supporting their use to prevent prolapse progression (11, 12).

Baden–Walker System for the Evaluation of Pelvic Organ Prolapse on Physical Examination

Grade posterior urethral descent, lowest part other sites

Grade 0: Normal position for each respective site

Grade 1: Descent halfway to the hymen

Grade 2: Descent to the hymen

Grade 3: Descent halfway past the hymen

Grade 4: Maximum possible descent for each site

Baden WF, Walker T. Fundamentals, symptoms and classification. In: Baden WF, Walker T, editors. Surgical repair of vaginal defects. Philadelphia (PA): J.B. Lippincott; 1992. p. 14.

Symptom-directed therapy with observation of prolapse (watchful waiting) can be recommended for women with low-stage prolapse (ie, stage I and stage II, especially when descent is still above the hymen) and nonspecific symptoms. The POP-Q stages of pelvic organ prolapse are shown in the box. Women with prolapse who are asymptomatic or mildly symptomatic can be observed at regular intervals, which can be conveniently combined with annual well-woman care unless new bothersome symptoms develop between visits. Although estrogen receptors are plentiful throughout the pelvis, their role in pelvic support is not fully understood, and there is no evidence currently to support the pharmacologic use of estrogen to prevent or treat prolapse.

Stages of Pelvic Organ Prolapse

Stages are based on the maximal extent of prolapse relative to the hymen, in one or more compartments.

Stage 0: No prolapse; anterior and posterior points are all −3 cm, and C (cervix) or D (posterior fornix) is between −TVL (total vaginal length) and −(TVL − 2) cm.

Stage I: The criteria for stage 0 are not met, and the most distal prolapse is more than 1 cm above the level of the hymen (less than −1 cm).

Stage II: The most distal prolapse is between 1 cm above and 1 cm below the hymen (at least one point is −1, 0, or +1).

Stage III: The most distal prolapse is more than 1 cm below the hymen but no further than 2 cm less than TVL.

Stage IV: Represents complete procidentia or vault eversion; the most distal prolapse protrudes to at least (TVL − 2) cm.

Pelvic Organ Prolapse Quantification System

Six vaginal sites used in staging prolapse:

Points Aa and Ba anteriorly

Points Ap and Bp posteriorly

Point C for the cervix or vaginal apex

Point D for the posterior fornix (not measured after hysterectomy)

Three additional measurements:

GH – genital hiatus

PB – perineal body

TVL – total vaginal length

Bump RC, Mattiasson A, Bo K, Brubaker LP, DeLancey JO, Klarskov P, et al. The standardization of terminology of female pelvic organ prolapse and pelvic floor dysfunction. Am J Obstet Gynecol 1996; 175:10–7.

Pessaries

Traditional indications for pessary treatment include pregnancy and specific medical contraindications to surgery in elderly and debilitated patients; however, pessaries also can be used in all circumstances when women prefer a nonsurgical alternative. Pessaries can be fitted in most women with prolapse, regardless of prolapse stage or site of predominant prolapse, and are used by 75% of urogynecologists as first-line therapy for prolapse (13). Pessary devices are available in various shapes and sizes, and can be categorized as supportive (such as a ring pessary) or space-occupying (such as a donut pessary). Pessaries commonly used for prolapse include ring pessaries (with and without support) and Gellhorn, donut, and cube pessaries.

In most patients (range, 50–73%), an appropriately sized pessary can be fitted successfully in one or two office visits; however, a lower percentage (range, 41–67%) maintain pessary use after fitting (14–19). Although some clinicians use pessaries less frequently for advanced prolapse, recent studies have not found an association between prolapse stage and the outcome of a pessary trial (16, 19). Other factors related to successful pessary fitting or continued pessary use are not consistent across studies (Tables 1 and 2). However, the type of pessary that can be fitted is probably related to the severity of prolapse. In one study protocol, ring pessaries were inserted first, followed by Gellhorn pessaries if the rings did not stay in place. Ring pessaries were used more successfully with stage II (100%) and stage III (71%) prolapse, and stage IV prolapse more frequently required Gellhorn pessaries (64%) (16). For women who can be fitted and whose pelvic organ support can be maintained with a pessary, treatment has a high likelihood of benefit. In one study, 2 months after successful fitting, 92% of patients were satisfied with pessary management, nearly all prolapse symptoms had resolved, and 50% of urinary problems were reduced (17). Neither stage of prolapse (19) nor sexual activity (18) contraindicates pessary use. Clinicians should discuss the option of pessary use with all women who have prolapse that warrants treatment based on symptoms. In particular, pessary use should be considered before surgical intervention in women with symptomatic prolapse.

Symptom-Directed Therapy

Therapy may include weight loss and exercise, in addition to therapy targeted at specific symptoms. Although weight loss and exercises (either aerobic exercise or pelvic floor muscle exercises) have not been proved beneficial specifically for prolapse treatment or prevention, such recommendations are appropriate as general health

Table 1. Factors Affecting Pessary Fitting for Pelvic Organ Prolapse

Author Percent of Study Population With Successful Pessary Fit	Factors Associated With Successful Pessary Fitting	Factors Not Associated With Successful Pessary Fitting
Clemons et al, 2004*: 73 of 100 women (73%)	Longer vaginal length (more than 7 cm) Narrower vaginal introitus (less than four finger-breadths)	Age Parity Estrogen use Sexually active Previous hysterectomy Previous prolapse surgery Pelvic organ prolapse stage Predominant prolapse compartment Genital hiatus size
Mutone et al, 2005†: 288 of 407 women (71%)	(not stated)	(not stated)

*Clemons JL, Aguilar VC, Tillinghast TA, Jackson ND, Myers DL. Risk factors associated with an unsuccessful pessary fitting trial in women with pelvic organ prolapse. Am J Obstet Gynecol 2004;190:345–50.

†Mutone MF, Terry C, Hale D, Benson JT. Factors which influence the short-term success of pessary management of pelvic organ prolapse. Am J Obstet Gynecol 2005:193:89–94.

Table 2. Factors Affecting Continued Pessary Use for Pelvic Organ Prolapse

Author Percent of Study Population With Continued Pessary Use	Factors Associated With Continued Pessary Use	Factors Not Associated With Continued Pessary Use
Brincat et al, 2004*: 82 of 136 women (60%)	Sexually active (vs not sexually active) Pessary use for prolapse (vs for stress incontinence)	Age Parity Menopausal status Surgical history
Mutone et al, 2005†: 168 of 407 women (41%)	No previous hysterectomy No previous surgery for prolapse Normal weight (vs obesity)	Age Levator ani strength Pelvic organ prolapse stage Predominant prolapse compartment Genital hiatus size Perineal body length Total vaginal length

*Brincat C, Kenton K, Fitzgerald MP, Brubaker L. Sexual activity predicts continued pessary use. Am J Obstet Gynecol 2004;191:198–200.

†Mutone MF, Terry C, Hale D, Benson JT. Factors which influence the short-term success of pessary management of pelvic organ prolapse. Am J Obstet Gynecol 2005:193:89–94.

guidelines. In addition, symptoms related to altered voiding or defecatory habits should be addressed. For example, patients with defecatory problems, such as incomplete emptying and straining, often benefit from behavior training (such as establishing a scheduled time to facilitate regular bowel habits), dietary modification (such as increased dietary fiber or fiber supplements as needed), and splinting or laxative or enema use to permit evacuation without straining. Women with urinary incontinence as their primary symptom can be treated with behavior modification (timed voiding), fluid intake alterations,

pelvic muscle training and exercise (see the following section), and medication as first steps.

Pelvic Floor Muscle Rehabilitation

Pelvic muscle training (Kegel exercises) is a simple, noninvasive intervention that may improve pelvic function. Whether Kegel exercises can resolve prolapse has not been studied since Kegel's original articles (20). Nevertheless, the benefit of pelvic floor muscle training has been clearly demonstrated for women with urinary or fecal symptoms, especially incontinence. It is commonly recommended as adjunct therapy for women with prolapse and associated symptoms, often with symptom-directed therapy.

▶ *What are effective surgical treatments for uterine or vaginal vault prolapse?*

Hysterectomy is often the traditional surgical approach for women with uterine or uterovaginal prolapse. However, because the uterus plays only a passive role in prolapse, hysterectomy alone or hysterectomy with anterior or posterior colporrhaphy does not address the underlying problem of deficient apical support. When hysterectomy is performed for uterine prolapse, attention must be directed toward restoration of apical support once the uterus is removed. Surgical options for patients with apical prolapse (when hysterectomy has been performed remotely or as part of the current procedure) include abdominal sacral colpopexy and transvaginal suspension procedures using pelvic structures for fixation, such as the sacrospinous ligament(s), uterosacral ligaments, and iliococcygeus fascia or muscle.

Multiple case series on vaginal and abdominal approaches to apical prolapse have been summarized in extensive reviews (21, 22). These predominantly retrospective studies demonstrate a wide range of effectiveness for surgical treatment of prolapse at the vaginal apex, with failure rates ranging from 0% to 20% for each type of procedure (sacrospinous ligament fixation, uterosacral ligament suspension, endopelvic fascial suspension by vaginal approach, or abdominal sacral colpopexy by open or laparoscopic approach). Whether abdominal sacral colpopexy offers advantages in outcomes over vaginal approaches to prolapse repair is controversial.

A 2005 Cochrane review (6) of surgical management of prolapse concluded that, based on a synthesis of three randomized trials (23–25), compared with vaginal sacrospinous ligament fixation, abdominal sacral colpopexy has less apical failure and less postoperative dyspareunia and stress incontinence, but is also associated with more complications. The reported recurrence for vault prolapse was 3 in 84 abdominal sacral colpopexies versus 13 in 85 vaginal surgeries (relative risk [RR], 0.23; 95% confidence interval [CI], 0.07–0.77). However, operating time and patient recovery was longer with abdominal sacral colpopexy compared with vaginal sacrospinous ligament fixation. Short-term and long-term complications, particularly related to intraabdominal adhesions and small-bowel obstruction, may be more frequent after abdominal sacral colpopexy compared with vaginal prolapse repair. Therefore, clinicians should carefully consider each patient's risk for complications and potential for recurrent prolapse, along with the patient's preferences, when making recommendations for abdominal sacral colpopexy or vaginal sacrospinous ligament fixation.

Whether results are superior with uterosacral versus sacrospinous ligament suspension is unknown; the two procedures have never been compared in a controlled or randomized trial. From case series of sacrospinous and uterosacral ligament vaginal suspensions, risks common to surgery in general are similar probably because the two procedures share the vaginal approach. However, some risks are specific to each procedure. Ureteral injury rates as high as 11% have been reported with uterosacral ligament suspension (26). Cystoscopy should be performed intraoperatively to assess for bladder or ureteral damage after all prolapse or incontinence procedures during which the bladder or ureters may be at risk of injury. If promptly identified and treated, such injury usually requires only suture release and replacement to avoid serious morbidity. However, ureteral injury occasionally requires reimplantation, particularly if recognition of the injury is delayed. Hemorrhage from pudendal vessels injured in sacrospinous ligament suspension is rare but can be life-threatening and is technically challenging to address. Buttock pain after sacrospinous suspension occurs infrequently and usually is self-limited but may require reoperation for suture removal to resolve persistent pain.

Outcomes of laparoscopic sacral colpopexy have been reported in case series (27–29) and one comparative cohort study (30). Recurrent apical prolapse occurred in only 4–7%, but anterior or posterior vaginal prolapse recurred in up to 32%. Without randomized trials, it is not possible to draw conclusions of similar efficacy compared with abdominal sacral colpopexy, but it does seem that for surgeons with advanced laparoscopic skills, sacral colpopexy can be accomplished, thereby avoiding laparotomy. However, even in the hands of experienced laparoscopists, a protracted learning curve is described for laparoscopic sacral colpopexy (28), and average operative times are almost an hour longer than for open sacral colpopexy (30), although postoperative recovery may be shorter.

Reviews of several case series of uterosacral ligament suspension describe recurrent prolapse in 4–18% of patients after relatively short follow-up (up to 4 years), although conclusions are limited by the inherent weaknesses of uncontrolled studies (26, 31–35). In one study of 168 women, 11 (6.5%) had recurrent prolapse at follow-up from 6 months to 3 years (34). In 72 of those women monitored for a mean of 5.1 years (range, 3.5–7.5 years), 11 (15.3%) experienced symptomatic recurrent prolapse of stage II or greater, although only two women (3%) had apical prolapse (36). Alternative sites for apical support, such as sacrospinous ligament(s) or iliococcygeus fascia, can be used when the uterosacral ligaments are not easily accessible or are attenuated and unable to provide adequate support. Use of the iliococcygeus fascia during vaginal surgery has been reported in case series (37, 38).

▶ *What management options are recommended for women who are poor surgical candidates and who present with complete eversion of the vagina, with or without a uterus?*

In some cases, including women who are at such high risk of surgical or anesthetic complications that surgery is contraindicated, nonsurgical treatment will be first-line therapy. Expectant management, nonsurgical therapy, and surgery have not been directly compared for any patient population, including older or medically compromised women with advanced prolapse. In general, perioperative risk is increased in patients with concomitant medical problems. However, if surgery becomes necessary, limited data support its relative safety; morbidity occurs frequently but mortality is rare.

In 267 women aged 75 years or older, after primarily vaginal urogynecologic surgery, 26% had perioperative complications, most commonly blood loss, pulmonary edema, and congestive heart failure (39). In a study reviewing an administrative database of inpatient urogynecologic procedures in 264,340 women (40), mortality was increased in a nonlinear pattern with each decade of life: 1 in 10,000 for women younger than 60 years; 5 in 10,000 for women aged 60–69 years; 9 in 10,000 for those aged 70–79 years; and 28 per 10,000 for women aged 80 years and older. Complications were more frequent in women aged 80 years and older and in women who had reconstructive rather than obliterative surgery.

Colpocleisis (or colpectomy) can be offered to women who are at high risk for complications with reconstructive procedures and who do not desire vaginal intercourse. In a recent review, colpocleisis was reported as successful for prolapse repair in close to 100% of patients in modern retrospective series (41). However, the rate of reoperation for stress incontinence or recurrent prolapse after colpocleisis is unknown. Although complications are relatively common in this group of predominantly older patients, serious morbidity or mortality is uncommon. Concomitant hysterectomy is associated with increased blood loss, blood transfusion, and length of hospital stay, without known benefit. Few studies systematically assess pelvic symptoms, either before or after surgery. The Manchester procedure (amputation of the cervix combined with anterior and posterior colporrha-

phy) has been considered another option for older, frail women with prolapse, but it has been little used since the mid-1970s.

▶ *Are effective surgical treatments available for a woman with pelvic organ prolapse who prefers to avoid hysterectomy?*

For women who choose surgical management and who prefer uterine conservation (which may or may not include interest in further childbearing), the same procedures performed for vaginal suspension (after either remote or concomitant hysterectomy) can be performed without hysterectomy: uterosacral or sacrospinous ligament fixation by the vaginal approach, or sacral hysteropexy by the abdominal approach. Limited data on pregnancy outcomes (42, 43) and even fewer data on prolapse outcomes are available. Ideally, childbearing should be complete before considering surgery for prolapse to avoid the theoretical but plausible risk of recurrent prolapse after subsequent pregnancy and delivery. For women who become pregnant after prolapse repair, decisions regarding mode of delivery should be made on a case-by-case basis; evidence to guide such decisions is lacking.

Hysteropexy

In retrospective series review, prolapse recurrence ranges from 6.6% to 23.5% after sacral hysteropexy or sacral colpopexy (abdominal attachment of the lower uterus or upper vagina to the sacral promontory with synthetic mesh) (44, 45), and up to 30% for sacrospinous hysteropexy (43, 46). Complications include hemorrhage, hematoma, wound infection, small-bowel obstruction, incisional hernia, and mesh erosion. The laparoscopic approach has been used for hysteropexy, but data are limited (47, 48). Hysteropexy should not be performed by using the ventral abdominal wall for support because of the high risk for recurrent prolapse, particularly enterocele.

Round Ligament Suspension

Round ligament suspension is not effective in treating uterine or vaginal prolapse. A retrospective case series review on laparoscopic suspension to the round ligament found that 90% of patients had already experienced recurrent prolapse by 3 months postoperatively (49).

Colpocleisis

Some patients do not desire vaginal function for sexual activity or future childbearing and prefer to avoid hysterectomy. For these women, colpocleisis is an option.

▶ *Are effective surgical treatments available for a woman with anterior or posterior vaginal prolapse or both (ie, cystocele or rectocele or both)?*

Anterior vaginal prolapse (cystocele) may be repaired with traditional midline anterior colporrhaphy, with or without the addition of mesh or graft material, or by paravaginal repair, which can be accomplished vaginally or retropubically by open or laparoscopic access. No data are available on the effectiveness of laparoscopic paravaginal repair primarily for prolapse. Retrospective case series review regarding open retropubic and vaginal paravaginal repairs (in combination with other procedures for prolapse and often stress incontinence) show recurrent prolapse in 15–37% with relatively short follow-up up to 3 years (50–53). Controlled studies comparing open retropubic repair with vaginal paravaginal repair or studies comparing paravaginal repair by any approach with anterior colporrhaphy are lacking.

Posterior vaginal prolapse (rectocele) has traditionally been treated surgically by posterior colporrhaphy, with midline plication of the subepithelial vaginal tissue. Although in the past plication of the medial portion of the levator ani often was performed as an adjunct to posterior repair, its use has been largely abandoned because of postoperative dyspareunia except when postoperative sexual activity is not anticipated. Site-specific repair also can be accomplished, in which a specific "defect" in the vaginal muscularis or adventitia is visualized and repaired. Abdominal and laparoscopic approaches also have been suggested, usually in conjunction with sacral colpopexy, where mesh is placed along the posterior vagina, sometimes all the way to the perineal body (sacral colpoperineopexy).

No randomized trials compare posterior colporrhaphy with site-specific defect repairs; in one uncontrolled comparison (54), after site-specific repairs, prolapse recurred more frequently (33%) than after traditional midline plication (14%) within 1 year of follow-up. Dyspareunia remains a frequent and difficult postoperative problem, even when introital narrowing is avoided (55).

Colorectal surgeons have advocated the transanal approach to rectocele repair, with plication of redundant rectal mucosa and anterior rectal muscle. However, in a trial comparing transanal and transvaginal approaches (6, 56), transvaginal repair was more effective for subjective symptom relief and objective recurrence of posterior vaginal prolapse (rectocele and enterocele). The vaginal approach was associated with a smaller mean rectocele depth determined by defecography, and postoperative enterocele was less common, compared with the transanal approach (6). Therefore, transvaginal posterior colporrhaphy is recommended over transanal repair for posterior vaginal prolapse.

▶ *What can be recommended regarding currently available graft materials for use in prolapse surgery?*

Biologic and synthetic graft materials have been used to augment traditional prolapse repairs, such as anterior and posterior colporrhaphy, as a substitute or reinforcement for the original vaginal tissue. For apical prolapse, new techniques use materials mounted on trocars to bypass native supportive structures (eg, uterosacral–cardinal ligament complex) in order to provide vaginal support. Despite the lack of risk–benefit information, many new techniques and products are being incorporated rapidly into clinical practice, even while continuous modifications are taking place in an attempt to reduce complications, particularly those related to mesh erosion, contraction (resulting in vaginal shortening and narrowing), and fistula. Given the pace of change with new techniques and products, any publication attempting to provide a comprehensive list will be outdated even before publication. Clinicians should follow the emerging literature closely to remain knowledgeable about which techniques and products should be avoided and which are ultimately proved to be of benefit to patients. The topic of graft materials is well covered in a review by Silva and Karram (57).

Although synthetic mesh used in early reports of abdominal sacral colpopexy was associated with good prolapse outcomes, mesh erosion occurred in some cases. Most cases of mesh erosion can be managed successfully with limited vaginal excision, incurring minimal morbidity; however, in rare cases, the entire mesh must be removed via laparotomy, often in the setting of refractory peritoneal infection, severe adhesions, and high likelihood of bowel complications. In an effort to reduce the risk of mesh erosion, some surgeons switched from synthetic mesh to allograft (cadaveric) fascia for abdominal sacral colpopexy. However, high rates of prolapse recurrence after abdominal sacral colpopexy using cadaveric fascia were initially reported in case series review (58–60), followed by randomized trial evidence (61). The use of cadaveric fascia for abdominal sacral colpopexy should be abandoned.

When choosing the best material for specific procedures, it is critically important that surgeons understand how certain characteristics of materials play a key role in the risk–benefit ratio for various types of surgery. Pore size in surgical mesh is one of the most important factors in determining risk of postoperative infection. In addition, chemical coatings of materials can markedly influence the risk of complications. For example, silicone-coated synthetic mesh was used in sacral colpopexy with an unacceptably high rate of erosion, 24% (62), even after high erosion rates were reported in slings of similar material (63). It should be noted that some synthetic materials when used in abdominal surgery, such as abdominal sacral colpopexy, have a low rate of complications such as erosion, compared with their use in vaginal surgery, where the complication rate may be higher.

Following the success of the new generation of midurethral slings (in which synthetic material, mounted on trocars, was put in place through tiny incisions with minimal dissection), several new products have been introduced to augment or replace traditional prolapse procedures. Analogous to abdominal sacral colpopexy in which synthetic material is used to bypass native supports, products designed for use in treating apical prolapse are intended to replace deficient apical support with synthetic or biologic material.

In 2001, investigators reported 75 cases of infracoccygeal sacropexy (also known as posterior intravaginal slingplasty), a technique that initially used nylon mesh inserted via the ischiorectal fossa into the posterior vaginal fornices, to treat vaginal vault prolapse (64). Despite encouraging initial results reported by the inventor, subsequent case series review has shown high rates of recurrent prolapse (65) and mesh complications (66) even after the material was changed to polypropylene.

Other devices for the placement of mesh to provide apical support have been developed and are currently being marketed in the United States. Long-term data are insufficient to make recommendations concerning these products.

Other products have been introduced for use with repair of anterior and posterior vaginal prolapse. Biologic graft material (xenograft or allograft) or synthetic material (absorbable or permanent) can be used in place of or in addition to traditional colporrhaphy (67). However, as with apical support materials, data are insufficient to determine risks or benefits. In one study of 312 patients undergoing vaginal surgery for prolapse repair, 98 (31.4%) with graft use did not have better prolapse outcomes than those without graft use, but complications (such as vaginal or graft infection) occurred much more frequently (68). A high rate of early failures has been reported after vaginal prolapse repair with porcine xenograft (69, 70). Although several studies have evaluated anterior colporrhaphy with and without mesh or graft materials of different types (71–79),

because of heterogeneity of material studied, small sample sizes, and short-term follow-up, it is not possible to draw definitive conclusions about the risk versus the benefit of absorbable or permanent synthetic materials in anterior colporrhaphy.

Given the limited data and frequent changes in the marketed products for vaginal surgery for prolapse repair (particularly with regard to type of mesh material itself, which is associated with several of the postoperative risks, especially mesh erosion), patients should consent to surgery with an understanding of the postoperative risks and complications and lack of long-term outcomes data.

▶ *Can the occurrence of stress urinary incontinence after surgery for pelvic organ prolapse be anticipated and avoided?*

Many women with advanced prolapse, particularly prolapse involving the anterior vagina, will not have symptoms of stress urinary incontinence, either because the urethral sphincteric mechanism is in fact competent or because the advanced prolapse kinks the urethra, causing obstruction. Some of these stress-continent women will become stress incontinent after prolapse surgery. Subjectively stress-continent women with positive reduction stress test results (prolapse reduced) more frequently have stress urinary incontinence after prolapse repair if no antiincontinence procedure is performed; in small case series review, this ranges widely, from 8% to 60%. Until recently, clinicians were faced with a dilemma in trying to balance potential risks of an antiincontinence procedure without strong evidence of benefit. However, randomized trial evidence is now available to guide management decisions for apparently stress-continent women with prolapse.

In two randomized trials of women undergoing prolapse repair, postoperative stress incontinence was reduced significantly by the inclusion of an antiincontinence procedure. Improvement in stress incontinence was obtained without a concomitant worsening of voiding symptoms or impaired bladder emptying. In one trial of 50 women with a positive stress test result with prolapse reduction, tension-free vaginal tape (TVT) or suburethral plication was added to vaginal prolapse repair (80). With median follow-up of approximately 2 years, the TVT group had less stress incontinence, both subjectively (96% versus 64%) and objectively (92% versus 56%). For women with positive prolapse reduction stress test results who are planning vaginal prolapse repair, the TVT midurethral sling (rather than suburethral fascial plication) appears to offer better prevention from postoperative stress incontinence.

In the second trial, the Colpopexy and Urinary Reduction Efforts (CARE) trial, 322 women were randomly assigned to undergo either the Burch procedure or no antiincontinence procedure at the time of abdominal sacral colpopexy (81). Three months after surgery, fewer women in the Burch group (23.8%) had stress incontinence than in the no-Burch group (44.1%). In addition, among women with stress incontinence after surgery, fewer women in the Burch group were bothered (6.1%) by their symptoms, compared with 24.5% of women in the no-Burch group.

Although long-term data are not yet available, it seems evident that subjectively stress-continent women with positive stress test results (with prolapse reduced) benefit from the addition of an antiincontinence procedure at the time of prolapse repair. In making recommendations to women planning prolapse repair, clinicians should discuss the potential risks and benefits of adding an antiincontinence procedure, keeping in mind that prophylaxis against postoperative stress incontinence is not perfectly effective (just as anti-incontinence procedures used for treatment are not perfectly effective). Even when antiincontinence procedures are performed, some women continue to have incontinence symptoms (both stress and urge) after surgery. Further study is needed to determine how to better prevent incontinence symptoms after prolapse repair, and whether more selective application of anti-incontinence procedures will improve the risk–benefit ratio.

Women with negative stress test results despite prolapse reduction also may benefit from the addition of an antiincontinence procedure at the time of prolapse repair. In the CARE trial, women with negative stress test results (prolapse reduced) benefited from the addition of Burch colposuspension (20.8% with stress incontinence 3 months after surgery in the Burch group, compared with 38.2% in the no-Burch group). However, a smaller trial of women undergoing vaginal prolapse repair did not show a benefit from the addition of pubourethral ligament plication (82). Including only women with negative stress test results (prolapse reduced), 102 patients were randomly assigned to receive vaginal prolapse repair with or without pubourethral ligament plication. After 1 year, the proportion of women with stress incontinence was the same in both groups (8%). Until further data become available, clinicians should discuss with women the potential advantages and disadvantages of adding an antiincontinence procedure to prolapse repair when results of preoperative prolapse reduction stress testing are negative.

Summary of Recommendations and Conclusions

The following recommendations and conclusions are based on good and consistent scientific evidence (Level A):

▶ The only symptom specific to prolapse is the awareness of a vaginal bulge or protrusion. For all other pelvic symptoms, resolution with prolapse treatment cannot be assumed.

▶ Pessaries can be fitted in most women with prolapse, regardless of prolapse stage or site of predominant prolapse.

▶ Cadaveric fascia should not be used as graft material for abdominal sacral colpopexy because of a substantially higher risk of recurrent prolapse than with synthetic mesh.

▶ Stress-continent women with positive stress test results (prolapse reduced) are at higher risk for developing postoperative stress incontinence after prolapse repair alone compared with women with negative stress test results (prolapse reduced).

▶ For stress-continent women planning abdominal sacral colpopexy, regardless of the results of preoperative stress testing, the addition of the Burch procedure substantially reduces the likelihood of postoperative stress incontinence without increasing urgency symptoms or obstructed voiding.

▶ For women with positive prolapse reduction stress test results who are planning vaginal prolapse repair, TVT midurethral sling (rather than suburethral fascial plication) appears to offer better prevention from postoperative stress incontinence.

The following recommendations and conclusions are based on limited or inconsistent scientific evidence (Level B):

▶ Clinicians should discuss the option of pessary use with all women who have prolapse that warrants treatment based on symptoms. In particular, pessary use should be considered before surgical intervention in women with symptomatic prolapse.

▶ Alternative operations for uterine preservation in women with prolapse include uterosacral or sacrospinous ligament fixation by the vaginal approach, or sacral hysteropexy by the abdominal approach.

▶ Hysteropexy should not be performed by using the ventral abdominal wall for support because of the high risk for recurrent prolapse, particularly enterocele.

▶ Round ligament suspension is not effective in treating uterine or vaginal prolapse.

▶ Compared with vaginal sacrospinous ligament fixation, abdominal sacral colpopexy has less apical failure and less postoperative dyspareunia and stress incontinence, but is also associated with more complications.

▶ Transvaginal posterior colporrhaphy is recommended over transanal repair for posterior vaginal prolapse.

The following recommendations are based primarily on consensus and expert opinion (Level C):

▶ Clinicians should discuss with women the potential risks and benefits in performing a prophylactic anti-incontinence procedure at the time of prolapse repair.

▶ Women with prolapse who are asymptomatic or mildly symptomatic can be observed at regular intervals, unless new bothersome symptoms develop.

▶ For women who are at high risk for complications with reconstructive procedures and who no longer desire vaginal intercourse, colpocleisis can be offered.

▶ Cystoscopy should be performed intraoperatively to assess for bladder or ureteral damage after all prolapse or incontinence procedures during which the bladder or ureters may be at risk of injury.

Proposed Performance Measure

The percentage of women with diagnosed symptomatic pelvic organ prolapse who are offered pessary use as first-line treatment

References

1. Olsen AL, Smith VJ, Bergstrom JO, Colling JC, Clark AL. Epidemiology of surgically managed pelvic organ prolapse and urinary incontinence. Obstet Gynecol 1997; 89:501–6. (Level II-3)

2. Boyles SH, Weber AM, Meyn L. Procedures for pelvic organ prolapse in the United States, 1979–1997. Am J Obstet Gynecol 2003;188:108–15. (Level II-3)

3. Wilcox LS, Koonin LM, Pokras R, Strauss LT, Xia Z, Peterson HB. Hysterectomy in the United States, 1988–1990. Obstet Gynecol 1994;83:549–55. (Level II-3)

4. Samuelsson EC, Victor FT, Tibblin G, Svardsudd KF. Signs of genital prolapse in a Swedish population of women 20 to 59 years of age and possible related factors. Am J Obstet Gynecol 1999;180:299–305. (Level II-3)

5. Mant J, Painter R, Vessey M. Epidemiology of genital prolapse: observations from the Oxford Family Planning Association Study. Br J Obstet Gynaecol 1997;104: 579–85. (Level II-2)

6. Maher C, Baessler K. Surgical management of posterior vaginal wall prolapse: an evidence based literature review. Int Urogynecol J 2005;17:84–8. (Level III)

7. Weber AM, Richter HE. Pelvic organ prolapse. Obstet Gynecol 2005;106:615–34. (Level III)

8. Thakar R, Ayers S, Clarkson P, Stanton S, Manyonda I. Outcomes after total versus subtotal abdominal hysterectomy. N Engl J Med 2002;347:1318–25. (Level I)

9. Learman LA, Summitt RL, Varner RE, McNeeley SG, Goodman-Gruen D, Richter HE, et al. A randomized comparison of total or supracervical hysterectomy: surgical complications and clinical outcomes. Total or Supracervical Hysterectomy (TOSH) Research Group. Obstet Gynecol 2003;102:453–62. (Level I)

10. Bump RC, Mattiasson A, Bo K, Brubaker LP, Delancey JO, Klarskov P, et al. The standardization of terminology of female pelvic organ prolapse and pelvic floor dysfunction. Am J Obstet Gynecol 1996;175:10–7. (Level III)

11. Adams E, Thomson A, Maher C, Hagen S. Mechanical devices for pelvic organ prolapse in women. The Cochrane Database of Systematic Reviews 2004, Issue 2. Art. No.: CD004010. DOI: 10.1002/14651858. CD004010.pub2. (Level III)

12. Hagen S, Stark D, Maher C, Adams E. Conservative management of pelvic organ prolapse in women. The Cochrane Database of Systematic Reviews 2004, Issue 2. Art No.: CD003882. DOI:10.1002/14651858.CD003882. pub2. (Level III)

13. Cundiff GW, Weidner AC, Visco AG, Bump RC, Addison WA. A survey of pessary use by members of the American Urogynecologic Society. Obstet Gynecol 2000;95:931–5. (Level III)

14. Sulak PJ, Kuehl TJ, Shull BL. Vaginal pessaries and their use in pelvic relaxation. J Reprod Med 1993;38:919–23. (Level III)

15. Wu V, Farrell SA, Baskett TF, Flowerdew G. A simplified protocol for pessary management. Obstet Gynecol 1997; 90:990–4. (Level II-3)

16. Clemons JL, Aguilar VC, Tillinghast TA, Jackson ND, Myers DL. Patient satisfaction and changes in prolapse and urinary symptoms in women who were fitted successfully with a pessary for pelvic organ prolapse. Am J Obstet Gynecol 2004;190:1025–9. (Level III)

17. Clemons JL, Aguilar VC, Tillinghast TA, Jackson ND, Myers DL. Risk factors associated with an unsuccessful pessary fitting trial in women with pelvic organ prolapse. Am J Obstet Gynecol 2004;190:345–50. (Level II-3)

18. Brincat C, Kenton K, Fitzgerald MP, Brubaker L. Sexual activity predicts continued pessary use. Am J Obstet Gynecol 2004;191:198–200. (Level II-3)

19. Mutone MF, Terry C, Hale D, Benson JT. Factors which influence the short-term success of pessary management of pelvic organ prolapse. Am J Obstet Gynecol 2005:193: 89–94. (Level II-3)

20. Kegel AH. Early genital relaxation: new technic of diagnosis and nonsurgical treatment. Obstet Gynecol 1956;8: 545–50. (Level III)

21. Sze EH, Karram MM. Transvaginal repair of vault prolapse: a review. Obstet Gynecol 1997;89:466–75. (Level III)

22. Nygaard IE, McCreery R, Brubaker L, Connolly AM, Cundiff G, Weber AM, et al. Abdominal sacrocolpopexy: a comprehensive review. Pelvic Floor Disorders Network. Obstet Gynecol 2004;104:805–23. (Level III)

23. Benson JT, Lucente V, McClellan E. Vaginal versus abdominal reconstructive surgery for the treatment of pelvic support defects: a prospective randomized study with long-term outcome evaluation. Am J Obstet Gynecol 1996;175:1418–21; discussion 1421–2. (Level I)

24. Lo TS, Wang AC. Abdominal colposacropexy and sacrospinous ligament suspension for severe uterovaginal prolapse: a comparison. J Gynecol Surg 1998;14:59–64. (Level I)

25. Maher CF, Qatawneh AM, Dwyer PL, Carey MP, Cornish A, Schluter P. Abdominal sacral colpopexy or vaginal sacrospinous colpopexy for vaginal vault prolapse: a prospective randomized study. Am J Obstet Gynecol 2004;190:20–6. (Level I)

26. Barber MD, Visco AG, Weidner AC, Amundsen CL, Bump RC. Bilateral uterosacral ligament vaginal vault suspension with site-specific endopelvic fascia defect repair for treatment of pelvic organ prolapse. Am J Obstet Gynecol 2000;183:1402–10; discussion 1410–1. (Level III)

27. Higgs PJ, Chua HL, Smith AR. Long term review of laparoscopic sacrocolpopexy. BJOG 2005;112:1134–8. (Level III)

28. Ross JW, Preston M. Laparoscopic sacrocolpopexy for severe vaginal vault prolapse: five-year outcome. J Minim Invasive Gynecol 2005;12:221–6. (Level III)

29. Rozet F, Mandron E, Arroyo C, Andrews H, Cathelineau X, Mombet A, et al. Laparoscopic sacral colpopexy approach for genitourinary prolapse: experience with 363 cases. Eur Urol 2005;47:230–6. (Level III)

30. Paraiso MF, Walters MD, Rackley RR, Melek S, Hugney C. Laparoscopic and abdominal sacral colpopexies: a comparative cohort study. Am J Obstet Gynecol 2005; 192:1752–8. (Level II-2)

31. Jenkins VR 2nd. Uterosacral ligament fixation for vaginal vault suspension in uterine and vaginal vault prolapse. Am J Obstet Gynecol 1997;177:1337–43; discussion 1343–4. (Level III)

32. Miklos JR, Kohli N, Lucente V, Saye WB. Site-specific fascial defects in the diagnosis and surgical management of enterocele. Am J Obstet Gynecol 1998;179:1418–22; discussion 1422–3. (Level III)

33. Shull BL, Bachofen C, Coates KW, Kuehl TJ. A transvaginal approach to repair of apical and other associated sites of pelvic organ prolapse with uterosacral ligaments. Am J Obstet Gynecol 2000;183:1365–73; discussion 1373–4. (Level II-3)

34. Karram M, Goldwasser S, Kleeman S, Steele A, Vassallo B, Walsh P. High uterosacral vaginal vault suspension with fascial reconstruction for vaginal repair of enterocele and vaginal vault prolapse. Am J Obstet Gynecol 2001; 185:1339–42; discussion 1342–3. (Level III)

35. Amundsen CL, Flynn BJ, Webster GD. Anatomical correction of vaginal vault prolapse by uterosacral ligament fixation in women who also require a pubovaginal sling. J Urol 2003;169:1770–4. (Level II-2)

36. Silva WA, Pauls RN, Segal JL, Rooney CM, Kleeman SD, Karram MM. Uterosacral ligament vault suspension: five-year outcomes. Obstet Gynecol 2006;108:255–63. (Level II-3)

37. Koyama M, Yoshida S, Koyama S, Ogita K, Kimura T, Shimoya K, et al. Surgical reinforcement of support for the vagina in pelvic organ prolapse: concurrent ilio coccygeus fascia colpopexy (Inmon technique). Int Urogynecol J Pelvic Floor Dysfunct 2005;16:197–202. (Level III)

38. Meeks GR, Washburne JF, McGehee RP, Wiser WL. Repair of vaginal vault prolapse by suspension of the vagina to iliococcygeus (prespinous) fascia. Am J Obstet Gynecol 1994;171:1444–52; discussion 1452–4. (Level III)

39. Stepp KJ, Barber MD, Yoo EH, Whiteside JL, Paraiso MF, Walters MD. Incidence of perioperative complications of urogynecologic surgery in elderly women. Am J Obstet Gynecol 2005;192:1630–6. (Level II-3)

40. Sung VW, Weitzen S, Sokol ER, Rardin CR, Myers DL. Effect of patient age on increasing morbidity and mortality following urogynecologic surgery. Am J Obstet Gynecol 2006;194:1411–7. (Level II-2)

41. FitzGerald MP, Richter HE, Siddique S, Thompson P, Zyczynski H, Weber A. Colpocleisis: a review. Pelvic Floor Disorders Network. Int Urogynecol J Pelvic Floor Dysfunct 2006;17:261–71. (Level III)

42. Kovac SR, Cruikshank SH. Successful pregnancies and vaginal deliveries after sacrospinous uterosacral fixation in five of nineteen patients. Am J Obstet Gynecol 1993; 168:1778–83; discussion 1783–6. (Level II-3)

43. Maher CF, Cary MP, Slack MC, Murray CJ, Milligan M, Schluter P. Uterine preservation or hysterectomy at sacrospinous colpopexy for uterovaginal prolapse? Int Urogynecol J Pelvic Floor Dysfunct 2001;12:381–4; discussion 384–5. (Level III)

44. Barranger E, Fritel X, Pigne A. Abdominal sacrohysteropexy in young women with uterovaginal prolapse: long-term follow-up. Am J Obstet Gynecol 2003; 189:1245–50. (Level III)

45. Costantini E, Mearini L, Bini V, Zucchi A, Mearini E, Porena M. Uterus preservation in surgical correction of urogenital prolapse. Eur Urol 2005;48:642–9. (Level II-2)

46. Van Brummen HJ, van de Pol G, Aalders CI, Heintz AP, van der Vaart CH. Sacrospinous hysteropexy compared to vaginal hysterectomy as primary surgical treatment for a descensus uteri: effects on urinary symptoms. Int Urogynecol J Pelvic Floor Dysfunct 2003;14:350–5; discussion 355. (Level II-3)

47. Diwan A, Rardin CR, Strohsnitter WC, Weld A, Rosenblatt P, Kohli N. Laparoscopic uterosacral ligament uterine suspension compared with vaginal hysterectomy with vaginal vault suspension for uterovaginal prolapse. Int Urogynecol J Pelvic Floor Dysfunct 2005;17:79–83. (Level II-2)

48. Lin LL, Ho MH, Haessler AL, Betson LH, Alinsod RM, Liu CY, et al. A review of laparoscopic uterine suspension procedures for uterine preservation. Curr Opin Obstet Gynecol 2005;17:541–6. (Level III)

49. O'Brien PM, Ibrahim J. Failure of laparoscopic uterine suspension to provide a lasting cure for uterovaginal prolapse. Br J Obstet Gynaecol 1994;101:707–8. (Level III)

50. Young SB, Daman JJ, Bony LG. Vaginal paravaginal repair: one-year outcomes. Am J Obstet Gynecol 2001; 185:1360–6; discussion 1366–7. (Level III)

51. Mallipeddi PK, Steele AC, Kohli N, Karram MM. Anatomic and functional outcome of vaginal paravaginal repair in the correction of anterior vaginal wall prolapse. Int Urogynecol J Pelvic Floor Dysfunct 2001;12:83–8. (Level III)

52. Bruce RG, El-Galley RE, Galloway NT. Paravaginal defect repair in the treatment of female stress urinary incontinence and cystocele. Urology 1999;54:647–51. (Level III)

53. Scotti RJ, Garely AD, Greston WM, Flora RF, Olson TR. Paravaginal repair of lateral vaginal wall defects by fixation to the ischial periosteum and obturator membrane. Am J Obstet Gynecol 1998;179:1436–45. (Level III)

54. Abramov Y, Gandhi S, Goldberg RP, Botros SM, Kwon C, Sand PK. Site-specific rectocele repair compared with standard posterior colporrhaphy. Obstet Gynecol 2005; 105:314–8. (Level II-3)

55. Weber AM, Walters MD, Piedmonte MR. Sexual function and vaginal anatomy in women before and after surgery for pelvic organ prolapse and urinary incontinence. Am J Obstet Gynecol 2000;182:1610–5. (Level II-3)

56. Nieminen K, Hiltunen KM, Laitinen J, Oksala J, Heinonen PK. Transanal or vaginal approach to rectocele repair: a prospective, randomized pilot study. Dis Colon Rectum 2004;47:1636–42. (Level I)

57. Silva WA, Karram MM. Scientific basis for use of grafts during vaginal reconstructive procedures. Curr Opin Obstet Gynecol 2005;17:519–29. (Level III)

58. FitzGerald MP, Mollenhauer J, Bitterman P, Brubaker L. Functional failure of fascia lata allografts. Am J Obstet Gynecol 1999;181:1339–44; discussion 1344–6. (Level III)

59. FitzGerald MP, Edwards SR, Fenner D. Medium-term follow-up on use of freeze-dried, irradiated donor fascia for sacrocolpopexy and sling procedures. Int Urogynecol J Pelvic Floor Dysfunct 2004;15:238–42. (Level III)

60. Gregory WT, Otto LN, Bergstrom JO, Clark AL. Surgical outcome of abdominal sacrocolpopexy with synthetic mesh versus abdominal sacrocolpopexy with cadaveric fascia lata. Int Urogynecol J Pelvic Floor Dysfunct 2005;16:369–74. (Level II-3)

61. Culligan PJ, Blackwell L, Goldsmith LJ, Graham CA, Rogers A, Heit MH. A randomized controlled trial comparing fascia lata and synthetic mesh for sacral colpopexy. Obstet Gynecol 2005;106:29–37. (Level I)

62. Govier FE, Kobashi KC, Kozlowski PM, Kuznetsov DD, Begley SJ, McGonigle KF, et al. High complication rate identified in sacrocolpopexy patients attributed to silicone mesh. Urology 2005;65:1099–103. (Level III)

63. Duckett JR, Constantine G. Complications of silicone sling insertion for stress urinary incontinence. J Urol 2000;163:1835–7. (Level III)

64. Petros PE. Vault prolapse II: Restoration of dynamic vaginal supports by infracoccygeal sacropexy, an axial daycase vaginal procedure. Int Urogynecol J Pelvic Floor Dysfunct 2001;12:296–303. (Level III)

65. Mattox TF, Moore S, Stanford EJ, Mills BB. Posterior vaginal sling experience in elderly patients yields poor results. Am J Obstet Gynecol 2006;194:1462–6. (Level III)

66. Baessler K, Hewson AD, Tunn R, Schuessler B, Maher CF. Severe mesh complications following intravaginal slingplasty. Obstet Gynecol 2005;106:713–6. (Level III)

67. Altman D, Mellgren A, Zetterstrom J. Rectocele repair using biomaterial augmentation: current documentation and clinical experience. Obstet Gynecol Surv 2005;60: 753–60. (Level III)

68. Vakili B, Huynh T, Loesch H, Franco N, Chesson RR. Outcomes of vaginal reconstructive surgery with and without graft material. Am J Obstet Gynecol 2005;193: 2126–32. (Level II-2)

69. Altman D, Zetterstrom J, Mellgren A, Gustafsson C, Anzen B, Lopez A. A three-year prospective assessment of rectocele repair using porcine xenograft. Obstet Gynecol 2006;107:59–65. (Level II-3)

70. Wheeler TL 2nd, Richter HE, Duke AG, Burgio KL, Redden DT, Varner RE. Outcomes with porcine graft placement in the anterior vaginal compartment in patients who undergo high vaginal uterosacral suspension and cystocele repair. Am J Obstet Gynecol 2006;194:1486–91. (Level III)

71. Julian TM. The efficacy of Marlex mesh in the repair of severe, recurrent vaginal prolapse of the anterior midvaginal wall. Am J Obstet Gynecol 1996;175:1472–5. (Level II-3)

72. Sand PK, Koduri S, Lobel RW, Winkler HA, Tomezsko J, Culligan PJ, et al. Prospective randomized trial of polyglactin 910 mesh to prevent recurrence of cystoceles and rectoceles. Am J Obstet Gynecol 2001;184:1357–62; discussion 1362–4. (Level I)

73. Weber AM, Walters MD, Piedmonte MR, Ballard LA. Anterior colporrhaphy: a randomized trial of three surgical techniques. Am J Obstet Gynecol 2001;185:1299–304; discussion 1304–6. (Level I)

74. Gandhi S, Goldberg RP, Kwon C, Koduri S, Beaumont JL, Abramov Y, et al. A prospective randomized trial using solvent dehydrated fascia lata for the prevention of recurrent anterior vaginal wall prolapse. Am J Obstet Gynecol 2005;192:1649–54. (Level I)

75. Migliari R, Usai E. Treatment results using a mixed fiber mesh in patients with Grade IV cystocele. J Urol 1999; 161:1255–8. (Level III)

76. Migliari R, De Angelis M, Madeddu G, Verdacchi T. Tension-free vaginal mesh repair for anterior vaginal wall prolapse. Eur Urol 2000;38:151–5. (Level III)

77. De Tayrac R, Gervaise A, Chauveaud-Lambling A, Fernandez H. Combined genital prolapse repair reinforced with a polypropylene mesh and tension-free vaginal tape in women with genital prolapse and stress urinary incontinence: a retrospective case-control study with short-term follow-up. Acta Obstet Gynecol Scand 2004; 83:950–4. (Level II-2)

78. Hung MJ, Liu FS, Shen PS, Chen GD, Lin LY, Ho ES. Factors that affect recurrence after anterior colporrhaphy procedure reinforced with four-corner anchored polypropylene mesh. Int Urogynecol J Pelvic Floor Dysfunct 2004;15:399–406. (Level III)

79. De Tayrac R, Gervaise A, Chauveaud A, Fernandez H. Tension-free polypropylene mesh for vaginal repair of anterior vaginal wall prolapse. J Reprod Med 2005;50: 75–80. (Level III)

80. Meschia M, Pifarotti P, Spennacchio M, Buonaguidi A, Gattei U, Somigliana E. A randomized comparison of tension-free vaginal tape and endopelvic fascia plication in women with genital prolapse and occult stress urinary incontinence. Am J Obstet Gynecol 2004;190:609–13. (Level I)

81. Brubaker L, Cundiff GW, Fine P, Nygaard I, Richter HE, Visco AG, et al. Abdominal sacrocolpopexy with Burch colposuspension to reduce urinary stress incontinence. Pelvic Floor Disorders Network. N Engl J Med 2006; 354;1557–66. (Level I)

82. Colombo M, Maggioni A, Zanetta G, Vignali M, Milani R. Prevention of postoperative urinary stress incontinence after surgery for genitourinary prolapse. Obstet Gynecol 1996;87:266–71. (Level I)

The MEDLINE database, the Cochrane Library, and ACOG's own internal resources and documents were used to conduct a literature search to locate relevant articles published between January 1985 and August 2006. The search was restricted to articles published in the English language. Priority was given to articles reporting results of original research, although review articles and commentaries also were consulted. Abstracts of research presented at symposia and scientific conferences were not considered adequate for inclusion in this document. Guidelines published by organizations or institutions such as the National Institutes of Health and the American College of Obstetricians and Gynecologists were reviewed, and additional studies were located by reviewing bibliographies of identified articles. When reliable research was not available, expert opinions from obstetrician–gynecologists were used.

Studies were reviewed and evaluated for quality according to the method outlined by the U.S. Preventive Services Task Force:

I   Evidence obtained from at least one properly designed randomized controlled trial.

II-1 Evidence obtained from well-designed controlled trials without randomization.

II-2 Evidence obtained from well-designed cohort or case–control analytic studies, preferably from more than one center or research group.

II-3 Evidence obtained from multiple time series with or without the intervention. Dramatic results in uncontrolled experiments also could be regarded as this type of evidence.

III   Opinions of respected authorities, based on clinical experience, descriptive studies, or reports of expert committees.

Based on the highest level of evidence found in the data, recommendations are provided and graded according to the following categories:

Level A—Recommendations are based on good and consistent scientific evidence.

Level B—Recommendations are based on limited or inconsistent scientific evidence.

Level C—Recommendations are based primarily on consensus and expert opinion.

ISSN 1099-3630

The American College of Obstetricians and Gynecologists
409 12th Street, SW, PO Box 96920, Washington, DC 20090-6920

Pelvic organ prolapse. ACOG Practice Bulletin No. 85. American College of Obstetricians and Gynecologists. Obstet Gynecol 2007; 110:717–29.

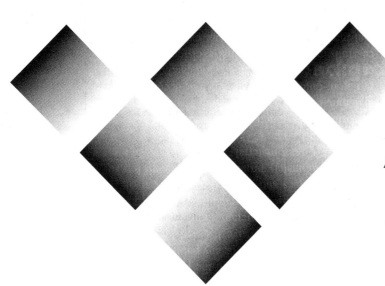

ACOG PRACTICE BULLETIN

CLINICAL MANAGEMENT GUIDELINES FOR
OBSTETRICIAN–GYNECOLOGISTS

NUMBER 89, JANUARY 2008

(Replaces Practice Bulletin Number 7, September 1999)

This Practice Bulletin was developed by the ACOG Committee on Practice Bulletins—Gynecology with the assistance of Elizabeth Swisher, MD, and Susan Reed, MD, MPH. The information is designed to aid practitioners in making decisions about appropriate obstetric and gynecologic care. These guidelines should not be construed as dictating an exclusive course of treatment or procedure. Variations in practice may be warranted based on the needs of the individual patient, resources, and limitations unique to the institution or type of practice.

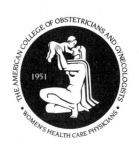

Elective and Risk-Reducing Salpingo-oophorectomy

In the United States, 600,000 hysterectomies are performed annually, of which one half include salpingo-oophorectomy (1). Salpingo-oophorectomy is performed electively at the time of hysterectomy to decrease the risk of ovarian cancer and to avoid possible morbidities and future surgery related to benign ovarian neoplasms, endometriosis, and pelvic pain.

There is a subset of women with an elevated risk of ovarian carcinoma and breast carcinoma recurrence who are candidates for risk-reducing salpingo-oophorectomy performed for the primary purpose of reducing breast, ovarian, and fallopian tube carcinoma risks. The purpose of this document is to provide a framework for counseling women about the benefits and risks of elective salpingo-oophorectomy at the time of hysterectomy and to provide some guidelines for risk-reducing salpingo-oophorectomy.

Background

Risk-reducing and elective salpingo-oophorectomies are the removal of the ovaries for the potential benefit of preventing long-term morbidity and mortality. The term risk-reducing salpingo-oophorectomy implies that the ovaries are normal at the time of removal. Salpingo-oophorectomy can be performed either alone as a planned surgical procedure or in conjunction with other planned surgical procedures such as hysterectomy or colectomy. Elective salpingo-oophorectomy is a term commonly used when the ovaries are removed at the time of another indicated surgical procedure, and this term should not be used interchangeably with risk-reducing salpingo-oophorectomy.

Ovarian Physiology in Premenopause and Natural and Surgical Menopause

The mean age at which menopause occurs in developed countries is 51.4 years (2). After menopause, estradiol production decreases by 90% (3, 4) because of follicular atresia, and estrone becomes the dominant estrogen. Estrone produced after menopause comes primarily from peripheral conversion of adrenal androstenedione by aromatase, primarily in adipose tissues. After menopause, small concentrations of progesterone continue to be produced by the adrenal gland. However, with natural menopause, the transition from a premenopausal profile to postmenopausal profile occurs over 4 years, on average (5).

As reproductive aging progresses, serum levels of androgens decrease, but not to the extent that estrogen levels diminish. Androstenedione levels decrease by approximately 50% because of declines in ovarian production (3, 6, 7) while adrenal output remains relatively constant. Testosterone continues to be secreted by the ovarian stroma but decreases by approximately 30% (3, 6, 7). Serum concentrations of the adrenal androgen precursor dehydroepiandrosterone (DHEA) decrease with biological aging, beginning before the final menstrual period (7).

The reproductive hormone profile observed with surgical menopause is quite similar to that of a postmenopausal woman. In premenopausal women, the mean reductions in serum testosterone and estradiol concentrations following oophorectomy are 50% and 80%, respectively (8).

Cancer Prevention

The American Cancer Society estimates that 22,430 new cases of ovarian cancer will be diagnosed in 2007 in the United States, with an estimated 15,280 deaths from ovarian cancer (9). The lifetime risk of developing ovarian cancer in the general population is 1 in 70 or 1.4%. Current methods of ovarian cancer screening have not been found to enable early diagnosis of invasive ovarian carcinomas, much less decrease morbidity and mortality from ovarian cancer. Transvaginal ultrasonography and serum CA 125 measurement are not recommended for screening in the general population.

The most effective method of preventing ovarian cancer is surgical removal of the ovaries and fallopian tubes. It is estimated that approximately 1,000 cases of ovarian cancer could be prevented each year if elective salpingo-oophorectomy was performed in all women undergoing hysterectomy at 40 years or older in the United States (10). Approximately 5–10% of women with ovarian cancer have had a previous hysterectomy at age 40 years or older (11). The potential benefit in cancer risk reduction for premenopausal women at average risk of ovarian cancer must be balanced with the consequences of premature loss of estrogen production.

Identification of women with a genetically increased risk of ovarian carcinoma is important in identifying those who would benefit from risk-reducing salpingo-oophorectomy (see box "Oophorectomy Versus Ovarian Preservation at the Time of Hysterectomy"). Women with this increased risk account for 10–15% of all ovarian carcinomas that could be effectively prevented if risk were identified (12–14). Other factors that increase the risk of ovarian carcinoma include nulligravidity, decreased fertility, age, and family history of ovarian carcinoma (15). Data from the Women's Health Initiative are not mature enough to determine if the risk of ovarian carcinoma is significantly increased by the use of estrogen therapy (16). The use of ovulation induction agents is not clearly linked to an increased risk of ovarian carcinoma (17).

In addition to pregnancy, factors that are protective against ovarian carcinoma include bilateral tubal ligation, hysterectomy with ovarian preservation, and use of oral contraceptives (15, 18–20).

Recognizing women with a genetically increased risk of ovarian cancer may provide the opportunity of preventing most hereditary ovarian carcinomas. This approach has the potential to prevent more total cases of

---

Oophorectomy Versus Ovarian Preservation at the Time of Hysterectomy

Factors favoring oophorectomy

- Genetic susceptibility for ovarian carcinoma based on family history or genetic testing
- Bilateral ovarian neoplasms
- Severe endometriosis
- Pelvic inflammatory disease or bilateral tuboovarian abscesses
- Postmenopausal status

Factors favoring ovarian preservation

- Premenopausal status
- Desire for fertility
- Impact on sexual function, libido, and quality of life in young women
- Osteopenia, osteoporosis, or risk factors for osteoporosis (if premenopausal)

ovarian carcinoma, with far fewer oophorectomies, than if elective oophorectomy were performed at the time of hysterectomy in all average-risk women older than 40 years.

Inherited susceptibility to ovarian cancer has the greatest impact of all ovarian cancer risk factors. Women with the highest risk of ovarian carcinoma are those with hereditary breast and ovarian cancer, followed by women with hereditary nonpolyposis colorectal cancer (HNPCC). Suggestive family histories of hereditary cancer risk include cancer occurring at young ages; cancer in first-degree relatives; cancer in multiple generations; bilateral, metachronous, or synchronous cancer in one individual; and clustering of cancer on one side of the family (see box "Criteria for Referral for *BRCA* Testing").

The types of cancer suggestive of hereditary breast and ovarian cancer include early-onset (before age 50 years) or bilateral breast cancer, epithelial ovarian cancer (at any age), male breast cancer, pancreatic cancer, and early-onset prostate cancer. If a *BRCA1* or *BRCA2* mutation comes from the paternal side of the family or from a lineage containing few females, cancer histories may be subtle or absent (21). Most hereditary breast and ovarian cancer are caused by inherited mutations in the *BRCA1* or *BRCA2* genes, which lead to lifetime risks of ovarian cancer of 20–50% and of breast cancer of 60–85% (21, 22). Inherited mutations in *BRCA1* and *BRCA2* account for 10–15% of all ovarian carcinomas (12, 14). Mucinous and borderline ovarian neoplasms are not suggestive of *BRCA1* or *BRCA2* mutations. The *BRCA* mutation carrier rate is higher in certain populations because of the presence of founder mutations. Three founder mutations in *BRCA1* and *BRCA2* are present in 2–2.5% of Ashkenazi individuals (23, 24). Consequently, in Ashkenazim, a higher proportion of breast and ovarian cancers (12% and 40%, respectively) are associated with inherited mutations in *BRCA1* or *BRCA2* (21, 23, 25, 26).

Types of cancer associated with HNPCC include those of the colon or rectum, endometrium, biliary tract, stomach, brain, and urinary tract. Because HNPCC leads to cancer equally in both sexes, women with HNPCC are more likely to have a positive family history than are those women with hereditary breast and ovarian cancer. Criteria for diagnosis of HNPCC have been modified to include gynecologic and other noncolonic cancer (27) (see box "Criteria for Referral for *BRCA* Testing" and box "Revised Diagnostic Criteria for Hereditary Nonpolyposis Colorectal Cancer"). Hereditary nonpolyposis colorectal cancer or Lynch syndrome is caused by inherited mutations in the DNA mismatch repair genes *MSH2*, *MLH1*, *PMS2*, and *MSH6*. The most common types of cancer in women with HNPCC are colon and endometrial cancer. Women with HNPCC have a 40–60% lifetime risk of endometrial cancer and an 8–10% risk of ovarian cancer (28, 29).

Criteria for Referral for *BRCA* Testing

For non-Ashkenazi Jewish women:

- Two first-degree relatives with breast cancer, one relative in whom breast cancer was diagnosed when younger than 50 years
- A combination of three or more first- or second-degree relatives with breast cancer at any age
- A combination of both breast and ovarian cancer among first- and second-degree relatives
- A first-degree relative with bilateral breast cancer
- A combination of two or more first- or second-degree relatives with ovarian cancer at any age
- A first- or second-degree relative with both breast and ovarian cancer at any age
- A male relative with breast cancer

For women of Ashkenazi Jewish heritage:

- Any first-degree relative with breast or ovarian cancer
- Two second-degree relatives on the same side of the family with breast or ovarian cancer

U.S. Preventive Services Task Force. Genetic risk assessment and BRCA mutation testing for breast and ovarian cancer susceptibility: recommendation statement. Ann Intern Med 2005;143:355–61.

Revised Diagnostic Criteria for Hereditary Nonpolyposis Colorectal Cancer

- Three or more relatives have an HNPCC-associated cancer, including cancer of the colon, endometrium, small bowel, ureter, or renal pelvis.
- Two or more successive generations are affected.
- Cancer is diagnosed in at least one individual who is younger than 50 years.
- Familial adenomatosis polyposis should be excluded in any colorectal cancers.

Adapted from Vasen HF, Watson P, Mecklin JP, et al. New clinical criteria for hereditary nonpolyposis colorectal cancer (HNPCC, Lynch syndrome) proposed by the International Collaborative group on HNPCC. Gastroenterology 1999;116:1453–6.

Clinical Considerations and Recommendations

▶ *What factors should be considered when deciding on elective salpingo-oophorectomy versus ovarian preservation at the time of hysterectomy?*

Multiple factors should be considered, including the age of the woman, genetic risk of ovarian carcinoma (see boxes, "Criteria for Referral for *BRCA* Testing" and "Revised Diagnostic Criteria for Hereditary Nonpolyposis Colorectal Cancer"), atherosclerosis, osteoporosis predisposition, risk of subsequent ovarian surgery if the ovaries are retained, and issues related to quality of life. Age is probably the most important factor to consider. Only approximately 4% of women who are ovulatory at age 40 years become menopausal by age 45 years (30); consequently, the positive effects of ongoing production of estrogen by the ovaries versus potential nonadherence with estrogen therapy should be considered before removal of the ovaries in premenopausal women. Strong consideration should be given to retaining normal ovaries in premenopausal women who are not at increased genetic risk of ovarian cancer. However, given the risk of ovarian cancer in postmenopausal women, ovarian removal at the time of hysterectomy should be considered for these women. There are no studies evaluating differences in surgical complications with the addition of salpingo-oophorectomy to abdominal or laparoscopic hysterectomy.

▶ *What is the effect of salpingo-oophorectomy on long-term survival?*

Epidemiologic studies have suggested that premature menopause (natural or surgical) without estrogen therapy is associated with a subsequent increased risk of heart disease, fractures, cognitive impairment, dementia, parkinsonism, and decreased long-term survival (31–38). Prospective population-based studies show that age of menopause, either natural or surgical (without subsequent use of estrogen therapy), is the most important determinant of long-term survival (31, 34, 39, 40). The findings of these studies showed that in general, women with menopause after age 50 years have a lower all-cause mortality rate than do women age 50 years or younger. In one study, the overall survival was determined predominantly by the decreased risk for ischemic heart disease (hazard ratio = 0.98 per year [95% confidence interval, 0.97–0.99]) and less so by the increased risk for fatal uterine and ovarian cancer (hazard ratio = 1.07 per year [95% confidence interval, 1.01–1.12]) (34).

A study using decision analysis to calculate the optimal age for elective salpingo-oophorectomy at hysterectomy for benign disease concluded that ovarian conservation through age 65 years benefited long-term survival in women who had an average risk of ovarian carcinoma (41). The results of this decision analysis are controversial and are not supported by evidence from large prospective cohort studies (31, 40, 42).

▶ *How often will ovarian preservation result in reoperation?*

The frequency of repeat surgery for ovarian pathology is reported to be twice as high in women who had one ovary retained versus both (7.6% versus 3.6%). Most of these repeat surgical procedures are performed because of pelvic pain or a pelvic mass and occur within 5 years of the hysterectomy. Women with endometriosis, pelvic inflammatory disease, and chronic pelvic pain are at higher risk of reoperation if the ovaries are retained. The risk of subsequent ovarian surgery should be weighed against the benefit of ovarian retention in these patients.

▶ *Should estrogen therapy be recommended for women undergoing oophorectomy?*

Use of estrogen therapy in women younger than 50 years has not been examined in randomized controlled trials. In women ages 50–79 years (average age, 63 years) who have had a hysterectomy, use of estrogen therapy has shown no increased risk of breast cancer or heart disease with up to 7.2 years of use (42, 43). However, an increased risk of thromboembolic disease and stroke was observed (42, 43).

▶ *How will salpingo-oophorectomy or ovarian preservation affect the patient's quality of life?*

The primary disadvantage of salpingo-oophorectomy is loss of natural ovarian hormone secretion. Estrogen therapy may relieve most of the clinical symptoms related to oophorectomy (eg, hot flushes, vaginal dryness, irritability, mood swings). Other possible disadvantages include changes in self-image and decreased libido attributed to loss of ovarian androgen production, but androgen replacement has been shown to improve mood, libido, and bone mineral density (44–48). Several studies performed in general populations of premenopausal women show overall sexual function was unaltered after oophorectomy, despite lower concentrations of ovarian sex steroids (49).

Potential benefits of testosterone therapy need to be weighed against possible increased risk for breast cancer and cardiovascular disease. Studies to date suggest that testosterone therapy and progestin therapy may be the determining factor in breast cancer risk with post-menopausal hormone therapy (50, 51).

▶ What are contraindications to ovarian preservation?

Women at very high risk of ovarian carcinoma—specifically, women with documented hereditary breast and ovarian cancer susceptibility or hereditary nonpolyposis colorectal cancer (HNPCC or Lynch syndrome)—are not candidates for ovarian preservation. Referral to a certified genetic counselor can help clarify risk of ovarian cancer in women with suggestive personal or family histories. Other contraindications to ovarian preservation include invasive ovarian or endometrial carcinomas. Malignant germ cell tumors, stromal tumors, and borderline ovarian tumors do not mandate bilateral salpingo-oophorectomy in women desiring fertility preservation.

▶ What is the role of genetic counseling and testing for women who are considering risk-reducing salpingo-oophorectomy?

The U.S. Preventive Services Task Force has recommended that women with family histories suggestive of *BRCA1* and *BRCA2* mutations be referred for genetic counseling and evaluation for *BRCA* testing (52) (see box "Criteria for Referral for *BRCA* Testing"). Both maternal and paternal family histories are important. Approximately 2% of U.S. women would meet these criteria for referral, and obstetrician–gynecologists play a critical role in identifying these women before their peak age of cancer risk.

Genetic testing can clarify ovarian carcinoma risk as well as risk of cancer to other organs. Women with an increased risk of ovarian carcinoma secondary to hereditary breast and ovarian cancer or HNPCC are at risk of cancer in other organs and qualify for more intensive surveillance or prevention measures. Women with hereditary breast and ovarian cancer should be offered surveillance for breast cancer with breast magnetic resonance imaging in addition to mammography and should be counseled about the option of prophylactic mastectomy (53–57). Women with HNPCC should have annual colonoscopies with removal of any polyps (57). Ovarian cancer risk should not be addressed in isolation without consideration of other cancer risks.

Genetic testing also provides the opportunity to clarify risk to other unaffected family members, targeting truly high-risk individuals for intensive surveillance or prevention measures and freeing relatives who have not inherited the familial risk from additional interventions.

▶ How effective is risk-reducing salpingo-oophorectomy?

Carriers of the *BRCA1* and *BRCA2* mutations who undergo salpingo-oophorectomy achieve an 80–90% ovarian cancer risk reduction (13, 58), as well as an approximate 50–60% decrease in breast cancer risk if surgery is performed before menopause. Therefore, bilateral salpingo-oophorectomy should be offered to women with *BRCA1* and *BRCA2* mutations after completion of childbearing, preferably by age 40 years. After salpingo-oophorectomy, women remain at risk of primary peritoneal carcinoma. Findings of a large registry study indicated a 4.3% risk of primary peritoneal cancer at 20 years after risk-reducing salpingo-oophorectomy in *BRCA* mutation carriers. Many cases of primary peritoneal cancer occur within 2 years of risk-reducing salpingo-oophorectomy, suggesting that an occult cancer may have been missed at the time of risk-reducing salpingo-oophorectomy (58). Additionally, primary peritoneal cancer risk appears to be higher after risk-reducing salpingo-oophorectomy when salpingectomy is not performed, suggesting that occult cancer in fallopian tubes may seed the peritoneal cavity (59).

Hysterectomy with bilateral salpingo-oophorectomy effectively reduces endometrial and ovarian cancer risk in women with HNPCC and should be offered after completion of childbearing (57, 60).

▶ When is salpingo-oophorectomy indicated in women with breast cancer?

Salpingo-oophorectomy may be indicated for breast cancer survivors who have a high risk of ovarian cancer. Less than 5% of women with breast cancer harbor a germline *BRCA1* mutation, but *BRCA1* mutations are more frequently observed in younger women with breast cancer and those with family histories of breast and ovarian cancer. Families that are affected only by breast cancer and that test negative for *BRCA1* and *BRCA2* mutations do not have an appreciable increased risk of ovarian cancer (61). Those women with breast cancer who are identified with a *BRCA1* or *BRCA2* mutation have a 20–50% lifetime risk of ovarian cancer and a 40–60% risk of developing a second breast cancer (62, 63). For this reason, genetic counseling with consideration of genetic testing should be offered to all Ashkenazi women with breast cancer at any age, non-Ashkenazi women with invasive breast cancer younger than 40 years, and women with breast cancer and significant maternal or paternal family histories of breast or ovarian cancer.

Salpingo-oophorectomy also may be indicated for hormonal therapy of breast cancer. Salpingo-oophorectomy appears to be more effective than tamoxifen alone as adjuvant therapy in premenopausal women with hormone-sensitive breast cancer (64). Whether there is an added benefit to salpingo-oophorectomy in premenopausal women undergoing chemotherapy is less certain (64). In premenopausal women who are undergoing chemotherapy and are older than 40 years, induced menopause may negate any additional benefit of salpingo-oophorectomy (65). Ovarian ablation may be beneficial in women younger than 35 years who are treated with chemotherapy for hormone-sensitive breast cancer (66).

Estrogen receptor-positive metastatic breast cancer is treated first with aggressive hormonal therapy that may include suppressing the ovaries either medically or surgically (67, 68). Increasingly, aromatase inhibitors are used in the adjuvant therapy of estrogen-sensitive breast cancer (69). Aromatase inhibitors stimulate ovarian function in premenopausal women, resulting in high circulating estradiol levels. Premenopausal women taking aromatase inhibitors for breast cancer need concurrent suppression of ovarian function, and salpingo-oophorectomy may be a cost-effective alternative to long-term ovarian suppression using gonadotropin-releasing hormone (GnRH) agonists. In premenopausal women who become amenorrheic during chemotherapy, aromatase inhibitors may stimulate residual ovarian function. Monitoring serum estradiol levels in these women is important in recognizing ovarian stimulation and identifying the possible need for ovarian suppression or ablation.

▶ *Can women who undergo risk-reducing salpingo-oophorectomy for hereditary breast and ovarian cancer use postmenopausal estrogen therapy?*

The use of short-term estrogen without progestins does not mitigate the sharp reduction in breast cancer risk achieved by premenopausal women with *BRCA1* and *BRCA2* mutations who undergo risk-reducing salpingo-oophorectomy (70). However, the ideal dose, duration of therapy, estrogen compound, and delivery method that maximizes quality of life while minimizing breast cancer risk in women with mutations in *BRCA1* and *BRCA2* have not been determined. The safety of progestins in this population has not been established. Because estrogen and progestin combination therapy is less favorable than estrogen alone for breast cancer risk in the general population (42, 50), it seems prudent to minimize combination hormone therapy in *BRCA* mutation carriers with intact breast tissue.

▶ *At what age should risk-reducing salpingo-oophorectomy be performed?*

Ovarian cancer diagnoses are rare before age 40 years in women with hereditary breast and ovarian cancer (12, 14,

71, 72). The average age of ovarian cancer diagnosis is 52 years for women with *BRCA1* mutations and 60 years for those with *BRCA2* mutations (12, 14, 71). It is recommended that women with *BRCA1* or *BRCA2* mutations consider risk-reducing salpingo-oophorectomy between ages 35 years and 40 years if they have completed their childbearing. When risk-reducing salpingo-oophorectomy is performed before age 40 years in *BRCA1* mutation carriers, there is a 64% reduction in breast cancer risk, compared with a 50% reduction if performed between ages 40 years and 50 years (73).

There are no established guidelines for age of risk-reducing surgery in women with HNPCC mutations. In women with HNPCC, the average age of ovarian cancer diagnosis is 42 years and the average age of endometrial cancer diagnosis is 50 years (28, 29, 74). Thus, it is also reasonable to consider prophylactic surgery in women with HNPCC between ages 35 and 40 years if childbearing is no longer desired (57).

▶ *Are surgical techniques for risk-reducing salpingo-oophorectomy different from standard techniques?*

Performing risk-reducing salpingo-oophorectomy in women at an increased risk of ovarian cancer necessitates complete removal of the ovaries and fallopian tubes. Risk-reducing salpingo-oophorectomy for these women should include careful inspection of the peritoneal cavity, pelvic washings, removal of the fallopian tubes, and ligation of the ovarian vessels at the pelvic brim. If hysterectomy is not performed, care must be taken to completely remove the fallopian tubes to the level of the cornu.

In women with *BRCA1* and *BRCA2* mutations, 5–12% will have an occult neoplasm of the ovary, peritoneum, or fallopian tube identified at risk-reducing salpingo-oophorectomy if thorough pathologic evaluation is performed (75–79). Appropriate evaluation includes serial sectioning at 2–3-mm intervals of the entire ovaries and fallopian tubes. Most of the earliest microscopic neoplasms originate in the fallopian tube when careful sectioning is performed (77, 79, 80). Both age and mutation status are predictors of occult neoplasm, and women with *BRCA1* mutations who are 45 years or older have a 20% risk of occult neoplasm (77, 79).

▶ *Should hysterectomy be performed at the time of risk-reducing salpingo-oophorectomy for hereditary breast and ovarian cancer?*

When salpingo-oophorectomy is performed primarily for prevention of ovarian cancer or for the hormonal therapy of breast cancer, hysterectomy is not required. Women with *BRCA1* or *BRCA2* mutations do not have a known increased risk of endometrial cancer (81). Theoretically, hysterectomy allows more complete removal of the fallopian tube, a target of neoplasia in *BRCA1* or *BRCA2* mutation carriers. However, the interstitial component of the fallopian tube is not a known location of tubal cancer, and its removal may not be essential (82). Furthermore, there are no data to suggest that uterine preservation results in higher cancer risks in *BRCA1* or *BRCA2* mutation carriers. Careful consideration of the benefits and risks of elective hysterectomy in conjunction with risk-reducing salpingo-oophorectomy should be made with each woman, including individual risk factors for endometrial and cervical cancer, such as tamoxifen use, body mass index, and history of cervical dysplasia. In younger women undergoing risk-reducing salpingo-oophorectomy who want to use hormones after surgery, hysterectomy allows the use of estrogen without progestins, a regimen shown to be safe in high-risk women for short-term therapy (70).

Summary of Recommendations and Conclusions

The following conclusion is based on good and consistent scientific evidence (Level A):

▶ In women ages 50–79 years who have had a hysterectomy, use of estrogen therapy has shown no increased risk of breast cancer or heart disease with up to 7.2 years of use.

The following recommendation is based on limited or inconsistent scientific evidence (Level B):

▶ Bilateral salpingo-oophorectomy should be offered to women with *BRCA1* and *BRCA2* mutations after completion of childbearing.

The following recommendations are based primarily on consensus and expert opinion (Level C):

▶ Women with family histories suggestive of *BRCA1* and *BRCA2* mutations should be referred for genetic counseling and evaluation for *BRCA* testing.

▶ For women with an increased risk of ovarian cancer, risk-reducing salpingo-oophorectomy should include careful inspection of the peritoneal cavity, pelvic washings, removal of the fallopian tubes, and ligation of the ovarian vessels at the pelvic brim.

▶ Strong consideration should be made for retaining normal ovaries in premenopausal women who are not at increased genetic risk of ovarian cancer.

▶ Given the risk of ovarian cancer in postmenopausal women, ovarian removal at the time of hysterectomy should be considered for these women.

▶ Women with endometriosis, pelvic inflammatory disease, and chronic pelvic pain are at higher risk of reoperation; consequently, the risk of subsequent ovarian surgery if the ovaries are retained should be weighed against the benefit of ovarian retention in these patients.

References

1. Lepine LA, Hillis SD, Marchbanks PA, Koonin LM, Morrow B, Kieke BA, et al. Hysterectomy surveillance—United States, 1980-1993. MMWR CDC Surveill Summ 1997;46(SS-4):1–15. (Level II-3)

2. Santoro N, Brockwell S, Johnston J, Crawford SL, Gold EB, Harlow SD, et al. Helping midlife women predict the onset of the final menses: SWAN, the Study of Women's Health Across the Nation. Menopause 2007;14:415–24. (Level II-2)

3. Burger HG, Dudley EC, Cui J, Dennerstein L, Hopper JL. A prospective longitudinal study of serum testosterone, dehydroepiandrosterone sulfate, and sex hormone-binding globulin levels through the menopause transition. J Clin Endocrinol Metab 2000;85:2832–8. (Level III)

4. Rannevik G, Jeppsson S, Johnell O, Bjerre B, Laurell-Borulf Y, Svanberg L. A longitudinal study of the perimenopausal transition: altered profiles of steroid and pituitary hormones, SHBG and bone mineral density. Maturitas 1995;21:103–13. (Level III)

5. Kronenberg F. Hot flashes: epidemiology and physiology. Ann N Y Acad Sci 1990;592:52–86; discussion 123–33. (Level III)

6. Labrie F, Belanger A, Cusan L, Gomez JL, Candas B. Marked decline in serum concentrations of adrenal C19 sex steroid precursors and conjugated androgen metabolites during aging. J Clin Endocrinol Metab 1997; 82:2396–402. (Level III)

7. Zumoff B, Strain GW, Miller LK, Rosner W. Twenty-four-hour mean plasma testosterone concentration declines with age in normal premenopausal women. J Clin Endocrinol Metab 1995;80:1429–30. (Level III)

8. Guzick DS, Hoeger K. Sex, hormones, and hysterectomies. N Engl J Med 2000;343:730–1. (Level III)

9. Jemal A, Siegel R, Ward E, Murray T, Xu J, Thun MJ. Cancer statistics, 2007. CA Cancer J Clin 2007;57:43–66. (Level III)

10. Sightler SE, Boike GM, Estape RE, Averette HE. Ovarian cancer in women with prior hysterectomy: a 14-year experience at the University of Miami. Obstet Gynecol 1991; 78:681–4. (Level III)

11. Piver MS. Prophylactic oophorectomy: reducing the U.S. death rate from epithelial ovarian cancer. A continuing debate. Oncologist 1996;1:326–30. (Level III)

12. Pal T, Permuth-Wey J, Betts JA, Krischer JP, Fiorica J, Arango H, et al. BRCA1 and BRCA2 mutations account for a large proportion of ovarian carcinoma cases. Cancer 2005;104:2807–16. (Level II-3)

13. Rebbeck TR, Lynch HT, Neuhausen SL, Narod SA, Van't Veer L, Garber JE, et al. Prophylactic oophorectomy in carriers of BRCA1 or BRCA2 mutations. Prevention and Observation of Surgical End Points Study Group. N Engl J Med 2002;346:1616–22. (Level II-2)

14. Risch HA, McLaughlin JR, Cole DE, Rosen B, Bradley L, Kwan E, et al. Prevalence and penetrance of germline BRCA1 and BRCA2 mutations in a population series of 649 women with ovarian cancer. Am J Hum Genet 2001;68:700–10. (Level II-3)

15. Whittemore AS, Harris R, Itnyre J. Characteristics relating to ovarian cancer risk: collaborative analysis of 12 US case-control studies. II. Invasive epithelial ovarian cancers in white women. Collaborative Ovarian Cancer Group. Am J Epidemiol 1992;136:1184–203. (Level III)

16. Anderson GL, Judd HL, Kaunitz AM, Barad DH, Beresford SA, Pettinger M, et al. Effects of estrogen plus progestin on gynecologic cancers and associated diagnostic procedures: the Women's Health Initiative randomized trial. Women's Health Initiative Investigators. JAMA 2003;290:1739–48. (Level I)

17. Rossing MA, Tang MT, Flagg EW, Weiss LK, Wicklund KG, Weiss NS. Body size and risk of epithelial ovarian cancer (United States). Cancer Causes Control 2006; 17:713–20. (Level II-2)

18. Kumle M, Weiderpass E, Braaten T, Adami HO, Lund E. Risk for invasive and borderline epithelial ovarian neoplasias following use of hormonal contraceptives: the Norwegian-Swedish Women's Lifestyle and Health Cohort Study. Norwegian-Swedish Women's Lifestyle and Health Cohort Study. Br J Cancer 2004;90:1386–91. (Level II-2)

19. Ness RB, Grisso JA, Vergona R, Klapper J, Morgan M, Wheeler JE. Oral contraceptives, other methods of contraception, and risk reduction for ovarian cancer. Study of Health and Reproduction (SHARE) Study Group. Epidemiology 2001;12:307–12. (Level II-2)

20. Narod SA, Risch H, Moslehi R, Dorum A, Neuhausen S, Olsson H, et al. Oral contraceptives and the risk of hereditary ovarian cancer. Hereditary Ovarian Cancer Clinical Study Group. N Engl J Med 1998;339:424–8. (Level II-2)

21. King MC, Marks JH, Mandell JB. Breast and ovarian cancer risks due to inherited mutations in BRCA1 and BRCA2. New York Breast Cancer Study Group. Science 2003;302:643–6. (Level II-3)

22. Ford D, Easton DF, Stratton M, Narod S, Goldgar D, Devilee P, et al. Genetic heterogeneity and penetrance analysis of the BRCA1 and BRCA2 genes in breast cancer families. The Breast Cancer Linkage Consortium. Am J Hum Genet 1998;62:676–89. (Level II-3)

23. Levy-Lahad E, Catane R, Eisenberg S, Kaufman B, Hornreich G, Lishinsky E, et al. Founder BRCA1 and BRCA2 mutations in Ashkenazi Jews in Israel: frequency and differential penetrance in ovarian cancer and in breast-ovarian cancer families. Am J Hum Genet 1997; 60:1059–67. (Level III)

24. Roa BB, Boyd AA, Volcik K, Richards CS. Ashkenazi Jewish population frequencies for common mutations in BRCA1 and BRCA2. Nat Genet 1996;14:185–7. (Level III)

25. Abeliovich D, Kaduri L, Lerer I, Weinberg N, Amir G, Sagi M, et al. The founder mutations 185delAG and 5382insC in BRCA1 and 6174delT in BRCA2 appear in 60% of ovarian cancer and 30% of early-onset breast cancer patients among Ashkenazi women. Am J Hum Genet 1997;60:505–14. (Level III)

26. Moslehi R, Chu W, Karlan B, Fishman D, Risch H, Fields A, et al. BRCA1 and BRCA2 mutation analysis of 208 Ashkenazi Jewish women with ovarian cancer. Am J Hum Genet 2000;66:1259–72. (Level II-2)

27. Vasen, HF, Watson P, Mecklin JP, Lynch HT. New clinical criteria for hereditary nonpolyposis colorectal cancer (HNPCC, Lynch syndrome) proposed by the International Collaborative group on HNPCC. Gastroenterology 1999;116:1453–6. (Level III)

28. Aarnio M, Sankila R, Pukkala E, Salovaara R, Aaltonen LA, de la Chapelle A, et al. Cancer risk in mutation carriers of DNA-mismatch-repair genes. Int J Cancer 1999; 81:214–8. (Level III)

29. Dunlop MG, Farrington SM, Carothers AD, Wyllie AH, Sharp L, Burn J, et al. Cancer risk associated with germline DNA mismatch repair gene mutations. Hum Mol Genet 1997;6:105–10. (Level III)

30. Coulam CB, Adamson SC, Annegers JF. Incidence of premature ovarian failure. Obstet Gynecol 1986;67:604–6. (Level II-2)

31. Colditz GA, Willett WC, Stampfer MJ, Rosner B, Speizer FE, Hennekens CH. Menopause and the risk of coronary heart disease in women. N Engl J Med 1987;316: 1105–10. (Level II-2)

32. Cooper GS, Ephross SA, Weinberg CR, Baird DD, Whelan EA, Sandler DP. Menstrual and reproductive risk factors for ischemic heart disease. Epidemiology 1999; 10:255–9. (Level II-3)

33. Mack WJ, Slater CC, Xiang M, Shoupe D, Lobo RA, Hodis HN. Elevated subclinical atherosclerosis associated with oophorectomy is related to time since menopause rather than type of menopause. Fertil Steril 2004;82: 391–7. (Level II-2)

34. Ossewaarde ME, Bots ML, Verbeek AL, Peeters PH, van der Graaf Y, Grobbee DE, et al. Age at menopause, cause-specific mortality and total life expectancy. Epidemiology 2005;16:556–62. (Level II-2)

35. Stampfer MJ, Colditz GA, Willett WC. Menopause and heart disease. A review. Ann N Y Acad Sci 1990;592: 193–203; discussion 257–62. (Level III)

36. van Der Voort DJ, van Der Weijer PH, Barentsen R. Early menopause: increased fracture risk at older age. Osteoporos Int 2003;14:525–30. (Level II-3)

37. Rocca WA, Bower JH, Maraganore DM, Ahlskog JE, Grossardt BR, de Andrade M, et al. Increased risk of parkinsonism in women who underwent oophorectomy before menopause. Neurology, August 29, 2007. DOI: 10.1212/01.wnl.0000280573.30975.6a. (Level II-2)

38. Rocca WA, Bower JH, Maraganore DM, Ahlskog JE, Grossardt BR, de Andrade M, et al. Increased risk of cognitive impairment or dementia in women who underwent oophorectomy before menopause. Neurology 2007;69:1074–83. (Level II-2)

39. Jansen SC, Temme EH, Schouten EG. Lifetime estrogen exposure versus age at menopause as mortality predictor. Maturitas 2002;43:105–12. (Level II-2)

40. Rocca WA, Grossardt BR, de Andrade M, Malkasian GD, Melton LJ 3rd. Survival patterns after oophorectomy in premenopausal women: a population-based cohort study. Lancet Oncol 2006;7:821–8. (Level II-2)

41. Parker WH, Broder MS, Liu Z, Shoupe D, Farquhar C, Berek JS. Ovarian conservation at the time of hysterectomy for benign disease. Obstet Gynecol 2005;106:219–26. (Level III)

42. Anderson GL, Limacher M, Assaf AR, Bassford T, Beresford SA, Black H, et al. Effects of conjugated equine estrogen in postmenopausal women with hysterectomy: the Women's Health Initiative randomized controlled trial. Women's Health Initiative Steering Committee. JAMA 2004;291:1701–12. (Level I)

43. Manson JE, Allison MA, Rossouw JE, Carr JJ, Langer RD, Hsia J, et al. Estrogen therapy and coronary-artery calcification. WHI and WHI-CACS Investigators. N Engl J Med 2007;356:2591–602. (Level I)

44. Barrett-Connor E, Young R, Notelovitz M, Sullivan J, Wiita B, Yang HM, et al. A two-year, double-blind comparison of estrogen-androgen and conjugated estrogens in surgically menopausal women. Effects on bone mineral density, symptoms and lipid profiles. J Reprod Med 1999;44:1012–20. (Level I)

45. Davis SR, McCloud P, Strauss BJ, Burger H. Testosterone enhances estradiol's effects on postmenopausal bone density and sexuality. Maturitas 1995;21:227–36. (Level I)

46. Raisz LG, Wiita B, Artis A, Bowen A, Schwartz S, Trahiotis M, et al. Comparison of the effects of estrogen alone and estrogen plus androgen on biochemical markers of bone formation and resorption in postmenopausal women. J Clin Endocrinol Metab 1996;81:37–43. (Level I)

47. Shifren JL, Braunstein GD, Simon JA, Casson PR, Buster JE, Redmond GP, et al. Transdermal testosterone treatment in women with impaired sexual function after oophorectomy. N Engl J Med 2000;343:682–8. (Level II-3)

48. Dennerstein L, Koochaki P, Barton I, Graziottin A. Hypoactive sexual desire disorder in menopausal women: a survey of Western European women. J Sex Med 2006;3:212–22. (Level II-3)

49. Aziz A, Bergquist C, Brannstrom M, Nordholm L, Silfverstolpe G. Differences in aspects of personality and sexuality between perimenopausal women making different choices regarding prophylactic oophorectomy at elective hysterectomy. Acta Obstet Gynecol Scand 2005;84:854–9. (Level II-3)

50. Chlebowski RT, Hendrix SL, Langer RD, Stefanick ML, Gass M, Lane D, et al. Influence of estrogen plus progestin on breast cancer and mammography in healthy postmenopausal women: the Women's Health Initiative Randomized Trial. WHI Investigators. JAMA 2003;289:3243–53. (Level I)

51. Tamimi RM, Hankinson SE, Chen WY, Rosner B, Colditz GA. Combined estrogen and testosterone use and risk of breast cancer in postmenopausal women. Arch Intern Med 2006;166:1483–9. (Level II-2)

52. U.S. Preventive Services Task Force. Genetic risk assessment and BRCA mutation testing for breast and ovarian cancer susceptibility: recommendation statement. Ann Intern Med 2005;143:355–61. (Level III)

53. Hartmann LC, Sellers TA, Schaid DJ, Frank TS, Soderberg CL, Sitta DL, et al. Efficacy of bilateral prophylactic mastectomy in *BRCA1* and *BRCA2* gene mutation carriers. J Natl Cancer Inst 2001;93:1633–7. (Level III)

54. Kuhl CK, Schmutzler RK, Leutner CC, Kempe A, Wardelmann E, Hocke A, et al. Breast MR imaging screening in 192 women proved or suspected to be carriers of a breast cancer susceptibility gene: preliminary results. Radiology 2000;215:267–79. (Level II-3)

55. Leach MO, Boggis CR, Dixon AK, Easton DF, Eeles RA, Evans DG, et al. Screening with magnetic resonance imaging and mammography of a UK population at high familial risk of breast cancer: a prospective multicentre cohort study (MARIBS). MARIBS study group [published erratum appears in Lancet 2005;365:1848]. Lancet 2005;365:1769–78. (Level II-3)

56. Warner E, Plewes DB, Hill KA, Causer PA, Zubovits JT, Jong RA, et al. Surveillance of *BRCA1* and *BRCA2* mutation carriers with magnetic resonance imaging, ultrasound, mammography, and clinical breast examination. JAMA 2004;292:1317–25. (Level II-3)

57. Lindor NM, Petersen GM, Hadley DW, Kinney AY, Miesfeldt S, Lu KH, et al. Recommendations for the care of individuals with an inherited predisposition to Lynch syndrome: a systematic review. JAMA 2006;296:1507–17. (Level III)

58. Finch A, Beiner M, Lubinski J, Lynch HT, Moller P, Rosen B, et al. Salpingo-oophorectomy and the risk of ovarian, fallopian tube, and peritoneal cancers in women with a *BRCA1* or *BRCA2* mutation. Hereditary Ovarian Cancer Clinical Study Group. JAMA 2006;296:185–92. (Level II-2)

59. Olivier RI, van Beurden M, Lubsen MA, Rookus MA, Mooij TM, van de Vijver MJ, et al. Clinical outcome of prophylactic oophorectomy in *BRCA1/BRCA2* mutation carriers and events during follow-up. Br J Cancer 2004;90:1492–7. (Level III)

60. Schmeler KM, Lynch HT, Chen LM, Munsell MF, Soliman PT, Clark MB, et al. Prophylactic surgery to reduce the risk of gynecologic cancers in the Lynch syndrome. N Engl J Med 2006;354:261–9. (Level II-2)

61. Kauff ND, Mitra N, Robson ME, Hurley KE, Chuai S, Goldfrank D, et al. Risk of ovarian cancer in *BRCA1* and *BRCA2* mutation-negative hereditary breast cancer families. J Natl Cancer Inst 2005;97:1382–4. (Level II-3)

62. Ford D, Easton DF, Bishop DT, Narod SA, Goldgar DE. Risks of cancer in *BRCA1*-mutation carriers. Breast Cancer Linkage Consortium. Lancet 1994;343:692–5. (Level III)

63. Haffty BG, Harrold E, Khan AJ, Pathare P, Smith TE, Turner BC, et al. Outcome of conservatively managed early-onset breast cancer by BRCA1/2 status. Lancet 2002;359:1471–7. (Level II-3)

64. Emens LA, Davidson NE. Adjuvant hormonal therapy for premenopausal women with breast cancer. Clin Cancer Res 2003;9(suppl):486S–94S. (Level III)

65. Bines J, Oleske DM, Cobleigh MA. Ovarian function in premenopausal women treated with adjuvant chemotherapy for breast cancer. J Clin Oncol 1996;14:1718–29. (Level III)

66. Aebi S, Gelber S, Castiglione-Gertsch M, Gelber RD, Collins J, Thurlimann B, et al. Is chemotherapy alone adequate for young women with oestrogen-receptor-positive breast cancer? Lancet 2000;355:1869–74. (Level II-2)

67. Michaud LB, Buzdar AU. Complete estrogen blockade for the treatment of metastatic and early stage breast cancer. Drugs Aging 2000;16:261–71. (Level III)

68. Pritchard KI. Endocrine therapy of advanced disease: analysis and implications of the existing data. Clin Cancer Res 2003;9(suppl):460S–7S. (Level III)

69. Winer EP, Hudis C, Burstein HJ, Wolff AC, Pritchard KI, Ingle JN, et al. American Society of Clinical Oncology technology assessment on the use of aromatase inhibitors as adjuvant therapy for postmenopausal women with hormone receptor-positive breast cancer: status report 2004. J Clin Oncol 2005;23:619–29. (Level III)

70. Rebbeck TR, Friebel T, Wagner T, Lynch HT, Garber JE, Daly MB, et al. Effect of short-term hormone replacement therapy on breast cancer risk reduction after bilateral prophylactic oophorectomy in *BRCA1* and *BRCA2* mutation carriers: the PROSE Study Group. PROSE Study Group. J Clin Oncol 2005;23:7804–10. (Level II-2)

71. Boyd J, Sonoda Y, Federici MG, Bogomolniy F, Rhei E, Maresco DL, et al. Clinicopathologic features of BRCA-linked and sporadic ovarian cancer. JAMA 2000;283:2260–5. (Level II-2)

72. Stratton JF, Thompson D, Bobrow L, Dalal N, Gore M, Bishop DT, et al. The genetic epidemiology of early-onset epithelial ovarian cancer: a population-based study. Am J Hum Genet 1999;65:1725–32. (Level II-2)

73. Eisen A, Lubinski J, Klijn J, Moller P, Lynch HT, Offit K, et al. Breast cancer risk following bilateral oophorectomy in *BRCA1* and *BRCA2* mutation carriers: an international case-control study. J Clin Oncol 2005;23:7491–6. (Level II-2)

74. Watson P, Butzow R, Lynch HT, Mecklin JP, Jarvinen HJ, Vasen HF, et al. The clinical features of ovarian cancer in hereditary nonpolyposis colorectal cancer. International Collaborative Group on HNPCC. Gynecol Oncol 2001; 82:223–8. (Level III)

75. Colgan TJ, Murphy J, Cole DE, Narod S, Rosen B. Occult carcinoma in prophylactic oophorectomy specimens: prevalence and association with BRCA germline mutation status. Am J Surg Pathol 2001;25:1283–9. (Level III)

76. Finch A, Shaw P, Rosen B, Murphy J, Narod SA, Colgan TJ. Clinical and pathologic findings of prophylactic salpingo-oophorectomies in 159 BRCA1 and BRCA2 carriers. Gynecol Oncol 2006;100:58–64. (Level III)

77. Lamb JD, Garcia RL, Goff BA, Paley PJ, Swisher EM. Predictors of occult neoplasia in women undergoing risk-reducing salpingo-oophorectomy. Am J Obstet Gynecol 2006;194:1702–9. (Level III)

78. Lu KH, Garber JE, Cramer DW, Welch WR, Niloff J, Schrag D, et al. Occult ovarian tumors in women with BRCA1 or BRCA2 mutations undergoing prophylactic oophorectomy. J Clin Oncol 2000;18:2728–32. (Level III)

79. Powell CB, Kenley E, Chen LM, Crawford B, McLennan J, Zaloudek C, et al. Risk-reducing salpingo-oophorectomy in BRCA mutation carriers: role of serial sectioning in the detection of occult malignancy. J Clin Oncol 2005;23:127–32. (Level III)

80. Carcangiu ML, Peissel B, Pasini B, Spatti G, Radice P, Manoukian S. Incidental carcinomas in prophylactic specimens in BRCA1 and BRCA2 germ-line mutation carriers, with emphasis on fallopian tube lesions: report of 6 cases and review of the literature. Am J Surg Pathol 2006;30:1222–30. (Level III)

81. Levine DA, Lin O, Barakat RR, Robson ME, McDermott D, Cohen L, et al. Risk of endometrial carcinoma associated with BRCA mutation. Gynecol Oncol 2001;80:395–8. (Level II-3)

82. Cass I, Holschneider C, Datta N, Barbuto D, Walts AE, Karlan BY. BRCA-mutation-associated fallopian tube carcinoma: a distinct clinical phenotype? Obstet Gynecol 2005;106:1327–34. (Level III)

The MEDLINE database, the Cochrane Library, and ACOG's own internal resources and documents were used to conduct a literature search to locate relevant articles published between January 1985 and June 2007. The search was restricted to articles published in the English language. Priority was given to articles reporting results of original research, although review articles and commentaries also were consulted. Abstracts of research presented at symposia and scientific conferences were not considered adequate for inclusion in this document. Guidelines published by organizations or institutions such as the National Institutes of Health and the American College of Obstetricians and Gynecologists were reviewed, and additional studies were located by reviewing bibliographies of identified articles. When reliable research was not available, expert opinions from obstetrician–gynecologists were used.

Studies were reviewed and evaluated for quality according to the method outlined by the U.S. Preventive Services Task Force:

I   Evidence obtained from at least one properly designed randomized controlled trial.
II-1 Evidence obtained from well-designed controlled trials without randomization.
II-2 Evidence obtained from well-designed cohort or case–control analytic studies, preferably from more than one center or research group.
II-3 Evidence obtained from multiple time series with or without the intervention. Dramatic results in uncontrolled experiments also could be regarded as this type of evidence.
III Opinions of respected authorities, based on clinical experience, descriptive studies, or reports of expert committees.

Based on the highest level of evidence found in the data, recommendations are provided and graded according to the following categories:

Level A—Recommendations are based on good and consistent scientific evidence.

Level B—Recommendations are based on limited or inconsistent scientific evidence.

Level C—Recommendations are based primarily on consensus and expert opinion.

ISSN 1099-3630

The American College of Obstetricians and Gynecologists
409 12th Street, SW, PO Box 96920, Washington, DC 20090-6920

Elective and risk-reducing salpingo-oophorectomy. ACOG Practice Bulletin No. 89. American College of Obstetricians and Gynecologists. Obstet Gynecol 2008;111:231–41.

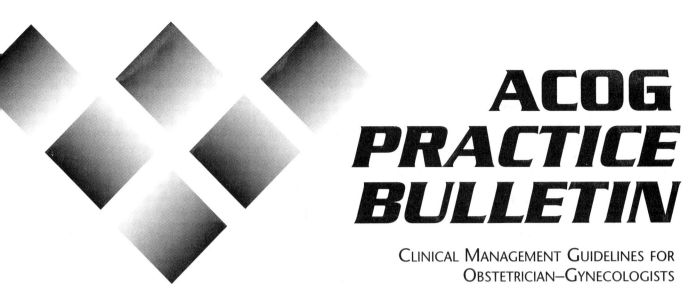

ACOG PRACTICE BULLETIN

CLINICAL MANAGEMENT GUIDELINES FOR
OBSTETRICIAN–GYNECOLOGISTS
NUMBER 91, MARCH 2008

This Practice Bulletin was developed by the ACOG Committee on Practice Bulletins— Gynecology with the assistance of Jeanne Sheffield, MD. The information is designed to aid practitioners in making decisions about appropriate obstetric and gynecologic care. These guidelines should not be construed as dictating an exclusive course of treatment or procedure. Variations in practice may be warranted based on the needs of the individual patient, resources, and limitations unique to the institution or type of practice.

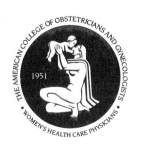

Treatment of Urinary Tract Infections in Nonpregnant Women

An estimated 11% of U.S. women report at least one physician-diagnosed urinary tract infection (UTI) per year, and the lifetime probability that a woman will have a UTI is 60% (1, 2). Despite the frequency of UTIs, there is confusion about diagnostic strategies, and changes in antimicrobial resistance among uropathogens require alterations in traditional treatment regimens. The purpose of this bulletin is to address the diagnosis, treatment, and prevention of uncomplicated acute bacterial cystitis and acute bacterial pyelonephritis in nonpregnant women. Complicated UTIs (eg, in patients with diabetes mellitus, abnormal anatomy, prior urologic surgery, a history of renal stones, an indwelling catheter, spinal cord injury, immunocompromise, or in pregnant patients) are a heterogeneous group of conditions beyond the scope of this bulletin.

Background

Definitions

Urinary tract infections are among the most common bacterial infections in adults and may involve the lower or upper urinary tract or both. *Asymptomatic bacteriuria* refers to considerable bacteriuria in a woman with no symptoms. When the infection is limited to the lower urinary tract and occurs with symptoms of dysuria and frequent and urgent urination and, occasionally, suprapubic tenderness, it is termed *cystitis*. *Acute pyelonephritis* is defined as infection of the renal parenchyma and pelvicaliceal system accompanied by significant bacteriuria, usually occurring with fever and flank pain. Recurrent UTI with the same organism after adequate therapy is termed a *relapse*. *Reinfection* is a recurrent UTI caused by bacteria previously isolated after treatment and a negative intervening urine culture result or a recurrent UTI caused by a second isolate.

Prevalence and Epidemiology

The burden from UTIs on both the clinical and financial aspects of health care in the United State is immense. Approximately 62.7 million adults aged 20 years and older have reported at least one episode of a UTI or cystitis (3), 50.8 million (81%) of whom were women. In 2000, there were an estimated 11 million office and outpatient hospital visits by patients aged 20 years and older with a UTI (approximately 9 million visits by women). The cost to the health care system in 2000 was estimated to be 3.5 billion dollars for evaluation and treatment (2, 3). More than one half of women will have at least one UTI during their lifetime (1), and 3–5% of all women will have multiple recurrences (4). The prevalence of asymptomatic bacteriuria also is higher in women than men; 5–6 % in young, sexually active, nonpregnant women, compared with less than 0.1% in young men. The prevalence increases to 20% in women older than 65 years (5).

Pathophysiology and Microbiology

Urinary tract infections result from interactions between host biologic and behavioral factors and microorganism virulence. Most cases are caused by ascending infection from the urethra into the bladder. The female urethra is short, and the external one third is often colonized by pathogens from normal vaginal and enteric flora. Bacteria travel up the urethra during urethral massage, sexual intercourse, or mechanical instrumentation. Once in the bladder, bacterial factors play a major role in colonization and infection. Although UTIs are caused by many species of microorganisms, most (80–90%) are caused by uropathogenic *Escherichia coli* (predominantly O, K, and H antigen serotypes) (1, 4–6). These *E coli* serogroups have a number of virulence factors that facilitate colonization and invasion of the vagina and urinary tract. Specific virulence factors, such as Type 1 fimbria, P-fimbria, and S-fimbria, enhance binding to vaginal and uroepithelial cells. Virulence factors also increase resistance to serum bactericidal activity and resistance to host phagocytic activity. Certain *E coli* subgroups also are associated with ascending infection into the renal parenchyma, causing pyelonephritis (predominantly P-fimbriated *E coli*).

The remaining 10–20% of UTIs are caused by other microorganisms, occasionally colonizing the vagina and periurethral area (1, 4–6). *Staphylococcus saprophyticus* frequently causes lower UTIs and has been isolated in 3% of nonpregnant, sexually active, reproductive-aged women with pyelonephritis (7). *Proteus, Pseudomonas, Klebsiella,* and *Enterobacter* species all have been isolated in women with cystitis or pyelonephritis, and these frequently are associated with structural abnormalities of the urinary tract, indwelling catheters, and renal calculi (5, 6). *Enterococcus* species also have been isolated in women with structural abnormalities. Gram-positive isolates, including group B streptococci, are increasingly isolated along with fungal infections in women with indwelling catheters (6). Anaerobic organisms and mycoplasmas are uncommonly isolated from UTIs and probably have a minor role in urinary tract pathogenesis.

Although ascending infection is the predominant route of infection in the urinary tract, occasionally infection may arise from hematogenous or lymphatic spread. Bloodborne pathogens may seed the renal parenchyma during episodes of bacteremia. Renal abscesses may arise from bacterial endocarditis bacteremia from *Staphylococcus aureus*. Rare cases of pyelonephritis, caused by fungemia from *Candida* species in hospitalized patients, have been reported. Although lymphatic connections are present along the ureters and kidneys and reverse lymphatic flow into the kidneys has been reported, lymphatic spread of microorganisms leading to UTI is rare (8).

Risk Factors

Risk factors for UTI in women vary among the different age groups. In school-aged girls, common risk factors include congenital abnormalities and new onset of sexual activity. Risk factors for premenopausal and postmenopausal women are listed in the box. With advancing age, the rate of UTI increases, likely because of the hypoestrogenic state and vaginal epithelium atrophy, impaired voiding, and changes in hygiene (7, 9). A lifetime history of UTIs also is an important predictor of UTIs in postmenopausal women (10).

Diagnosis

Clinical History and Examination

Acute bacterial cystitis usually presents clinically as dysuria, with symptoms of frequent and urgent urination, secondary to irritation of the urethral and bladder mucosa. Women also may experience suprapubic pain or pressure and rarely have hematuria. Fever is uncommon in women with uncomplicated lower UTI. Acute urethritis secondary to infection from *Neisseria gonorrhoeae* and *Chlamydia trachomatis* or pain secondary to genital herpes simplex virus type 1 and herpes simplex virus type 2 may occur with similar clinical symptoms and should be ruled out.

In contrast, upper UTI or acute pyelonephritis frequently occurs with a combination of fever and chills, flank pain, and varying degrees of dysuria, urgency, and frequency. Severe flank pain radiating to the groin is

---

Risk Factors For Urinary Tract Infection in Premenopausal and Postmenopausal Women

Premenopausal Women

- History of urinary tract infection
- Frequent or recent sexual activity
- Diaphragm contraception use
- Use of spermicidal agents
- Increasing parity
- Diabetes mellitus
- Obesity
- Sickle cell trait
- Anatomic congenital abnormalities
- Urinary tract calculi
- Neurologic disorders or medical conditions requiring indwelling or repetitive bladder catheterization

Postmenopausal Women

- Vaginal atrophy
- Incomplete bladder emptying
- Poor perineal hygiene
- Rectocele, cystocele, urethrocele, or uterovaginal prolapse
- Lifetime history of urinary tract infection
- Type 1 diabetes mellitus

---

more indicative of renal calculi. Occasionally, renal pain may radiate to other abdominal areas, necessitating evaluation for cholelithiasis, cholecystitis, pelvic inflammatory disease, gastric ulcers, and appendicitis. Older women with UTI may be asymptomatic, present moribund from septic shock (urosepsis), have symptoms only of urinary incontinence, or have any combination of these symptoms.

Laboratory Evaluation

Bacteriuria is diagnosed using a clean-voided midstream urine sample. Traditionally, 100,000 single isolate bacteria per milliliter has been used to define significant bacteriuria, with excellent specificity, but a sensitivity of 50% (1). To diagnose bacteriuria, decreasing the colony count to 1,000–10,000 bacteria per milliliter in symptomatic patients will improve the sensitivity without significantly compromising specificity. Urine dipstick testing for leukocyte esterase or nitrite is a rapid and inexpensive method with a sensitivity of 75% and specificity of 82% (1, 11). It is a good screening test, but women with negative test results and symptoms should still have

a urine culture or urinalysis or both performed because false-negative results are common. A standard urinalysis will detect pyuria, defined as 10 leukocytes per milliliter, but pyuria alone is not a reliable predictor of infection. However, pyuria and bacteriuria together on microscopic examination results markedly increases the probability of UTI. The use of a postvoid residual volume measure, urodynamic testing, cystourethroscopy, or radiologic imaging is not cost-effective in women unless they have evidence of a complicated infection or renal calculi. These are rarely necessary to diagnose acute uncomplicated cystitis and pyelonephritis.

Antimicrobial Resistance

A major consequence of indiscriminate prescribing practices of common antibiotics is the emergence of antimicrobial resistance. Data from areas reporting antimicrobial susceptibility profiles have shown an alarming increase in the prevalence of resistance to amoxicillin and trimethoprim–sulfamethoxazole, as high as 30% in some populations (12, 13). Particularly for acute pyelonephritis, urine culture and susceptibility testing can help tailor antimicrobial choices. If available, local community or hospital surveillance data should be reviewed to guide empirical therapy for UTIs. These data should be periodically updated as susceptibility patterns change over time. Resistance rates higher than 15–20% necessitate a change in antibiotic class.

General Principles of Treatment

Uncomplicated Acute Bacterial Cystitis

In the past, uncomplicated acute cystitis has been treated with 7–10 days of antimicrobial therapy. However, recent data have shown that 3 days of therapy is equivalent in efficacy to longer duration of therapy, with eradication rates exceeding 90%. Recommended agents for the 3-day therapy are detailed in the next section and in Table 1. Of note, β-lactams, such as first-generation cephalosporins and amoxicillin, are less effective in the treatment of uncomplicated acute cystitis than those antimicrobials listed in Table 1. This is because of increasing resistance among the common uropathogens, rapid excretion from the urinary tract, and the inability to completely clear gram-negative rods from the vagina, increasing the risk for recurrence (5, 14).

Acute Pyelonephritis

Acute pyelonephritis traditionally has been treated with hospitalization and parenteral antibiotics. However, there has been a recent shift to outpatient management, when possible, with an emphasis on cost-savings,

Table 1. Treatment Regimens for Uncomplicated Acute Bacterial Cystitis

Antimicrobial Agent	Dose	Adverse Events
Trimethoprim–sulfamethoxazole	One tablet (160 mg trimethoprim–800 mg sulfamethoxazole), twice daily for 3 days	Fever, rash, photosensitivity, neutropenia, thrombocytopenia, anorexia, nausea and vomiting, pruritus, headache, urticaria, Stevens–Johnson syndrome, and toxic epidermal necrosis
Trimethoprim	100 mg, twice daily for 3 days	Rash, pruritus, photosensitivity, exfoliative dermatitis, Stevens–Johnson syndrome, toxic epidermal necrosis, and aseptic meningitis
Ciprofloxacin	250 mg, twice daily for 3 days	Rash, confusion, seizures, restlessness, headache, severe hypersensitivity, hypoglycemia, hyperglycemia, and Achilles tendon rupture (in patients older than 60 years)
Levofloxacin	250 mg, once daily for 3 days	Same as for ciprofloxacin
Norfloxacin	400 mg, twice daily for 3 days	Same as for ciprofloxacin
Gatifloxacin	200 mg, once daily for 3 days	Same as for ciprofloxacin
Nitrofurantoin macrocrystals	50–100 mg, four times daily for 7 days	Anorexia, nausea, vomiting, hypersensitivity, peripheral neuropathy, hepatitis, hemolytic anemia, and pulmonary reactions
Nitrofurantoin monohydrate macrocrystals	100 mg, twice daily for 7 days	Same as for nitrofurantoin macrocrystals
Fosfomycin tromethamine	3 g dose (powder) single dose	Diarrhea, nausea, vomiting, rash, and hypersensitivity

although this management scheme is based on results from few large treatment trials (14). In otherwise healthy women who are clinically stable and able to tolerate oral antimicrobial agents and fluids, outpatient management is acceptable and has similar efficacy (14). The reliability of the patient and the social situation also should be taken into account when determining inpatient versus outpatient management. A urine culture is performed and empiric antibiotic therapy initiated as detailed in the next section. As in acute cystitis, β-lactams are not first-line therapy in most cases. There is a high rate of ampicillin resistance in organisms causing pyelonephritis and a high rate of recurrence in those women treated with β-lactams. The exception to this is if a gram-positive organism is the causative agent. Amoxicillin or amoxicillin combined with clavulanic acid may then be used. Regardless of management scheme, 14 days of oral or parenteral antibiotics or both is now standard, with cure rates approaching 100%. Outcomes after a 2-week course are equivalent to the traditional 6-week parenteral course, with no differences in recurrence rates. A substantial clinical response should be evident by 48–72 hours after initiating therapy. A urine culture test of cure usually is performed when the 2-week course of antibiotics is completed.

Recurrent Urinary Tract Infection

Recurrent UTIs are common in women, occurring in up to 25–50% within 1 year of initial infection. Of all women, 3–5% will have multiple recurrences over many years (1, 4). Management of recurrent UTIs should start with a search for known risk factors associated with recurrence. These include frequent intercourse, long-term spermicide use, diaphragm use, a new sexual partner, young age at first UTI, and a maternal history of UTI (15, 16). Behavioral changes, such as using a different form of contraception instead of spermicide, should be advised. Antimicrobial treatment of recurrent UTIs is based on patient desire and frequency of recurrences. A 3-day course of one of the antimicrobial regimens listed in Table 1 is started to clear the infection. A urine culture test of cure 1–2 weeks later to confirm clearance is suggested.

For women with frequent recurrences, continuous prophylaxis with once-daily treatment with nitrofurantoin, norfloxacin, ciprofloxacin, trimethoprim, trimethoprim–sulfamethoxazole, or another agent listed in Table 1 has been shown to decrease the risk of recurrence by 95% (4). This can be continued for 6–12 months and then reassessed. Women with recurrences associated with sexual activity may benefit from postcoital prophylaxis—a single dose of one of the agents listed in Table 1, taken after sexual intercourse, is effective in decreasing recurrences (1, 17, 18).

Urinary Tract Infections in Postmenopausal Women

Antimicrobial therapy for UTIs in postmenopausal women is influenced by a number of factors. The organisms causing UTIs in this population differ from the causative agents in younger women. *Staphylococcus saprophyticus* rarely is isolated; however, gram-negative bacteria and enterococci are common (*E coli* remains the most common causative organism). Pharmacokinetic and pharmacodynamic changes also influence medication choices to limit drug toxicity and interactions (19, 20). Despite these differences, few studies have adequately evaluated treatment options in these women. In a meta-analysis that evaluated 13 trials, including a total of 1,435 older women with UTIs, it was concluded that 3–6 days of antibiotic treatment was equivalent to longer courses of treatment (7–14 days), with fewer adverse events (20). Single-dose therapy was not as effective as longer treatment regimens and should not be used. Another randomized, controlled trial assessing the optimal duration of antibiotic therapy for uncomplicated UTIs in women aged 65 years or older concluded that the 3-day regimen was equally effective but better tolerated than a 7-day course (21).

Patient-Initiated Therapy

Many women with recurrent UTIs are aware of symptom onset. As the cost of office and hospital emergency room visits continues to increase, patient-initiated therapy has become a viable option for treatment. Women are given a prescription for one of the 3-day dosage regimens listed in Table 1 and should be instructed to start therapy when symptoms develop. Some clinicians also will give the women urine dipsticks and use pyuria as well as symptoms as an indication to initiate treatment. If symptoms do not improve in 48 hours, clinical evaluation should be performed. Patient-initiated therapy has been found to be safe, effective, and economical (22–24).

Clinical Considerations and Recommendations

▶ *Is empiric treatment of urinary tract infection without performing urinalysis appropriate?*

It is a common practice among primary care physicians to empirically treat women with symptoms of a lower UTI without performing laboratory analyses. It has been considered a cost-effective strategy, decreasing the number of diagnostic tests and office visits (25, 26). However, many women, especially postmenopausal women, without a laboratory-proven UTI have symptoms of intermittent dysuria or urgent or frequent urination. Empiric treatment of these women leads to unnecessary antibiotic use and the development of antimicrobial resistance. Testing for pyuria, by urinalysis or by uri-

nary dipstick testing, improves the likelihood of identifying infection by 25% or more (1, 27–29). Thus, in women without a history of a laboratory-confirmed UTI, an office visit for urinalysis or dipstick testing is appropriate. Women with frequent recurrences and prior confirmation by diagnostic tests who are aware of their symptoms may be empirically treated without recurrent testing for pyuria.

▶ *When is urine culture necessary?*

The initial treatment of a symptomatic lower UTI with pyuria or bacteriuria does not require a urine culture. However, if clinical improvement does not occur within 48 hours or in the case of recurrence, a urine culture is useful to help tailor treatment. A urine culture should be performed in all cases of upper UTIs.

▶ *In what situations do patients require further evaluation?*

Imaging of the urinary tract rarely is required in women—it is not cost-effective nor does it provide useful information in the setting of uncomplicated lower or upper UTIs. Women with infections that do not respond to appropriate antimicrobial therapy or in whom the clinical status worsens require further evaluation. Renal ultrasonography is the best noninvasive method to evaluate renal collecting system obstruction. An intravenous pyelography also may be useful in this situation. Contrast-enhanced computed tomography or magnetic resonance imaging is useful to obtain an image of the renal parenchyma in order to rule out a perinephric abscess or phlegmon.

▶ *How should uncomplicated acute bacterial cystitis in women be treated?*

A 3-day antimicrobial regimen is now the recommended treatment for uncomplicated acute bacterial cystitis in women, with bacterial eradication rates consistently higher than 90%. Table 1 lists the current recommended regimens for treatment, both 3-day and 7-day courses. Use of trimethoprim–sulfamethoxazole for 3 days is considered the preferred therapy, with a 94% bacterial eradication rate. However, in areas where resistance to this antimicrobial agent exceeds 15–20%, another one of the listed regimens should be chosen. The other medications that have shown equivalency include trimethoprim alone, ciprofloxacin, levofloxacin, norfloxacin, and gatifloxacin. The fluoroquinolones, although highly effective, should not be used as a first-line agent in areas where resistance prevalence to trimethoprim–sulfamethoxazole is low—currently resistance to the fluoroquinolones is uncommon, and overuse will likely hinder the ability to effectively use this class of antimicrobials in patients with complicated UTIs and those patients with respiratory and other non–urinary tract infections. Most experts now agree that use of sulfonamides, ampicillin, and amoxicillin is less effective than use of trimethoprim–sulfamethoxazole and the fluoroquinolones (see previous section) and should not be used as first-line therapy.

Use of nitrofurantoin, a drug frequently used in the pregnant population, is not well studied in nonpregnant women with acute cystitis. It is not recommended for use in a 3-day regimen but has been found to be effective in a 7-day antimicrobial regimen and is listed in Table 1. Resistance to nitrofurantoin remains low (less than 5%) (1). The low prevalence of resistance and its ability to concentrate in urine continue to make nitrofurantoin a useful medication in the treatment of uncomplicated cystitis, particularly in areas where resistance rates to the first-line medications are high. It is ineffective against *Proteus mirabilis*. Of note, nitrofurantoin can rarely induce hemolytic anemia in patients with glucose-6-phosphate dehydrogenase deficiency, and use should be avoided in these patients (30). Compared with the nitrofurantoin macrocrystal formulation, which requires frequent dosing (four times per day) and has a high likelihood of gastrointestinal side effects, monohydrate macrocrystal formu-lation is given twice daily, so side effects occur less frequently.

▶ *How should uncomplicated acute pyelonephritis be treated?*

Women who present with acute pyelonephritis should have an initial urine culture and susceptibility testing before the initiation of antimicrobial therapy. Intravenous hydration should be started while the clinical assessment is being performed. Women who are severely ill, have complications, are unable to tolerate oral medications or fluids, or who the clinician suspects will be noncompliant with outpatient therapy should be hospitalized and receive empiric broad-spectrum parenteral antibiotics. Knowledge of specific antimicrobial resistance in the community should influence the choice of initial antimicrobial agent. Once the urine and susceptibility culture results are available, therapy is altered as needed. Most women can be treated on an outpatient basis initially or given intravenous fluids and one parenteral dose of an antibiotic before being discharged and given a regimen of oral therapy.

The initial antimicrobial regimen is empiric. If a gram-positive organism is identified on a Gram stain, amoxicillin or ampicillin are acceptable treatment choices. Gram-positive organisms in clusters (probable Staphylococci) maybe treated initially with cephalosporin. In all other

cases, β-lactam agents no longer are recommended (14). First-line therapy now is use of a fluoroquinolone for 14 days. In areas where resistance rates are low, trimethoprim–sulfamethoxazole use is an acceptable alternative (31). For women with severe illness or urosepsis who require hospitalization, the broad-spectrum parenteral antibiotics available include aminoglycosides plus ampicillin, piperacillin or first-generation cephalosporins, aztreonam, third-generation cephalosporins, piperacillin-tazobactam, or parenteral fluoroquinolones used alone or in combination, depending on the individual case. In all cases of acute pyelonephritis, whether the patient is treated on an inpatient or outpatient basis, 14 days of total antimicrobial therapy should be completed. Treatment of severe complications associated with pyelonephritis, such as septic shock, acute respiratory distress syndrome, and multiorgan failure, is beyond the scope of this bulletin.

A notable clinical response should be evident by 48–72 hours. If no improvement is noted or if the patient's status worsens, it may be necessary to change therapy based on results of available susceptibility testing of the initial isolate. Routine imaging studies are not recommended in women with uncomplicated acute pyelonephritis.

▶ *Is single-dose therapy as effective as therapy of longer duration for uncomplicated acute bacterial cystitis?*

Antimicrobials recommended for single-dose therapy produce inhibitory concentrations of antibiotics for 12–24 hours. The benefits of a single-dose course include cost, directly observed therapy so compliance is not an issue, fewer side effects, and a potentially decreased chance of resistance. If used, single-dose therapy should be reserved for young, sexually active women with a normal urinary tract who have had symptoms for no more than 1 week. However, single-dose therapy generally is considered less effective than the same antimicrobials used in a 3-day course of treatment with regards to bacterial eradication and clinical cure rates (14, 20, 32, 33). In a few recent trials that evaluated the use of single-dose gatifloxacin, fosfomycin tromethamine, rufloxacin, and pefloxacin, early promise has been shown, using clinical cure rates as the outcome measure, but questions of adverse side effects and higher recurrence rates necessitate further study (14, 34, 35).

▶ *How effective are interventions to prevent recurrence of cystitis?*

The first-line intervention for the prevention of the recurrence of cystitis is prophylactic or intermittent antimicrobial therapy, as discussed previously. Recurrences are prevented in 95% of cases (4). However, multiple other nonmedical and medical interventions have been suggested. There is little evidence that aggressive hydration to prevent recurrences has any major effect, and this practice can theoretically worsen urinary retention issues, decrease urinary pH affecting the antibacterial activity of urine itself, and dilute antimicrobial concentrations in the urinary tract. It currently is not recommended for prevention of UTI recurrence. Likewise, postcoital voiding has not been proved effective (1, 36), nor have douching or wiping techniques (1). The benefit of vaginal lactobacilli application also remains unproven (37).

Drinking cranberry juice has been shown to decrease symptomatic UTIs. This is because of the proanthocyanidin-inhibiting attachment of urinary pathogens to the urinary tract epithelial cells (38, 39). In a recent meta-analysis addressing the effectiveness of drinking cranberry juice and taking other formulations, it was reported that taking cranberry formulations was more effective compared with taking placebo (40). In one of the studies in the meta-analysis, it was reported that both drinking cranberry juice and taking cranberry tablets significantly decreased the number of women with at least one symptomatic UTI per year to 18% and 20%, respectively, compared with 32% for those taking placebo (41). However, there are insufficient data to determine the length of therapy and the concentration required to prevent recurrence long term.

Methenamine salts (methenamine hippurate and methenamine mandelate) have long been used for the prevention of UTI. They produce formaldehyde, which acts as a bacteriostatic agent (42). In a meta-analysis reviewing 11 trials using methenamine hippurate, it was found that, although well tolerated, there was not enough evidence to conclusively support this use for urinary prophylaxis (43).

Recurrence rates are high among postmenopausal women. The hypoestrogenic state with associated genitourinary atrophy likely contributes to the increased prevalence. Oral and vaginal exogenous estrogens have been studied with varying results. Estrogen-releasing pessaries and rings have had some success in decreasing UTI recurrences (44, 45), as have topical estrogen creams (46). Although in one study a benefit from oral estrogen therapy was found (47), in other larger studies no reduction in UTI frequency in postmenopausal women receiving oral estrogen was shown (48, 49). Large, randomized trials are required before exogenous estrogen therapy can be conclusively recommended for UTI recurrence prevention.

Vaginal mucosal vaccines have been proposed to improve long-term resistance to recurrent UTIs. Vaccine targets include the Type I and Type II pili. One study has shown some promise (50), but currently no vaccines are available for clinical use.

▶ *When should asymptomatic bacteriuria be treated?*

Screening for and treatment of asymptomatic bacteriuria is not recommended in nonpregnant, premenopausal women. Asymptomatic bacteriuria has not been shown to be harmful in this population, nor does treatment of asymptomatic bacteriuria decrease the frequency of symptomatic infections (51). The current Infectious Diseases Society of America guidelines for the diagnosis and treatment of asymptomatic bacteriuria in adults, released in 2005, list specific groups in whom treatment of asymptomatic bacteriuria is recommended. These include all pregnant women, women undergoing a urologic procedure in which mucosal bleeding is anticipated, and women in whom catheter-acquired bacteriuria persists 48 hours after catheter removal. They do not recommend treatment of asymptomatic bacteriuria in women with diabetes mellitus, older institutionalized patients, older patients living in a community setting, patients with spinal cord injuries, or patients with indwelling catheters (51).

Summary of Recommendations and Conclusions

The following recommendations and conclusions are based on good and consistent scientific evidence (Level A):

▶ Screening for and treatment of asymptomatic bacteriuria is not recommended in nonpregnant, premenopausal women.

▶ Resistance rates higher than 15–20% necessitate a change in antibiotic class.

▶ In all cases of acute pyelonephritis, whether treatment is on an inpatient or outpatient basis, 14 days of total antimicrobial therapy should be completed.

▶ A 3-day antimicrobial regimen is the preferred treatment duration for uncomplicated acute bacterial cystitis in women, including women aged 65 years and older.

The following conclusion is based on limited or inconsistent evidence (Level B):

▶ The initial treatment of a symptomatic lower UTI with pyuria or bacteriuria or both does not require a urine culture.

The following conclusions are based primarily on consensus and expert opinion (Level C):

▶ Beta-lactams, such as first-generation cephalosporins and amoxicillin, are less effective in the treatment of acute uncomplicated cystitis than those antimicrobials listed in Table 1.

▶ To diagnose bacteriuria, decreasing the colony count to 1,000–10,000 bacteria per milliliter in symptomatic patients will improve the sensitivity without significantly compromising specificity.

Proposed Performance Measure

The percentage of women in whom acute pyelonephritis is diagnosed who are treated with 14 days of antimicrobial therapy

References

1. Fihn SD. Clinical practice. Acute uncomplicated urinary tract infection in women. N Engl J Med 2003;349: 259–66. (Level III)

2. Griebling TL. Urinary tract infection in women. In: National Institute of Diabetes and Digestive and Kidney Diseases. Urologic diseases in America. NIH Publication No. 07-5512. Washington, DC: Government Printing Office; 2007. p. 587–619. Available at: http://kidney.niddk.nih.gov/statistics/uda/Urinary_Tract_Infection_in_Women-Chapter18.pdf. Retrieved December 4, 2007. (Level III)

3. Griebling TL. Urinary tract infection in men. In: National Institute of Diabetes and Digestive and Kidney Diseases. Urologic diseases in America. NIH Publication No. 07-5512. Washington, DC: Government Printing Office; 2007. p. 621–45. Available at: http://kidney.niddk.nih.gov/statistics/uda/Urinary_Tract_Infection_in_Men-Chapter19.pdf. Retrieved December 4, 2007. (Level III)

4. Hooton TM. Recurrent urinary tract infection in women. Int J Antimicrob Agents 2001;17:259–68. (Level III)

5. Hooton TM, Stamm WE. The vaginal flora and urinary tract infections. In: Mobley HL, Warren JW. Urinary tract infections: molecular pathogenesis and clinical management. Washington, DC: American Society for Microbiology Press; 1996. p. 67–94. (Level III)

6. Ronald A. The etiology of urinary tract infection: traditional and emerging pathogens. Am J Med 2002;113 (suppl 1A):14S–19S. (Level III)

7. Scholes D, Hooton TM, Roberts PL, Gupta K, Stapleton AE, Stamm WE. Risk factors associated with acute pyelonephritis in healthy women. Ann Intern Med 2005;142:20–7. (Level II-2)

8. Sobel JD, Kaye D. Urinary tract infections. In: Mandell GL, Bennett JE, Dolin R. Mandell, Douglas, and Bennett's principles and practice of infectious diseases. 6th ed. Philadelphia (PA): Elsevier Churchill Livingstone; 2005. p. 875–905. (Level III)

9. Sheffield JS, Cunningham FG. Urinary tract infection in women. Obstet Gynecol 2005;106:1085–92. (Level III)

10. Jackson SL, Boyko EJ, Scholes D, Abraham L, Gupta K, Fihn SD. Predictors of urinary tract infection after menopause: a prospective study. Am J Med 2004; 117:903–11. (Level II-2)

11. Hurlbut TA 3rd, Littenberg B. The diagnostic accuracy of rapid dipstick tests to predict urinary tract infection. Am J Clin Pathol 1991;96:582–8. (Level III)

12. Hooton TM, Stamm WE. Diagnosis and treatment of uncomplicated urinary tract infection. Infect Dis Clin North Am 1997;11:551–81. (Level III)

13. Gupta K, Scholes D, Stamm WE. Increasing prevalence of antimicrobial resistance among uropathogens causing acute uncomplicated cystitis in women. JAMA 1999; 281:736–8. (Level II-3)

14. Warren JW, Abrutyn E, Hebel JR, Johnson JR, Schaeffer AJ, Stamm WE. Guidelines for antimicrobial treatment of uncomplicated acute bacterial cystitis and acute pyelonephritis in women. Infectious Diseases Society of America (IDSA). Clin Infect Dis 1999;29:745–58. (Level III)

15. Handley MA, Reingold AL, Shiboski S, Padian NS. Incidence of acute urinary tract infection in young women and use of male condoms with and without nonoxynol-9 spermicides. Epidemiology 2002;13:431–6. (Level II-2)

16. Scholes D, Hooton TM, Roberts PL, Stapleton AE, Gupta K, Stamm WE. Risk factors for recurrent urinary tract infection in young women. J Infect Dis 2000;182: 1177–82. (Level II-2)

17. Melekos MD, Asbach HW, Gerharz E, Zarakovitis IE, Weingaertner K, Naber KG. Postintercourse versus daily ciprofloxacin prophylaxis for recurrent urinary tract infections in premenopausal women. J Urol 1997;157:935–9. (Level II-2)

18. Pfau A, Sacks TG. Effective postcoital quinolone prophylaxis of recurrent urinary tract infections in women. J Urol 1994;152:136–8. (Level II-1)

19. Borrego F, Gleckman R. Principles of antibiotic prescribing in the elderly. Drugs Aging 1997;11:7–18. (Level III)

20. Lutters M, Vogt-Ferrier NB. Antibiotic duration for treating uncomplicated, symptomatic lower urinary tract infections in elderly women. Cochrane Database of Systematic Reviews 2002, Issue 3. Art. No.: CD001535. DOI: 10.1002/14651858.CD001535. (Level III)

21. Vogel T, Verreault R, Gourdeau M, Morin M, Grenier-Gosselin L, Rochette L. Optimal duration of antibiotic therapy for uncomplicated urinary tract infection in older women: a double-blind randomized controlled trial. CMAJ 2004;170:469–73. (Level I)

22. Gupta K, Hooton TM, Roberts PL, Stamm WE. Patient-initiated treatment of uncomplicated recurrent urinary tract infections in young women. Ann Intern Med 2001;135:9–16. (Level II-2)

23. Schaeffer AJ, Stuppy BA. Efficacy and safety of self-start therapy in women with recurrent urinary tract infections. J Urol 1999;161:207–11. (Level II-3)

24. Wong ES, McKevitt M, Running K, Counts GW, Turck M, Stamm WE. Management of recurrent urinary tract infections with patient-administered single-dose therapy. Ann Intern Med 1985;102:302–7. (Level II-1)

25. Barry HC, Ebell MH, Hickner J. Evaluation of suspected urinary tract infection in ambulatory women: a cost-utility analysis of office-based strategies. J Fam Pract 1997;44: 49–60. (Level III)

26. Fenwick EA, Briggs AH, Hawke CI. Management of urinary tract infection in general practice: a cost-effectiveness analysis. Br J Gen Pract 2000;50:635–9. (Level III)

27. Sultana RV, Zalstein S, Cameron P, Campbell D. Dipstick urinalysis and the accuracy of the clinical diagnosis of urinary tract infection. J Emerg Med 2001;20:13–9. (Level II-3)

28. Fahey T, Webb E, Montgomery AA, Heyderman RS. Clinical management of urinary tract infection in women: a prospective cohort study. Fam Pract 2003;20:1–6. (Level II-2)

29. McIsaac WJ, Low DE, Biringer A, Pimlott N, Evans M, Glazier R. The impact of empirical management of acute cystitis on unnecessary antibiotic use. Arch Intern Med 2002;162:600–5. (Level II-2)

30. Gait JE. Hemolytic reactions to nitrofurantoin in patients with glucose-6-phosphate dehydrogenase deficiency: theory and practice. DICP 1990;24:1210–3. (Level II-2)

31. Talan DA, Stamm WE, Hooton TM, Moran GJ, Burke T, Iravani A, et al. Comparison of ciprofloxacin (7 days) and trimethoprim-sulfamethoxazole (14 days) for acute uncomplicated pyelonephritis in women: a randomized trial. JAMA 2000;283:1583–90. (Level I)

32. Norrby SR. Short-term treatment of uncomplicated lower urinary tract infections in women. Rev Infect Dis 1990;12:458–67. (Level III)

33. Leibovici L, Wysenbeek AJ. Single-dose antibiotic treatment for symptomatic urinary tract infections in women: a meta-analysis of randomized trials. Q J Med 1991;78: 43–57. (Level III)

34. Stein GE. Comparison of single-dose fosfomycin and a 7-day course of nitrofurantoin in female patients with uncomplicated urinary tract infection. Clin Ther 1999; 21:1864–72. (Level I)

35. Richard GA, Mathew CP, Kirstein JM, Orchard D, Yang JY. Single-dose fluoroquinolone therapy of acute uncomplicated urinary tract infection in women: results from a randomized, double-blind, multicenter trial comparing single-dose to 3-day fluoroquinolone regimens. Urology 2002;59:334–9. (Level I)

36. Strom BL, Collins M, West SL, Kreisberg J, Weller S. Sexual activity, contraceptive use, and other risk factors for symptomatic and asymptomatic bacteriuria. A case–control study. Ann Intern Med;107:816–23. (Level II-2)

37. Baerheim A, Larsen E, Digranes A. Vaginal application of lactobacilli in the prophylaxis of recurrent lower urinary tract infection in women. Scand J Prim Health Care 1994;12:239–43. (Level II-1)

38. Sobota AE. Inhibition of bacterial adherence by cranberry juice: potential use for the treatment of urinary tract infections. J Urol 1984;131:1013–6. (Level III)

39. Schmidt DR, Sobota AE. An examination of the anti-adherence activity of cranberry juice on urinary and nonurinary bacterial isolates. Microbios 1988;55:173–81. (Level III)

40. Jepson RG, Mihaljevic L, Craig J. Cranberries for preventing urinary tract infections. Cochrane Database of Systematic Reviews 2004, Issue 2. Art. No.: CD001321. DOI: 10.1002/14651858.CD001321.pub3. (Level III)

41. Stothers L. A randomized trial to evaluate effectiveness and cost effectiveness of naturopathic cranberry products as prophylaxis against urinary tract infection in women. Can J Urol 2002;9:1558–62. (Level I)

42. Mayrer AR, Andriole VT. Urinary tract antiseptics. Med Clin North Am 1982;66:199–208. (Level III)

43. Lee BB, Simpson JM, Craig JC, Bhuta T. Methenamine hippurate for preventing urinary tract infections. Cochrane Database of Systematic Reviews 2007, Issue 4. Art. No.: CD003265. DOI: 10.1002/14651858.CD003265. pub2. (Level III)

44. Eriksen B. A randomized, open, parallel-group study on the preventive effect of an estradiol-releasing vaginal ring (Estring) on recurrent urinary tract infections in post-menopausal women. Am J Obstet Gynecol 1999;180: 1072–9. (Level I)

45. Raz R, Colodner R, Rohana Y, Battino S, Rottensterich E, Wasser I, et al. Effectiveness of estriol-containing vaginal pessaries and nitrofurantoin macrocrystal therapy in the prevention of recurrent urinary tract infection in post-menopausal women. Clin Infect Dis 2003;36:1362–8. (Level II-2)

46. Raz R, Stamm WE. A controlled trial of intravaginal estriol in postmenopausal women with recurrent urinary tract infections. N Engl J Med 1993;329:753–6. (Level I)

47. Kirkengen AL, Andersen P, Gjersoe E, Johannessen GR, Johnsen N, Bodd E. Oestriol in the prophylactic treatment of recurrent urinary tract infections in postmenopausal women. Scand J Prim Health Care 1992;10:139–42. (Level I)

48. Brown JS, Vittinghoff E, Kanaya AM, Agarwal SK, Hulley S, Foxman B. Urinary tract infections in post-menopausal women: effect of hormone therapy and risk factors. Heart and Estrogen/Progestin Replacement Study Research Group. Obstet Gynecol 2001;98:1045–52. (Level I)

49. Oliveria SA, Klein RA, Reed JI, Cirillo PA, Christos PJ, Walker AM. Estrogen replacement therapy and urinary tract infections in postmenopausal women aged 45–89. Menopause 1998;5:4–8. (Level II-2)

50. Uehling DT, Hopkins WJ, Elkahwaji JE, Schmidt DM, Leverson GE. Phase 2 clinical trial of a vaginal mucosal vaccine for urinary tract infections. J Urol 2003; 170:867–9. (Level I)

51. Nicolle LE, Bradley S, Colgan R, Rice JC, Schaeffer A, Hooton TM. Infectious Diseases Society of America guidelines for the diagnosis and treatment of asymptomatic bacteriuria in adults. Infectious Diseases Society of America; American Society of Nephrology; American Geriatric Society [published erratum appears in Clin Infect Dis 2005;40:1556]. Clin Infect Dis 2005;40: 643–54. (Level III)

The MEDLINE database, the Cochrane Library, and ACOG's own internal resources and documents were used to conduct a literature search to locate relevant articles published between January 1985 and April 2007. The search was restricted to articles published in the English language. Priority was given to articles reporting results of original research, although review articles and commentaries also were consulted. Abstracts of research presented at symposia and scientific conferences were not considered adequate for inclusion in this document. Guidelines published by organizations or institutions such as the National Institutes of Health and the American College of Obstetricians and Gynecologists were reviewed, and additional studies were located by reviewing bibliographies of identified articles. When reliable research was not available, expert opinions from obstetrician–gynecologists were used.

Studies were reviewed and evaluated for quality according to the method outlined by the U.S. Preventive Services Task Force:

I   Evidence obtained from at least one properly designed randomized controlled trial.

II-1   Evidence obtained from well-designed controlled trials without randomization.

II-2   Evidence obtained from well-designed cohort or case–control analytic studies, preferably from more than one center or research group.

II-3   Evidence obtained from multiple time series with or without the intervention. Dramatic results in uncontrolled experiments also could be regarded as this type of evidence.

III   Opinions of respected authorities, based on clinical experience, descriptive studies, or reports of expert committees.

Based on the highest level of evidence found in the data, recommendations are provided and graded according to the following categories:

Level A—Recommendations are based on good and consistent scientific evidence.

Level B—Recommendations are based on limited or inconsistent scientific evidence.

Level C—Recommendations are based primarily on consensus and expert opinion.

ISSN 1099-3630

The American College of Obstetricians and Gynecologists
409 12th Street, SW, PO Box 96920, Washington, DC 20090-6920

Treatment of urinary tract infections in nonpregnant women. ACOG Practice Bulletin No. 91. American College of Obstetricians and Gynecologists. Obstet Gynecol 2008;111:785–94.

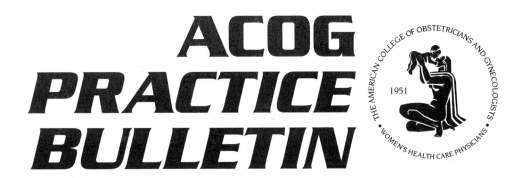

ACOG PRACTICE BULLETIN

CLINICAL MANAGEMENT GUIDELINES FOR OBSTETRICIAN–GYNECOLOGISTS

NUMBER 93, MAY 2008

This Practice Bulletin was developed by the ACOG Committee on Practice Bulletins—Gynecology with the assistance of Lori A. Boardman, MD, and Colleen M. Kennedy, MD. The information is designed to aid practitioners in making decisions about appropriate obstetric and gynecologic care. These guidelines should not be construed as dictating an exclusive course of treatment or procedure. Variations in practice may be warranted based on the needs of the individual patient, resources, and limitations unique to the institution or type of practice.

THE AMERICAN COLLEGE OF OBSTETRICIANS AND GYNECOLOGISTS

WOMEN'S HEALTH CARE PHYSICIANS

Diagnosis and Management of Vulvar Skin Disorders

Symptoms of vulvovaginal disorders are common, often chronic, and can significantly interfere with women's sexual function and sense of well-being. In the evaluation of women who report symptoms of vulvar disorders, the most common diagnoses are dermatologic conditions and vulvodynia (both generalized and localized forms) (1). The purpose of this document is to review diagnostic approaches and provide a structured framework for the management of vulvar disorders.

Background

Definition

Pruritus and pain are two of the most common presenting symptoms of vulvar disorders in women treated in clinics that provide specialized care for vulvar conditions (1–3). Pruritus and vulvar pain may occur in the presence of obvious dermatologic disease or in conditions with few visible skin changes. In evaluating vulvar pruritus, it can be helpful to group women into those with acute symptoms and those with chronic symptoms (see box, "Conditions Commonly Associated With Vulvar Pruritus"). Vulvodynia, defined as burning, stinging, rawness, or soreness, with or without pruritus, can be further characterized by the site of the pain, whether it is generalized or localized, and whether it is provoked, spontaneous, or both (4).

Examination and Evaluation

In cases of acute vulvar pruritus, common etiologies include vulvovaginal candidiasis and contact dermatitis. Chronic vulvar pruritus should prompt a search for underlying dermatoses, such as lichen sclerosus, lichen simplex chronicus, or psoriasis; neoplasia, including vulvar intraepithelial neoplasia, squamous cell carcinoma, and Paget disease of the vulva; or vulvar manifestations of systemic diseases, such as Crohn disease.

Patients presenting with pain should first be evaluated to rule out underlying organic causes, including inflammatory conditions, neoplasias, infections, or neurologic disorders. When organic causes are ruled out, the diagnosis of vulvodynia can be made, and attention should then be paid to more fully elucidating the nature of the pain disorder.

Chronic or recurrent forms of vulvovaginal disease can be difficult to diagnose and treat. When taking a medical history, it is important to ask about the onset, duration, location, and nature of vulvar symptoms (including the relationship of symptoms to the patient's menstrual cycle), as well as any possible precipitating or known risk factors. In the evaluation of infectious causes of vulvovaginal symptoms, microscopy using both

saline and potassium hydroxide preparations, in conjunction with vaginal pH determination, will help to guide the use of subsequent diagnostic tools. These additional diagnostic approaches include vaginal yeast culture, a variety of point-of-care tests approved by the U.S. Food and Drug Administration, culture or polymerase chain reaction for confirmation of herpes simplex virus, and specific serologic tests (5). For autoimmune disorders and suspected cases of neoplasia, biopsy is the preferred approach.

Vulvar Dermatoses

Dermatitis (or eczema), a poorly demarcated, erythematous, and usually itchy rash, has been reported to occur in 20–60% of patients with chronic vulvar symptoms (6). Contact dermatitis is one of the most frequently encountered and often avoidable problems seen in clinics that provide specialized care for vulvar disorders. Many seemingly innocuous behaviors, such as bathing, the use of sanitary or incontinence pads, or exposure to known irritants or allergens in numerous topical medications (see box, "Common Vulvar Irritants and Allergens"), have the potential to initiate contact dermatitis (7, 8). Avoiding allergens can reduce the occurrence of both contact dermatitis and lichen simplex chronicus. On examination, clinical signs can range from mild erythema, swelling, and scaling to marked erythema, fissures, skin thickening, erosions, and ulcers (8). The evaluation of dermatoses also should include assessment to rule out candidiasis.

Vulvar lichen simplex chronicus is a chronic eczematous disease characterized by scaling and lichenified plaque with intense and unrelenting itching, which may result in sleep disruption. Although lichen simplex chronicus occurs primarily in mid- to late-adult life, it can occur in children. From 65% to 75% of patients will report a history of atopic disease, and lichen simplex chronicus can be seen as a localized variant of atopic dermatitis. Lichen simplex chronicus represents an end-stage response to a wide variety of possible initiating processes, including environmental factors (eg, heat, excessive sweating, and irritation from clothing or topically applied products) and dermatologic disease (eg, candidiasis, lichen sclerosus) (9). In long-standing disease, the skin appears thickened and leathery, and areas of hyperpigmentation and hypopigmentation may be present. Erosions and ulcers also can develop, most commonly from chronic scratching. Vaginal yeast cultures are helpful in identifying the presence of an underlying condition on which lichen simplex chronicus is superimposed.

Lichen sclerosus, a chronic disorder of the skin, is most commonly seen on the vulva, with extragenital lesions reported in up to 13% of women with vulvar dis-

---

Conditions Commonly Associated With Vulvar Pruritus

Acute

Infections

- Fungal, including candidiasis and tinea cruris
- Trichomoniasis
- Vulvovaginal candidiasis
- Molluscum contagiosum
- Infestations, including scabies and pediculosis

Contact dermatitis (allergic or irritant)

Chronic

Dermatoses

- Atopic and contact dermatitis
- Lichen sclerosus, lichen planus, lichen simplex chronicus
- Psoriasis
- Genital atrophy

Neoplasia

- Vulvar intraepithelial neoplasia, vulvar cancer
- Paget disease

Infection

- Human papillomavirus infection

Vulvar manifestations of systemic disease

- Crohn disease

Common Vulvar Irritants and Allergens

Adult or baby wipes

Antiseptics (eg, povidine iodine, hexachlorophene)

Body fluids (eg, semen or saliva)

Colored or scented toilet paper

Condoms (lubricant or spermicide containing)

Contraceptive creams, jellies, foams, nonoxynol-9, lubricants

Dyes

Emollients (eg, lanolin, jojoba oil, glycerin)

Laundry detergents, fabric softeners, and dryer sheets

Rubber products (including latex)

Sanitary products, including tampons, pads

Soaps, bubble bath and salts, shampoos, conditioners

Tea tree oil

Topical anesthetics (eg, benzocaine, lidocaine, dibucaine)

Topical antibacterials (eg, neomycin, bacitracin, polymyxin)

Topical antimycotics (eg, imidazoles, nystatin)

Topical corticosteroids

Topical medications, including trichloroacetic acid, 5-fluorouracil, podofilox or podophyllin

Vaginal hygiene products, including perfumes and deodorants

---

ease (10). The mean age of onset is in the fifth to sixth decade, but it may occur at any age, including prepuberty (11). The exact etiology of this condition is unclear, although an autoimmune process or possible genetic link is likely (12, 13). Patients presenting with lichen sclerosus most commonly report pruritus, followed by irritation, burning, dyspareunia, and tearing. The prevalence of this condition remains unknown because lichen sclerosus may be asymptomatic.

On examination, typical lesions of lichen sclerosus are porcelain-white papules and plaques, often with areas of ecchymosis or purpura. The skin commonly appears thinned, whitened, and crinkling (leading to the description "cigarette paper"). Although the vaginal epithelium is largely spared from lichen sclerosus, involvement of the mucocutaneous junctions may lead to introital narrowing. Perianal involvement can create the classic "figure of eight" or hourglass shape. Other findings include fusion of the labia minora, phimosis of the clitoral hood, and fissures (14). Because other vulvar diseases can mimic lichen sclerosus, a biopsy is necessary to confirm the diagnosis, except in a prepubertal child (15, 16).

Lichen planus, an inflammatory disorder of the genital mucosa most likely related to cell-mediated immunity, exhibits a wide range of morphologies. The most common form and the most difficult to treat is the erosive form, which can lead to significant scarring and pain. Most commonly recognized on the skin or oral mucosa, this condition may affect the lower genital tract. Approximately 1% of the population has oral lichen planus, and of women with oral disease (17), approximately 20–25% have genital vulvovaginal disease (18). The classic presentation of lichen planus on mucous membranes, including the buccal mucosa, is that of white, reticulate, lacy, or fernlike striae (Wickham striae). On occasion, the skin may appear uniformly white, and thus lichen planus can be confused with lichen sclerosus. Pruritic, purple, shiny papules are typically associated with lichen planus. However, if papules are found on the genital skin, they appear dusky pink in color, without an apparent scale, and less well demarcated.

In erosive lichen planus, deep, painful, erythematous erosions appear in the posterior vestibule and often extend to the labia minora, resulting in agglutination and resorption of the labial architecture. The vaginal epithelium can become erythematous, eroded, acutely inflamed, and denuded of epithelium. Erosive patches, if present, are extremely friable. Over time, these eroded surfaces may adhere, resulting in synechiae and, eventually, complete obliteration of the vaginal space (19, 20). Symptoms commonly reported by patients with erosive vulvar lichen planus include dyspareunia, burning, and increased vaginal discharge (21).

Erosive lichen planus often is labeled as desquamative inflammatory vaginitis when vaginal discharge reveals predominance of inflammatory cells and immature parabasal and basal epithelial cells (these will appear small and round, with relatively large nuclei). The vaginal pH is increased, usually in the range of 5–6. Whether desquamative inflammatory vaginitis is a type of erosive lichen planus or a distinct type of vaginitis is controversial (19, 20). Biopsy of the affected area, which reveals a bandlike infiltrate of lymphocytes and colloid bodies in the basal layers of the epidermis, may be relatively nonspecific because of the complete loss of the epithelium. However, a histologic specimen can help rule out immunobullous diseases, such as cicatricial pemphigoid, bullous pemphigoid, and pemphigus vulgaris, which may mimic lichen planus (22).

Vulvar Atrophy

Estimates indicate that up to 50% of all postmenopausal women will experience vulvovaginal irritation, soreness, and dryness, lower urinary tract problems, and dyspareunia (23, 24). The onset of symptoms can occur long after other menopausal symptoms (eg, hot flushes) resolve. However, perimenopausal women who do not have visible signs of vulvovaginal atrophy also can experience symptoms of vulvar irritation and dryness (25). Finally, despite the use of systemic hormone therapy, approximately 10–25% of users will continue to experience symptoms of urogenital atrophy despite improvement in other symptoms associated with estrogen deficiency (26).

As women approach menopause, vulvar tissue becomes increasingly sensitive to irritants (27), and in the absence of estrogen, the vaginal mucosa becomes pale, thin, and often dry. Vaginal secretions are reduced, the vaginal pH becomes more alkaline, and the vaginal flora is altered (28, 29). Activities that once were not associated with discomfort may become so. The genital area becomes increasingly susceptible to trauma, chemical irritants, and bacterial overgrowth. In severe atrophic vaginitis, a purulent, noninfectious discharge may develop, along with fissuring of the vestibule. The diagnosis is based on an elevated vaginal pH (range of 6.0–7.5) and the presence of parabasal or intermediate cells on microscopy. An amine test result will be negative in this setting (although bacterial vaginosis continues to be a problem in this population as well) (30).

Other Considerations

In assessing vulvar pruritus and pain, the common causes of vulvovaginitis (candidiasis, bacterial vaginosis, and trichomoniasis), particularly in their more complicated forms, must be included in the differential diagnosis. For example, non-*albicans* candidal infections typically present with burning, not itching, and minimal evidence of inflammation. Because most atypical species do not form hyphae or pseudohyphae, microscopy is not helpful and, therefore, culture is warranted (31, 32). Negative yeast cultures, in the setting of persistent vulvar burning with no other identifiable organic cause, also will help establish a diagnosis of vulvodynia (33, 34).

Genital human papillomavirus (HPV), the most common sexually transmitted viral infection, is associated with a number of vulvar epithelial disorders, including genital warts, vulvar intraepithelial neoplasia (VIN), and some vulvar carcinomas. Distinguishing warts from vulvar neoplasia on the basis of appearance alone is not always possible because VIN can present as red, white, dark, raised, or eroded lesions. In general, a biopsy should be performed on hyperpigmented, indurated, fixed, or ulcerative lesions, or lesions that do not respond to treatment or worsen during treatment.

If the patient is immunocompromised or the diagnosis is uncertain (eg, Paget disease can present as multiple bright red, scaly, eczematoid plaques [35], whereas melanoma can range in color from brown to bluish-black [36]), biopsy should be undertaken. Because multicentric disease is commonly encountered, particularly in younger women, a complete examination should include the cervix, vagina, and perianal area. Up to 50% of women with VIN will have antecedent or concomitant lower genital tract neoplasia, usually cervical or vaginal intraepithelial neoplasia (5).

In addition to contact irritation from the array of treatments used to alleviate vulvar symptoms, many patients with underlying chronic vulvar skin disorders, including lichen sclerosus, lichen planus, and psoriasis, are also at risk of developing steroid rebound dermatitis, also called steroid rosacea. Withdrawing from use of a moderate- to high-potency topical steroid can result in rebound vasodilation, accompanied by burning and irritation.

Clinical Considerations and Recommendations

▶ *When and how should a vulvar biopsy be performed?*

The threshold for biopsy of the vulva should be low except in the pediatric population. Changes on the vulva often are subtle and can be overlooked. Findings such as thickening, pebbling, hypopigmentation, or thinning of the epithelium indicate a possible dermatologic process, and biopsy will aid in diagnosis and management. Biopsy of hyperpigmented or exophytic lesions, lesions with changes in vascular patterns, or unresolving lesions is particularly important and should be performed in order to rule out carcinoma. Diagnostic delays in identifying vulvar cancer are exceedingly common and have been linked to failures or procrastination in the performance of biopsies of abnormal-appearing vulvar skin (37).

Anesthesia is recommended for vulvar biopsy; combination lidocaine and prilocaine cream or 4% liposomal lidocaine cream can be placed on the proposed biopsy site before inserting the anesthesia needle (38). A systematic review of topical anesthetics for dermatologic procedures found both medications to be effective, but liposomal lidocaine had a more rapid onset (30 minutes versus 60 minutes with combination lidocaine and prilocaine cream) and lower cost (39). To minimize discomfort, a solution of 8.4% sodium bicarbonate can be added to the lidocaine (1:10 ratio). Onset of action occurs within 2–5 minutes; if epinephrine is used with either of these anesthetics, the onset of action will be delayed, but the duration of effect will be increased (40).

Choice of biopsy instrument depends on the location and nature of the lesions. For most inflammatory diseases, ulcers, pigmented lesions, or suspected tumors, a punch biopsy is the preferred method because establishing the depth of such lesions is critical (41). Small lesions often can be completely excised, and lesions involving the submucosal or subcutaneous tissue should be adequately sampled. When sampling ulcerative areas, a biopsy of the edge of the ulcer is preferred; when sampling hyperpigmented areas, a biopsy of the thickest region is recommended (42).

One of the most common methods of biopsy involves the use of a 3–5-mm Keyes punch. A shave or snip biopsy works best for sampling more superficial disorders, such as lichen sclerosus or lichen planus, or for sampling bullous lesions. Although both shave and snip samples will extend into the dermis, they should not go through the dermis. A stitch or topical solution can be used to control bleeding (43).

▶ *How should labial adhesions be treated?*

Labial adhesions are not uncommon in prepubertal girls and typically resolve spontaneously by menarche. Labial adhesions should be observed unless they are symptomatic (eg, urinary obstructive symptom). Topical estrogen cream is considered first-line medical treatment for the separation of labial adhesions (44). Girls should be monitored for side effects of estrogen therapy, including breast budding and vaginal bleeding. To decrease the risk of recurrence and to prevent reagglutination of raw opposing skin surfaces, an emollient can be applied nightly for at least 1 month. Manual separation in the office setting should only be performed with adequate anesthesia, and surgical excision should be reserved for acute urinary obstruction (45). One small trial showed success with topical steroids as a potential alternative to the use of estrogen (46).

▶ *In what circumstances is estrogen or testosterone cream an appropriate treatment?*

The use of estrogen treatment for vaginal atrophy has been well documented and can be accomplished with a variety of locally applied estrogen preparations (24). However, some differences have been demonstrated between forms of local therapies. When compared in randomized controlled trials with either estrogen tablets or with the estrogen ring, conjugated equine estrogen cream was found to be significantly associated with adverse effects, including bleeding, breast pain, and per-

ineal pain (47–49). All forms of topical estrogen therapy increase the possibility of endometrial hyperplasia and overstimulation. However, it is currently unknown whether women receiving long-term therapy with topical estrogen require prophylactic therapy with progesterone (24). It should be noted that systemic estrogen therapy, although efficacious, raises concerns for many women and may still not be sufficient to relieve the symptoms of urogenital atrophy (50).

Whether or not estrogen use improves the function of vulvar epithelium in vulvar atrophy (including clitoral circulation and fibrosis) remains controversial. Small studies have demonstrated improvement in circulation and sexual function in women following localized or systemic estrogen use (51, 52).

Topical estrogen therapy also has been reported for the treatment of symptomatic labial adhesions (53, 54). The use of estrogen for other vaginal disorders is less well documented, and includes treatment for radiation injury (55) and treatment of vaginal mucosa burn injury following misapplication of 100% acetic acid (56).

Indications for the use of testosterone cream in the treatment of vulvar or vaginal disorders remain controversial. Historically, testosterone cream was used in the treatment of lichen sclerosus. Subsequently, studies were undertaken comparing testosterone with topical steroids in the treatment of vulvar lichen sclerosus and resulted in two findings, a lack of clear effect with testosterone and the superiority of topical steroids (12, 57–59). Thus, given the undesirable side effects of masculinization and virilization associated with the use of testosterone, and unproven therapeutic benefit, it should not be used in the primary treatment of lichen sclerosus.

▶ *How should vulvar atrophy be treated?*

As noted previously, the data specifically addressing vulvar atrophy are limited. Studies assessing the benefits of a variety of therapies, including hormones, focus on patient symptoms such as vulvovaginal dryness, burning, pruritus, and dyspareunia, with the distinction between vulvar and vaginal symptoms not clearly made.

Management options for urogenital atrophy in adult women include lifestyle modification strategies, the use of vaginal moisturizers, and low-dose topical estradiol preparations. Maintaining regular vaginal intercourse provides protection from urogenital atrophy by increasing blood flow to the pelvic organs (60), an effect that also may occur through masturbation (61). The use of a nonhormonal vaginal moisturizer has been shown through prospective randomized studies to exert a beneficial effect similar to that of local hormone therapy (49, 62), although the same cannot be said of vaginal lubricants (25).

▶ *What is the appropriate treatment for lichen sclerosus?*

The recommended treatment for lichen sclerosus is use of a high-potency topical steroid, the most studied of which is clobetasol propionate (59, 63, 64). In one prospective cohort study of patients with lichen sclerosus treated with ultrapotent topical steroids, 96% experienced complete or partial relief of their vulvar symptoms, 23% demonstrated complete resolution of the vulvar skin to normal texture and color, and 68% showed partial resolution of the hyperkeratosis, purpura, fissuring, and erosions associated with this disorder (65). Although no randomized controlled trials provide evidence of the most effective steroid regimen, a reasonable approach is to begin with once-daily application of ultrapotent topical steroids for 4 weeks, tapering to alternate days for 4 weeks, followed by 4 weeks of twice weekly application (16). Although some practitioners recommend twice-daily application, pharmacodynamic studies have clearly demonstrated that once-daily application of an ultrapotent steroid is sufficient (66). Topical steroid therapy is not without complications, including the possibility of contact sensitization, skin changes, and secondary infection. However, studies have shown that long-term maintenance therapy with either a moderate or ultrapotent topical steroid did not lead to steroid-induced atrophy, telangiectasia, striae, or secondary infection (67). In general, a 30-g tube of an ultrapotent topical steroid should last approximately 3–6 months (16).

There is conflicting evidence on the need for ongoing maintenance therapy. Some experts recommend discontinuation of therapy following the initial regimen described previously and reuse of therapy for flares or recurrent symptoms (16). However, others recommend an ongoing maintenance regimen of twice-weekly application of either an ultrapotent or moderate strength steroid (68). Monitoring at 3 months and 6 months following initial therapy is recommended to assess the patient's response to therapy and to ensure proper application of the medication. Annual examinations are suggested for patients whose lichen sclerosus is well controlled, and more frequent visits for those with poorly controlled disease (for whom intralesional steroid injections also may be beneficial) (69). Patients should be advised to return for visits if persistent ulcerations or new growths appear. Biopsy of such lesions, as well as of erosions, hyperkeratotic, or hyperpigmented areas, is important to exclude intraepithelial neoplasia or invasive squamous cell cancer. Whether long-term topical treatment with a potent steroid cream can reduce the risk of malignant evolution (68) remains unclear pending results from larger follow-up studies.

In small, uncontrolled studies, other therapies found to be of use in the treatment of complicated lichen sclerosus (eg, unresponsive to topical steroids) include retinoids (70, 71), potassium para-aminobenzoate (72), cryotherapy (73), and photodynamic therapy with topical 5-aminolaevulinic acid (74). Topical cyclosporine failed to show benefit in the treatment of five cases of vulvar lichen sclerosus (75). Management with hormonal topical therapies, including estrogen, testosterone (57, 61, 63, 76), and progesterone (63, 77), has inconsistently resulted in improvement in lichen sclerosus and has been associated with significant side effects (eg, hyperandrogenism). The use of the topical macrolide immunosuppressants (eg, pimecrolimus, tacrolimus) was proposed initially as a therapeutic option for lichen sclerosus, given that these medications do not cause dermal atrophy. Although promising in the treatment of lichen sclerosus (78–80), these immunosuppressants are considered by most experts to be second-line agents for treatment of patients unresponsive to or intolerant of other treatment. Surgery, although not curative, is reserved for the treatment of malignancy and postinflammatory sequelae (eg, release of labial adhesions or introital stenosis) (81).

▶ *What is the appropriate treatment for lichen planus?*

The prognosis for spontaneous remission of vulvovaginal lichen planus is poor. As with vulvovaginal atrophy and lichen sclerosus, lifestyle modifications are important in maintaining function as well as providing comfort. Treatment options are numerous and include topical and systemic corticosteroids, topical and oral cyclosporine, topical tacrolimus, hydroxychloroquine, oral retinoids, methotrexate, azathioprine, and cyclophosphamide. Although symptomatic improvement is possible (21), patients should be advised that complete control is not the norm (20). Rather, vulvovaginal lichen planus is a frustrating, chronic, and recurring disease that requires long-term maintenance.

Evidence supporting treatment options for vulvovaginal lichen planus have come largely from retrospective case reports and case series (82–85). The most frequently recommended treatment for vulvovaginal lichen planus is the use of high-potency topical steroids, with the evidence for this recommendation based on small studies of oral rather than genital disease (84). Given the potential for significant side effects with the use of systemic immunosuppressants, methotrexate, cyclosporine, azathioprine, and hydroxychloroquine sulfate should be used only after local treatments have failed. Furthermore, study results of systemic therapies have been inconsistent, likely related to selection of those patients with more severe disease (85).

As with lichen sclerosus, surgery is reserved for the treatment of postinflammatory sequelae, including vaginal coaptation and release of labial adhesions. Finally, although squamous cell carcinomas are rarely encountered, women with lichen planus should be routinely monitored (85, 86).

▶ *What other conditions should be investigated in women presenting with vulvar disease (eg, lichen planus, lichen sclerosus, or Paget disease)?*

Diseases with vulvar and perianal involvement include not only dermatologic processes (eg, lichen sclerosus and psoriasis) but also systemic diseases such as Crohn disease. Approximately one third of women with Crohn disease present with gynecologic complications, including enteric fistulas to both the upper and lower genital tract, granulomatous salpingitis and oophoritis, and vulvar inflammation, edema, granulomas, abscesses, and ulcerations (87).

Numerous studies have now demonstrated a strong association, particularly in women, between lichen sclerosus and a variety of autoimmune-related disorders, including alopecia, vitiligo, thyrotoxicosis, hypothyroidism, and pernicious anemia (12). In a recent case series of women with vulvovaginal lichen planus, 55% had a personal or family history of an autoimmune disorder (88). Despite the strong association between lichen sclerosus and autoimmune-related disorders, there are no recommendations regarding evaluation for coexisting autoimmune-related disorders in women with lichen sclerosus beyond a brief examination for alopecia areata and vitiligo and consideration of thyroid function tests (89). In women, there is also an association of vulvar lichen sclerosus with squamous cell carcinoma, with up to a 5% incidence of malignancy (12). Therefore, close follow-up is recommended with biopsy of any concerning lesions, although the recommended follow-up interval has not been determined (eg, 6 months, 12 months, or other). Additionally, although the concern of malignancy is greater in poorly controlled lichen sclerosus, there is no clear evidence that optimal control of lichen sclerosus symptoms reduces the risk of malignancy.

Paget disease of the vulva is a rare form of intraepithelial neoplasia characterized by adenocarcinomatous cells and accounts for approximately 2% of vulvar neoplasms. Although most cases of extramammary vulvar Paget disease are primary rather than associated with underlying adenocarcinoma, approximately 25% of cases are associated with neoplastic disease (90). When associated disease is present, it is typically local (adenocarcinoma in the skin adnexa or Bartholin gland) but also may be distant (most commonly, of the breast, but also of the genital, urinary, or intestinal tract). In contrast, perianal extramammary Paget disease is associated with underlying colorectal adenocarcinoma in up to 80% of cases (90). Thus, when Paget disease is confirmed by biopsy, evaluation including breast, genitourinary tract, and gastrointestinal tract should be undertaken.

Summary of Recommendations

The following recommendation is based on limited or inconsistent scientific evidence (Level B):

▶ The recommended treatment for lichen sclerosus is an ultrapotent topical corticosteroid, such as clobetasol propionate.

The following recommendations are based primarily on consensus and expert opinion (Level C):

▶ Biopsy of hyperpigmented or exophytic lesions, lesions with changes in vascular patterns, or unresolving lesions is particularly important and should be performed to rule out carcinoma.

▶ For patients with biopsy-confirmed Paget disease, further evaluation of the breast, genitourinary tract, and gastrointestinal tract should be undertaken.

Proposed Performance Measure

The percentage of women with lichen sclerosus who are offered high-potency topical corticosteroids as first-line treatment

References

1. Hansen A, Carr K, Jensen JT. Characteristics and initial diagnoses in women presenting to a referral center for vulvovaginal disorders in 1996-2000. J Reprod Med 2002; 47:854–60. (Level III)

2. Bornstein J, Pascal B, Abramovici H. The common problem of vulvar pruritus. Obstet Gynecol Surv 1993;48: 111–8. (Level III)

3. Kehoe S, Luesley D. Pathology and management of vulval pain and pruritus. Curr Opin Obstet Gynecol 1995; 7:16–9. (Level III)

4. Moyal-Barracco M, Lynch PJ. 2003 ISSVD terminology and classification of vulvodynia: a historical perspective. J Reprod Med 2004;49:772–7. (Level III)

5. Workowski KA, Berman SM. Sexually transmitted diseases treatment guidelines, 2006. Centers for Disease Control and Prevention [published erratum appears in MMWR Recomm Rep 2006;55:997]. MMWR Recomm Rep 2006;55(RR-11):1–94. (Level III)

6. Crone AM, Stewart EJ, Wojnarowska F, Powell SM. Aetiological factors in vulvar dermatitis. J Eur Acad Dermatol Venereol 2000;14:181–6. (Level III)

7. Marren P, Wojnarowska F, Powell S. Allergic contact dermatitis and vulvar dermatoses. Br J Dermatol 1992; 126:52–6. (Level III)

8. Margesson LJ. Contact dermatitis of the vulva. Dermatol Ther 2004;17:20–7. (Level III)

9. Virgili A, Bacilieri S, Corazza M. Managing vulvar lichen simplex chronicus. J Reprod Med 2001;46:343–6. (Level III)

10. Thomas RH, Ridley CM, McGibbon DH, Black MM. Anogenital lichen sclerosus in women. J R Soc Med 1996;89:694–8. (Level III)

11. Pokorny SF. Prepubertal vulvovaginopathies. Obstet Gynecol Clin North Am 1992;19:39–58. (Level III)

12. Smith YR, Haefner HK. Vulvar lichen sclerosus: pathophysiology and treatment. Am J Clin Dermatol 2004; 5:105–25. (Level III)

13. Val I, Almeida G. An overview of lichen sclerosus. Clin Obstet Gynecol 2005;48:808–17. (Level III)

14. Funaro D. Lichen sclerosus: a review and practical approach. Dermatol Ther 2004;17:28–37. (Level III)

15. O'Keefe RJ, Scurry JP, Dennerstein G, Sfameni S, Brenan J. Audit of 114 non-neoplastic vulvar biopsies. Br J Obstet Gynaecol 1995;102:780–6. (Level I)

16. Neill SM, Tatnall FM, Cox NH. Guidelines for the management of lichen sclerosus. British Association of Dermatologists. Br J Dermatol 2002;147:640–9. (Level III)

17. Eisen D. The clinical features, malignant potential, and systemic associations of oral lichen planus: a study of 723 patients. J Am Acad Dermatol 2002;46:207–14. (Level III)

18. Eisen D. The evaluation of cutaneous, genital, scalp, nail, esophageal, and ocular involvement in patients with oral lichen planus. Oral Surg Oral Med Oral Pathol Oral Radiol Endod 1999;88:431–6. (Level III)

19. Rogers RS 3rd, Eisen D. Erosive oral lichen planus with genital lesions: the vulvovaginal-gingival syndrome and the peno-gingival syndrome. Dermatol Clin 2003;21: 91–8, vi–vii. (Level III)

20. Moyal-Barracco M, Edwards L. Diagnosis and therapy of anogenital lichen planus. Dermatol Ther 2004;17:38–46. (Level III)

21. Kennedy CM, Galask RP. Erosive vulvar lichen planus: retrospective review of characteristics and outcomes in 113 patients seen in a vulvar specialty clinic. J Reprod Med 2007;52:43–7. (Level III)

22. Ramer MA, Altchek A, Deligdisch L, Phelps R, Montazem A, Buonocore PM. Lichen planus and the vulvovaginal-gingival syndrome. J Periodontol 2003;74: 1385–93. (Level III)

23. Greendale GA, Judd HL. The menopause: health implications and clinical management. J Am Geriatr Soc 1993;41:426–36. (Level III)

24. Suckling J, Lethaby A, Kennedy R. Local oestrogen for vaginal atrophy in postmenopausal women. Cochrane Database of Systematic Reviews 2006, Issue 4. Art. No.: CD001500. DOI: 10.1002/14651858.CD001500.pub2. (Level III)

25. Johnston SL, Farrell SA, Bouchard C, Farrell SA, Beckerson LA, Comeau M, et al. The detection and management of vaginal atrophy. SOGC Joint Committee-Clinical Practice Gynaecology and Urogynaecology. J Obstet Gynaecol Can 2004;26:503–15. (Level III)

26. Smith RN, Studd JW. Recent advances in hormone replacement therapy. Br J Hosp Med 1993;49:799–808. (Level III)

27. Bohl TG. Overview of vulvar pruritus through the life cycle. Clin Obstet Gynecol 2005;48:786–807. (Level III)

28. Hillier SL, Lau RJ. Vaginal microflora in postmenopausal women who have not received estrogen replacement therapy. Clin Infect Dis 1997;25(suppl 2):S123–6. (Level III)

29. Farage M, Maibach H. Lifetime changes in the vulva and vagina. Arch Gynecol Obstet 2006;273:195–202. (Level III)

30. Ballagh SA. Vaginal hormone therapy for urogenital and menopausal symptoms. Semin Reprod Med 2005;23: 126–40. (Level III)

31. Fidel PL Jr, Vazquez JA, Sobel JD. Candida glabrata: review of epidemiology, pathogenesis, and clinical disease with comparison to C. albicans. Clin Microbiol Rev 1999;12:80–96. (Level III)

32. Sobel JD, Wiesenfeld HC, Martens M, Danna P, Hooton TM, Rompalo A, et al. Maintenance fluconazole therapy for recurrent vulvovaginal candidiasis. N Engl J Med 2004;351:876–83. (Level I)

33. Vulvodynia. ACOG Committee Opinion No. 345. American College of Obstetricians and Gynecologists. Obstet Gynecol 2006;108:1049–52. (Level III)

34. Bachmann GA, Rosen R, Pinn VW, Utian WH, Ayers C, Basson R, et al. Vulvodynia: a state-of-the-art consensus on definitions, diagnosis and management. J Reprod Med 2006;51:447–56. (Level III)

35. Parker LP, Parker JR, Bodurka-Bevers D, Deavers M, Bevers MW, Shen-Gunther J, et al. Paget's disease of the vulva: pathology, pattern of involvement, and prognosis. Gynecol Oncol 2000;77:183–9. (Level II-3)

36. Finan MA, Barre G. Bartholin's gland carcinoma, malignant melanoma and other rare tumours of the vulva. Best Pract Res Clin Obstet Gynaecol 2003;17:609–33. (Level III)

37. Jones RW, Joura EA. Analyzing prior clinical events at presentation in 102 women with vulvar carcinoma. Evidence of diagnostic delays. J Reprod Med 1999;44: 766–8. (Level II-2)

38. Kundu S, Achar S. Principles of office anesthesia: part II. Topical anesthesia. Am Fam Physician 2002;66:99–102. (Level III)

39. Eidelman A, Weiss JM, Lau J, Carr DB. Topical anesthetics for dermal instrumentation: a systematic review of randomized, controlled trials. Ann Emerg Med 2005;46: 343–51. (Level III)

40. Achar S, Kundu S. Principles of office anesthesia: part I. Infiltrative anesthesia. Am Fam Physician 2002;66:91–4. (Level III)

41. Zuber TJ. Punch biopsy of the skin. Am Fam Physician 2002;65:1155–8, 1161–2, 1164, 1167–8. (Level III)

42. Mirowski G, Edwards L. Diagnostic and therapeutic procedures. In: Edwards L, editor. Genital dermatology atlas. Philadelphia (PA): Lippincott Williams & Wilkins; 2004. p. 9–17. (Level III)

43. Alguire PC, Mathes BM. Skin biopsy techniques for the internist. J Gen Intern Med 1998;13:46–54. (Level III)

44. Tebruegge M, Misra I, Nerminathan V. Is the topical application of oestrogen cream an effective intervention in girls suffering from labial adhesions? Arch Dis Child 2007;92:268–71. (Level III)

45. Bacon JL. Prepubertal labial adhesions: evaluation of a referral population. Am J Obstet Gynecol 2002;187: 327–31; discussion 332. (Level II-3)

46. Myers JB, Sorensen CM, Wisner BP, Furness PD 3rd, Passamaneck M, Koyle MA. Betamethasone cream for the treatment of pre-pubertal labial adhesions. J Pediatr Adolesc Gynecol 2006;19:407–11. (Level II-3)

47. Rioux JE, Devlin C, Gelfand MM, Steinberg WM, Hepburn DS. 17beta-estradiol vaginal tablet versus conjugated equine estrogen vaginal cream to relieve menopausal atrophic vaginitis. Menopause 2000;7:156–61. (Level I)

48. Ayton RA, Darling GM, Murkies AL, Farrell EA, Weisberg E, Selinus I, et al. A comparative study of safety and efficacy of continuous low dose oestradiol released from a vaginal ring compared with conjugated equine oestrogen vaginal cream in the treatment of postmenopausal urogenital atrophy. Br J Obstet Gynaecol 1996;103:351–8. (Level I)

49. Nachtigall LE. Comparative study: Replens versus local estrogen in menopausal women. Fertil Steril 1994; 61:178–80. (Level III)

50. Cardozo L, Bachmann G, McClish D, Fonda D, Birgerson L. Meta-analysis of estrogen therapy in the management of urogenital atrophy in postmenopausal women: second report of the Hormones and Urogenital Therapy Committee. Obstet Gynecol 1998;92:722–7. (Level III)

51. Foster DC. Vulvar disease. Obstet Gynecol 2002;100: 145–63. (Level III)

52. Nappi RE, Ferdeghini F, Sampaolo P, Vaccaro P, De Leonardis C, Albani F, et al. Clitoral circulation in post-menopausal women with sexual dysfunction: a pilot randomized study with hormone therapy. Maturitas 2006;55:288–95. (Level II-1)

53. Girton S, Kennedy CM, Galask RP. Characteristics and outcomes of 16 patients with symptomatic labial adhesion. Internet J Gynecol Obstet 2007;7(1). Available at: http://www.ispub.com/ostia/index.php?xmlFilePath=journals/ijgo/vol7n1/labial.xml. Retrieved January 10, 2008. (Level III)

54. Schober J, Dulabon L, Martin-Alguacil N, Kow LM, Pfaff D. Significance of topical estrogens to labial fusion and vaginal introital integrity. J Pediatr Adolesc Gynecol 2006;19:337–9. (Level III)

55. Grigsby PW, Russell A, Bruner D, Eifel P, Koh WJ, Spanos W, et al. Late injury of cancer therapy on the female reproductive tract. Int J Radiat Oncol Biol Phys 1995;31:1281–99. (Level III)

56. Ou KY, Chen YC, Hsu SC, Tsai EM. Topical vaginal oestrogen cream used for treatment of burn injury of vaginal mucosa after misapplication of 100% acetic acid in a perimenopausal woman: a case report. Aust N Z J Obstet Gynaecol 2007;47:345–6. (Level III).

57. Sideri M, Origoni M, Spinaci L, Ferrari A. Topical testosterone in the treatment of vulvar lichen sclerosus. Int J Gynaecol Obstet 1994;46:53–6. (Level III)

58. Cattaneo A, Carli P, De Marco A, Sonni L, Bracco G, De Magnis A, et al. Testosterone maintenance therapy. Effects on vulvar lichen sclerosus treated with clobetasol propionate. J Reprod Med 1996;41:99–102. (Level I)

59. Bornstein J, Heifetz S, Kellner Y, Stolar Z, Abramovici H. Clobetasol dipropionate 0.05% versus testosterone propionate 2% topical application for severe vulvar lichen sclerosus. Am J Obstet Gynecol 1998;178:80–4. (Level II-3)

60. Leiblum S, Bachmann G, Kemmann E, Colburn D, Swartzman L. Vaginal atrophy in the postmenopausal woman. The importance of sexual activity and hormones. JAMA 1983;249:2195–8. (Level II-3)

61. Laan E, van Lunsen RH. Hormones and sexuality in postmenopausal women: a psychophysiological study. J Psychosom Obstet Gynaecol 1997;18:126–33. (Level II-3)

62. Bygdeman M, Swahn ML. Replens versus dienoestrol cream in the symptomatic treatment of vaginal atrophy in postmenopausal women. Maturitas 1996;23:259–63. (Level I)

63. Bracco GL, Carli P, Sonni L, Maestrini G, De Marco A, Taddei GL, et al. Clinical and histologic effects of topical treatments of vulval lichen sclerosus. A critical evaluation. J Reprod Med 1993;38:37–40. (Level II-3)

64. Lorenz B, Kaufman RH, Kutzner SK. Lichen sclerosus. Therapy with clobetasol propionate. J Reprod Med 1998; 43:790–4. (Level III)

65. Cooper SM, Gao XH, Powell JJ, Wojnarowska F. Does treatment of vulvar lichen sclerosus influence its prognosis? Arch Dermatol 2004;140:702–6. (Level II-2)

66. Lagos BR, Maibach HI. Frequency of application of topical corticosteroids: an overview. Br J Dermatol 1998; 139:763–6. (Level III)

67. Dalziel KL, Wojnarowska F. Long-term control of vulval lichen sclerosus after treatment with a potent topical steroid cream. J Reprod Med 1993;38:25–7. (Level III)

68. Renaud-Vilmer C, Cavelier-Balloy B, Porcher R, Dubertret L. Vulvar lichen sclerosus: effect of long-term topical application of a potent steroid on the course of the disease. Arch Dermatol 2004;140:709–12. (Level II-2)

69. Baggish MS, Ventolini G. Lichen sclerosus: subdermal steroid injection therapy. A large, long-term follow-up study. J Gynecol Surg 2006,22:137–41. (Level III)

70. Bousema MT, Romppanen U, Geiger JM, Baudin M, Vaha-Eskeli K, Vartiainen J, et al. Acitretin in the treatment of severe lichen sclerosus et atrophicus of the vulva: a double-blind, placebo-controlled study. J Am Acad Dermatol 1994;30:225–31. (Level I)

71. Virgili A, Corazza M, Bianchi A, Mollica G, Califano A. Open study of topical 0.025% tretinoin in the treatment of vulvar lichen sclerosus. One year of therapy. J Reprod Med 1995;40:614–8. (Level III)

72. Penneys NS. Treatment of lichen sclerosus with potassium para-aminobenzoate. J Am Acad Dermatol 1984;10:1039–42. (Level III)

73. August PJ, Milward TM. Cryosurgery in the treatment of lichen sclerosus et atrophicus of the vulva. Br J Dermatol 1980;103:667–70. (Level III)

74. Hillemanns P, Untch M, Prove F, Baumgartner R, Hillemanns M, Korell M. Photodynamic therapy of vulvar lichen sclerosus with 5-aminolevulinic acid. Obstet Gynecol 1999;93:71–4. (Level III)

75. Carli P, Cattaneo A, Taddei G, Giannotti B. Topical cyclosporine in the treatment of vulvar lichen sclerosus: clinical, histologic, and immunohistochemical findings. Arch Dermatol 1992;128:1548–9. (Level III)

76. Joura EA, Zeisler H, Bancher-Todesca D, Sator MO, Schneider B, Gitsch G. Short-term effects of topical testosterone in vulvar lichen sclerosus. Obstet Gynecol 1997;89:297–9. (Level II-3)

77. Leone M, Gerbaldo D, Caldana A, Leone MM, Capitanio GL. Progesterone topically administered influences epidermal growth factor immunoreactivity in vulvar tissue from patients with lichen sclerosus. Cervix Low Female Genital Tract 1993;11:25–7. (Level III)

78. Bohm M, Frieling U, Luger TA, Bonsmann G. Successful treatment of anogenital lichen sclerosus with topical tacrolimus. Arch Dermatol 2003;139:922–4. (Level III)

79. Goldstein AT, Marinoff SC, Christopher K. Pimecrolimus for the treatment of vulvar lichen sclerosus: a report of 4 cases. J Reprod Med 2004;49:778–80. (Level III)

80. Hengge UR, Krause W, Hofmann H, Stadler R, Gross G, Meurer M, et al. Multicentre, phase II trial on the safety and efficacy of topical tacrolimus ointment for the treatment of lichen sclerosus. Br J Dermatol 2006;155:1021–8. (Level II-3)

81. Rouzier R, Haddad B, Deyrolle C, Pelisse M, Moyal-Barracco M, Paniel BJ. Perineoplasty for the treatment of introital stenosis related to vulvar lichen sclerosus. Am J Obstet Gynecol 2002;186:49–52. (Level III)

82. Anderson M, Kutzner S, Kaufman RH. Treatment of vulvovaginal lichen planus with vaginal hydrocortisone suppositories. Obstet Gynecol 2002;100:359–62. (Level III)

83. Byrd JA, Davis MD, Rogers RS 3rd. Recalcitrant symptomatic vulvar lichen planus: response to topical tacrolimus. Arch Dermatol 2004;140:715–20. (Level III)

84. Jensen JT, Bird M, Leclair CM. Patient satisfaction after the treatment of vulvovaginal erosive lichen planus with topical clobetasol and tacrolimus: a survey study. Am J Obstet Gynecol 2004;190:1759–63; discussion 1763–5. (Level III)

85. Cooper SM, Wojnarowska F. Influence of treatment of erosive lichen planus of the vulva on its prognosis. Arch Dermatol 2006;142:289–94. (Level II-2)

86. Lewis FM. Vulval lichen planus. Br J Dermatol 1998;138:569–75. (Level III)

87. Gunthert AR, Hinney B, Nesselhut K, Hanf V, Emons G. Vulvitis granulomatosa and unilateral hypertrophy of the vulva related to Crohn's disease: a case report. Am J Obstet Gynecol 2004;191:1719–20. (Level III)

88. Setterfield JF, Neill S, Shirlaw PJ, Theron J, Vaughan R, Escudier M, et al. The vulvovaginal gingival syndrome: a severe subgroup of lichen planus with characteristic clinical features and a novel association with the class II HLA DQB1*0201 allele. J Am Acad Dermatol 2006;55:98–113. (Level II-2)

89. Lynch PJ, Edwards L. White patches and plaques. In: Genital dermatology. New York (NY): Churchill Livingstone; 1994. p. 149–62. (Level III)

90. Lloyd J, Flanagan AM. Mammary and extramammary Paget's disease. J Clin Pathol 2000;53:742–9. (Level III)

The MEDLINE database, the Cochrane Library, and ACOG's own internal resources and documents were used to conduct a literature search to locate relevant articles published between January 1985 and August 2007. The search was restricted to articles published in the English language. Priority was given to articles reporting results of original research, although review articles and commentaries also were consulted. Abstracts of research presented at symposia and scientific conferences were not considered adequate for inclusion in this document. Guidelines published by organizations or institutions such as the National Institutes of Health and the American College of Obstetricians and Gynecologists were reviewed, and additional studies were located by reviewing bibliographies of identified articles. When reliable research was not available, expert opinions from obstetrician–gynecologists were used.

Studies were reviewed and evaluated for quality according to the method outlined by the U.S. Preventive Services Task Force:

I Evidence obtained from at least one properly designed randomized controlled trial.

II-1 Evidence obtained from well-designed controlled trials without randomization.

II-2 Evidence obtained from well-designed cohort or case–control analytic studies, preferably from more than one center or research group.

II-3 Evidence obtained from multiple time series with or without the intervention. Dramatic results in uncontrolled experiments also could be regarded as this type of evidence.

III Opinions of respected authorities, based on clinical experience, descriptive studies, or reports of expert committees.

Based on the highest level of evidence found in the data, recommendations are provided and graded according to the following categories:

Level A—Recommendations are based on good and consistent scientific evidence.

Level B—Recommendations are based on limited or inconsistent scientific evidence.

Level C—Recommendations are based primarily on consensus and expert opinion.

The American College of Obstetricians and Gynecologists
409 12th Street, SW, PO Box 96920, Washington, DC 20090-6920

Diagnosis and management of vulvar skin disorders. ACOG Practice Bulletin No. 93. American College of Obstetricians and Gynecologists. Obstet Gynecol 2008;111:1243–53.

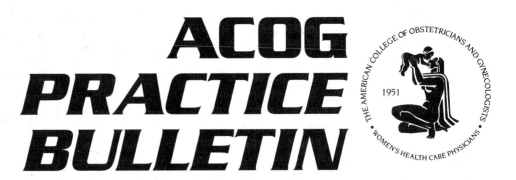

CLINICAL MANAGEMENT GUIDELINES FOR OBSTETRICIAN–GYNECOLOGISTS

NUMBER 94, JUNE 2008

(Replaces Practice Bulletin Number 3, December 1998)

This Practice Bulletin was developed by the ACOG Committee on Practice Bulletins—Gynecology with the assistance of Donald Fylstra, MD. The information is designed to aid practitioners in making decisions about appropriate obstetric and gynecologic care. These guidelines should not be construed as dictating an exclusive course of treatment or procedure. Variations in practice may be warranted based on the needs of the individual patient, resources, and limitations unique to the institution or type of practice.

THE AMERICAN COLLEGE OF OBSTETRICIANS AND GYNECOLOGISTS

WOMEN'S HEALTH CARE PHYSICIANS

Medical Management of Ectopic Pregnancy

In the United States, ectopic pregnancy accounts for 2% of all first-trimester pregnancies and 6% of all pregnancy-related deaths; it is the leading cause of maternal death in the first trimester (1). Early detection of ectopic pregnancy can lead to successful management without surgery. Methotrexate, a folic acid antagonist, can be used successfully to treat early, nonruptured ectopic pregnancy. The purpose of this document is to review the risks and benefits of the use of methotrexate in the management of ectopic pregnancy.

Background

Incidence

The true incidence of ectopic pregnancy is difficult to estimate because many patients are treated in an outpatient setting. In 1992, ectopic pregnancies accounted for 2% of pregnancies (2). The prevalence of ectopic pregnancy among women presenting to an emergency department with first-trimester vaginal bleeding, abdominal pain, or both has been reported to be as high as 18% (3).

Etiology

Nearly all ectopic pregnancies (97%) are implanted within the fallopian tube, although implantation can occur within the abdomen, cervix, ovary, or uterine cornua. One common factor for the development of an ectopic pregnancy is a pathologic fallopian tube. Causes for such pathology include tubal surgery, genital tract infections leading to pelvic inflammatory disease, previous ectopic pregnancy, and in utero exposure to diethylstilbestrol (4). One third of pregnancies that occur after sterilization failure are ectopic implantations (5, 6), and such pregnancies account for 10% of all ectopic pregnancies (7). Additionally, one third of pregnancies after an ectopic pregnancy are also ectopic implantations (7). Other risk factors for the development of ectopic pregnancy include infertility, use of assisted reproductive technologies, previous pelvic or abdominal surgery, and smoking.

Diagnosis

Traditionally, the diagnosis of ectopic pregnancy has been based on the clinical signs and physical symptoms of tubal rupture. However, if ectopic pregnancy is diagnosed before rupture, conservative treatment is an option. By measuring serial human chorionic gonadotropin (hCG) levels and using serial ultrasonography, ectopic pregnancy can be diagnosed before rupture. At least one half of women in whom ectopic pregnancy is diagnosed have no identifiable risk factors or initial definitive physical findings. Early diagnosis is aided by a high index of suspicion. Every sexually active reproductive-aged woman who presents with abdominal pain or vaginal bleeding should be screened for pregnancy (8, 9).

Transvaginal ultrasonography should be considered for all women with suspected early gestational pathology. An initial transvaginal ultrasound examination can be used to visualize an intrauterine pregnancy or a definite extrauterine gestation, or it can be nondiagnostic (10). The woman with a nondiagnostic ultrasound examination result (nothing seen to confirm a gestation inside or outside the uterus) requires further evaluation, including measurement of serum hCG levels. Accurate gestational age calculation, rather than an absolute level of hCG, is the best determinant of when a normal pregnancy should be seen within the uterus with transvaginal ultrasonography. Therefore, if the precise gestational age is known, as in the case of patients conceiving with ovulation induction or embryo transfer, the failure to detect a gestational sac within the uterus by 24 days or later after conception is presumptive evidence of an abnormal pregnancy (13). Without such precise gestational dating, the serum level of hCG must be used in order to interpret a nondiagnostic ultrasonogram. The "discriminatory zone" of hCG is that level of hCG, generalized 1,500–2,000 mIU/mL (International Reference Preparation) (11, 12), which when reached is associated with the appearance, on transvaginal ultrasonography, of a normal singleton intrauterine gestation.

Historically, detection of an intrauterine sac has led to the presumptive exclusion of ectopic pregnancy. However, the incidence of heterotopic pregnancy appears to have increased with the use of assisted reproductive techniques. It has been reported to be as high as 1% in some series (14), although the overall incidence of heterotopic pregnancy probably is much lower.

If the hCG level is higher than the discriminatory zone, and the transvaginal ultrasound examination result is nondiagnostic, ectopic pregnancy is likely (15). However, multiple gestations have higher hCG levels than singletons at any given gestational age and may lead to hCG levels well above 2,000 mIU/mL before ultrasound recognition (13). Therefore, if a multiple gestation is likely, such as in a woman who has conceived with assisted reproductive technology, the discriminatory zone should be reevaluated.

Serum progesterone level determination may help confirm an ectopic pregnancy diagnosis. Serum progesterone values are independent of hCG levels, and an abnormal progesterone level is consistent with an abnormal, failing pregnancy but does not identify the site of the pregnancy (failed intrauterine or ectopic pregnancy). A serum progesterone level less than 5 ng/mL has a specificity of 100% in confirming an abnormal pregnancy (16). Serum progesterone levels higher than 20 ng/mL usually are associated with normal intrauterine pregnancies, and levels between 5 ng/mL and 20 ng/mL are considered equivocal. Most ectopic pregnancies are associated with a serum progesterone level between 10 ng/mL and 20 ng/mL, limiting the clinical utility of this assessment.

In the absence of a diagnostic ultrasound examination result or a low serum progesterone level consistent with a failed pregnancy, serial hCG levels must be used to evaluate an ongoing pregnancy. With 99% sensitivity in early pregnancy, an increase in serum hCG of less than 53% in 48 hours confirms an abnormal pregnancy (17). Therefore, a nondiagnostic ultrasound examination result with a serum progesterone level less than 5 ng/mL and an inappropriate increase in hCG are each associated with an abnormal pregnancy. If necessary, endometrial sampling can be used to differentiate between a failed intrauterine pregnancy and ectopic pregnancy by confirming the presence or absence of intrauterine chorionic villi.

If a woman has an initial nondiagnostic ultrasound examination result, an equivocal or normal serum progesterone level, and an appropriately increasing hCG level, and she remains clinically stable, a transvaginal ultrasound examination should be repeated when the hCG reaches the discriminatory zone. The same diagnostic possibilities then should be considered.

Methotrexate

Methotrexate is an antimetabolite that binds to the catalytic site of dihydrofolate reductase, interrupting the synthesis of purine nucleotides and the amino acids serine and methionine, thus inhibiting DNA synthesis and repair and cell replication. Methotrexate affects actively proliferating tissues such as bone marrow, buccal and intestinal mucosa, respiratory epithelium, malignant cells, and trophoblastic tissue. Systemic methotrexate has been used to treat gestational trophoblastic disease since 1956 and was first used to treat ectopic pregnancy in 1982 (18). The overall success for treatment of ectopic pregnancy using systemic methotrexate in observational studies ranges from 71.2% to 94.2% (7, 19). Success depends on the treatment regimen used, gestational age, and hCG level. A systematic review of several observational studies reported a failure rate of 14.3% or higher with single-dose methotrexate when pretreatment hCG levels are higher than 5,000 mIU/mL, compared with a 3.7% failure rate for hCG levels less than 5,000 mIU/mL (20). If hCG levels are higher than 5,000 mIU/mL, multiple doses may be appropriate (21).

Clinical Considerations and Recommendations

▶ *Who are candidates for treatment with methotrexate?*

Methotrexate therapy can be considered for those women with a confirmed, or high clinical suspicion of, ectopic pregnancy who are hemodynamically stable with an unruptured mass. A candidate for methotrexate treatment must be able to comply with follow-up surveillance. Because methotrexate affects all rapidly dividing tissues within the body, including bone marrow, the gastrointestinal mucosa, and the respiratory epithelium, it should not be given to women with blood dyscrasias or active gastrointestinal and respiratory disease. Methotrexate is directly toxic to the hepatocytes and is cleared from the body by renal excretion; therefore, it should not be used in women with liver or kidney disease. Contraindications for the use of methotrexate are listed in the box, "Contraindications to Methotrexate Therapy." Before administering methotrexate, a woman should have a confirmed normal serum creatinine level, normal liver transaminases, and no bone marrow dysfunction indicated by significant anemia, leucopenia, or thrombocytopenia. Typically, these laboratory tests are repeated 1 week after administering methotrexate to evaluate any possible impact on renal, hepatic, and hematologic function.

▶ *How is methotrexate used in the management of ectopic pregnancy?*

Three protocols are published for the administration of methotrexate to treat ectopic pregnancy: 1) single dose,

---

Contraindications to Medical Therapy

Absolute contraindications

Breastfeeding

Overt or laboratory evidence of immunodeficiency

Alcoholism, alcoholic liver disease, or other chronic liver disease

Preexisting blood dyscrasias, such as bone marrow hypoplasia, leukopenia, thrombocytopenia, or significant anemia

Known sensitivity to methotrexate

Active pulmonary disease

Peptic ulcer disease

Hepatic, renal, or hematologic dysfunction

Relative contraindications

Gestational sac larger than 3.5 cm

Embryonic cardiac motion

Methotrexate Treatment Protocols

Single-dose regimen:*

Single dose MTX 50 mg/m^2 IM day 1

Measure hCG level on posttreatment days 4 and 7

Check for 15% hCG decrease between days 4 and 7.

Then measure hCG level weekly until reaching the nonpregnant level.

If results are less than the expected 15% decrease, readminister MTX 50 mg/m^2 and repeat hCG measurement on days 4 and 7 after second dose. This can be repeated as necessary.

If, during follow-up, hCG levels plateau or increase, consider repeating MTX.

Two-dose regimen:†

Administer 50 mg/m^2 IM on day 0.

Repeat 50 mg/m^2 IM on day 4.

Measure hCG levels on days 4 and 7, and expect a 15% decrease between days 4 and 7.

If the decrease is greater than 15%, measure hCG levels weekly until reaching nonpregnant level.

If less than a 15% decrease in hCG levels, readminister MTX 50 mg/m^2 on days 7 and 11, measuring hCG levels.

(continued)

2) two dose, and 3) fixed multidose (see the box, "Methotrexate Treatment Protocols"). The single 50 mg/m² dose regimen is the simplest and has been shown by some to be as effective as the fixed multidose regimen, eliminating the need for folinic acid rescue to minimize side effects (22). However, a recent meta-analysis has shown the fixed multidose regimen to be more effective, especially in treating women with more advanced gestations and those with embryonic cardiac activity (19). A recent prospective study evaluating a two-dose regimen found high patient satisfaction, few side effects, and 87% treatment success (23).

Methotrexate also can be used after surgical management of an ectopic pregnancy. Treatment failure (persistent ectopic pregnancy) ranges from 2% to 11% after laparotomy and salpingostomy, and from 5% to 20% after laparoscopic salpingostomy (7). A nonruptured, persistent ectopic pregnancy after salpingostomy diagnosed by monitoring serial hCG levels almost uniformly resolves with a single dose of methotrexate. In one randomized trial, the empiric administration of a single dose of methotrexate immediately after laparoscopic salpingostomy essentially eliminated the risk of subsequent persistent ectopic pregnancy (24). However, many women would need to be treated with methotrexate to prevent one persistent ectopic pregnancy; therefore, monitoring with serum hCG levels may be more useful (25).

▶ *What surveillance is needed after methotrexate treatment?*

With any conservative surgical or medical treatment of ectopic pregnancy, women require close monitoring to ensure disappearance of trophoblastic activity and elimination of the possibility of persistent ectopic pregnancy after treatment with methotrexate. Persistent trophoblastic activity is confirmed by serially measuring hCG levels. The hCG level may increase initially to levels higher than the pretreatment level, but then should progressively decrease to reach a nonpregnant level (26). Failure of the hCG level to decrease by at least 15% from day 4 to day 7 after methotrexate administration is considered treatment failure. Therapy with either additional methotrexate administration or surgical intervention is required. Posttreatment hCG levels should be monitored until a nonpregnancy level is reached.

▶ *What are the potential side effects from systemic methotrexate administration?*

Methotrexate morbidity usually is dose and treatment duration dependent. Because methotrexate affects rapidly dividing tissues, gastrointestinal side effects, such as nausea, vomiting, and stomatitis, are the most common. Therefore, women treated with methotrexate should be advised not to use alcohol and nonsteroidal antiinflammatory drugs (NSAIDs). Elevation of liver enzymes usually is seen only with multidose regimens and resolves after discontinuing methotrexate use or increasing the rescue dose of folinic acid (27). Alopecia is a rare side effect with the doses used to treat ectopic pregnancy. Women should report any fever or respiratory symptoms because pneumonitis has been reported.

It is not unusual for women treated with methotrexate to experience abdominal pain 2–3 days after administration, presumably from the cytotoxic effect of the drug on the trophoblast tissue, causing tubal abortion. In the absence of signs and symptoms of overt tubal rupture and significant hemoperitoneum, this pain usually can be managed expectantly by monitoring a woman's hemoglobin level and intraperitoneal fluid amount with transvaginal ultrasonography.

> ▶ *How should women be counseled regarding immediate and long-term treatment effects of methotrexate?*

Patients should receive information about the types of side effects they might experience and about activity restrictions during treatment. They should be informed of the ongoing risk of tubal rupture during treatment. It is important to educate patients about symptoms of tubal rupture and to emphasize the need to seek immediate medical attention if these symptoms occur. The patient should be advised during therapy not to use folic acid supplements, NSAIDs, or alcohol, to avoid sunlight exposure, and to refrain from sexual intercourse or vigorous physical activity (27).

Methotrexate is one of the most studied drugs in pregnant women, with an extensive history of use in treating gestational trophoblastic disease. Methotrexate therapy has not been associated with any additional congenital anomalies in future offspring. Comparing systemic methotrexate with tube-sparing laparoscopic surgery, randomized trials have shown no difference in overall tubal preservation, tubal patency, repeat ectopic pregnancy, or future pregnancies (25).

> ▶ *Is there a role for expectant management of ectopic pregnancy?*

Distinguishing patients who are experiencing spontaneous resolution of their ectopic pregnancies from patients who have proliferating ectopic pregnancies and require active intervention is difficult. Candidates for successful expectant management must be willing to accept the potential risks of tubal rupture and hemorrhage; they should be asymptomatic and have objective evidence of resolution (generally manifested by decreasing hCG levels). In general, patients with early tubal gestations with lower hCG levels are the best candidates for observation. Approximately 20–30% of ectopic pregnancies are associated with decreasing hCG levels at the time of presentation (28). If the initial hCG level is less than 200 mU/mL, 88% of patients experience spontaneous resolution, and lower spontaneous resolution rates can be anticipated with higher hCG levels (29). Reasons for abandoning expectant management include intractable or significantly increased pain, failure of hCG levels to decrease, and tubal rupture with hemoperitoneum.

Summary of Recommendations and Conclusions

The following conclusion is based on good and consistent evidence (Level A):

▶ In comparing systemic methotrexate with tube-sparing laparoscopic surgery, randomized trials have shown no difference in overall tubal preservation, tubal patency, repeat ectopic pregnancy, or future pregnancies.

The following recommendations and conclusions are based on limited or inconsistent evidence (Level B):

▶ An increase in serum hCG of less than 53% in 48 hours confirms an abnormal pregnancy.

▶ With an hCG level of 5,000 mIU/mL or higher, multiple doses of methotrexate may be appropriate.

▶ Methotrexate can be considered in those women with a confirmed, or high clinical suspicion of, ectopic pregnancy who are hemodynamically stable with an unruptured mass.

▶ Failure of the hCG level to decrease by at least 15% from day 4 to day 7 after methotrexate administration is considered treatment failure requiring therapy with either additional methotrexate administration or surgical intervention.

▶ Posttreatment hCG levels should be monitored until a nonpregnancy level is reached.

The following conclusion is based primarily on consensus and expert opinion (Level C):

▶ If the initial hCG level is less than 200 mU/mL, 88% of patients experience spontaneous resolution.

Performance Measure

Percentage of women with an ectopic pregnancy in whom hCG levels are monitored to a nonpregnant level

References

1. Chang J, Elam-Evans LD, Berg CJ, Herndon J, Flowers L, Seed KA, et al. Pregnancy-related mortality surveillance—United States, 1991—1999. MMWR Surveill Summ 2003;52:1–8. (Level II-3)

2. Ectopic pregnancy—United States, 1990-1992. Centers for Disease Control and Prevention (CDC). MMWR Morb Mortal Wkly Rep 1995;44:46–8. (Level III)

3. Barnhart KT, Sammel MD, Gracia CR, Chittams J, Hummel AC, Shaunik A. Risk factors for ectopic pregnancy in women with symptomatic first-trimester pregnancies. Fertil Steril 2006;86:36–43. (Level II-2)

4. Ankum WM, Mol BW, Van der Veen F, Bossuyt PM. Risk factors for ectopic pregnancy: a meta-analysis. Fertil Steril 1996;65:1093–9. (Level III)

5. Peterson HB, Xia Z, Hughes JM, Wilcox LS, Tylor LR, Trussell J. The risk of pregnancy after tubal sterilization: findings from the U.S. Collaborative Review of Sterilization. Am J Obstet Gynecol 1996;174:1161–8; discussion 1168–70. (Level II-2)

6. Peterson HB, Xia Z, Hughes JM, Wilcox LS, Tylor LR, Trussell J. The risk of ectopic pregnancy after tubal sterilization. U.S. Collaborative Review of Sterilization Working Group. N Engl J Med 1997;336:762–7. (Level II-2)

7. Fylstra DL. Tubal pregnancy: a review of current diagnosis and treatment. Obstet Gynecol Surv 1998;53:320–8. (Level III)

8. Abbott J, Emmans LS, Lowenstein SR. Ectopic pregnancy: ten common pitfalls in diagnosis. Am J Emerg Med 1990;8:515–22. (Level II-3)

9. Dart RG, Kaplan B, Varaklis K. Predictive value of history and physical examination in patients with suspected ectopic pregnancy. Ann Emerg Med 1999;33:283–90. (Level II-2)

10. Gracia CR, Barnhart KT. Diagnosing ectopic pregnancy: decision analysis comparing six strategies. Obstet Gynecol 2001;97:464–70. (Level III)

11. Kadar N, Bohrer M, Kemmann E, Shelden R. The discriminatory human chorionic gonadotropin zone for endovaginal sonography: a prospective, randomized study. Fertil Steril 1994;61:1016–20. (Level I)

12. Fossum GT, Davajan V, Kletzky OA. Early detection of pregnancy with transvaginal ultrasound. Fertil Steril 1988;49:788–91. (Level III)

13. Goldstein SR, Snyder JR, Watson C, Danon M. Very early pregnancy detection with endovaginal ultrasound. Obstet Gynecol 1988;72:200–4. (Level III)

14. Svare J, Norup P, Grove Thomsen S, Hornnes P, Maigaard S, Helm P, et al. Heterotopic pregnancies after in-vitro fertilization and embryo transfer—a Danish survey. Hum Reprod 1993;8:116–8. (Level III)

15. Condous G, Kirk E, Lu C, Van Huffel S, Gevaert O, De Moor B, et al. Diagnostic accuracy of varying discriminatory zones for the prediction of ectopic pregnancy in women with a pregnancy of unknown location. Ultrasound Obstet Gynecol 2005;26:770–5. (Level II-3)

16. Stovall TG, Ling FW, Carson SA, Buster JE. Serum progesterone and uterine curettage in differential diagnosis of ectopic pregnancy. Fertil Steril 1992;57:456–7. (Level III)

17. Barnhart KT, Sammel MD, Rinaudo PF, Zhou L, Hummel AC, Guo W. Symptomatic patients with an early viable intrauterine pregnancy: HCG curves redefined. Obstet Gynecol 2004;104:50–5. (Level II-2)

18. Tanaka T, Hayashi H, Kutsuzawa T, Fujimoto S, Ichinoe K. Treatment of interstitial ectopic pregnancy with methotrexate: report of a successful case. Fertil Steril 1982;37:851–2. (Level III)

19. Barnhart KT, Gosman G, Ashby R, Sammel M. The medical management of ectopic pregnancy: a meta-analysis comparing "single dose" and "multidose" regimens. Obstet Gynecol 2003;101:778–84. (Level II-2)

20. Menon S, Colins J, Barnhart KT. Establishing a human chorionic gonadotropin cutoff to guide methotrexate treatment of ectopic pregnancy: a systematic review. Fertil Steril 2007;87:481–4. (Level III)

21. Alleyassin A, Khademi A, Aghahosseini M, Safdarian L, Badenoosh B, Hamed EA. Comparison of success rates in the medical management of ectopic pregnancy with single-dose and multiple-dose administration of methotrexate: a prospective, randomized clinical trial. Fertil Steril 2006;85:1661–6. (Level I)

22. Alexander JM, Rouse DJ, Varner E, Austin JM Jr. Treatment of the small unruptured ectopic pregnancy: a cost analysis of methotrexate versus laparoscopy. Obstet Gynecol 1996;88:123–7. (Level III)

23. Barnhart K, Hummel AC, Sammel MD, Menon S, Jain J, Chakhtoura N. Use of "2-dose" regimen of methotrexate to treat ectopic pregnancy. Fertil Steril 2007;87:250–6. (Level III)

24. Graczykowski JW, Mishell DR Jr. Methotrexate prophylaxis for persistent ectopic pregnancy after conservative treatment by salpingostomy. Obstet Gynecol 1997;89:118–22. (Level I)

25. Hajenius PJ, Mol F, Mol BWJ, Bossuyt PMM, Ankum WM, van der Veen F. Interventions for tubal ectopic pregnancy. Cochrane Database of Systematic Reviews 2007, Issue 1. Art. No.: CD000324. DOI: 10.1002/14651858.CD000324.pub2. (Level III)

26. Stovall TG, Ling FW. Single-dose methotrexate: an expanded clinical trial. Am J Obstet Gynecol 1993;168:1759–62; discussion 1762–5. (Level II-3)

27. Pisarska MD, Carson SA, Buster JE. Ectopic pregnancy. Lancet 1998;351:1115–20. (Level III)

28. Shalev E, Peleg D, Tsabari A, Romono S, Bustan M. Spontaneous resolution of ectopic tubal pregnancy: natural history. Fertil Steril 1995;63:15–9. (Level II-3)

29. Korhonen J, Stenman UH, Ylotalo P. Serum human chorionic gonadotropin dynamics during spontaneous resolution of ectopic pregnancy. Fertil Steril 1994;61:632–6. (Level III)

The MEDLINE database, the Cochrane Library, and ACOG's own internal resources and documents were used to conduct a literature search to locate relevant articles published between January 1985 and May 2007. The search was restricted to articles published in the English language. Priority was given to articles reporting results of original research, although review articles and commentaries also were consulted. Abstracts of research presented at symposia and scientific conferences were not considered adequate for inclusion in this document. Guidelines published by organizations or institutions such as the National Institutes of Health and the American College of Obstetricians and Gynecologists were reviewed, and additional studies were located by reviewing bibliographies of identified articles. When reliable research was not available, expert opinions from obstetrician–gynecologists were used.

Studies were reviewed and evaluated for quality according to the method outlined by the U.S. Preventive Services Task Force:

I   Evidence obtained from at least one properly designed randomized controlled trial.

II-1   Evidence obtained from well-designed controlled trials without randomization.

II-2   Evidence obtained from well-designed cohort or case–control analytic studies, preferably from more than one center or research group.

II-3   Evidence obtained from multiple time series with or without the intervention. Dramatic results in uncontrolled experiments also could be regarded as this type of evidence.

III   Opinions of respected authorities, based on clinical experience, descriptive studies, or reports of expert committees.

Based on the highest level of evidence found in the data, recommendations are provided and graded according to the following categories:

Level A—Recommendations are based on good and consistent scientific evidence.

Level B—Recommendations are based on limited or inconsistent scientific evidence.

Level C—Recommendations are based primarily on consensus and expert opinion.

The American College of Obstetricians and Gynecologists
409 12th Street, SW, PO Box 96920, Washington, DC 20090-6920

Medical management of ectopic pregnancy. ACOG Practice Bulletin No. 94. American College of Obstetricians and Gynecologists. Obstet Gynecol 2008;111:1479–85.

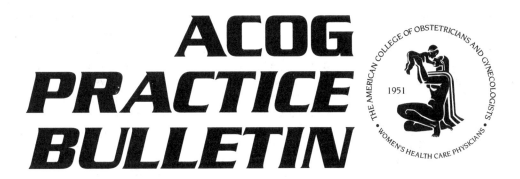

ACOG PRACTICE BULLETIN

CLINICAL MANAGEMENT GUIDELINES FOR OBSTETRICIAN–GYNECOLOGISTS

NUMBER 96, AUGUST 2008

Replaces Practice Bulletin Number 16, May 2000 and Committee Opinion Number 293, February 2004

Alternatives to Hysterectomy in the Management of Leiomyomas

This Practice Bulletin was developed by the ACOG Committee on Practice Bulletins—Gynecology with the assistance of Elizabeth A. Stewart, MD. The information is designed to aid practitioners in making decisions about appropriate obstetric and gynecologic care. These guidelines should not be construed as dictating an exclusive course of treatment or procedure. Variations in practice may be warranted based on the needs of the individual patient, resources, and limitations unique to the institution or type of practice.

Uterine leiomyomas (also called fibroids) are the most common solid pelvic tumors in women and the leading indication for hysterectomy. Although many women with uterine leiomyomas are asymptomatic and can be monitored without treatment, some will require more active measures. Hysterectomy remains the most common surgical treatment for leiomyomas because it is the only definitive treatment and eliminates the possibility of recurrence. Many women seek an alternative to hysterectomy because they desire future childbearing or wish to retain their uteri even if they have completed childbearing. As alternatives to hysterectomy become increasingly available, the efficacies and risks of these treatments are important to delineate. The purpose of this bulletin is to review the literature about medical and surgical alternatives to hysterectomy and to offer treatment recommendations.

Background

The two most common symptoms of uterine leiomyomas for which women seek treatment are abnormal uterine bleeding and pelvic pressure. The most common kind of abnormal uterine bleeding associated with leiomyomas is heavy or prolonged menstrual bleeding, which frequently results in iron deficiency anemia (1). This heavy flow may result in significant disruption of a woman's daily activities. However, not all bleeding is caused by leiomyomas; therefore, other causes of abnormal bleeding should be ruled out. The pelvic and abdominal discomfort that women experience with leiomyomas often is described as pressure. In addition to pelvic pressure, leiomyomas may interfere

THE AMERICAN COLLEGE OF OBSTETRICIANS AND GYNECOLOGISTS
WOMEN'S HEALTH CARE PHYSICIANS

with adjacent structures, leading to dyspareunia and difficulty with urination or defecation.

Uterine leiomyomas are very common, with some studies reporting leiomyomas in 70% of white women and more than 80% of black women by age 50 years (2). Leiomyomas can vary greatly in size and may be present in subserosal, submucosal, intramural, pedunculated, or combined locations. Symptoms and treatment options are affected by the size, number, and location of the leiomyomas. The lack of a simple, inexpensive, and safe long-term medical treatment means that most symptomatic leiomyomas are still managed surgically.

Alternatives to Hysterectomy

In choosing an alternative to hysterectomy, both safety and efficacy need to be considered for each treatment. It must be recognized that all alternatives to hysterectomy allow the possibility for new leiomyomas to form, and preexisting small or undetected leiomyomas may exhibit significant growth, necessitating another treatment. The risk of recurrence must be balanced against the potential benefits of uterine-sparing procedures, such as decreased rates of morbidity and continued fertility. However, procedural complications may rarely lead to an unanticipated hysterectomy.

Medication

Contraceptive Steroids and Nonsteroidal Antiinflammatory Drugs

Contraceptive steroids (estrogen and progestin combinations and progestin alone) are widely used for the control of abnormalities of menstruation. These agents often are first-line therapy for control of abnormal bleeding and painful menstruation in women with and without leiomyomas. However, evidence-based reviews suggest that current medical therapies tend to give only short-term relief, and the crossover rate to surgical therapies is high (3).

Data are limited about the effects of estrogen and progestin treatment of leiomyomas. Estrogen and progestin treatment, usually with oral contraceptives, may control bleeding symptoms without stimulating further leiomyoma growth. However, studies of progestin therapy have demonstrated mixed results. Although several small studies have shown a decrease in leiomyoma size during progestin therapy (4, 5), other studies using progestin therapy alone or in conjunction with a gonadotropin-releasing hormone (GnRH) agonist identify an increase in leiomyoma volume or uterine volume during therapy (6–10). Therefore, when contraceptive steroid therapy is initiated, close monitoring of both leiomyoma

and uterine size is recommended. Epidemiologic studies also suggest that both combined oral contraceptives and progestin-only contraceptives also may decrease the risk of developing clinically significant leiomyomas (11, 12). Nonsteroidal antiinflammatory drugs are effective in reducing dysmenorrhea, but there are no studies that document improvement in women with dysmenorrhea caused by leiomyomas.

The levonorgestrel intrauterine system leads to minimal systemic effects, and the localized endometrial effect is beneficial for treatment of menorrhagia (3). Small studies suggest that the levonorgestrel intrauterine system may be effective for treatment of heavy uterine bleeding in women with leiomyomas (13). However, these women may have a higher rate of expulsion and vaginal spotting.

Gonadotropin-Releasing Hormone Agonists

Gonadotropin-releasing hormone agonists lead to amenorrhea in most women and provide a 35–65% reduction in leiomyoma volume within 3 months of treatment (14). The GnRH agonist leuprolide acetate is approved by the U.S. Food and Drug Administration (FDA) for preoperative therapy in women with anemia in conjunction with supplemental iron, and it is most useful in women with large leiomyomas. The effects of GnRH agonists are temporary, with gradual recurrent growth of leiomyomas to previous size within several months after cessation of treatment. In addition, the significant symptoms of pseudomenopause and adverse impact of the induced hypoestrogenism on bone density limit their suggested use to no more than 6 months without hormonal add-back therapy.

If treatment is continued for more than 6 months, low-dose steroidal add-back therapy should be considered to minimize continued bone loss and vasomotor symptoms. Whereas contraceptive steroid add-back therapy can be used for some diseases, for leiomyomas only low-dose preparations, equivalent to menopausal hormonal therapy, have been studied. It also appears that using a sequential regimen, in which a GnRH agonist is first used to achieve down regulation to which steroids are added after 1–3 months of therapy, gives maximal results. However, the addition of progestin add-back therapy results in an increase in mean uterine volume to 95% of baseline within 24 months (9).

Aromatase Inhibitors

Aromatase inhibitors block ovarian and peripheral estrogen production and decrease estradiol levels after 1 day of treatment (15). Based on their mechanism of action, these agents may have fewer side effects than GnRH analogues, with the benefit of a rapid effect. Several small studies and case reports have identified reductions in leiomyoma size and symptoms with the use of aromatase inhibitors (16–18). Overall, little data exist about the use of aromatase inhibitors to treat uterine leiomyomas, and further research is necessary to elucidate their clinical use. These medications are not FDA approved for the treatment of leiomyomas.

Progesterone Modulators

Antiprogesterone agents act at the level of the progesterone receptors found in high concentration in leiomyomatous uteri (19, 20). Mifepristone is the most extensively studied progesterone-modulating compound; recent studies have shown its usefulness in controlling leiomyoma symptoms (21, 22). Several studies of high-dose mifepristone have reported a reduction of leiomyoma volume of 26–74% (23, 24). This reduction is comparable to those achieved through the use of analogues, and leiomyomas appear to have a slower rate of recurrent growth after cessation of mifepristone treatment (23). Amenorrhea also is a common result of mifepristone use, with rates up to 90%, coupled with stable bone mineral density and improvements in pelvic pressure (21, 23).

Potential side effects of mifepristone include endometrial hyperplasia without atypia (14–28%) and transient elevations in transaminase levels (4%) necessitating liver-function monitoring (23, 25). In addition, mifepristone requires a compounding pharmacy to produce clinically relevant doses and, thus, has limited availability. Significantly lower doses may be effective without increasing the risk of atypical hyperplasia (21, 22). Antiprogesterone agents may have a short-term role in the preoperative management of leiomyomas, but further study is needed.

Myomectomy

For women who desire uterine preservation, myomectomy may be an option. The goal of a myomectomy procedure is to remove the visible and accessible leiomyomas and then reconstruct the uterus. Traditionally, most myomectomies have been performed by laparotomy; however, endoscopic options increasingly are being used.

Abdominal Myomectomy

Although early studies suggested that the rate of morbidity associated with myomectomy was increased compared with hysterectomy, subsequent research suggests that the risks of the two procedures are similar (26–28). Clinical experience and pooled results of numerous small studies suggest that abdominal myomectomy significantly improves menorrhagia symptoms (overall 81% resolution; range 40–93%), with similar results for resolution of pelvic pressure (29). Therefore, abdominal myomectomy is a safe and effective option for treatment of women with symptomatic leiomyomas.

However, women choosing myomectomy face the risk of recurrence of leiomyomas. A number of studies have examined the use of ultrasonography to assess the recurrence risk of leiomyomas after abdominal myomectomy, but the accuracy of the estimate depends on the sensitivity of the measuring instrument (10, 30–32). Studies have indicated that women who experience childbirth after a myomectomy appear to have a decreased recurrence risk (30, 31). There have been conflicting reports over whether the preoperative use of GnRH agonists affects recurrence risk (10, 32).

The clinically relevant endpoint is whether a second surgical procedure is needed after conservative surgery. In a relatively large series (125 patients monitored at least 5 years and up to 23 years), there was evidence that recurrence depended on the number of leiomyomas present. Of those women who had a single leiomyoma, 27% had recurrent tumors and 11% required hysterectomy. Of those women who had multiple leiomyomas, 59% experienced recurrent tumors. Of the women in the multiple leiomyoma group, 26% required repeat myomectomy, hysterectomy, or both procedures (33).

Another risk of myomectomy is the possibility of undergoing an unexpected hysterectomy because of intraoperative complications. This risk appears to be low (less than 1%) even when uterine size is substantial (28, 34–37). Blood loss and the risk of transfusion may be increased in women with larger uteri (28, 37).

Laparoscopic Myomectomy

Endoscopic myomectomy is a treatment option for some women (38). Laparoscopic myomectomy minimizes the size of the abdominal incision, resulting in a quicker postoperative recovery. Because of the complex nature of laparoscopic dissection and suturing, special surgical expertise typically is required.

There are a number of case series of laparoscopic myomectomies, the largest reporting on more than 2,000 patients over a 6-year period (39). These cohorts report overall complication rates between 8% and 11%, with subsequent pregnancy rates between 57% and 69% (39, 40).

Two randomized controlled trials including a total of 284 patients have compared laparoscopic myomectomy with a minilaparotomy myomectomy (41, 42). The first trial demonstrated shorter operating room duration for minilaparotomy. Laparoscopic myomectomy resulted in less blood loss, reduced length of postoperative ileus, a shorter time to hospital discharge, reduced analgesic requirements, and a more rapid recuperation (41). A second trial compared minilaparotomic myomectomy and laparoscopic myomectomy in patients with unexplained infertility and concluded that both techniques improve reproductive outcomes to a similar degree (42).

Recommendations differ regarding cases amenable to a laparoscopic approach. Previous recommendations have suggested avoiding laparoscopy for leiomyomas larger than 5–8 cm, multiple leiomyomas, or the presence of deep intramural leiomyomas (43, 44). A prospective study compared laparoscopic myomectomy for the management of leiomyomas greater than 80 g with laparoscopic myomectomy in those smaller than 80 g. Operative time (121 minutes versus 79 minutes) and estimated blood loss (346 mL versus 123 mL) were significantly greater in the group with the larger uterine leiomyomas. However, no difference was seen in length of stay or overall complication rates (45).

A large retrospective series of 512 patients reported a leiomyoma recurrence rate of 11.7% after 1 year and up to 84.4% after 8 years, but a reoperation rate for recurrence of 6.7% at 5 years and 16% at 8 years (46). A case series described a 33% recurrence risk at 27 months (47). Successful outcomes from laparoscopic myomectomy have been reported primarily by surgeons with expertise and advanced laparoscopic skills, including laparoscopic myomectomy, and may not be generalizable to surgeons with less laparoscopic experience.

Robot-assisted laparoscopic surgery also has been used to perform myomectomy (48). It may have the advantage of improved optics, including a three-dimensional view, and enhanced surgeon dexterity. Disadvantages with robot-assisted surgery in general include diminished haptic (tactile) sensation, additional operating room time, and increased cost. Further studies, including randomized clinical trials, are needed to better determine clinical outcomes and cost-effectiveness.

Hysteroscopic Myomectomy

Hysteroscopic myomectomy is an accepted method for the management of abnormal uterine bleeding caused by submucous leiomyomas. Submucosal leiomyomas are estimated to be the cause of 5–10% of cases of abnormal uterine bleeding, pain, and subfertility and infertility (4). Submucous leiomyomas are classified based on the amount of leiomyoma within the uterine cavity, with type 0 leiomyomas completely intracavitary, type I leiomyomas less than 50% intramural, and type II leiomyomas more than 50% intramural (49). This classi-

fication has been shown to be predictive of the likelihood of complete surgical resection, which is the most predictive indicator of surgical success. Uterine size and the number of leiomyomas also have been shown to be independent prognostic variables for recurrence (50).

Studies have shown successful removal of the leiomyoma at the initial hysteroscopy at a rate of 65–100%, with most ranging from 85–95% (51). Subsequent surgery is needed in approximately 5–15% of cases, and most of these cases involve a second hysteroscopic procedure. As with abdominal leiomyomectomy, the effectiveness of the procedure decreases over time. One study of 274 procedures, with follow-up of more than 5 years, reported a success rate of 94.6% at 1 year, which decreased to 76.3% at 5 years (52).

Leiomyoma classification is an important predictor of the ability to achieve complete resection, although there have been some reports of success with type II leiomyomas. One retrospective study of 235 patients reported a 95% rate of complete leiomyoma resection in a population that included 70% type II leiomyomas. The 3-year success rate was reported as 97%; however, 36% underwent concomitant endometrial ablation (52).

The reported complication rate for hysteroscopic myomectomy ranges between 1% and 12%, with rates of 1–5% reported in most studies (51). Potential surgical complications include fluid overload with secondary hyponatremia, pulmonary edema, cerebral edema, intraoperative and postoperative bleeding, uterine perforation, gas embolism, and infection.

Uterine Artery Embolization

Uterine artery embolization for the treatment of leiomyoma, performed primarily by interventional radiologists, is a procedure in which the uterine arteries are embolized via a transcutaneous femoral artery approach, resulting in uterine leiomyoma devascularization and involution. The uterine arteries are embolized using polyvinyl alcohol particles of trisacryl gelatin microspheres. Supplemental metal coils also may be used to assist with vascular occlusion.

A large multicenter study of more than 500 patients undergoing uterine artery embolization reported favorable 3-month outcomes for dominant leiomyoma volume reduction (42%) and decreased median leiomyoma life-impact scores, mean menstrual duration, dysmenorrhea, and urinary frequency or urgency (53). The Uterine Artery Embolization in the Treatment of Symptomatic Uterine Fibroid Tumors (EMMY) randomized trial compared uterine artery embolization to total abdominal hysterectomy. In this trial, patients undergoing uterine artery embolization had significantly less pain during the first

24 hours postoperatively and returned to work sooner (28.1 versus 63.4 days) than patients who underwent hysterectomy (54). The rates of major complications were similar, 4.9% for uterine artery embolization and 2.7% for hysterectomy. Minor complications, such as vaginal discharge, leiomyoma expulsion, and hematoma were higher in the group that had uterine artery embolization compared with those that had hysterectomy (58% versus 40%) as well as higher readmission rates for those undergoing uterine artery embolization (11.1% versus 0%) (55). Similar clinical findings were reported in a multicenter trial of uterine artery embolization versus myomectomy (56). Analysis of three randomized clinical trials comparing uterine artery embolization with myomectomy and hysterectomy confirmed that the uterine artery embolization resulted in shorter hospital stay, quicker return to activities, and a higher minor complication rate after discharge (57). The overall complication rates for uterine artery embolization have been reported to be approximately 5% (58).

Long-term outcomes have been reported in several studies. One case–control study comparing uterine artery embolization with myomectomy reported a higher reoperation rate of 29% in the uterine artery embolization group (15 of 51) compared with 3% (1 of 30) in the myomectomy group (59). However, when subjective variables, such as symptom worsening and patient dissatisfaction, were considered, 39% (20 of 51) in the uterine artery embolization group were considered clinical failures, compared with 30% (9 of 30) in the myomectomy group. In 5-year follow-up results of 200 patients treated with uterine artery embolization, a 20% reoperation rate (hysterectomy 13.7%, myomectomy 4.4%, repeat embolization 1.6%) and failure to control symptoms in 25% were documented (60). Another trial reported a reintervention rate of 6% in the myomectomy group, compared with a rate of 33% for those undergoing uterine artery embolization (61). Based on long- and short-term outcomes, uterine artery embolization is a safe and effective option for appropriately selected women who wish to retain their uteri. Women who wish to undergo uterine artery embolization should have a thorough evaluation with an obstetrician–gynecologist to help facilitate optimal collaboration with the interventional radiologists and to ensure the appropriateness of therapy, taking into account the reproductive wishes of the patient.

Magnetic Resonance Imaging-Guided Focused Ultrasound Surgery

In 2004, the FDA granted approval for the use of a magnetic resonance imaging (MRI)-guided system for the localization and treatment of uterine leiomyomas with focused ultrasound therapy. This noninvasive approach uses high-intensity ultrasound waves directed into a focal volume of a leiomyoma. The ultrasound energy penetrates soft tissue and produces well-defined regions of protein denaturation, irreversible cell damage, and coagulative necrosis.

Outcomes of 109 patients undergoing MRI-guided focused ultrasound surgery were reported at 6 months and 12 months (62, 63). Although only modest uterine volume reductions were noted (13.5% at 6 months and 9.4% at 12 months, using intention to treat analysis), 71% of patients reported symptom reduction at 6 months. At 12 months, 51% had symptom reduction. Adverse events included heavy menses, requiring transfusion (5); persistent pain and bleeding (1); hospitalization for nausea (1); and leg and buttock pain caused by sonification of the sciatic nerve in the far field (1), which eventually resolved. Case series suggest that improvement in symptoms at 12 months and 24 months is related to the thoroughness of treatment and that adverse events decrease with increasing experience (64–66). Whereas short-term studies show safety and efficacy, long-term studies are needed to discern whether the minimally invasive advantage of MRI-guided focused ultrasound surgery will lead to durable results beyond 24 months. Protocols for treating larger leiomyoma volumes are being studied.

Clinical Considerations and Recommendations

▶ *In women with leiomyomas who are candidates for surgery, does the use of adjunctive medical treatment result in better outcomes?*

Preoperative Adjuvants

Gonadotropin-releasing hormone agonists have been used widely for preoperative treatment of uterine leiomyomas, both for myomectomy and hysterectomy. They may be beneficial when a significant reduction in uterine volume could change the surgical approach, such as allowing a transverse incision, an endoscopic procedure, or a vaginal hysterectomy.

By inducing amenorrhea, GnRH agonists have been shown to improve hematologic parameters, shorten hospital stay, and decrease blood loss, operating time, and postoperative pain when given for 2–3 months preoperatively (67–69). However, no study has shown a significant decrease in transfusion risk or improvement in quality of life, and the cost of these medications is substantial. Therefore, the benefits of preoperative use of GnRH agonists should be weighed against their cost and side effects for individual patients. It also is worth noting that in a study that achieved hematologic improvement with GnRH agonist treatment in 74% of women, there was a 46% improvement rate in the placebo group with iron supplementation alone (68). One surgical disadvantage to preoperative GnRH agonist therapy is that it may make the leiomyomas softer and the surgical planes less distinct. Although many studies find the operative time equivalent for laparotomies, one study of laparoscopic myomectomies found that overall operating time decreased after GnRH agonist treatment. However, in the subgroup in which the largest leiomyoma was hypoechoic, operative time was longer because of the difficulty in dissection (69).

Gonadotropin-releasing hormone antagonists are now available and have the advantage of not inducing an initial steroidal flare as seen with GnRH agonists. The rapid effect of the antagonist allows a shorter duration of side effects with presurgical treatment. The antagonist has been shown to reduce leiomyoma volume by 25–40% in 19 days, thereby allowing surgery to be scheduled sooner (70). As with the agonist, the reduction of leiomyoma and uterine volumes are transient. Although GnRH antagonists are not currently FDA approved for preoperative treatment of leiomyomas, they may be beneficial.

Intraoperative Adjuvants

Several studies suggest that the infiltration of vasopressin into the myometrium decreases blood loss at the time of myomectomy. A study of 20 patients demonstrated that vasopressin significantly decreased blood loss compared with saline injection in a randomized myomectomy study (71). Two studies compared the use of physical vascular compression, primarily a tourniquet around the lower uterine segment, with pharmacologic vasoconstriction (vasopressin administration). In one study that used a Penrose drain tourniquet and vascular clamps, there was no significant difference between the two techniques (37). The other study, which compared the use of a Foley catheter tourniquet with vasopressin administration, found significantly greater blood loss in the tourniquet group (72). There are no studies that compare tourniquet use with placebo. Additionally, one study demonstrated that injection of vasopressin into the cervix at the time of operative hysteroscopy decreased blood loss, fluid intravasation, and operative time (73).

▶ *In pregnant women who have undergone a myomectomy, does a planned cesarean delivery versus a trial of labor help prevent uterine rupture?*

A trial of labor is not recommended in patients at high risk of uterine rupture, including those with previous classical or T-shaped uterine incisions or extensive transfundal uterine surgery. Because myomectomy also can produce a transmural incision in the uterus, it often has been treated in an analogous way. There are no clinical trials that specifically address this issue; however, one study reports no uterine ruptures in 212 deliveries (83% vaginal) after myomectomy (74).

Pooled data from several case series of laparoscopic myomectomy involving more than 750 pregnancies identified one case of uterine rupture (39, 40, 75–77). Other case reports have described the occurrence of uterine rupture before and during labor (78–80), including rare case reports of uterine rupture remote from term after traditional abdominal myomectomy (81, 82). Most obstetricians allow women who underwent hysteroscopic myomectomy for type O or type I leiomyomas to go through labor and give birth vaginally; however, there are case reports of uterine rupture in women who experienced uterine perforation during hysteroscopy (83–85). It appears that the risk of uterine rupture in pregnancy after laparoscopic or hysteroscopic myomectomy is low. However, because of the serious nature of this complication, a high index of suspicion must be maintained when managing pregnancies after this procedure.

▶ *In women with leiomyomas who desire to become pregnant, does surgical removal of leiomyomas increase the pregnancy rate?*

As with any woman with asymptomatic leiomyomas, those who desire future fertility should be managed expectantly because they have no indication for surgery. For mildly symptomatic women, given the risk of recurrence, intervening as close to the desired pregnancy as practical is desirable. For symptomatic women, prior treatment history should be considered, as well as possible benefit of normalization of the endometrial cavity, the particular fertility consequences of each technique, and the risk of pregnancy complications with untreated leiomyomas.

The contribution of leiomyomas to infertility is difficult to assess because of the high prevalence of leiomyomas in the general population and because the incidence of leiomyomas increases with age, as does infertility. Furthermore, many women with uterine leiomyomas conceive and have uncomplicated pregnancies. Leiomyomas are present in approximately 5–10% of women with infertility and are the sole factor identified in 1–2.4% of women with infertility (29, 86, 87). However, leiomyomas should not be considered the cause of infertility, or significant component of infertility, without completing a basic fertility evaluation to assess the woman and her partner.

Intramural and submucosal leiomyomas can cause distortion of the uterine cavity or obstruction of the tubal ostia or cervical canal and, thus, may affect fertility or lead to pregnancy complications (88–90). When abdominal myomectomies have been performed on women with otherwise unexplained infertility, the subsequent pregnancy rates have been reported to be 40–60% after 1–2 years (29, 91–93). Studies of the effect of laparoscopic or hysteroscopic myomectomy on fertility have shown similar results (94–96). However, the use of additional fertility treatments may have contributed to these marked positive effects.

Several studies have investigated the effect of leiomyomas on reproductive outcomes after in vitro fertilization (IVF). In the setting of an abnormal, distorted uterine cavity caused by leiomyomas (submucosal or intramural), significantly lower IVF pregnancy rates were identified (90–98). In addition, after myomectomy was performed for submucosal leiomyomas, pregnancy rates markedly increased (90). Subserosal leiomyomas have not been shown to have an impact on reproductive outcomes (90). However, in the setting of a nondistorted uterine cavity, the impact of intramural leiomyomas on IVF outcomes remains unclear. Intramural, nondistorting leiomyomas may have a subtle impact on IVF outcomes (97), but there are no definitive data supporting routine prophylactic myomectomy before IVF for women with leiomyomas and normal uterine cavities (98). It should be noted that most studies included women with leiomyomas of 5 cm or less, and women with larger leiomyomas were often excluded from these studies (99). Therefore, although leiomyomas that distort the uterine cavity clearly affect reproductive outcomes, further data about leiomyoma size and reproductive outcomes are needed.

Some surgeons believe that a prophylactic myomectomy may be appropriate for select women with large leiomyomas who wish to preserve future fertility. With a skilled surgeon, the evidence demonstrates that the myomectomy complication rate is low even with substantial uterine size; thus, surgery may be reasonable (28, 30, 31, 34, 36). However, the high risk of recurrent leiomyomas makes this procedure a less effective treatment (30, 31). Additionally, myomectomy can lead to pelvic adhesive disease, which could cause tubal impairment or obstruction and, hence, infertility (100).

When assessing a woman with infertility and leiomyomas, targeted evaluation of the uterus and endometrial cavity to assess leiomyoma location, size, and number is indicated. The data suggest that before infertility treatment, surgical treatment for a distorted uterine cavity caused by leiomyomas is indicated. In addition, myomectomy should be considered for a woman with uterine leiomyomas who has undergone several unsuccessful IVF cycles despite appropriate ovarian response and good quality embryos. There are potential adverse effects of nondistorting leiomyomas on IVF outcomes, although these effects are unconfirmed.

▶ *In women with leiomyomas planning future pregnancies, what is the impact on future fertility of uterine artery embolization and magnetic resonance imaging-guided focused ultrasonography?*

Successful pregnancies can occur following uterine artery embolization (101). Notably, early series demonstrated successful term pregnancies in women who would be expected to have a high rate of infertility (102). There are two issues of specific concern related to uterine artery embolization for women intending to become pregnant. The first is that there appears to be an age-related risk of impairment of ovarian function, as demonstrated by amenorrhea (53). Originally, this risk was attributed only to the circumstances of misembolization, but an understanding of the collateral blood supply of the uterus suggests this can occur with technically correct uterine artery embolization. Although this risk is low in young women (3%), given the prevalence of decreased ovarian reserve as an infertility factor, long-term studies are necessary. A recent report of antimüllerian hormone in women participating in a randomized clinical trial of uterine artery embolization versus hysterectomy suggests that both procedures cause similar impairment of ovarian reserve (103).

There are case reports of pregnancy complications after uterine artery embolization, but this may represent publication bias. However, the most significant data come from the Ontario cohort that includes close follow-up (104). In this case series of 24 pregnancies occurring in women with prior uterine artery embolization, there was a 12% risk of placentation problems (two placenta previa and one placenta accreta), and all occurred in nulliparous patients who were otherwise unlikely to have this type of complication. Thus, because there is biologic plausibility of uterine artery embolization causing compromised endometrial perfusion resulting in abnormal placentation in women not otherwise at risk, this approach should be used with caution for women who are pursuing pregnancy. The effect of uterine artery embolization on pregnancy remains understudied.

Case reports of pregnancy with term delivery have been reported after MRI-guided focused ultrasonography (65, 105–107). However, larger experience is necessary before drawing conclusions.

▶ *In menopausal women with leiomyomas, what is the effect of hormone therapy on leiomyoma growth, bleeding, and pain?*

For many years, health care providers have counseled patients that leiomyomas are a self-limiting problem that will resolve when a woman completes the transition to menopause. Because leiomyomas are responsive to estrogen, the hypoestrogenism of menopause results in uterine shrinkage for most women. However, for women electing hormone therapy, there is the possibility that symptoms associated with leiomyomas may persist into menopause.

There is some evidence that women with leiomyomas who take hormone therapy are more likely to have abnormal bleeding. In a study using hysteroscopy to evaluate women with abnormal bleeding who were taking hormone therapy (using women with no abnormal bleeding as controls), women with structural abnormalities of the cavity, including endometrial polyps and submucosal leiomyomas, had an increased likelihood of abnormal bleeding (108).

A small pilot study examined whether hormone therapy during menopause caused an increase in size of asymptomatic leiomyomas (109). This study showed a significant increase in leiomyoma dimension after 1 year of transdermal hormone therapy but no increase with oral conjugated estrogens. Hormone therapy may cause some modest increase in uterine leiomyoma size, but it does not appear to have an impact on clinical symptoms. Therefore, this treatment option should not be withheld from women who desire or need such therapy.

▶ *In asymptomatic women with leiomyomas, does expectant management produce a better outcome than surgical treatment in relation to long-term morbidity?*

Expectant management in an asymptomatic patient should be the norm, but in some instances an asymptomatic leiomyomatous uterus might require treatment. Historically, it has been argued that uterine size alone should be an indication for hysterectomy. The argument usually has been twofold. The first issue was that a large leiomyomatous uterus made assessment of the ovaries and early surveillance for ovarian cancer impossible. However, the National Institutes of Health and National Cancer Institute Consensus Conference acknowledged the futility of routine pelvic examinations in the identification of early ovarian cancer (110).

Second, the argument is made that, because of the increased rate of morbidity during surgery for a large uterus, surgery is a safer option when the uterus is smaller.

Although some studies have shown increased rates of morbidity, others show no differences in perioperative complications (9, 27, 28, 111). This currently does not appear to be a cogent argument for intervention.

In rare circumstances, the uterus causes significant compression of the ureters that could lead to compromised renal function. A small retrospective review demonstrated ureteral dilation in 56% of patients with uterine size greater or equal to 12 weeks, but no dilation in patients with uterine size less than 12 weeks (112). However, in no studies have the effects of uterine size on renal function been evaluated.

If there is concern that the mass is not a leiomyoma but instead a sarcoma, further evaluation is warranted. Traditionally, the major clinical sign used to make this distinction was rapid growth in uterine size. However, in a study of 1,332 hysterectomy specimens for which the preoperative diagnosis was uterine leiomyomas, sarcomas were rare (2–3/1,000) and no more common in the subgroup of women who had experienced rapidly enlarging uterine size (113). The clinical diagnosis of rapidly growing leiomyomas should not be used as an indication for myomectomy or hysterectomy.

If a comparison is made between the prevalence of leiomyosarcomas discovered incidentally (1/2,000) and the mortality rate for hysterectomy for benign disease (1–1.6/1,000 for premenopausal women), the decision to proceed to hysterectomy to find potential sarcomas should be made cautiously (111). Other risk factors for sarcomas, including increasing age, a history of prior pelvic radiation, tamoxifen use, or having a rare genetic predisposition resulting in hereditary leiomyomatosis and renal cell carcinoma syndrome may influence this decision (114). Alternatively, both endometrial biopsy and MRI appear to be useful in diagnosing sarcomas and differentiating them from other intrauterine lesions (115–117).

In conclusion, there is insufficient evidence to support hysterectomy for asymptomatic leiomyomas solely to improve detection of adnexal masses, to prevent impairment of renal function, or to rule out malignancy.

Summary of Recommendations

The following recommendations and conclusions are based on good and consistent scientific evidence (Level A):

▶ Abdominal myomectomy is a safe and effective alternative to hysterectomy for treatment of women with symptomatic leiomyomas.

▶ Based on long- and short-term outcomes, uterine artery embolization is a safe and effective option for appropriately selected women who wish to retain their uteri.

▶ Gonadotropin-releasing hormone agonists have been shown to improve hematologic parameters, shorten hospital stay, and decrease blood loss, operating time, and postoperative pain when given for 2–3 months preoperatively. Benefits of preoperative use of GnRH agonists should be weighed against their cost and side effects for individual patients.

▶ Several studies suggest that the infiltration of vasopressin into the myometrium decreases blood loss at the time of myomectomy.

The following recommendations are based on limited or inconsistent scientific evidence (Level B):

▶ The clinical diagnosis of rapidly growing leiomyomas should not be used as an indication for myomectomy or hysterectomy.

▶ Hysteroscopic myomectomy is an accepted method for the management of abnormal uterine bleeding caused by submucosal leiomyomas.

The following recommendations and conclusions are based primarily on consensus and expert opinion (Level C):

▶ There is insufficient evidence to support hysterectomy for asymptomatic leiomyomas solely to improve detection of adnexal masses, to prevent impairment of renal function, or to rule out malignancy.

▶ Leiomyomas should not be considered the cause of infertility, or significant component of infertility, without completing a basic fertility evaluation to assess the woman and her partner.

▶ Hormone therapy may cause some modest increase in uterine leiomyoma size but does not appear to have an impact on clinical symptoms. Therefore, this treatment option should not be withheld from women who desire or need such therapy.

▶ The effect of uterine artery embolization on pregnancy remains understudied.

References

1. Fraser IS, Critchley HO, Munro MG, Broder M. A process designed to lead to international agreement on terminologies and definitions used to describe abnormalities of menstrual bleeding. Writing Group for this Menstrual Agreement Process. Fertil Steril 2007;87: 466–76. (Level III)

2. Day Baird D, Dunson DB, Hill MC, Cousins D, Schectman JM. High cumulative incidence of uterine leiomyoma in black and white women: ultrasound evidence. Am J Obstet Gynecol 2003;188:100–7. (Level II-3)

3. Marjoribanks J, Lethaby A, Farquhar C. Surgery versus medical therapy for heavy menstrual bleeding. Cochrane Database of Systematic Reviews 2006, Issue 2. Art. No.: CD003855. DOI: 10.1002/14651858.CD003855.pub2. (Level III)

4. Wallach EE, Vlahos NF. Uterine myomas: an overview of development, clinical features, and management. Obstet Gynecol 2004;104:393–406. (Level III)

5. Venkatachalam S, Bagratee JS, Moodley J. Medical management of uterine fibroids with medroxyprogesterone acetate (Depo Provera): a pilot study. J Obstet Gynaecol 2004;24:798–800. (Level III)

6. Harrison-Woolrych M, Robinson R. Fibroid growth in response to high-dose progestogen. Fertil Steril 1995; 64:191–2. (Level III)

7. Mixson WT, Hammond DO. Response of fibromyomas to a progestin. Am J Obstet Gynecol 1961;82:754–60. (Level III)

8. Carr BR, Marshburn PB, Weatherall PT, Bradshaw KD, Breslau NA, Byrd W, et al. An evaluation of the effect of gonadotropin-releasing hormone analogs and medroxyprogesterone acetate on uterine leiomyomata volume by magnetic resonance imaging: a prospective, randomized, double blind, placebo-controlled, crossover trial. J Clin Endocrinol Metab 1993;76:1217–23. (Level II-3)

9. Friedman AJ, Haas ST. Should uterine size be an indication for surgical intervention in women with myomas? Am J Obstet Gynecol 1993;168:751–5. (Level III)

10. Friedman AJ, Daly M, Juneau-Norcross M, Fine C, Rein MS. Recurrence of myomas after myomectomy in women pretreated with leuprolide acetate depot or placebo. Fertil Steril 1992;58:205–8. (Level III)

11. Marshall LM, Spiegelman D, Goldman MB, Manson JE, Colditz GA, Barbieri RL, et al. A prospective study of reproductive factors and oral contraceptive use in relation to the risk of uterine leiomyomata. Fertil Steril 1998;70:432–9. (Level II-2)

12. Wise LA, Palmer JR, Harlow BL, Spiegelman D, Stewart EA, Adams-Campbell LL, et al. Reproductive factors, hormonal contraception, and risk of uterine leiomyomata in African-American women: a prospective study. Am J Epidemiol 2004;159:113–23. (Level II-2)

13. Mercorio F, De Simone R, Di Spiezio Sardo A, Cerrota G, Bifulco G, Vanacore F, et al. The effect of a levonorgestrel-releasing intrauterine device in the treatment of myoma-related menorrhagia. Contraception 2003; 67:277–80. (Level III)

14. Olive DL, Lindheim SR, Pritts EA. Non-surgical management of leiomyoma: impact on fertility. Curr Opin Obstet Gynecol 2004;16:239–43. (Level III)

15. Iveson TJ, Smith IE, Ahern J, Smithers DA, Trunet PF, Dowsett M. Phase I study of the oral nonsteroidal aromatase inhibitor CGS 20267 in healthy postmenopausal women. J Clin Endocrinol Metab 1993;77:324–31. (Level I)

16. Shozu M, Murakami K, Segawa T, Kasai T, Inoue M. Successful treatment of a symptomatic uterine leiomyoma in a perimenopausal woman with a nonsteroidal aromatase inhibitor. Fertil Steril 2003;79:628–31. (Level III)

17. Attilakos G, Fox R. Regression of tamoxifen-stimulated massive uterine fibroid after conversion to anastrozole. J Obstet Gynaecol 2005;25:609–10. (Level III)

18. Varelas FK, Papanicolaou AN, Vavatsi-Christaki N, Makedos GA, Vlassis GD. The effect of anastrazole on symptomatic uterine leiomyomata. Obstet Gynecol 2007; 110:643–9. (Level III)

19. Englund K, Blanck A, Gustavsson I, Lundkvist U, Sjoblom P, Norgren A, et al. Sex steroid receptors in human myometrium and fibroids: changes during the menstrual cycle and gonadotropin-releasing hormone treatment. J Clin Endocrinol Metab 1998;83:4092–6. (Level III)

20. Nisolle M, Gillerot S, Casanas-Roux F, Squifflet J, Berliere M, Donnez J. Immunohistochemical study of the proliferation index, oestrogen receptors and progesterone receptors A and B in leiomyomata and normal myometrium during the menstrual cycle and under gonadotrophin-releasing hormone agonist therapy. Hum Reprod 1999; 14:2844–50. (Level II-3)

21. Fiscella K, Eisinger SH, Meldrum S, Feng C, Fisher SG, Guzick DS. Effect of mifepristone for symptomatic leiomyomata on quality of life and uterine size: a randomized controlled trial. Obstet Gynecol 2006;108: 1381–7. (Level I)

22. Eisinger SH, Bonfiglio T, Fiscella K, Meldrum S, Guzick DS. Twelve-month safety and efficacy of low-dose mifepristone for uterine myomas. J Minim Invasive Gynecol 2005;12:227–33. (Level II-2)

23. Steinauer J, Pritts EA, Jackson R, Jacoby AF. Systematic review of mifepristone for the treatment of uterine leiomyomata. Obstet Gynecol 2004;103:1331–6. (Level III)

24. Murphy AA, Kettel LM, Morales AJ, Roberts VJ, Yen SS. Regression of uterine leiomyomata in response to the antiprogesterone RU 486. J Clin Endocrinol Metab 1993;76:513–7 (Level III)

25. Eisinger SH, Meldrum S, Fiscella K, le Roux HD, Guzick DS. Low-dose mifepristone for uterine leiomyomata. Obstet Gynecol 2003;101:243–50. (Level I)

26. Hillis SD, Marchbanks PA, Peterson HB. Uterine size and risk of complications among women undergoing abdominal hysterectomy for leiomyomas. Obstet Gynecol 1996;87:539–43. (Level II-2)

27. Iverson RE Jr, Chelmow D, Strohbehn K, Waldman L, Evantash EG. Relative morbidity of abdominal hysterectomy and myomectomy for management of uterine leiomyomas. Obstet Gynecol 1996;88:415–9. (Level II-2)

28. Ecker JL, Foster JT, Friedman AJ. Abdominal hysterectomy or abdominal myomectomy for symptomatic leiomyoma: a comparison of preoperative demography and postoperative morbidity. J Gynecol Surg 1995;11: 11–7. (Level III)

29. Buttram VC Jr, Reiter RC. Uterine leiomyomata: etiology, symptomatology, and management. Fertil Steril 1981;36:433–45. (Level III)

30. Candiani GB, Fedele L, Parazzini F, Villa L. Risk of recurrence after myomectomy. Br J Obstet Gynaecol 1991;98:385–9. (Level II-3)

31. Fedele L, Parazzini F, Luchini L, Mezzopane R, Tozzi L, Villa L. Recurrence of fibroids after myomectomy: a transvaginal ultrasonographic study. Hum Reprod 1995; 10:1795–6. (Level I)

32. Fedele L, Vercellini P, Bianchi S, Brioschi D, Dorta M. Treatment with GnRH agonists before myomectomy and the risk of short-term myoma recurrence. Br J Obstet Gynaecol 1990;97:393–6. (Level I)

33. Malone LJ. Myomectomy: recurrence after removal of solitary and multiple myomas. Obstet Gynecol 1969; 34:200–3. (Level III)

34. Smith DC, Uhlir JK. Myomectomy as a reproductive procedure. Am J Obstet Gynecol 1990;162:1476–9; discussion 1479–82. (Level III)

35. Chong RK, Thong PH, Tan SL, Thong PW, Salmon YM. Myomectomy: indications, results of surgery and relation to fertility. Singapore Med J 1988;29:35–7. (Level III)

36. LaMorte AI, Lalwani S, Diamond MP. Morbidity associated with abdominal myomectomy. Obstet Gynecol 1993;82:897–900. (Level III)

37. Ginsburg ES, Benson CB, Garfield JM, Gleason RE, Friedman AJ. The effect of operative technique and uterine size on blood loss during myomectomy: a prospective randomized study. Fertil Steril 1993;60:956–62. (Level I)

38. Lefebvre G, Vilos G, Allaire C, Jeffrey J, Arneja J, Birch C, et al. The management of uterine leiomyomas. J Obstet Gynaecol Can 2003;25:396,418; quiz 419–22. (Level III)

39. Sizzi O, Rossetti A, Malzoni M, Minelli L, La Grotta F, Soranna L, et al. Italian multicenter study on complications of laparoscopic myomectomy. J Minim Invasive Gynecol 2007;14:453–62. (Level II-2)

40. Altgassen C, Kuss S, Berger U, Loning M, Diedrich K, Schneider A. Complications in laparoscopic myomectomy. Surg Endosc 2006;20:614–8. (Level II-3)

41. Alessandri F, Lijoi D, Mistrangelo E, Ferrero S, Ragni N. Randomized study of laparoscopic versus minilaparotomic myomectomy for uterine myomas. J Minim Invasive Gynecol 2006;13:92–7. (Level I)

42. Palomba S, Zupi E, Falbo A, Russo T, Marconi D, Tolino A, et al. A multicenter randomized, controlled study comparing laparoscopic versus minilaparotomic myomectomy: reproductive outcomes. Fertil Steril 2007;88: 933–41. (Level I)

43. Dubisson JB, Chapron C, Levy J. Difficulties and complications of laparoscopic myomectomy. J Gynecol Surg 1996;12:159–65. (Level III)

44. Seinera P, Arisio R, Decko A, Farina C, Crana F. Laparoscopic myomectomy: indications, surgical technique and complications. Hum Reprod 1997;12: 1927–30. (Level III)

45. Wang CJ, Yuen LT, Lee CL, Kay N, Soong YK. Laparoscopic myomectomy for large uterine fibroids. A comparative study. Surg Endosc 2006;20:1427–30. (Level II-1)

46. Yoo EH, Lee PI, Huh CY, Kim DH, Lee BS, Lee JK, et al. Predictors of leiomyoma recurrence after laparoscopic myomectomy. J Minim Invasive Gynecol 2007; 14: 690–7. (Level II-2)

47. Nezhat FR, Roemisch M, Nezhat CH, Seidman DS, Nezhat CR. Recurrence rate after laparoscopic myomectomy. J Am Assoc Gynecol Laparosc 1998;5:237–40. (Level II-3)

48. Advincula AP, Song A, Burke W, Reynolds RK. Preliminary experience with robot-assisted laparoscopic myomectomy. J Am Assoc Gyecol Lapaosc 2004;11: 511–8. (Level III)

49. Wamsteker K, de Blok S, Galilnat A, Lueken RP. Fibroids. In: Lewis BV, Magos AL, editors. Endometrial ablation. New York (NY): Churchill Livingstone; 1992. p.161–81. (Level III)

50. Emanuel MH, Wamsteker K, Hart AA, Metz G, Lammes FB. Long-term results of hysteroscopic myomectomy for abnormal uterine bleeding. Obstet Gynecol 1999;93: 743–8. (Level II-3)

51. Jenkins TR. Hysteroscopic myomectomy: a review. Female Patient 2006;31:37–44. (Level III)

52. Polena V, Mergui JL, Perrot N, Poncelet C, Barranger E, Uzan S. Long-term results of hysteroscopic myomectomy in 235 patients. Eur J Obstet Gynecol Reprod Biol 2007;130:232–7. (Level II-2)

53. Pron G, Bennett J, Common A, Wall J, Asch M, Sniderman K. The Ontario Uterine Fibroid Embolization Trial. Part 2. Uterine fibroid reduction and symptom relief after uterine artery embolization for fibroids. Ontario Uterine Fibroid Embolization Collaboration Group. Fertil Steril 2003;79:120–7. (Level II-3)

54. Hehenkamp WJ, Volkers NA, Birnie E, Reekers JA, Ankum WM. Pain and return to daily activities after uterine artery embolization and hysterectomy in the treatment of symptomatic uterine fibroids: results from the randomized EMMY trial. Cardiovasc Intervent Radiol 2006;29:179–87. (Level I)

55. Hehenkamp WJ, Volkers NA, Donderwinkel PF, de Blok S, Birnie E, Ankum WM, et al. Uterine artery embolization versus hysterectomy in the treatment of symptomatic uterine fibroids (EMMY trial): peri- and postprocedural results from a randomized controlled trial. Am J Obstet Gynecol 2005;193:1618–29. (Level I)

56. Goodwin SC, Bradley LD, Lipman JC, Stewart EA, Nosher JL, Sterling KM, et al. Uterine artery embolization versus myomectomy: a multicenter comparative study. Fertil Steril 2006;85:14–21. (Level II-2)

57. Gupta JK, Sinha AS, Lumsden MA, Hickey M. Uterine artery embolization for symptomatic uterine fibroids. Cochrane Database of Systematic Reviews 2006, Issue 1. Art. No.: CD005073. DOI: 10.1002/14651858. CD005073.pub2. (Level III)

58. Spies JB, Spector A, Roth AR, Baker CM, Mauro L, Murphy-Skrynarz K. Complications after uterine artery embolization for leiomyomas. Obstet Gynecol 2002; 100:873–80. (Level III)

59. Broder MS, Goodwin S, Chen G, Tang LJ, Costantino MM, Nguyen MH, et al. Comparison of long-term outcomes of myomectomy and uterine artery embolization. Obstet Gynecol 2002;100:864–8. (Level II-2)

60. Spies JB, Bruno J, Czeyda-Pommersheim F, Magee ST, Ascher SA, Jha RC. Long-term outcome of uterine artery embolization of leiomyomata. Obstet Gynecol 2005;106:933–9. (Level II-3)

61. Mara M, Fucikova Z, Maskova J, Kuzel D, Haakova L. Uterine fibroid embolization versus myomectomy in women wishing to preserve fertility: preliminary results of a randomized controlled trial. Eur J Obstet Gynecol Reprod Biol 2006;126:226–33. (Level I)

62. Hindley J, Gedroyc WM, Regan L, Stewart E, Tempany C, Hynyen K, et al. MRI guidance of focused ultrasound therapy of uterine fibroids: early results. AJR Am J Roentgenol 2004;183:1713–9. (Level III)

63. Stewart EA, Rabinovici J, Tempany CM, Inbar Y, Regan L, Gostout B, et al. Clinical outcomes of focused ultrasound surgery for the treatment of uterine fibroids [published erratum appears in Fertil Steril 2006;85:1072]. Fertil Steril 2006;85:22–9. (Level III)

64. Fennessy FM, Tempany CM, McDannold NJ, So MJ, Hesley G, Gostout B, et al. Uterine leiomyomas: MR imaging-guided focused ultrasound surgery—results of different treatment protocols. Radiology 2007;243: 885–93. (Level I)

65. Morita Y, Ito N, Ohashi H. Pregnancy following MR-guided focused ultrasound surgery for a uterine fibroid. Int J Gynaecol Obstet 2007;99:56–7. (Level III)

66. Stewart EA, Gostout B, Rabinovici J, Kim HS, Regan L, Tempany CM. Sustained relief of leiomyoma symptoms by using focused ultrasound surgery. Obstet Gynecol 2007;110:279–87. (Level III)

67. Gerris J, Degueldre M, Peters AA, Romao F, Stjernquist M, al-Taher H. The place of Zoladex in deferred surgery for uterine fibroids. Zoladex Myoma Study Group. Horm Res 1996;45:279–84. (Level I)

68. Stovall TG, Muneyyirci-Delale O, Summitt RL Jr, Scialli AR. GnRH agonist and iron versus placebo and iron in the anemic patient before surgery for leiomyomas: a randomized controlled trial. Leuprolide Acetate Study Group. Obstet Gynecol 1995;86:65–71. (Level I)

69. Zullo F, Pellicano M, De Stefano R, Zupi E, Mastrantonio P. A prospective randomized study to evaluate leuprolide acetate treatment before laparoscopic myomectomy: efficacy and ultrasonographic predictors. Am J Obstet Gynecol 1998;178:108–12. (Level I)

70. Flierman PA, Oberye JJ, van der Hulst VP, de Blok S. Rapid reduction of leiomyoma volume during treatment with the GnRH antagonist ganirelix. BJOG 2005;112: 638–42. (Level III)

71. Frederick J, Fletcher H, Simeon D, Mullings A, Hardie M. Intramyometrial vasopressin as a haemostatic agent during myomectomy. Br J Obstet Gynaecol 1994;101:435–7. (Level I-2)

72. Fletcher H, Frederick J, Hardie M, Simeon D. A randomized comparison of vasopressin and tourniquet as hemostatic agents during myomectomy. Obstet Gynecol 1996;87:1014–8. (Level II-1)

73. Phillips DR, Nathanson HG, Milim SJ, Haselkorn JS, Khapra A, Ross PL. The effect of dilute vasopressin solution on blood loss during operative hysteroscopy: a randomized controlled trial. Obstet Gynecol 1996;88:761–6. (Level I)

74. Garnet JD. Uterine rupture during pregnancy. An analysis of 133 patients. Obstet Gynecol 1964;23:898–905. (Level III)

75. Paul PG, Koshy AK, Thomas T. Pregnancy outcomes following laparoscopic myomectomy and single-layer myometrial closure. Hum Reprod 2006;21:3278–81. (Level III)

76. Seracchioli R, Rossi S, Govoni F, Rossi E, Venturoli S, Bulletti C, et al. Fertility and obstetric outcome after laparoscopic myomectomy of large myomata: a randomized comparison with abdominal myomectomy. Hum Reprod 2000;15:2663–8. (Level I)

77. Kumakiri J, Takeuchi H, Kitade M, Kikuchi I, Shimanuki H, Itoh S, et al. Pregnancy and delivery after laparoscopic myomectomy. J Minim Invasive Gynecol 2005;12:241–6. (Level II-2)

78. Parker WH, Iacampo K, Long T. Uterine rupture after laparoscopic removal of a pedunculated myoma. J Minim Invasive Gynecol 2007;14:362–4. (Level III)

79. Banas T, Klimek M, Fugiel A, Skotniczny K. Spontaneous uterine rupture at 35 weeks' gestation, 3 years after laparoscopic myomectomy, without signs of fetal distress. J Obstet Gynaecol Res 2005;31:527–30. (Level III)

80. Grande N, Catalano GF, Ferrari S, Marana R. Spontaneous uterine rupture at 27 weeks of pregnancy after laparoscopic myomectomy. J Minim Invasive Gynecol 2005;12:301. (Level III)

81. Golan D, Aharoni A, Gonen R, Boss Y, Sharf M. Early spontaneous rupture of the post myomectomy gravid uterus. Int J Gynaecol Obstet 1990;31:167–70. (Level III)

82. Ozeren M, Ulusoy M, Uyanik E. First-trimester spontaneous uterine rupture after traditional myomectomy: case report. Isr J Med Sci 1997;33:752–3. (Level III)

83. Hart R, Molnar BG, Magos A. Long term follow up of hysteroscopic myomectomy assessed by survival analysis. Br J Obstet Gynaecol 1999;106:700–5. (Level II-3)

84. Abbas A, Irvine LM. Uterine rupture during labour after hysteroscopic myomectomy. Gynaecol Endosc 1997;6:245–6. (Level III)

85. Yaron Y, Shenhav M, Jaffa AJ, Lessing JB, Peyser MR. Uterine rupture at 33 weeks' gestation subsequent to hysteroscopic uterine perforation. Am J Obstet Gynecol 1994;170:786–7. (Level III)

86. Manyonda I, Sinthamoney E, Belli AM. Controversies and challenges in the modern management of uterine fibroids. BJOG 2004;111:95–102. (Level III)

87. Olufowobi O, Sharif K, Papaionnou S, Neelakantan D, Mohammed H, Afnan M. Are the anticipated benefits of myomectomy achieved in women of reproductive age? A 5-year review of the results at a UK tertiary hospital. J Obstet Gynaecol 2004;24:434–40. (Level III)

88. Garcia CR, Tureck RW. Submucosal leiomyomas and infertility. Fertil Steril 1984;42:16–9. (Level III)

89. Rice JP, Kay HH, Mahony BS. The clinical significance of uterine leiomyomas in pregnancy. Am J Obstet Gynecol 1989;160:1212–6. (Level II-3)

90. Pritts EA. Fibroids and infertility: a systematic review of the evidence. Obstet Gynecol Surv 2001;56:483–91. (Level I)

91. Babakhnia A, Rock JA, Jones HW Jr. Pregnancy success following abdominal myomectomy for infertility. Fertil Steril 1978;30:644–7. (Level III)

92. Gehlbach DL, Sousa RC, Carpenter SE, Rock JA. Abdominal myomectomy in the treatment of infertility. Int J Gynaecol Obstet 1993;40:45–50. (Level III)

93. Sudik R, Husch K, Steller J, Daume E. Fertility and pregnancy outcome after myomectomy in sterility patients. Eur J Obstet Gynecol Reprod Biol 1996;65:209–14. (Level II-2)

94. Ubaldi F, Tournaye H, Camus M, Van der Pas H, Gepts E, Devroey P. Fertility after hysteroscopic myomectomy. Hum Reprod Update 1995;1:81–90. (Level III)

95. Dubuisson JB, Fauconnier A, Chapron C, Kreiker G, Norgaard C. Reproductive outcome after laparoscopic myomectomy in infertile women. J Reprod Med 2000;45:23–30. (Level III)

96. Campo S, Campo V, Gambadauro P. Reproductive outcome before and after laparoscopic or abdominal myomectomy for subserous or intramural myomas. Eur J Obstet Gynecol Reprod Biol 2003;110:215–9. (Level II-3)

97. Donnez J, Jadoul P. What are the implications of myomas on fertility? A need for a debate? Hum Reprod 2002;17:1424–30. (Level III)

98. Surrey ES, Lietz AK, Schoolcraft WB. Impact of intramural leiomyomata in patients with a normal endometrial cavity on in vitro fertilization-embryo transfer cycle outcome. Fertil Steril 2001;75:405–10. (Level II-2)

99. Rackow BW, Arici A. Fibroids and in-vitro fertilization: which comes first? Curr Opin Obstet Gynecol 2005;17:225–31. (Level III)

100. Tulandi T, Murray C, Guralnick M. Adhesion formation and reproductive outcome after myomectomy and second-look laparoscopy. Obstet Gynecol 1993;82:213–5. (Level III)

101. Dutton S, Hirst A, McPherson K, Nicholson T, Maresh M. A UK multicentre retrospective cohort study comparing hysterectomy and uterine artery embolisation for the treatment of symptomatic uterine fibroids (HOPEFUL study): main results on medium-term safety and efficacy. BJOG 2007;114:1340–51. (Level II-2)

102. Ravina JH, Vigneron NC, Aymard A, Le Dref O, Merland JJ. Pregnancy after embolization of uterine myoma: report of 12 cases. Fertil Steril 2000;73:1241–3. (Level III)

103. Hehenkamp WJ, Volkers NA, Brokemans FJ, de Jong FH, Themmen AP, Birnie E, et al. Loss of ovarian reserve after uterine artery embolization: a randomized comparison with hysterectomy. Hum Reprod 2007;22: 1996–2005. (Level I)

104. Pron G, Mocarski E, Bennett J, Vilos G, Common A, Vanderburgh L, et al. Pregnancy after uterine artery embolization for leiomyomata: the Ontario multicenter trial. Obstet Gynecol 2005;105:67–76. (Level II-3)

105. Rabinovici J, Inbar Y, Eylon SC, Schiff E, Hananel A, Freundlich D. Pregnancy and live birth after focused ultrasound surgery for symptomatic focal adenomyosis: a case report. Hum Reprod 2006;21:1255–9. (Level III)

106. Gavrilova-Jordan LP, Rose CH, Traynor KD, Brost BC, Gostout BS. Successful term pregnancy following MR-guided focused ultrasound treatment of uterine leiomyoma. J Perinatol 2007;27:59–61. (Level III)

107. Hanstede MM, Tempany CM, Stewart EA. Focused ultrasound surgery of intramural leiomyomas may facilitate fertility: a case report. Fertil Steril 2007;88: 497.e5–7. (Level III)

108. Akkad AA, Habiba MA, Ismail N, Abrams K, al-Azzawi F. Abnormal uterine bleeding on hormone replacement: the importance of intrauterine structural abnormalities. Obstet Gynecol 1995;86:330–4. (Level II-2)

109. Sener AB, Seckin NC, Ozmen S, Gokmen O, Dogu N, Ekici E. The effects of hormone replacement therapy on uterine fibroids in postmenopausal women. Fertil Steril 1996;65:354–7. (Level I)

110. Seltzer V. Screening for ovarian cancer: An overview of the screening recommendations of the 1994 NIH Consensus Conference. Prim Care Update Ob Gyns 1995;2:132–4. (Level III)

111. Reiter RC, Wagner PL, Gambone JC. Routine hysterectomy for large asymptomatic uterine leiomyomata: a reappraisal. Obstet Gynecol 1992;79:481–4. (Level III)

112. Piscitelli JT, Simel DL, Addison WA. Who should have intravenous pyelograms before hysterectomy for benign disease? Obstet Gynecol 1987;69:541–5. (Level III)

113. Parker WH, Fu YS, Berek JS. Uterine sarcoma in patients operated on for presumed leiomyoma and rapidly growing leiomyoma. Obstet Gynecol 1994;83:414–8. (Level III)

114. Stewart EA, Morton CC. The genetics of uterine leiomyomata: what clinicians need to know. Obstet Gynecol 2006;107:917–21. (Level III)

115. Schwartz LB, Diamond MP, Schwartz PE. Leiomyosarcomas: clinical presentation. Am J Obstet Gynecol 1993;168:180–3. (Level III)

116. Goto A, Takeuchi S, Sugimura K, Maruo T. Usefulness of Gd-DTPA contrast-enhanced dynamic MRI and serum determination of LDH and its isozymes in the differential diagnosis of leiomyosarcoma from degenerated leiomyoma of the uterus. Int J Gynecol Cancer 2002; 12:354–61. (Level II-1)

117. Tanaka YO, Nishida M, Tsunoda H, Okamoto Y, Yoshikawa H. Smooth muscle tumors of uncertain malignant potential and leiomyosarcomas of the uterus: MR findings. J Magn Reson Imaging 2004;20:998–1007. (Level III)

The MEDLINE database, the Cochrane Library, and ACOG's own internal resources and documents were used to conduct a literature search to locate relevant articles published between January 1985 and December 2007. The search was restricted to articles published in the English language. Priority was given to articles reporting results of original research, although review articles and commentaries also were consulted. Abstracts of research presented at symposia and scientific conferences were not considered adequate for inclusion in this document. Guidelines published by organizations or institutions such as the National Institutes of Health and the American College of Obstetricians and Gynecologists were reviewed, and additional studies were located by reviewing bibliographies of identified articles. When reliable research was not available, expert opinions from obstetrician–gynecologists were used.

Studies were reviewed and evaluated for quality according to the method outlined by the U.S. Preventive Services Task Force:

I   Evidence obtained from at least one properly designed randomized controlled trial.

II-1   Evidence obtained from well-designed controlled trials without randomization.

II-2   Evidence obtained from well-designed cohort or case–control analytic studies, preferably from more than one center or research group.

II-3   Evidence obtained from multiple time series with or without the intervention. Dramatic results in uncontrolled experiments also could be regarded as this type of evidence.

III   Opinions of respected authorities, based on clinical experience, descriptive studies, or reports of expert committees.

Based on the highest level of evidence found in the data, recommendations are provided and graded according to the following categories:

Level A—Recommendations are based on good and consistent scientific evidence.

Level B—Recommendations are based on limited or inconsistent scientific evidence.

Level C—Recommendations are based primarily on consensus and expert opinion.

ISSN 1099-3630

The American College of Obstetricians and Gynecologists
409 12th Street, SW, PO Box 96920, Washington, DC 20090-6920

Alternatives to hysterectomy in the management of leiomyomas. ACOG Practice Bulletin No. 96. American College of Obstetricians and Gynecologists. Obstet Gynecol 2008;112:387–400.

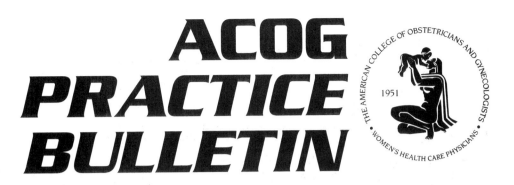

ACOG PRACTICE BULLETIN

THE AMERICAN COLLEGE OF OBSTETRICIANS AND GYNECOLOGISTS · 1951 · WOMEN'S HEALTH CARE PHYSICIANS

CLINICAL MANAGEMENT GUIDELINES FOR OBSTETRICIAN–GYNECOLOGISTS

NUMBER 99, DECEMBER 2008

Replaces Practice Bulletin Number 66, September 2005

This Practice Bulletin was developed by the ACOG Committee on Practice Bulletins—Gynecology with the assistance of Mark Spitzer, MD. The information is designed to aid practitioners in making decisions about appropriate obstetric and gynecologic care. These guidelines should not be construed as dictating an exclusive course of treatment or procedure. Variations in practice may be warranted based on the needs of the individual patient, resources, and limitations unique to the institution or type of practice.

THE AMERICAN COLLEGE OF OBSTETRICIANS AND GYNECOLOGISTS
WOMEN'S HEALTH CARE PHYSICIANS

Management of Abnormal Cervical Cytology and Histology

Recent evidence has shown that the risk of malignant and premalignant cervical disease and human papillomavirus (HPV) infections varies significantly with age (1, 2). Furthermore, evidence now shows that treatment for cervical disease carries significant risk for future pregnancies (3–7). These factors have led to a re-evaluation of the guidelines for the management of premalignant cervical disease. The purpose of this document is to define strategies for diagnosis and management of abnormal cervical cytology and histology results. In this document, HPV refers to high-risk oncogenic forms of the virus.

Background
Cytology and Histology Findings and Interpretation

The 2001 Bethesda System terminology (see box) is used throughout this document to describe the categories of epithelial cell abnormalities, including atypical squamous cells (ASC), low-grade or high-grade squamous intraepithelial lesions (LSIL or HSIL), and glandular cell abnormalities, including atypical glandular cells (AGC) and adenocarcinoma in situ (AIS). Histology diagnoses of abnormalities are reported as cervical intraepithelial neoplasia (CIN) grades 1–3 (8).

The key to developing effective guidelines for the management of cervical abnormalities is to distinguish true cervical cancer precursors from benign cervical abnormalities with little premalignant potential. Both LSIL and CIN 1 reflect the cytologic and pathologic effects of infection with HPV. Most of these lesions will never progress to cancer. However, as many as 28% of women with cytologic LSIL harbor CIN 2 or CIN 3, approximately two thirds of which is identified by colposcopy (9). Cervical intraepithelial neoplasia grade 3 and AIS

The 2001 Bethesda System Terminology

Squamous Cell

- Atypical squamous cells
  - Of undetermined significance
  - Cannot exclude high-grade squamous intraepithelial lesions
- Low-grade squamous intraepithelial lesions–encompassing human papillomavirus, mild dysplasia, and CIN 1
- High-grade squamous intraepithelial lesions–encompassing moderate and severe dysplasia, carcinoma in situ, CIN 2, and CIN 3
- Squamous cell carcinoma

Glandular Cell

- Atypical glandular cells (specify endocervical, endometrial, or not otherwise specified)
- Atypical glandular cells, favors neoplasia (specify endocervical or not otherwise specified)
- Endocervical adenocarcinoma in situ
- Adenocarcinoma

Abbreviation: CIN indicates cervical intraepithelial neoplasia.

Modified from Solomon D, Davey D, Kurman R, Moriarty A, O'Connor D, Prey M, et al. The 2001 Bethesda System: terminology for reporting results of cervical cytology. Forum Group Members; Bethesda 2001 Workshop. JAMA 2002;287:2114–9. Copyright © 2002, American Medical Association. All rights reserved.

---

are cervical cancer precursors (10). Cervical intraepithelial neoplasia grade 2 lesions are more heterogeneous, and their significance is less clear than that of CIN 3. The reproducibility of a diagnosis of CIN 2 is poor, and many women will have either CIN 1 or CIN 3 (11). Cervical intraepithelial neoplasia grade 2 is more likely to progress to CIN 3 and cancer than CIN 1. However, many CIN 2 lesions will regress without therapy. Many pathologists do not attempt to distinguish between CIN 2 and CIN 3, instead reporting a composite diagnosis of CIN 2,3 or high-grade CIN (CIN 2,3+).

The guidelines discussed in this document follow the 2006 consensus guidelines published by the American Society for Colposcopy and Cervical Pathology (12, 13). These guidelines recognized that a small risk of failing to detect high-grade CIN and even cancer must be accepted. It is unreasonable for patients or clinicians to expect that the risk can be reduced to zero, and attempts to achieve zero risk will result in greater harm than good in the form of overtreatment. When providing care for an individual patient, guidelines define the evidence base

for most cases but are not a substitute for clinical judgment because it is impossible to develop guidelines that would apply to all situations (12, 13). Newer data show that cervical treatments, such as ablation or excisional procedures, may have adverse effects on pregnancy, including preterm delivery and low birth weight (7, 14); thus, risk–benefit assessment sometimes favors observation of CIN 2, especially among younger women (12).

Finally, there is increasing recognition that colposcopy is less sensitive than previously thought. A single colposcopy examination in women with positive low-grade cytology results identified only 60% of women with CIN 2,3 lesions and 54% of women with CIN 3 lesions who received their diagnoses within 2 years of study enrollment (9). Some lesions with metaplastic or low-grade features contain CIN 2,3, whereas some lesions with high-grade features contain CIN 1, condylomatous changes, or atypical metaplasia. Recent studies suggest that the correlation between colposcopy impression and biopsy grade is poor (15–17). The sensitivity of colposcopy is significantly greater when two or more biopsy specimens are obtained (18).

Natural History of Cervical Intraepithelial Neoplasia

Carriage of HPV DNA is quite common in the general population, reported in one study to occur at least once over a 3-year period in 60% of young women (19). The lifetime cumulative risk is at least 80% (20). Most women clear the virus or suppress it to levels not associated with CIN 2,3+, and for most women this occurs promptly (21, 22). The duration of HPV positivity is shorter and the likelihood of clearance is higher in younger women (23–25).

The presence of high-risk HPV is a marker for the risk of diagnosis of CIN 2,3+; only 1 in 10 to 1 in 30 HPV infections are associated with abnormal cervical cytology results (26–28), with an even smaller proportion associated with CIN 2,3+ (29). Among women with negative cytology test results and a positive HPV test result, only 15% will have abnormal cytology results within 5 years (30). However, high-risk HPV is necessary for the development and maintenance of CIN 3 (31). Persistent high-risk HPV is a necessary but not sufficient condition for the development of almost all types of invasive cervical cancer (32, 33). Conversely, the risk of cervical cancer in women who do not harbor oncogenic HPV is extremely low (34). The longer high-risk HPV is present and the older the patient, the greater the risk of CIN (35). When HPV is present, smoking doubles the risk of progression to CIN 3 (36).

From a clinical perspective, it is important to distinguish which intraepithelial neoplastic lesions will progress to invasive cancer if left untreated. However, the diagnostic categories currently available have only modest predictive value, and that value decreases as the lesions become less severe. The likelihood of progression to cancer is higher and the time to progression is shorter as the grade of dysplasia increases (37). Although expression of the presence of HPV as CIN can occur within months of viral acquisition (10), the time course from CIN 3 to invasive cancer averages between 8.1 years and 12.6 years (9, 38, 39). The slow pace of these changes in immunocompetent women means that accurate estimates of progression risk require long follow-up periods. Perhaps more relevant for clinical practice are estimates of regression to normal status. A review of the literature from 1950 to 1992 noted the likelihood of regression to be 60% for CIN 1 and 40% for CIN 2 (40, 41).

Cervical Cytology

Cervical cytology screening programs are associated with a reduction in the incidence of and mortality from invasive squamous cancer. Conventional cytology is reported to be 30–87% sensitive for dysplasia (42). A meta-analysis of conventional cervical cytology studies suggested a sensitivity of 58% when used for population screening (43). Another meta-analysis comparing the performance of ThinPrep® liquid-based cervical cytology screening with conventional cytology screening methods found sensitivity rates, relative to histology, were 68% (conventional) and 76% (ThinPrep®), and specificity rates were 79% (conventional) and 86% (ThinPrep®) (44).

Because the range of sensitivity (30–87%) is so broad, all abnormal cytology results must be evaluated, although the vast majority of results do not represent underlying CIN 2,3+ (25). Reproducibility among observers and among multiple readings by the same observer is quite modest, even under optimal research conditions (45–48). In the ASC-US LSIL Triage Study (ALTS), the quality control reviewer at the National Cancer Institute and the university-based cytopathologist at the study site agreed on an ASC result in 43% of 1,473 cases, on an LSIL result in 68% of 1,335 cases, and on an HSIL result in 47% of 433 cases (45).

Human Papillomavirus Testing

Testing for low-risk HPV types has no role in cervical cancer prevention. Low-risk HPV types are associated with genital warts and with some low-grade intraepithelial lesions of the cervix, vagina, and vulva (49).

For women 30 years and older, high-risk HPV testing can help predict whether CIN 2,3+ will be diagnosed in the next few years despite a normal cytology result

(10, 21, 50–52). As new tests are introduced, decisions about clinical practice implementation must be based on clinical sensitivity (relationship of the test result to CIN 2,3+), not analytic sensitivity (ability of the test to detect low levels of HPV).

Human papillomavirus DNA positivity is much more prevalent in women aged 18–22 years (71%) versus those older than 29 years (31%) (88). In the algorithms used in the management of abnormal cervical cytology results or CIN, persistent HPV positivity is used as evidence of persistent HPV infection and, therefore, a marker of disease. However, many adolescents experience multiple sequential HPV infections, so a repetitively positive HPV DNA test in this age group may represent consecutive incident infections rather than a single persistent infection. Consequently, HPV testing should not be used in this age group and if inadvertently performed, a positive result should not influence management.

Colposcopy With and Without Directed Biopsy

Colposcopy with directed biopsy has been the criterion of disease detection and remains the technique of choice for treatment decisions. Evaluation of colposcopy sensitivity has, until recently, focused on populations with identified lesions sufficient to produce abnormal cytology.

Some recent studies have used colposcopy with endocervical curettage and blind four-quadrant ectocervical biopsies or loop electrosurgical excision procedure (LEEP) as the diagnostic criteria (38, 53). This approach permits a more realistic evaluation of the sensitivity of colposcopy with directed biopsy. The presence of CIN 2,3+ was missed on directed biopsy but detected on the random four-quadrant biopsies in 18.6–31.6% of CIN 2,3+ cases (53, 54). These figures may underestimate the prevalence of CIN 2,3+ not diagnosed on colposcopy-directed biopsy because excisions were not performed in the entire population—many women had normal screening test results. Comparing directed biopsy to conization also demonstrates a significant rate of underdiagnosis of CIN 2 and CIN 3 (55, 56).

Similar conclusions are reported in ALTS. Women with a previous LSIL or ASC-US HPV-positive test result and a CIN 1 biopsy were offered LEEP after 2 years of follow-up (38). Of the 189 women with CIN 2,3+ diagnosed during the 2-year study in the "immediate colposcopy" arm of the trial, only 106 (56%) women received the diagnoses on the initial colposcopy. The other cases were identified after HSIL cytology, an exit colposcopy, or LEEP.

Results of these studies indicate that biopsies of all visible lesions are warranted, regardless of colposcopy impression, and that follow-up should include multiple colposcopy examinations over time for those women with abnormal cytology or histology results who have persistent low-grade abnormalities or persistently test positive for HPV.

Endocervical Sampling

Endocervical sampling may be conducted either with vigorous endocervical brushing or by traditional endocervical curettage with a sharp curette. Compared with curettage, the brush technique is at least as sensitive for endocervical dysplasia (57–61) and returns fewer reports of insufficient specimens (60, 61). The disadvantage is that the result can be equivocal, such as ASC, in which case the patient must be recalled for sharp curettage.

Endocervical sampling is not indicated in the pregnant patient. The following discussion of indications applies to the nonpregnant patient. In the evaluation of an ASC or LSIL cytology result with a satisfactory colposcopy result, endocervical sampling may be considered, although the identification of cancer cases is low (62, 63). Sampling should be performed if colposcopy results are unsatisfactory (64, 65) or if ablative treatment, such as cryotherapy or laser ablation, is contemplated. Higher rates of postablation CIN 2 or CIN 3 and cancer have been reported if pretreatment endocervical assessment is not done (66). Studies of the contribution of endocervical curettage to diagnosis of CIN 2,3+ at

colposcopy suggest that its addition to directed biopsy may be expected to add 5–9% to the total number of CIN 2,3+ diagnoses (65, 67–69). This percentage becomes more important as the risk of CIN 2,3+ increases with higher-grade abnormal cytology results. As a consequence, in women with ASC-H, HSIL, AGC, or AIS cytology results, endocervical sampling should be considered as part of the initial colposcopy evaluation (70), unless excision is planned. If an excision is planned, endocervical sampling may be omitted (64), although it may be performed at the time of the procedure after the excision to assess the completeness of the procedure.

Clinical Considerations and Recommendations

▶ *When the results of cervical cytology screening are normal but a concurrent HPV test result is positive, what is the appropriate follow-up?*

The best management approach for HPV-positive, cytology-negative women 30 years and older is to repeat cytology and HPV testing at 12 months (Figure 1). Women whose HPV result is still positive on repeat testing 12 months later or whose cytology result is ASC or greater should undergo colposcopy, whereas women

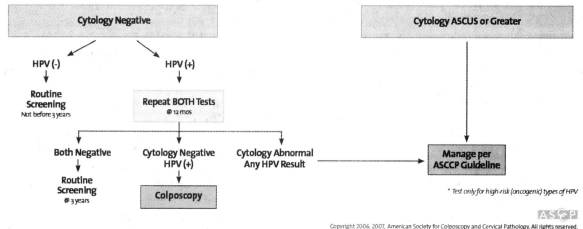

Use of HPV DNA Testing * as an Adjunct to Cytology for Cervical Cancer Screening in Women 30 Years and Older

* Test only for high-risk (oncogenic) types of HPV

Figure 1. Use of HPV DNA testing as an adjunct to cytology for cervical cancer screening in women 30 years and older. Abbreviations: ASCCP indicates American Society for Colposcopy and Cervical Cytology; ASCUS, atypical squamous cells of undetermined significance; HPV, human papillomavirus. Wright TC. Management of cervical cytologic abnormalities. J Low Genit Tract Dis 2007; 11:201–22. Reprinted from the Journal of Lower Genital Tract Disease Vol. 11 Issue 4, with the permission of ASCCP © American Society for Colposcopy and Cervical Pathology 2007. No copies of the algorithms may be made without the prior consent of ASCCP.

whose results are negative on both tests can defer screening for 3 years. Incorporating HPV testing into routine screening should be reserved for women aged 30 years and older (71, 72). In screening studies from North America and Europe, the sensitivity using a combination of HPV testing and cytology is significantly higher than that of either test alone with negative predictive values of 99–100% (73). Women who receive negative results from both initial cytology and HPV testing have a less than 1 in 1,000 risk of having CIN 2 or greater (CIN 2+), and prospective follow-up studies in both Europe and the United States have shown that the risk of developing CIN 3 over a 10-year period is less than 2% (71, 74, 75). Modeling studies demonstrate that in women 30 years and older, screening at 3-year intervals using a combination of cytology and HPV testing provides benefits equivalent or greater than those provided by annual screening with conventional cytology (76). Even in women 30 years and older, most HPV-positive women become HPV negative during follow-up (60% in a prospective study from France after a median follow-up of 6 months) (48). In a well-screened population, the risk of CIN 2+ in HPV-positive, cytology-negative women ranges from 2.4% to 5.1% (53, 77, 78).

▶ *When the results of cervical cytology are reported as atypical squamous cell of undetermined significance, how should they be managed?*

In the Bethesda 2001 guidelines, ASC is subcategorized into atypical squamous cells of undetermined significance (ASC-US) and atypical squamous cells, cannot exclude HSIL (ASC-H). The difference in the management guidelines for these two cytology findings relates to their inherent risk of CIN 2,3. Atypical squamous cells of undetermined significance is the most common cervical cytology abnormality, accounting for 4.4% of all Pap test results. Although the risk of cancer for any individual patient is very low (0.1–0.2%) (79, 80), and the risk of CIN 2,3+ also is low (6.4–11.9%) (38, 81, 82), because there are so many people with this cytology abnormality, it is the presenting cytology result for approximately one half of the women with CIN 2,3+. The first step in the evaluation of women with ASC-US is to triage those who are at higher risk to more intensive evaluation (colposcopy) and directing the rest to more routine follow-up. Premenopausal women 21 years and older with ASC-US cytology results may undergo immediate colposcopy or may undergo triage testing to determine whether they should be referred to colposcopy. Triage testing may be performed by a single test for high-risk (oncogenic) types of HPV or by repeat cytology screening at 6 months and 12 months. When the index cytology test specimen is obtained by liquid-based cytology or when an HPV specimen is co-collected, "reflex" HPV testing is the preferred approach (Figure 2). Data from ALTS demonstrated that two repeat cytology examinations at 6 months and 12 months at an

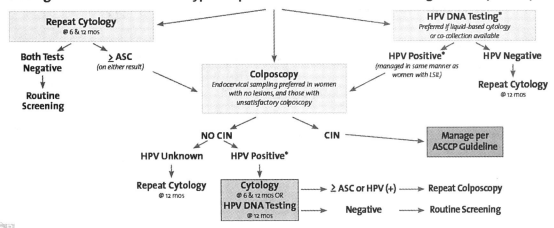

Management of Women with Atypical Squamous Cells of Undetermined Significance (ASC-US)

*Test only for high-risk (oncogenic) types of HPV

Figure 2. Management of women with atypical squamous cells of undetermined significance (ASC-US). Abbreviations: ASC indicates atypical squamous cells; ASCCP, American Society for Colposcopy and Cervical Cytology; CIN, cervical intraepithelial neoplasia; HPV, human papillomavirus; LSIL, low-grade squamous intraepithelial lesion. Wright TC. Management of cervical cytologic abnormalities. J Low Genit Tract Dis 2007;11:201–22. Reprinted from the Journal of Lower Genital Tract Disease Vol. 11 Issue 4, with the permission of ASCCP © American Society for Colposcopy and Cervical Pathology 2007. No copies of the algorithms may be made without the prior consent of ASCCP.

ASC-US threshold detected 88% of the CIN 2,3+ while referring 63.6% of the women to colposcopy. Human papillomavirus testing alone detected 92.2% of the CIN 2,3+ while referring 55% of the women to colposcopy.

The presence of ASC-US is less common in post-menopausal women, as is the risk of significant pathologic results (2, 83, 84). Human papillomavirus DNA positivity rates also decrease dramatically as women age (85, 86). This means that HPV testing actually is more efficient in older women because it refers a lower proportion of these women to colposcopy (87–89). The prevalence of CIN 2,3 is much higher among women with ASC-US than women with ASC-US, so ASC-H should be considered to represent equivocal HSIL.

▶ *What is the management of ASC-US for women 20 years or younger?*

Invasive cervical cancer is very rare in adolescent women before age 21 years. The National Cancer Institute's SEER program reported that from 1995 to 1999 the incidence rate of invasive cervical cancer was 0 per 100,000 per year for women aged 10–19 years and 1.7 per 100,000 per year for women aged 20–24 years (1). In contrast, minor grade cytology abnormalities (ASC and LSIL) are more common in women aged 15–19 years than in older women (2), and these HPV-associated abnormalities are of little long-term clinical significance (90). Human papillomavirus DNA positivity is much more prevalent in women aged 18–22 years

(71%) than those older than 29 years (31%) (85). Thus, using HPV DNA testing to triage adolescents and young women with ASC-US would refer large numbers of women to colposcopy who are at low risk for having cervical cancer. Also, many adolescents experience multiple sequential HPV infections, so a repetitively positive HPV DNA test in this age group may represent consecutive incident infections rather than a single persistent infection. In adolescents with ASC-US, follow-up with annual cytology testing is recommended. Human papillomavirus DNA testing and colposcopy are unacceptable for adolescents with ASC-US, and if HPV testing is inadvertently performed, a positive test result should not influence management. Also, in adolescents, the threshold for referral to colposcopy is different than in adult women (Figure 3). At the 12-month follow-up visit, only the patients with the diagnosis of HSIL or greater on the repeat cytology should be referred to colposcopy. At the 24-month follow-up, the patients with a diagnosis of ASC-US or greater should be referred to colposcopy (Figure 3).

▶ *When the results of cervical cytology are reported as atypical squamous cells, cannot exclude HSIL (ASC-H), how should they be managed?*

Women with ASC-H have a 20–50% risk of having a CIN 2,3 lesion and should be evaluated with immediate colposcopy (Figure 4). Most women with ASC-H are

Management of Adolescent Women with Either Atypical Squamous Cells of Undetermined Significance (ASC-US) or Low-grade Squamous Intraepithelial Lesion (LSIL)

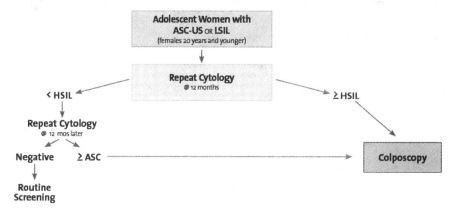

Figure 3. Management of adolescent women with either atypical squamous cells of undetermined significance (ASC-US) or low-grade squamous intraepithelial lesion (LSIL). Abbreviations: ASC indicates atypical squamous cells; ASC-US; atypical squamous cells of undetermined significance; HSIL, high-grade squamous intraepithelial lesion; LSIL, low-grade squamous intraepithelial lesion. Wright TC. Management of cervical cytologic abnormalities. J Low Genit Tract Dis 2007;11:201–22. Reprinted from the Journal of Lower Genital Tract Disease Vol. 11 Issue 4, with the permission of ASCCP © American Society for Colposcopy and Cervical Pathology 2007. No copies of the algorithms may be made without the prior consent of ASCCP.

HPV DNA positive (ranging from 67–84%) (91–93), so intermediate triage is inappropriate and HPV testing is not recommended. If CIN 2,3 is not identified by colposcopy, women aged 21 years and older should be monitored in a manner similar to HPV-positive women with ASC-US.

▶ *When the results of cervical cytology are reported as LSIL or ASC-US with HPV positive results, how should they be managed in patient 21 years and older?*

Although a cytology result of LSIL is thought to reflect the cytopathic effects of HPV infection rather than a true premalignant lesion, women with LSIL remain at moderate risk for having CIN 2+. In ALTS, 27.6% of women with LSIL were found to have CIN 2+ either on colposcopically directed biopsies or on close follow-up over the next 2 years (9). This rate is virtually identical to the rate of CIN 2+ in women who presented with HPV-positive ASC-US results in the same population (26.7%). Two thirds of the cases (17.9%) were identified on the initial colposcopy and the remainder at follow-up. Therefore, colposcopy is recommended in premenopausal women aged 21 years and older with ASC-US who are HPV positive, or have two consecutive ASC-US cytology results (Figure 2), or have LSIL (Figure 5).

Many studies have shown that the prevalence of both HPV DNA positivity and CIN 2,3 decreases with

age in women with LSIL (94, 95). Well-screened, postmenopausal women with previously negative results are likewise at low risk for invasive cervical cancer (96). This suggests that postmenopausal women with LSIL may be managed using HPV testing for triage in the same protocol as is used in reproductive-aged women with ASC-US.

▶ *When the results of colposcopy performed for the evaluation of ASC-US, ASC-H, or LSIL reveal no CIN 2,3, how should the patient's condition be managed?*

Because a single colposcopy examination can miss significant lesions, women who are referred for colposcopy and found not to have CIN 2,3 require some form of additional follow-up. In ALTS, the initial colposcopy identified only 58% of the CIN 2+ lesions. For the women not found to have CIN 2+ at the initial colposcopy, the rate of CIN 2+ during follow-up (approximately 10–13%) was unaffected by the findings at colposcopy (negative findings not worthy of biopsy, negative biopsy, or CIN 1 biopsy). The ASC-US–LSIL Triage Study evaluated different postcolposcopy follow-up strategies and found that HPV testing performed 12 months after the initial colposcopy and two repeat cytology examinations performed at 6-month intervals were equally effective (97). Because of the additional cost and lack of increased sensitivity, the strategy of

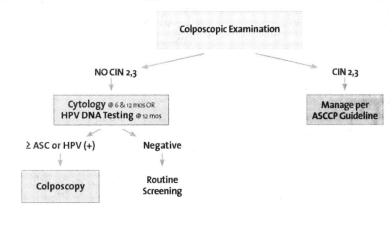

Management of Women with Atypical Squamous Cells: Cannot Exclude High-grade SIL (ASC - H)

Figure 4. Management of women with atypical squamous cells: cannot exclude high-grade SIL (ASC-H). Abbreviations: ASC indicates atypical squamous cells; ASCCP, American Society for Colposcopy and Cervical Pathology; ASC-H, atypical squamous cells—cannot exclude high-grade squamous intraepithelial lesion; CIN, cervical intraepithelial neoplasia; DNA deoxyribonucleic acid; HPV, human papillomavirus; SIL, squamous intraepithelial lesion. Wright TC. Management of cervical cytologic abnormalities. J Low Genit Tract Dis 2007;11:201–22. Reprinted from the Journal of Lower Genital Tract Disease Vol. 11 Issue 4, with the permission of ASCCP © American Society for Colposcopy and Cervical Pathology 2007. No copies of the algorithms may be made without the prior consent of ASCCP.

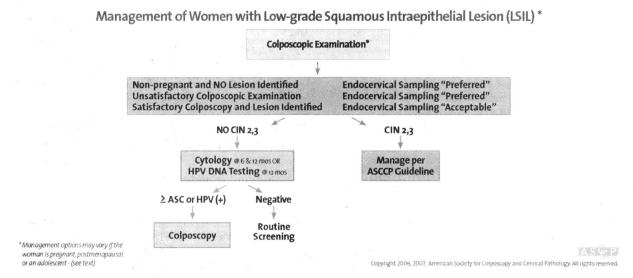

Figure 5. Management of women with low-grade squamous intraepithelial lesion (LSIL). Abbreviations: ASC indicates atypical squamous cells; ASCCP, American Society for Colposcopy and Cervical Pathology; CIN, cervical intraepithelial neoplasia; HPV, human papillomavirus. Wright TC. Management of cervical cytologic abnormalities. J Low Genit Tract Dis 2007;11:201–22. Reprinted from the Journal of Lower Genital Tract Disease Vol. 11 Issue 4, with the permission of ASCCP © American Society for Colposcopy and Cervical Pathology 2007. No copies of the algorithms may be made without the prior consent of ASCCP.

combined cytology plus HPV testing was discouraged. In the absence of CIN identified histologically, diagnostic excisional or ablative procedures are unacceptable for the initial management of patients with LSIL. Follow-up with either HPV testing at 12 months or cervical cytology at 6 months and 12 months (ASC-US threshold) is acceptable. If the HPV DNA test result is negative or if two consecutive repeat cytology test results are negative, return to routine screening is recommended. If either the HPV DNA test result is positive or if the result of repeat cytology is reported as ASC-US or greater, colposcopy is recommended (Figures 2, 4, and 5).

▶ *When the results of cervical cytology tests are reported as HSIL, how should these be managed in the adult patient?*

The mean reporting rate of HSIL in U.S. laboratories is 0.7% (98). The rate of HSIL varies with age. A cytology result of HSIL carries a high risk of significant cervical disease. A single colposcopy examination identifies CIN 2+ in 53–66% of women with HSIL, and CIN 2+ is diagnosed in 84–97% of women evaluated with LEEP (96, 99, 100). Traditionally, the management of HSIL cytology results has relied on the colposcopy identification of high-grade CIN, followed by treatment when lesions are found (101). This strategy has proved to be highly successful in reducing cervical cancer rates in developed countries. Because colposcopy can miss a significant number of CIN 2,3 lesions and most women with HSIL will eventually undergo a diagnostic exci-

sional procedure, a single-visit strategy (see and treat) is attractive in women in whom future fertility is not an issue (Figure 6). This strategy has been shown to be feasible and cost-effective (102–105). A diagnostic excisional procedure also is recommended for women with HSIL in whom the colposcopy examination is unsatisfactory, except in pregnant women. Because of the limited accuracy of colposcopy generally and of colposcopy grading particularly, colposcopy assessment is no longer required before immediate LEEP. Nevertheless, prudence would suggest that colposcopy is helpful to tailor the excision to the size of the lesion and the limits of the transformation zone.

Some CIN 2,3 lesions will regress spontaneously, especially in adolescents and young adults (11, 106). Therefore, in younger women in whom future fertility is an issue, colposcopy evaluation with endocervical assessment is more appropriate for initial evaluation (90, 107, 108).

▶ *When the initial evaluation of an HSIL cytology result is a diagnosis of CIN 1 or less, how should this condition be managed in the adult patient?*

An important consideration before treatment should be whether the high-grade cytology result is due to a vaginal lesion. Careful examination of the vagina using both 3–5% acetic acid and Lugol's solution may reveal a high-grade vaginal lesion. In such a case, although the cervix has no lesion, the cytology result is correctly pos-

Management of Women with High-grade Squamous Intraepithelial Lesion (HSIL) *
Immediate Loop Electrosurgical Excision+
OR
Colposcopic Examination
(with endocervical assessment)
NO CIN 2,3
Satisfactory Colposcopy
All three approaches are acceptable
CIN 2,3
Unsatisfactory Colposcopy
Observation with Colposcopy & Cytology
@ 6 mo intervals for 1 year
Diagnostic Excisional Procedure+
Review Material^
Change in Diagnosis
Diagnostic Excisional Procedure+
HSIL
@ either visit
Negative Cytology
@ both visits
Other Results
Manage per ASCCP Guideline
Routine Screening
+ Not if patient is pregnant or an adolescent
^ Includes referral cytology, colposcopic findings, and all biopsies
* Management options may vary if the woman is pregnant, postmenopausal, or an adolescent
Copyright 2006, 2007, American Society for Colposcopy and Cervical Pathology. All rights reserved.

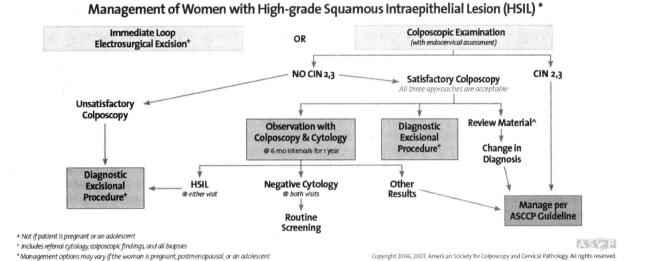

Figure 6. Management of women with high-grade squamous intraepithelial lesion (HSIL). Abbreviations: ASCCP indicates American Society for Colposcopy and Cervical Pathology; CIN, cervical intraepithelial neoplasia; HSIL, high-grade squamous intraepithelial lesion. Wright TC. Management of cervical cytologic abnormalities. J Low Genit Tract Dis 2007;11:201–22. Reprinted from the Journal of Lower Genital Tract Disease Vol. 11 Issue 4, with the permission of ASCCP © American Society for Colposcopy and Cervical Pathology 2007. No copies of the algorithms may be made without the prior consent of ASCCP.

Management of Adolescent Women (20 Years and Younger) with High-grade Squamous Intraepithelial Lesion (HSIL)
Colposcopic Examination
(immediate loop electrosurgical excision is unacceptable)
NO CIN 2,3
CIN 2,3
Two Consecutive Negative Paps AND NO High-grade Colposcopic Abnormality
Observation with Colposcopy & Cytology *
@ 6 mo intervals for up to 2 years
High-grade Colposcopic Lesion OR HSIL
Persists for 1 year
Routine Screening
Other Results
HSIL
Persists for 24 months with no CIN 2,3 identified
Biopsy
CIN 2,3
If NO CIN 2,3, continue observation
Manage per ASCCP Guideline
Diagnostic Excisional Procedure
Manage per ASCCP Guideline for Adolescents with CIN 2,3
* Preferred approach provided the colposcopic examination is satisfactory and endocervical sampling is negative. Otherwise a diagnostic excisional procedure should be performed.
Copyright 2006, 2007, American Society for Colposcopy and Cervical Pathology. All rights reserved.

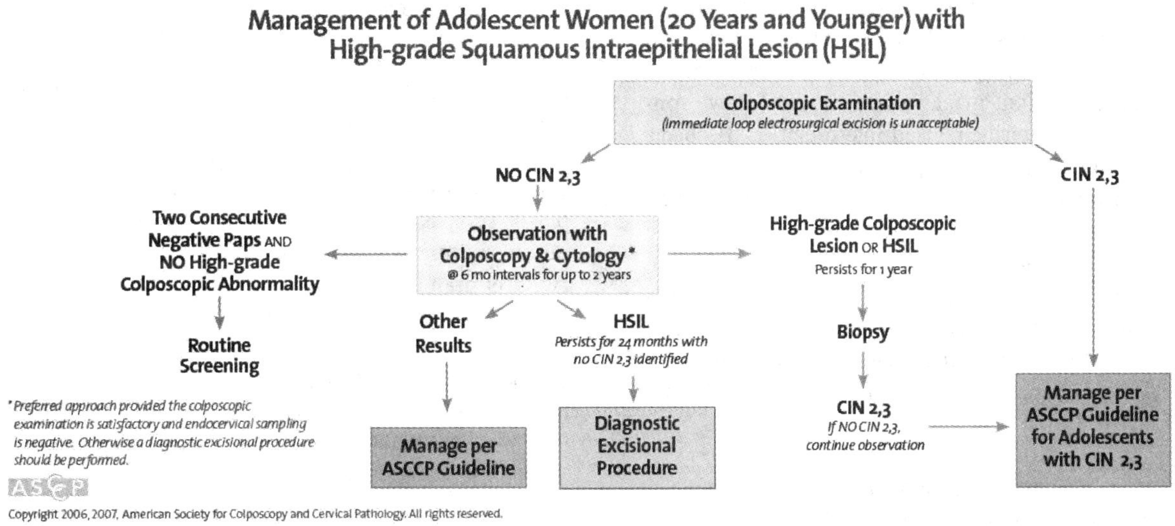

Figure 7. Management of adolescent women (20 years and younger) with high-grade squamous intraepithelial lesion (HSIL). Abbreviations: ASCCP indicates American Society for Colposcopy and Cerviccal Pathology; CIN, cervical intraepithelial neoplasia; HSIL, high-grade squamous intraepithelial lesion. Wright TC. Management of cervical cytologic abnormalities. J Low Genit Tract Dis 2007;11:201–22. Reprinted from the Journal of Lower Genital Tract Disease Vol. 11 Issue 4, with the permission of ASCCP © American Society for Colposcopy and Cervical Pathology 2007. No copies of the algorithms may be made without the prior consent of ASCCP.

itive, and the patient's disease can be cleared with appropriate therapy. Application of Lugol's solution to the cervix also may identify high-grade lesions not previously appreciated. However, the sensitivity of colposcopy is limited, and these women may harbor an unsuspected high-grade cervical lesion. A British study found that 44% of women with negative evaluations after moderate or severe dyskaryosis (HSIL) had CIN found during follow-up (109), whereas a Swedish study found that 22% of women with an HSIL cytology result had CIN during follow-up after negative colposcopy result (110). Women with an HSIL cytology result remain at significant risk for high-grade CIN not evident on their colposcopy or biopsy. However, the predictive value of an HSIL cytology result is limited, and some women with HSIL have CIN 1, subclinical HPV infections without colposcopically visible lesions, or even no disease. Finally, cytology interpretation is subjective, and women with HSIL diagnoses may not have HSIL. In a study of the reproducibility of cervical cytology, 27% of women with HSIL were found to have LSIL on review of their slides, whereas 23% had ASC-US, and 3% had negative results (45). Therefore, both the possibility of missed disease and the potential for overtreatment must be considered, and the management must be individualized based on the patient's needs. When CIN 2,3 is not identified histologically, either a diagnostic excisional procedure or observation with colposcopy and cytology at 6 months and 12 months is acceptable, provided in the latter case that the colposcopy examination is satisfactory and endocervical sampling is negative. A diagnostic excisional procedure is more appropriate in women not concerned about future fertility. However, because of the potential effect that treatment for cervical disease may have on future fertility and the possibility that these women may not have CIN 2,3, and that some CIN 2,3 lesions spontaneously regress, especially in adolescents and young adults (11, 106), the option of watchful waiting was added in the 2006 consensus guidelines. In this circumstance it also is acceptable to review the cytology, histology, and colposcopy findings; if the review yields a revised interpretation, management should follow consensus guidelines for the revised interpretation. If observation with cytology and colposcopy is elected, a diagnostic excisional procedure is recommended for women with the results of HSIL on repeat cytology at either the 6-month or 12-month visit. After 1 year of observation, women with two consecutive negative cytology results can return to routine screening. Ablation is unacceptable when CIN 2,3 is not identified histologically or the endocervical assessment identifies CIN of any grade (Figure 6).

▶ *When the results of cervical cytology tests are reported as HSIL in an adolescent (before age 21 years), how should they be managed?*

Because the likelihood of cancer in adolescents is quite small and the window of opportunity for identifying persistent high-grade cancer precursors is consequently longer, immediate excision is inappropriate, and colposcopy with biopsy of visible lesions is the recommended initial management for all adolescents and young women with HSIL cytology (Figure 7). In the 2006 consensus guidelines, the definition of young women was left deliberately vague but among the factors

that should be taken into consideration in applying this definition are the number of years since first intercourse and the woman's parity and desire for future fertility. When the colposcopy results are satisfactory, the endocervical sampling is negative and no lesion is identified, or when biopsies show either CIN 1 or no neoplasia, serial Pap testing and colposcopy at 6-month intervals for as long as 2 years are advised. If both Pap test results and colposcopy results are negative at two consecutive visits, then routine annual assessment can resume. Diagnostic excision is recommended when colposcopy results are unsatisfactory or when endocervical sampling yields CIN, but this should be unusual in young women. If during follow-up a high-grade colposcopy lesion is identified or a HSIL cytology result persists for 1 year, biopsy is recommended. However, if HSIL cytology result persists for 2 years, then a diagnostic excisional procedure is recommended. After two consecutive negative Pap test results, adolescents and young women without a high-grade colposcopy abnormality can return to routine screening.

▶ *When the results of cervical cytology tests are reported as AGC or AIS, how should they be managed?*

The results of AGC are relatively uncommon, with a mean reporting rate of only 0.4% in the United States in 2003 (98). Although AGC is frequently caused by benign conditions, such as reactive changes and polyps, it is sometimes associated with a significant underlying neoplasia, such as adenocarcinoma of the cervix, endometrium, ovary, or a fallopian tube. The risk associated with AGC is dramatically higher than that seen with ASC. The risk associated with glandular abnormalities increases as the description in the Bethesda classification system advances from AGC, not otherwise specified (NOS) to AGC, favors neoplasia and, finally, AIS. Recent series have reported that 9–38% of women with AGC have significant neoplasia (CIN 2,3, AIS, or cancer) and 3–17% have invasive cancer (111–113). The rate and type of significant findings in women with AGC varies with age (112). Women younger than 35 years with AGC are more likely to have CIN and less likely to have cancer, whereas in older women the risk of glandular lesions, including malignancies, is higher (111). Human papillomavirus testing, cervical cytology, and colposcopy are all suboptimal at detecting glandular disease (114, 115). Colposcopy with endocervical sampling is recommended for all women with all subcategories of AGC or AIS cytology results. In addition, endometrial sampling is recommended in women 35 years and older or in women younger than 35 years with clinical indications suggesting a risk of neoplastic endometrial lesions (eg, unexplained vaginal bleeding, chronic anovulation, or atypical endometrial cells). In the latter case, colposcopy can be deferred until the results of the initial biopsies are known.

The 2006 consensus guidelines recommend HPV DNA testing at the time of colposcopy in women with atypical endocervical, endometrial, or glandular cells, NOS (Figure 8). Knowledge of the HPV status in these women who do not have CIN 2,3 or glandular neoplasia identified histologically will allow expedited triage. Women with a positive HPV result would have their cytology and HPV test repeated at 6 months, and those with a negative HPV result would receive repeat cytology at 12 months. Those with a positive HPV result or an abnormal cytology result would be referred to colposcopy, and those in whom both tests are negative can return to routine screening. In contrast, if the HPV status is unknown, cervical cytology testing should be repeated every 6 months until there are four consecutive negative test results before the woman can return to routine screening (12). Because the risk of neoplasia (including invasive cancer) is high in women with AGC, favors neoplasia, AIS, or repeat AGC and the sensitivity of available diagnostic tests is poor, diagnostic excisional procedures are recommended for these women. Human papillomavirus testing is not useful in managing these patients (Figure 9). It is recommended that the type of diagnostic excisional procedure used in this setting pro-

vides an intact specimen with interpretable margins (12). In pregnant women, the initial evaluation of AGC should be identical to that of nonpregnant women, except that endocervical curettage and endometrial biopsy are unacceptable.

▶ *What is the significance of endometrial cells found in cervical cytology?*

In premenopausal women, benign-appearing endometrial cells or the presence of endometrial stromal cells or histiocytes is rarely associated with significant pathology (116). However, approximately 0.5–1.8% of cervical cytology specimens from women 40 years and older will have endometrial cells (116), and in postmenopausal women they may be associated with significant endometrial pathology (117). Benign-appearing glandular cells derived from small accessory ducts, foci of benign adenosis, or prolapse of the fallopian tube into the vagina are sometimes seen in cytology specimens after total hysterectomy and have no clinical significance.

For asymptomatic premenopausal women with benign endometrial cells, endometrial stromal cells, or histiocytes, no further evaluation is recommended. For postmenopausal women with benign endometrial cells, endometrial assessment is recommended regardless of symptoms. For posthysterectomy patients with a cytology report of benign glandular cells, no further evaluation is recommended.

Initial Workup of Women with Atypical Glandular Cells (AGC)

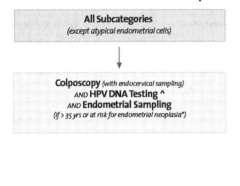

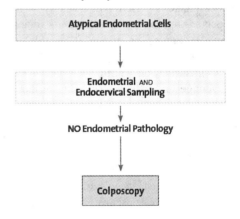

^ *If not already obtained. Test only for high-risk (oncogenic) types.*
* *Includes unexplained vaginal bleeding or conditions suggesting chronic anovulation.*

Figure 8. Initial workup of women with atypical glandular cells (AGC). Abbreviation: HPV indicates human papillomavirus. Wright TC. Management of cervical cytologic abnormalities. J Low Genit Tract Dis 2007;11:201–22. Reprinted from the Journal of Lower Genital Tract Disease Vol. 11 Issue 4, with the permission of ASCCP © American Society for Colposcopy and Cervical Pathology 2007. No copies of the algorithms may be made without the prior consent of ASCCP.

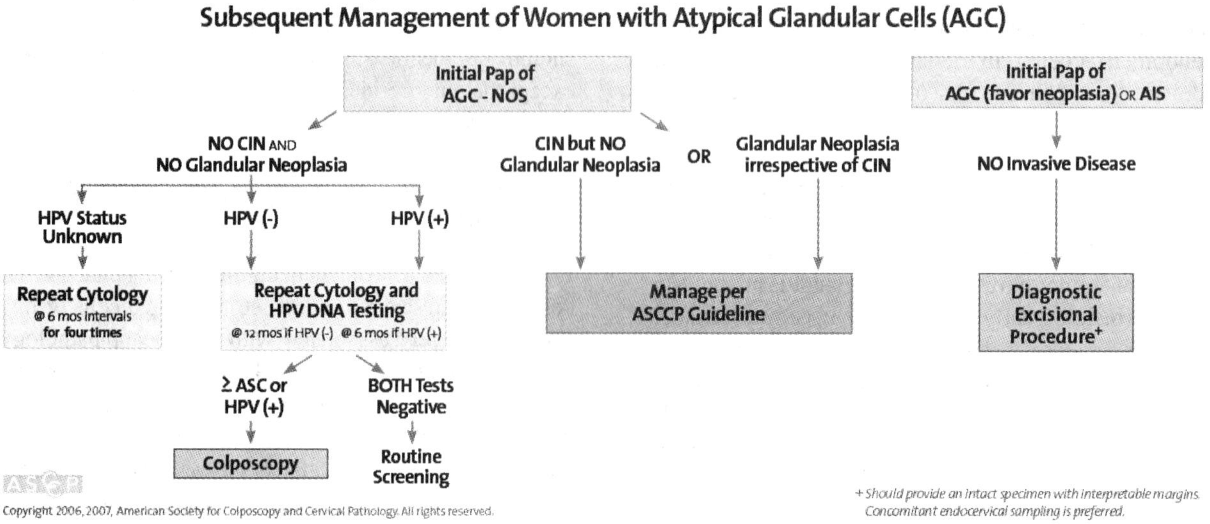

Subsequent Management of Women with Atypical Glandular Cells (AGC)

Figure 9. Subsequent management of women with atypical glandular cells (AGC). Abbreviations: AGC indicates atypical glandular cells; AGC-NOS, atypical glandular cells—not otherwise specified; AIS, adenocarcinoma in situ; ASC, atypical squamous cells; ASCCP, American Society for Colposcopy and Cervical Pathology; CIN, cervical intraepithelial neoplasia; HPV, human papillomavirus. Wright TC. Management of cervical cytologic abnormalities. J Low Genit Tract Dis 2007;11:201–22. Reprinted from the Journal of Lower Genital Tract Disease Vol. 11 Issue 4, with the permission of ASCCP © American Society for Colposcopy and Cervical Pathology 2007. No copies of the algorithms may be made without the prior consent of ASCCP.

▶ When should endocervical curettage be used in the colposcopy examination?

The value of routine endocervical curettage (ECC) is controversial. Endocervical sampling is preferred for nonpregnant women in whom no lesions are identified, women with an unsatisfactory colposcopy, and women who have follow-up colposcopy after a conization for CIN 2,3 with a positive endocervical margin. Endocervical curettage is preferred in cases where the results are expected to change the patient's management. Endocervical curettage is especially valuable for women 40 years and older. An analysis of ALTS data showed that ECC identified an additional 2.2% of CIN 2+ in women younger than 40 years, whereas it increased the detection by 13% in women 40 years and older (128). Endocervical curettage is recommended in women with a glandular abnormality on cytology and those who have any abnormal cytology result or HPV test result after cervical treatment. This procedure is unacceptable in pregnant women. However, in nonpregnant women with a satisfactory colposcopy result, a positive ECC result is most likely due to contamination that incorrectly indicates the need for a deeper excisional procedure rather than an ablative procedure or a shallower excision. Endocervical curettage may be especially helpful in such patients if ablative therapy is planned but may not change the management if excisional therapy is planned (119).

▶ If colposcopy is satisfactory and consistent with the results of cervical cytology, is biopsy necessary?

Colposcopy assessment may assist the examiner in identifying appropriate biopsy sites, but colposcopy assessment is not sufficiently accurate to eliminate the need for one or more biopsy procedures. A meta-analysis comparing colposcopy impression to colposcopy biopsy reported an average 48% sensitivity of colposcopy impression for separation of CIN 2,3+ from other diagnoses (120). Use of colposcopy impression alone could have caused 18–60% of patients to be treated incorrectly. Recent data suggest that taking additional biopsy specimens in other abnormal areas also may improve detection regardless of the colposcopist's level of experience (16). Biopsy of any visible lesion is an important component of a colposcopy examination, regardless of colposcopy impression. The only exceptions are women for whom a diagnostic excision is planned, and pregnant women without a colposcopically-diagnosed high-grade lesion.

▶ Is excision or ablation the better treatment for CIN?

Treatment modalities for CIN should be evaluated based on their effectiveness and appropriateness in treating CIN 2,3. The recommended management of CIN 1 is follow-up without treatment for at least 2 years during which regression of many of the lesions is expected. After 2 years, the patient may be treated, but continued follow-up is acceptable. Treatment options include cryotherapy, laser ablation, laser conization, knife conization, and loop electrosurgical excision. Although studies in general have been small and may have difficulty in distinguishing subtle differences among treatments, various treatments appear to be similarly efficacious in eradicating preinvasive disease (121–123). Selection of the appropriate treatment modality depends on the operator's experience, equipment availability, lesion size, and other factors. Alternatively, if the lesion extends onto the vagina, laser ablation may be more appropriate than other treatment because it can be tailored to encompass the entire lesion with excellent depth control. When microinvasive cancer or AIS is suspected, then conization provides a histology specimen for assessment.

Ablative treatments (eg, cryotherapy or laser vaporization) should be used only after rigorously excluding invasive cancer. When endocervical assessment shows CIN, the colposcopy result is not satisfactory, cytology or colposcopy examination suggests cancer, or after prior therapy, cancer may be present but unseen and ablative therapy is not appropriate (119, 124). Laser and loop electrosurgical excision minimize blood loss by thermal cautery during excision but may cause thermal artifact that impairs the interpretability of a specimen (125, 126). This may be clinically significant at a focus of possible microinvasion or AIS. In these cases, knife conization may be preferable.

▶ *How should CIN 1 be managed in women who present with HPV-positive ASC-US, ASC-H, or LSIL results?*

Most CIN 1 in ALTS regressed spontaneously and CIN 1 uncommonly progressed to CIN 2,3 (9). In ALTS, many of the CIN 2,3 lesions subsequently identified in women diagnosed with CIN 1 appeared to represent lesions that were missed during the initial colposcopy evaluation (9). The management of women with LSIL is dependent on their risk of CIN 2,3 and cancer that is in turn related to their presenting cytology. Among women enrolled in ALTS who presented with LSIL or HPV-positive ASC-US on cytology and were found to have CIN 1 on initial colposcopy, 13% were subsequently found to have CIN 2,3 (8.9% CIN 3) and none had cancer during the 24-month follow-up period. This rate of CIN 2,3 on follow-up was similar to women whose colposcopy results were completely negative and who had no biopsy (11.3%), and those whose biopsy specimens were negative for CIN (11.7%) (9). The rationale for

avoiding treatment in favor of more conservative follow-up is related to the cost, discomfort, and potential morbidity of commonly used treatment modalities. Recent studies have shown a significant risk of premature delivery and preterm premature rupture of membranes in pregnant women previously treated with LEEP (3, 4, 115). This is especially significant in young women with CIN 1, a group for whom future pregnancy complications are a concern and a group very likely to have spontaneous regression (127). Conservative management allows adequate time to identify cases that might have been initially misclassified or to allow identification of those that would progress to higher-grade lesions whereas the risk of developing cancer remains minimal.

Because the finding of CIN 1 on histology does not affect the risk of CIN 2,3 among women with HPV-positive ASC-US, ASC-H, or LSIL cytology results (compared with those in whom no disease was found), women 21 years and older with CIN 1 preceded by these cytology findings should be managed similarly with either HPV DNA testing every 12 months or repeat cervical cytology at 6 months and 12 months. The decision to treat is unaffected by whether the colposcopy result is satisfactory, and treatment during the first 2 years of follow-up is not recommended. Although persistence of CIN 1 beyond 2 years is associated with a higher risk of high-grade dysplasia and the likelihood of regression decreases the longer dysplasia persists, cancer can be effectively prevented with continued follow-up, and there are no data to preclude continued follow-up beyond 2 years. Thus, it is safe to monitor these patients with semi-annual cytology examinations or annual HPV DNA testing with colposcopy for women with positive high-risk HPV DNA testing or cytology of ASC-US or greater. If CIN 1 has not resolved after 2 years, treatment is acceptable with excision or ablation if the colposcopy result remains satisfactory (13).

If the decision has been made to treat the patient and the colposcopy result is unsatisfactory, the endocervical sampling contains CIN, or the patient has been previously treated, ablative procedures are unacceptable and a diagnostic excisional procedure is recommended.

The management of adolescents with CIN 1 is the same as that of adolescents with LSIL. The recommended management of histologically diagnosed CIN 1 in pregnant women is follow-up without treatment. Treatment of pregnant women for CIN 1 is unacceptable.

▶ *How should CIN 1 be managed in women who presented with HSIL or AGC-NOS?*

Either a diagnostic excisional procedure or observation with colposcopy and cytology at 6-month intervals for 1 year is acceptable for women 21 years or older with a histology diagnosis of CIN 1 preceded by an HSIL or AGC-NOS cytology result, provided in the latter case that the colposcopy examination is satisfactory and endocervical sampling is negative. A diagnostic excisional procedure is recommended for women with CIN 1 preceded by an HSIL or AGC-NOS cytology result in whom the colposcopy examination is unsatisfactory, except in pregnancy.

The risk of an undetected CIN 2,3 or an adenocarcinoma in situ lesion is expected to be greater in women with CIN 1 preceded by an HSIL or AGC cytology result than in women with CIN 1 preceded by an ASC or LSIL cytology result. Cervical intraepithelial neoplasia grade 2,3 is identified in 84–97% of women with HSIL cytology results evaluated with a LEEP (96, 99, 100). Therefore, separate recommendations are made for women with CIN 1 preceded by an HSIL or AGC cytology result.

▶ *How should CIN 2 and CIN 3 be managed?*

Cervical intraepithelial neoplasia grade 3 generally is considered to be a cancer precursor, although not all CIN 3 lesions will progress to cancer. The prevalence of CIN 3 peaks between ages 25 years and 30 years, and progression to cancer usually takes at least a decade longer (90). The risk of progression of CIN 3 is unclear because most experts consider the risk too high to justify observation. A biopsy diagnosis of CIN 3 may miss occult invasive cancer and apparent progression after a colposcopy biopsy diagnosis may reflect missed prevalent cancer. One review found that the likelihood of CIN 3 progressing to invasion was 12%, with 33% of patients regressing and the remainder having stable disease (10). Smaller lesions with fewer colposcopy features are more likely to regress, whereas larger lesions with coarse vascular changes are less likely to regress (128). Cervical intraepithelial neoplasia grade 2,3 lesions associated with HPV 16 genotype are less likely to regress, as are those in women with the HLA 201 phenotype (107). The significance of CIN 2 is unclear. The risk of progression to CIN 3 and cancer appears greater for women with CIN 2 than for women with CIN 1. However, many women with CIN 2 will have regression of their lesions without therapy. In one review, CIN 2 progressed to cancer in 5% of patients and to CIN 3 in 20% of patients, persisted in 40% of patients, and regressed in 40% of patients (10). No accepted tests are available to distinguish CIN 2 that reflects an exuberant HPV infection from that with true malignant potential. The cutoff between CIN 1 and CIN 2 and between CIN 2 and CIN 3 is arbitrary. Because of the moderate cancer risk associated with CIN 2, the decision among leaders in colposcopy and cervical cancer prevention in the United States has been to consider CIN 2 the threshold for treatment for most U.S. women.

However, there are exceptions. The risk of progression to invasive cancer is low before age 21 years, and some CIN 2,3 lesions regress, especially in younger women. For this reason, observation of adolescents and young women appears to be a safe and reasonable approach, provided cancer has been ruled out. When a histology diagnosis of CIN 2 is specified, observation is preferred. One study found unsuspected cancerous lesions in 8% of women undergoing hysterectomy for CIN 2,3, which suggests that prior conization is mandatory to exclude malignancy (129). For these reasons, hysterectomy is unacceptable as the primary therapy for CIN 2,3.

▶ *Does management of CIN 2 or CIN 3 differ for women who are HIV positive?*

Standard ablative or excisional treatment is recommended for women who are HIV positive with documented CIN 2 or CIN 3, regardless of HIV viral load. Effective treatment of CIN requires immunologic clearance or suppression of HPV to avoid recurrence (130). Women who are HIV positive have difficulty clearing HPV and, therefore, are at increased risk of recurrent disease in direct relation to their level of immunosuppression (131–134). Treatment of CIN should be pursued despite high recurrence rates (greater than 50% recurrence rate after standard treatment) because it can effectively interrupt progression to invasive cancer (131, 135–138). Women who are HIV positive also appear more likely to have positive surgical margins, which may contribute to increased recurrence rates (139). Because recent studies reported a lower prevalence of high-grade disease and HPV DNA positivity among immunosuppressed women, the 2006 consensus guidelines recommend that the management of these conditions be similar to that in the general population (140–142).

The role of highly active antiretroviral therapy in the management of precancerous cervical lesions remains unclear (143). Therefore, CIN 2 and CIN 3 should be treated similarly in women who are HIV positive regardless of their use of antiretroviral therapy.

▶ *How should AIS be managed? How should patients with AIS be monitored after treatment?*

Although the overall incidence of AIS is increasing, it remains relatively rare compared with CIN 2,3 (144). In 1991–1995, the overall incidence of squamous carcinoma in situ of the cervix among white women in the United States was 41.4 per 100,000, whereas the incidence of AIS was only 1.25 per 100,000 (144). Because cytology screening and colposcopy detection of AIS are so challenging and the clinical behavior of AIS is so different from CIN 2,3, the principles involved in the management of AIS differ from what is the norm for squamous disease. The colposcopy changes associated with AIS can be minimal or unfamiliar to most colposcopists. Adenocarcinoma in situ frequently is multifocal, may have "skip lesions," and frequently extends for a considerable distance into the endocervical canal, making complete excision difficult. Thus, negative margins on a diagnostic excisional specimen do not necessarily mean that the lesion has been completely excised.

Hysterectomy continues to be the treatment of choice for AIS in women who have completed childbearing. However, an excisional procedure is still curative in most of these patients. A comprehensive review of the published literature conducted in 2001 identified 16 studies that included a total of 296 women with AIS who were treated with a diagnostic excisional procedure (145). The overall failure rate was 8% (145). Margin status and endocervical sampling at the time of an excisional biopsy are clinically useful predictors of residual disease (146–149). Excisional biopsy is required in all women with AIS before making any subsequent management decisions. Conservative management is acceptable if future fertility is desired. If conservative management is planned and the margins of the specimen are involved or endocervical sampling obtained at the time of excision contains CIN or AIS, re-excision to increase the likelihood of complete excision is preferred. These women should be reevaluated at 6 months using a combination of cervical cytology, HPV DNA testing, and colposcopy with endocervical sampling. Long-term follow-up after treatment is recommended for all women with AIS.

▶ *How should inconclusive colposcopic biopsy results for early invasive cancer be managed?*

Colposcopic biopsy results that are inconclusive for cancer should be followed by excision to define whether cancer is present and to permit treatment planning. The management of early invasive cervical cancer depends on the depth of invasion and the presence or absence of lymph and vascular space invasion. Biopsy alone does not adequately provide this information. Cold-knife conization is preferred for this purpose because it maintains tissue orientation in a single specimen, which is essential to permit pathologic evaluation of depth of invasion and other variables that define stage and treatment (150). Loop and laser excisions are acceptable in experienced hands.

▶ *How should a patient's condition be monitored after treatment for CIN?*

Observation after treatment requires long-term surveillance. Although most recurrent or persistent CIN is found within the first 1–5 years, cases of cancer have been found as late as 20 years after initial therapy (151, 152). In one large study of women monitored after treatment for CIN 3, the sensitivity of cytology in identifying recurrent or persistent CIN was only 64%, whereas adding colposcopy improved the sensitivity to 91% but reduced specificity from 95% to 88% (153). The sensitivity of cytology improves with repeated testing, and whereas few women with CIN 2,3 present soon after treatment with invasive cancer, usually there is time for serial cytology assessment 6 months and 12 months after the treatment because the risk for persistence and recurrence is highest during the first year. The outcomes of treatment of recurrent or persistent disease are unaffected by a short delay in diagnosis as long as persistent disease is identified and eradicated before invasion occurs. Human papillomavirus testing alone is highly sensitive, and a single test at 1 year will detect most recurrences. A combination of HPV testing and cytology was only marginally more sensitive but was the least specific and most costly program for identifying persistent or recurrent CIN (154). Colposcopy with endocervical sampling is indicated with cytology results of ASC-US or greater or a positive HPV test result. If the HPV DNA test result is negative or if two consecutive repeat cytology tests yield negative results, routine screening commencing at 12 months is recommended for at least 20 years.

▶ *If LEEP or cone biopsy reveals a positive margin, how should management proceed?*

Most women with positive margins do not have residual disease, so although repeat conization to prevent recurrence is acceptable, it usually is not necessary. Observation without retreatment using cytology with endocervical sampling at 4–6 months after treatment is preferred in these women. Women with CIN 2,3 involving the excision margins of a conization specimen and those with CIN 2,3 at a postprocedure endocervical sampling are at increased risk for persistence of disease compared with those with clear margins (155–160). One center reporting on 5,386 women after conization for CIN 3 (two studies combined) found recurrence in 0.4% of women with clear margins and in 22% of women with involved margins, with cancerous lesions in 7% of recurrences (161, 162). In a meta-analysis of studies describing more than 35,000 women after an excision, the relative risk of CIN 2,3 after incomplete excision compared with complete excision was 6.09 (163). A positive excision margin is a convenient marker for recurrence, especially when the endocervical margin is involved. However, multiple studies have shown that margin involvement by CIN is not an independent marker for recurrence or persistence (155–157). Risk factors for recurrence or persistence of CIN include older age, larger lesions, and higher-grade disease, with risks as high as 50% for older women with large CIN 3 lesions.

Repeat diagnostic excisional procedures should be discouraged in adolescents because of the potential effect on future fertility. A hysterectomy for this indication is unacceptable in this population.

▶ *When is hysterectomy appropriate in women with CIN 2,3+?*

Hysterectomy in the absence of other indications, such as abnormal bleeding or uterine leiomyomas, usually is not required. However, one indication is in a patient with recurrent disease when the residual cervix is too small to allow safe repeat conization without risk of bladder and vaginal injury. A repeat diagnostic excision or hysterectomy is acceptable for women with a histology diagnosis of recurrent or persistent CIN 2,3. If excision is indicated, it should be performed (where possible) before hysterectomy to rule out invasive cancer. If hysterectomy is performed, the choice of either vaginal or abdominal approach should be dictated by other indications, such as the surgeon's experience and patient characteristics and preferences.

▶ *How do care and follow-up differ for women during pregnancy?*

In pregnancy, the only diagnosis that may alter management is invasive cancer. The presence of cancer may change treatment goals or change the route and timing of delivery. Therefore, colposcopy examination during pregnancy should have as its primary goal the exclusion of invasive cancer.

Management of LSIL and HPV-positive ASC-US results during pregnancy should be the same as in the nonpregnant state, although the evaluation of these conditions may be deferred until after delivery (Figure 10). If colposcopy is performed for LSIL during pregnancy, additional colposcopy examinations are not indicated. The practice of repeating the colposcopy once per trimester in pregnant women with LSIL is unacceptable unless CIN 2,3 is diagnosed. During pregnancy, limiting biopsy to lesions suspicious for CIN 2,3 or cancer is preferred, but biopsy of any lesion is acceptable. Biopsy during pregnancy has not been linked to fetal loss or preterm delivery, whereas failure to perform biopsy during pregnancy has been linked to missed invasive cancer (164–166). Pregnant adolescents should be treated in the same manner as nonpregnant adolescents.

All women with HSIL should undergo colposcopy, including those who are pregnant. The goal of cytology and colposcopy during pregnancy is to identify invasive cancer that requires treatment before or at the time of delivery. However, unless cancer is identified or suspected,

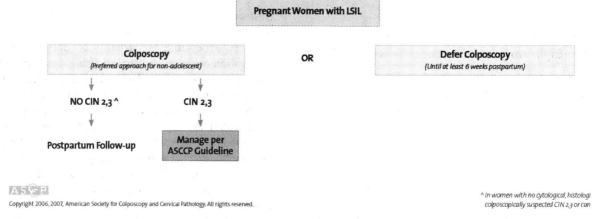

Management of Pregnant Women with Low-grade Squamous Intraepithelial Lesion (LSIL)

Figure 10. Management of pregnant women with low-grade squamous intraepithelial lesion (LSIL). Abbreviations: ASCCP indicates American Society for Colposcopy and Cervical Pathology; CIN, cervical intraepithelial neoplasia; LSIL, low-grade squamous intraepithelial lesion. Wright TC. Management of cervical cytologic abnormalities. J Low Genit Tract Dis 2007;11:201–22. Reprinted from the Journal of Lower Genital Tract Disease Vol. 11 Issue 4, with the permission of ASCCP © American Society for Colposcopy and Cervical Pathology 2007. No copies of the algorithms may be made without the prior consent of ASCCP.

treatment of CIN is contraindicated during pregnancy. Cervical intraepithelial neoplasia has no effect on the woman or fetus, whereas cervical treatments designed to eradicate CIN can result in fetal loss, preterm delivery, and maternal hemorrhage. Endocervical curettage may result in laceration of the soft cervix with consequent hemorrhage and it also may rupture the amniotic membranes. Endocervical curettage is contraindicated during pregnancy. Colposcopy during pregnancy is challenging because of cervical hyperemia, the development of prominent normal epithelial changes that mimic preinvasive disease colposcopically, obscuring mucus, contact bleeding, prolapsing vaginal walls, and bleeding after biopsy (167). Biopsy is important if the colposcopy impression is high grade, especially in older pregnant women at higher risk of invasive cancer. Once cancer has been excluded, cervical therapy can be deferred until postpartum. Cervical intraepithelial neoplasia may regress during the interval between antenatal cytology and a postpartum examination. In women with biopsy-proven CIN 2 during pregnancy, the risk of microinvasive cancer at the postpartum visit is negligible, whereas the risk after CIN 3 is substantially less than 10%, and deeply invasive cancers are rare (168, 169). For this reason, re-evaluation during pregnancy may prompt needless intervention that may jeopardize current and future pregnancies. Reassessment with cytology and colposcopy no sooner than 6 weeks after delivery is important in tailoring therapy.

Cervical intraepithelial neoplasia 2,3 rarely progresses to invasive cancer during the few months of pregnancy. For these reasons, observation of pregnant women appears a safe and reasonable approach, provided cancer has been ruled out.

Summary of Recommendations

The following recommendations are based on good and consistent scientific evidence (Level A):

▶ Premenopausal women 21 years and older with ASC-US cytology results may undergo immediate colposcopy or may undergo triage testing to determine which of them should be referred to colposcopy. Triage testing may be performed by a single test for high-risk (oncogenic) types of HPV or by repeat cytology screening at 6 months and 12 months. When the index cytology test specimen was obtained by liquid-based cytology or when an HPV specimen was co-collected, "reflex" HPV testing is the preferred approach.

▶ Colposcopy is recommended in premenopausal women 21 years and older with ASC-US who are HPV positive, those with two consecutive ASC-US cytology results or with LSIL, or women of any age with ASC-H.

▶ For premenopausal women 21 years and older with an HPV-positive ASC-US, or ASC-H or LSIL cytology result in whom CIN 2,3 is not identified, follow-up without treatment is recommended using either repeat cervical cytology tests at 6 months and 12 months or an HPV test at 12 month-intervals; a repeat colposcopy is indicated for a cytology result of ASC-US or higher-grade abnormality or a positive high-risk HPV test result. After two consecutive negative cytology results or one negative HPV result women can return to routine screening.

▶ In women 21 years and older with HSIL cytology results, immediate loop electrosurgical excision or colposcopy with endocervical assessment are both acceptable management options. In adolescents and pregnant women with HSIL cytology results, colposcopy is recommended. Immediate excision is not acceptable in adolescents and pregnant women. A diagnostic excisional procedure is recommended for all nonpregnant women with HSIL when colposcopy is unsatisfactory or when CIN of any grade is identified on endocervical assessment.

▶ Posttreatment management options for women 21 years and older who have CIN 2,3 include a single HPV DNA test at 6–12 months, cytology alone at 6-month intervals or a combination of cytology and colposcopy at 6-month intervals. For adolescents who have undergone treatment, cytology follow-up is preferred. Colposcopy with endocervical sampling is recommended for women who are HPV DNA positive or have a result of ASC-US or greater on repeat cytology. If the HPV DNA test is negative or if two consecutive repeat cytology test results are negative, routine screening commencing at 12 months is recommended for at least 20 years.

The following recommendations are based on limited and inconsistent scientific evidence (Level B):

▶ Women 21 years or older with ASC-US who test negative for HPV, or whose HPV status is unknown and who test negative for abnormalities using colposcopy, should have a repeat cytology test in 1 year. Women with ASC-US who have two negative results on repeat cytology at 6-month intervals can return to routine screening.

▶ In adolescents (before age 21 years) with ASC-US or LSIL cytology results, or CIN 1 histology results preceded by ASC-US or LSIL or AGC-NOS cytology results, follow-up is recommended at 12-month intervals. At the first follow-up visit (at 12 months), only adolescents with HSIL or greater on the repeat cytology should be referred to colposcopy. At the 24-month follow-up, those with an ASC-US or greater result should be referred to colposcopy. Human papillomavirus DNA testing is unacceptable for adolescents. If HPV testing is inadvertently performed, a positive result should not influence management.

▶ In nonpregnant women with ASC and LSIL cytology results who are undergoing colposcopy, endocervical sampling using a brush or curette is preferred for women in whom no lesions are identified and those with an unsatisfactory colposcopy results. Endocervical sampling is acceptable for women with satisfactory colposcopy results and a lesion identified in the transformation zone. Endo-cervical assessment either with colposcopy or by sampling is recommended for all nonpregnant women with HSIL cytology results. Endocervical curettage is unacceptable in pregnant women.

▶ The recommended management of pregnant women with a histology diagnosis of CIN 1 is follow-up without treatment. Treatment of pregnant women for CIN 1 is unacceptable.

▶ In a woman 21 years and older with CIN 1 that has persisted for at least 2 years, either continued follow-up or treatment is acceptable. If treatment is selected and the colposcopy result is satisfactory, either excision or ablation is acceptable. If treatment is selected and the colposcopy examination is unsatisfactory, the ECC is positive, or the woman has been previously treated, excision is recommended and ablative procedures are unacceptable.

▶ Pregnant women with biopsy-proven CIN 2 or CIN 3 in whom there is no suspicion of invasive cancer may postpone re-evaluation with cytology and colposcopy to no sooner than 6 weeks postpartum. Treatment during pregnancy is unacceptable unless invasion is suspected. When invasion is suspected, a diagnostic excisional procedure is recommended.

▶ For women 21 years and older, the preferred management of CIN 2,3 identified at the margins of a diagnostic excisional procedure or in an endocervical sample obtained at the end of the procedure is reassessment using cytology with endocervical sampling at 4–6 months following treatment. Perform-

ing a repeat diagnostic excisional procedure is acceptable, as is a hysterectomy if a repeat diagnostic procedure is not feasible and for women with a histology diagnosis of recurrent or persistent CIN 2,3.

▶ In nonpregnant women 21 years and older, both excision and ablation are acceptable treatment modalities in the presence of histology diagnoses of CIN 2,3 and satisfactory colposcopy results. Ablation is unacceptable when colposcopy has not been performed, the endocervical sampling is positive for any grade of CIN, the colposcopy result is unsatisfactory, or a woman has recurrent CIN 2,3.

▶ Colposcopy with endocervical sampling is recommended and HPV DNA testing is preferred for women with all subcategories of AGC and AIS. In addition, endometrial sampling is recommended in women 35 years and older and in women younger than 35 years with clinical indications suggesting they may be at risk of neoplastic endometrial lesions (eg, unexplained vaginal bleeding, chronic anovulation, or atypical endometrial cells). Colposcopy can be performed either at the initial evaluation or after the results are known. If no endometrial pathology is identified, colposcopy is recommended. Endometrial and endocervical sampling are unacceptable in pregnant women.

▶ Women 21 years and older with either atypical endocervical, endometrial, or glandular cells NOS who do not have CIN or glandular neoplasia identified histologically should receive repeat cytology testing combined with HPV DNA testing at 6 months if they are HPV DNA positive and at 12 months if they are HPV DNA negative. Referral to colposcopy is recommended for women who subsequently test positive for high-risk HPV DNA or who are found to have ASC-US or greater on their repeat cytology tests. If both tests are negative, women can return to routine cytology testing.

▶ Women with AGC, favors neoplasia or AIS cytology results should undergo a diagnostic excisional procedure unless invasive disease is identified during the initial colposcopy workup. The diagnostic excisional procedure used in this setting should provide an intact specimen with interpretable margins. Concomitant endocervical sampling is preferred, except in pregnant women.

▶ Hysterectomy is unacceptable as the primary therapy for CIN.

▶ Diagnostic ablation or excision is unacceptable as the initial management for ASC or LSIL.

The following recommendations are based primarily on consensus and expert opinion (Level C):

▶ In nonpregnant women 21 years and older with HSIL in whom CIN 2,3 has not been identified, three management options are acceptable: diagnostic excisional procedure; review of the cytology, histology, and colposcopy findings and management of the patient according to the revised interpretation; or if the colposcopy is satisfactory and endocervical sampling is negative, observation with colposcopy and cytology at 6 month-intervals for 1 year. A diagnostic excisional procedure is recommended for women with repeat HSIL cytology results at either the 6-month or 12-month visit. Women with two consecutive negative cytology results can return to routine screening.

▶ In adolescents (before age 21 years) with HSIL cytology results, a satisfactory colposcopy result, negative endocervical sampling, and no CIN 2,3 identified on colposcopy biopsy, follow-up is recommended at 6-month intervals with Pap testing and colposcopy for up to 24 months. If during follow-up a high grade colposcopy lesion is identified or HSIL cytology results persist for 1 year, biopsy is recommended. If HSIL persists for 24 months without identification of CIN 2,3, or if the colposcopy result is unsatisfactory, a diagnostic excisional procedure is recommended. After two consecutive negative cytology results, women can return to routine cytology testing.

▶ For adolescents and young women with a histology diagnosis of CIN 2,3 NOS and a satisfactory colposcopy result either treatment or observation for up to 24 months using both colposcopy and cytology at 6-month intervals is acceptable. When a histology diagnosis of CIN 2 is specified, observation is preferred. When a histology diagnosis of CIN 3 is specified or when the colposcopy result is unsatisfactory, treatment is recommended. If the colposcopy appearance of the lesion worsens or if an HSIL cytology result or a high-grade colposcopy lesion persists for 1 year, repeat biopsy is recommended. After two consecutive negative cytology results, women with normal colposcopy results can return to routine cytology screening. Treatment is recommended if CIN 3 is subsequently identified or if CIN 2,3 persists for 24 months.

▶ In nonpregnant women 21 years and older with HSIL or AGC-NOS cytology results in whom CIN 1 has been identified on colposcopy three management options are acceptable: diagnostic excisional procedure; review of the cytology, histology, and colposcopy findings and management of the patient according to the revised interpretation; or if the colposcopy is satisfactory and endocervical sampling is negative, observation with colposcopy and cytology at 6-month intervals for 1 year. A diagnostic excisional procedure is recommended for women with repeat HSIL cytology results at either the 6-month or 12-month visit. Women with two consecutive negative cytology results can return to routine cytology screening.

▶ In women 21 years and older with atypical endocervical, endometrial, or glandular cells NOS, HPV DNA testing is preferred at the time of colposcopy (if not already performed). For women of unknown HPV status who do not have CIN or glandular neoplasia identified histologically, the recommended postcolposcopy management is to repeat cytology testing at 6-month intervals. After four consecutive negative cytology results, women can return to routine cytology testing.

▶ Women with a cervical biopsy diagnosis of AIS should undergo excision to exclude invasive cancer. A conization technique that preserves specimen orientation and permits optimal interpretation of histology and margin status is recommended. After conization, hysterectomy is preferred for women who have completed childbearing. Conservative management is acceptable if the margins of the specimen and the postprocedure endocervical curettage results are negative and future fertility is desired. If conservative management is planned and the margins of the specimen are involved or the postprocedure endocervical curettage specimen contains CIN or AIS, re-excision is preferred. Reevaluation at 6 months using a combination of cervical cytology, HPV DNA testing, and colposcopy with endocervical sampling is acceptable in this circumstance. Long-term follow-up after treatment is recommended for all women with AIS.

References

1. Ries LA, Melbert D, Krapcho M, Stinchcomb DG, Howlader N, Horner MJ, et al, editors. SEER cancer statistics review, 1975-2005. Bethesda (MD): National Cancer Institute; 2008. Available at: http://seer.cancer.gov/csr/1975_2005. Retrieved July 14, 2008. (Level III)

2. Insinga RP, Glass AG, Rush BB. Diagnoses and outcomes in cervical cancer screening: a population-based study. Am J Obstet Gynecol 2004;191:105–13. (Level II-3)

3. Samson SL, Bentley JR, Fahey TJ, McKay DJ, Gill GH. The effect of loop electrosurgical excision procedure on

future pregnancy outcome. Obstet Gynecol 2005;105: 325–32. (Level II-2)

4. Sadler L, Saftlas A, Wang W, Exeter M, Whittaker J, McCowan L. Treatment for cervical intraepithelial neoplasia and risk of preterm delivery. JAMA 2004;291: 2100–6. (Level II-2)

5. Kyrgiou M, Koliopoulos G, Martin-Hirsch P, Arbyn M, Prendiville W, Paraskevaidis E. Obstetric outcomes after conservative treatment for intraepithelial or early invasive cervical lesions: systematic review and meta-analysis. Lancet 2006;367:489–98. (Level III)

6. Bruinsma F, Lumley J, Tan J, Quinn M. Precancerous changes in the cervix and risk of subsequent preterm birth. BJOG 2007;114:70–80. (Level II-3)

7. Jakobsson M, Gissler M, Sainio S, Paavonen J, Tapper AM. Preterm delivery after surgical treatment for cervical intraepithelial neoplasia. Obstet Gynecol 2007;109: 309–13. (Level II-2)

8. Solomon D, Davey D, Kurman R, Moriarty A, O'Connor D, Prey M, et al. The 2001 Bethesda System: terminology for reporting results of cervical cytology. Forum Group Members; Bethesda 2001 Workshop. JAMA 2002;287:2114–9. (Level III)

9. Cox JT, Schiffman M, Solomon D. Prospective follow-up suggests similar risk of subsequent cervical intraepithelial neoplasia grade 2 or 3 among women with cervical intraepithelial neoplasia grade 1 or negative colposcopy and directed biopsy. ASCUS-LSIL Triage Study (ALTS) Group. Am J Obstet Gynecol 2003;188:1406–12. (Level II-2)

10. Ostor AG. Natural history of cervical intraepithelial neoplasia: a critical review. Int J Gynecol Pathol 1993;12: 186–92. (Level III)

11. Eddy DM. Screening for cervical cancer. Ann Intern Med 1990;113:214–26. (Level III)

12. Wright TC Jr, Massad LS, Dunton CJ, Spitzer M, Wilkinson EJ, Solomon D. 2006 consensus guidelines for the management of women with abnormal cervical cancer screening tests. 2006 American Society for Colposcopy and Cervical Pathology-sponsored Consensus Conference. Am J Obstet Gynecol 2007;197:346–55. (Level III)

13. Wright TC Jr, Massad LS, Dunton CJ, Spitzer M, Wilkinson EJ, Solomon D. 2006 consensus guidelines for the management of women with cervical intraepithelial neoplasia or adenocarcinoma in situ. 2006 American Society for Colposcopy and Cervical Pathology-sponsored Consensus Conference. Am J Obstet Gynecol 2007;197:340–5. (Level III)

14. Crane JM. Pregnancy outcome after loop electrosurgical excision procedure: a systematic review. Obstet Gynecol 2003;102:1058–62. (Level III)

15. Ferris DG, Litaker MS. Prediction of cervical histologic results using an abbreviated Reid Colposcopic Index during ALTS. ALTS Group. Am J Obstet Gynecol 2006; 194:704–10. (Level II-3)

16. Massad LS, Collins YC. Strength of correlations between colposcopic impression and biopsy histology. Gynecol Oncol 2003;89:424–8. (Level II-3)

17. Jeronimo J, Schiffman M. Colposcopy at a crossroads. Am J Obstet Gynecol 2006;195:349–53. (Level III)

18. Gage JC, Hanson VW, Abbey K, Dippery S, Gardner S, Kubota J, et al. Number of cervical biopsies and sensitivity of colposcopy. ASCUS LSIL Triage Study (ALTS) Group. Obstet Gynecol 2006;108:264–72. (Level II-3)

19. Hildesheim A, Schiffman MH, Gravitt PE, Glass AG, Greer CE, Zhang T, et al. Persistence of type-specific human papillomavirus infection among cytologically normal women. J Infect Dis 1994;169:235–40. (Level II-2)

20. Herrero R, Munoz N. Human papillomavirus and cancer. Cancer Surv 1999;33:75–98. (Level III)

21. Moscicki AB, Shiboski S, Broering J, Powell K, Clayton L, Jay N, et al. The natural history of human papillomavirus infection as measured by repeated DNA testing in adolescent and young women. J Pediatr 1998;132: 277–84. (Level II-2)

22. Burk RD, Ho GY, Beardsley L, Lempa M, Peters M, Bierman R. Sexual behavior and partner characteristics are the predominant risk factors for genital human papillomavirus infection in young women. J Infect Dis 1996;174:679–89. (Level II-2)

23. Kotloff KL, Wasserman SS, Russ K, Shapiro S, Daniel R, Brown W, et al. Detection of genital human papillomavirus and associated cytological abnormalities among college women. Sex Transm Dis 1998;25:243–50. (Level II-2)

24. Bauer HM, Ting Y, Greer CE, Chambers JC, Tashiro CJ, Chimera J, et al. Genital human papillomavirus infection in female university students as determined by a PCR-based method. JAMA 1991;265:472–7. (Level II-3)

25. Kinney WK, Manos MM, Hurley LB, Ransley JE. Where's the high-grade cervical neoplasia? The importance of minimally abnormal Papanicolaou diagnoses. Obstet Gynecol 1998;91:973–6. (Level III)

26. Castle PE, Wacholder S, Sherman ME, Lorincz AT, Glass AG, Scott DR, et al. Absolute risk of a subsequent abnormal pap among oncogenic human papillomavirus DNA-positive, cytologically negative women. Cancer 2002;95: 2145–51. (Level II-2)

27. Nobbenhuis MA, Walboomers JM, Helmerhorst TJ, Rozendaal L, Remmink AJ, Risse EK, et al. Relation of human papillomavirus status to cervical lesions and consequences for cervical-cancer screening: a prospective study. Lancet 1999;354:20–5. (Level II-2)

28. Walboomers JM, Jacobs MV, Manos MM, Bosch FX, Kummer JA, Shah KV, et al. Human papillomavirus is a necessary cause of invasive cervical cancer worldwide. J Pathol 1999;189:12–9. (Level II-3)

29. Munoz N, Bosch FX, de Sanjose S, Herrero R, Castellsague X, Shah KV, et al. Epidemiologic classification of human papillomavirus types associated with cervical cancer. International Agency for Research on Cancer Multicenter Cervical Cancer Study Group. N Engl J Med 2003;348:518–27. (Level II-2)

30. Wright TC Jr, Schiffman M. Adding a test for human papillomavirus DNA to cervical-cancer screening. N Engl J Med 2003;348:489–90. (Level III)

31. Hopman EH, Rozendaal L, Voorhorst FJ, Walboomers JM, Kenemans P, Helmerhorst TJ. High risk human papillomavirus in women with normal cervical cytology prior to the development of abnormal cytology and colposcopy. BJOG 2000;107:600–4. (Level II-2)

32. Castle PE, Wacholder S, Lorincz AT, Scott DR, Sherman ME, Glass AG, et al. A prospective study of high-grade cervical neoplasia risk among human papillomavirus-infected women. J Natl Cancer Inst 2002;94:1406–14. (Level II-2)

33. Barron BA, Richart RM. A statistical model of the natural history of cervical carcinoma based on a prospective study of 557 cases. J Natl Cancer Inst 1968;41:1343–53. (Level III)

34. Koutsky LA, Holmes KK, Critchlow CW, Stevens CE, Paavonen J, Beckmann AM, et al. A cohort study of the risk of cervical intraepithelial neoplasia grade 2 or 3 in relation to papillomavirus infection. N Engl J Med 1992;327:1272–8. (Level II-2)

35. Boyes DA, Fidler HK, Lock DR. Significance of in situ carcinoma of the uterine cervix. Br Med J 1962;1:203–5. (Level III)

36. Dunn JE Jr, Martin PL. Morphogenesis of cervical cancer. Findings from San Diego County Cytology Registry. Cancer 1967;20:1899–906. (Level III)

37. Fidler HK, Boyes DA, Worth AJ. Cervical cancer detection in British Columbia. A progress report. J Obstet Gynaecol Br Commonw 1968;75:392–404. (Level II-3)

38. Solomon D, Schiffman M, Tarone R. Comparison of three management strategies for patients with atypical squamous cells of undetermined significance: baseline results from a randomized trial. ALTS Study group. J Natl Cancer Inst 2001;93:293–9. (Level I)

39. Nanda K, McCrory DC, Myers ER, Bastian LA, Hasselblad V, Hickey JD, et al. Accuracy of the Papanicolaou test in screening for and follow-up of cervical cytologic abnormalities: a systematic review. Ann Intern Med 2000;132:810–9. (Level III)

40. Fahey MT, Irwig L, Macaskill P. Meta-analysis of Pap test accuracy. Am J Epidemiol 1995;141:680–9. (Level III)

41. Kinney W, Sawaya GF, Sung HY, Kearney KA, Miller M, Hiatt RA. Stage at diagnosis and mortality in patients with adenocarcinoma and adenosquamous carcinoma of the uterine cervix diagnosed as a consequence of cytologic screening. Acta Cytol 2003;47:167–71. (Level II-3)

42. Smith AE, Sherman ME, Scott DR, Tabbara SO, Dworkin L, Olson J, et al. Review of the Bethesda System atlas does not improve reproducibility or accuracy in the classification of atypical squamous cells of undetermined significance smears. Cancer 2000;90:201–6. (Level II-3)

43. Quddus MR, Sung CJ, Steinhoff MM, Lauchlan SC, Singer DB, Hutchinson ML. Atypical squamous metaplastic cells: reproducibility, outcome, and diagnostic features on ThinPrep Pap test. Cancer 2001;93:16–22. (Level III)

44. Abulafia O, Pezzullo JC, Sherer DM. Performance of ThinPrep liquid-based cervical cytology in comparison with conventionally prepared Papanicolaou smears: a quantitative survey. Gynecol Oncol 2003;90:137–44. (Level III)

45. Stoler MH, Schiffman M. Interobserver reproducibility of cervical cytologic and histologic interpretations: realistic estimates from the ASCUS-LSIL Triage Study. Atypical Squamous Cells of Undetermined Significance-Low-grade Squamous Intraepithelial Lesion Triage Study (ALTS) Group. JAMA 2001;285:1500–5. (Level III)

46. Belinson J, Qiao YL, Pretorius R, Zhang WH, Elson P, Li L, et al. Shanxi Province Cervical Cancer Screening Study: a cross-sectional comparative trial of multiple techniques to detect cervical neoplasia [published erratum appears in Gynecol Oncol 2002;84:355]. Gynecol Oncol 2001;83:439–44. (Level II-3)

47. Belinson JL, Qiao YL, Pretorius RG, Zhang WH, Rong SD, Huang MN, et al. Shanxi Province cervical cancer screening study II: self-sampling for high-risk human papillomavirus compared to direct sampling for human papillomavirus and liquid based cervical cytology. Int J Gynecol Cancer 2003;13:819–26. (Level II-3)

48. Clavel C, Masure M, Bory JP, Putaud I, Mangeonjean C, Lorenzato M, et al. Human papillomavirus testing in primary screening for the detection of high-grade cervical lesions: a study of 7932 women. Br J Cancer 2001;84:1616–23. (Level II-3)

49. Cuzick J, Beverley E, Ho L, Terry G, Sapper H, Mielzynska I, et al. HPV testing in primary screening of older women. Br J Cancer 1999;81:554–8. (Level III)

50. Salmeron J, Lazcano-Ponce E, Lorincz A, Hernandez M, Hernandez P, Leyva A, et al. Comparison of HPV-based assays with Papanicolaou smears for cervical cancer screening in Morelos State, Mexico. Cancer Causes Control 2003;14:505–12. (Level II-3)

51. Schlecht NF, Kulaga S, Robitaille J, Ferreira S, Santos M, Miyamura RA, et al. Persistent human papillomavirus infection as a predictor of cervical intraepithelial neoplasia. JAMA 2001;286:3106–14. (Level II-2)

52. Woodman CB, Collins S, Winter H, Bailey A, Ellis J, Prior P, et al. Natural history of cervical human papillomavirus infection in young women: a longitudinal cohort study. Lancet 2001;357:1831–6. (Level II-2)

53. Cuzick J, Szarewski A, Cubie H, Hulman G, Kitchener H, Luesley D, et al. Management of women who test positive for high-risk types of human papillomavirus: the HART study. Lancet 2003;362:1871–6. (Level I)

54. Kjaer SK, van den Brule AJ, Paull G, Svare EI, Sherman ME, Thomsen BL, et al. Type specific persistence of high risk human papillomavirus (HPV) as indicator of high grade cervical squamous intraepithelial lesions in young women: population based prospective follow up study. BMJ 2002;325:572. (Level II-2)

55. Bonardi R, Cecchini S, Grazzini G, Ciatto S. Loop electrosurgical excision procedure of the transformation zone and colposcopically directed punch biopsy in the diagnosis of cervical lesions. Obstet Gynecol 1992;80:1020–2. (Level III)

56. Buxton EJ, Luesley DM, Shafi MI, Rollason M. Colposcopically directed punch biopsy: a potentially

misleading investigation. Br J Obstet Gynaecol 1991;98:1273–6. (Level III)

57. Andersen W, Frierson H, Barber S, Tabbarah S, Taylor P, Underwood P. Sensitivity and specificity of endocervical curettage and the endocervical brush for the evaluation of the endocervical canal. Am J Obstet Gynecol 1988;159:702–7. (Level II-3)

58. Hoffman MS, Sterghos S Jr, Gordy LW, Gunasekaran S, Cavanagh D. Evaluation of the cervical canal with the endocervical brush. Obstet Gynecol 1993;82:573–7. (Level II-3)

59. Klam S, Arseneau J, Mansour N, Franco E, Ferenczy A. Comparison of endocervical curettage and endocervical brushing. Obstet Gynecol 2000;96:90–4. (Level I)

60. Mogensen ST, Bak M, Dueholm M, Frost L, Knoblauch NO, Praest J, et al. Cytobrush and endocervical curettage in the diagnosis of dysplasia and malignancy of the uterine cervix. Acta Obstet Gynecol Scand 1997;76:69–73. (Level I)

61. Tate KM, Strickland JL. A randomized controlled trial to evaluate the use of the endocervical brush after endocervical curettage. Obstet Gynecol 1997;90:715–7. (Level I)

62. Naumann RW, Crispens MA, Alvarez RD, Partridge EE, Shingleton HM, Kilgore LC. Treatment of cervical dysplasia with large loop excision of the transformation zone: is endocervical curettage necessary? South Med J 1996;89:961–5. (Level III)

63. Williams DL, Dietrich C, McBroom J. Endocervical curettage when colposcopic examination is satisfactory and normal. Obstet Gynecol 2000;95:801–3. (Level III)

64. Drescher CW, Peters WA 3rd, Roberts JA. Contribution of endocervical curettage in evaluating abnormal cervical cytology. Obstet Gynecol 1983;62:343–7. (Level III)

65. Moniak CW, Kutzner S, Adam E, Harden J, Kaufman RH. Endocervical curettage in evaluating abnormal cervical cytology. J Reprod Med 2000;45:285–92. (Level III)

66. Fine BA, Feinstein GI, Sabella V. The pre- and postoperative value of endocervical curettage in the detection of cervical intraepithelial neoplasia and invasive cervical cancer. Gynecol Oncol 1998;71:46–9. (Level II-3)

67. Massad LS, Collins YC. Using history and colposcopy to select women for endocervical curettage. Results from 2,287 cases. J Reprod Med 2003;48:1–6. (Level II-3)

68. Pretorius RG, Zhang WH, Belinson JL, Huang MN, Wu LY, Zhang X, et al. Colposcopically directed biopsy, random cervical biopsy, and endocervical curettage in the diagnosis of cervical intraepthelial neoplasia II or worse. Am J Obstet Gynecol 2004;191:430–4. (Level II-3)

69. Spitzer M, Chernys AE, Shifrin A, Ryskin M. Indications for cone biopsy: pathologic correlation. Am J Obstet Gynecol 1998;178:74–9. (Level III)

70. Denehy TR, Gregori CA, Breen JL. Endocervical curettage, cone margins, and residual adenocarcinoma in situ of the cervix. Obstet Gynecol 1997;90:1–6. (Level III)

71. Wright TC Jr, Schiffman M, Solomon D, Cox JT, Garcia F, Goldie S, et al. Interim guidance for the use of human papillomavirus DNA testing as an adjunct to cervical cytology for screening. Obstet Gynecol 2004;103:304–9. (Level III)

72. Saslow D, Runowicz CD, Solomon D, Moscicki AB, Smith RA, Eyre HJ, et al. American Cancer Society guideline for the early detection of cervical neoplasia and cancer. American Cancer Society. CA Cancer J Clin 2002;52:342–62. (Level III)

73. Cuzick J, Clavel C, Petry KU, Meijer CJ, Hoyer H, Ratnam S, et al. Overview of the European and North American studies on HPV testing in primary cervical cancer screening. Int J Cancer 2006;119:1095–101. (Level III)

74. Kjaer S, Hogdall E, Frederiksen K, Munk C, van den Brule A, Svare E, et al. The absolute risk of cervical abnormalities in high-risk human papillomavirus-positive, cytologically normal women over a 10-year period. Cancer Res 2006;66:10630–6. (Level II-2)

75. Khan MJ, Castle PE, Lorincz AT, Wacholder S, Sherman M, Scott DR, et al. The elevated 10-year risk of cervical precancer and cancer in women with human papillomavirus (HPV) type 16 or 18 and the possible utility of type-specific HPV testing in clinical practice. J Natl Cancer Inst 2005;97:1072–9. (Level II-3)

76. Goldie SJ, Kim JJ, Wright TC. Cost-effectiveness of human papillomavirus DNA testing for cervical cancer screening in women aged 30 years or more. Obstet Gynecol 2004;103:619–31. (Level III)

77. Ronco G, Segnan N, Giorgi-Rossi P, Zappa M, Casadei GP, Carozzi F, et al. Human papillomavirus testing and liquid-based cytology: results at recruitment from the new technologies for cervical cancer randomized controlled trial. New Technologies for Cervical Cancer Working Group. J Natl Cancer Inst 2006;98:765–74. (Level I)

78. Bigras G, de Marval F. The probability for a Pap test to be abnormal is directly proportional to HPV viral load: results from a Swiss study comparing HPV testing and liquid-based cytology to detect cervical cancer precursors in 13,842 women. Br J Cancer 2005;93:575–81. (Level II-3)

79. Jones BA, Davey DD. Quality management in gynecologic cytology using interlaboratory comparison. Arch Pathol Lab Med 2000;124:672–81. (Level III)

80. Lonky NM, Sadeghi M, Tsadik GW, Petitti D. The clinical significance of the poor correlation of cervical dysplasia and cervical malignancy with referral cytologic results. Am J Obstet Gynecol 1999;181:560–6. (Level II-3)

81. Cox JT, Lorincz AT, Schiffman MH, Sherman ME, Cullen A, Kurman RJ. Human papillomavirus testing by hybrid capture appears to be useful in triaging women with a cytologic diagnosis of atypical squamous cells of undetermined significance. Am J Obstet Gynecol 1995;172:946–54. (Level II-3)

82. Manos MM, Kinney WK, Hurley LB, Sherman ME, Shieh-Ngai J, Kurman RJ, et al. Identifying women with cervical neoplasia: using human papillomavirus DNA testing for equivocal Papanicolaou results. JAMA 1999;281:1605–10. (Level II-3)

83. Dunn TS, Bajaj JE, Stamm CA, Beaty B. Management of the minimally abnormal Papanicolaou smear in pregnancy. J Low Genit Tract Dis 2001;5:133–7. (Level II-3)

84. Sawaya GF, Kerlikowske K, Lee NC, Gildengorin G, Washington AE. Frequency of cervical smear abnormalities within 3 years of normal cytology. Obstet Gynecol 2000;96:219–23. (Level III)

85. Boardman LA, Stanko C, Weitzen S, Sung CJ. Atypical squamous cells of undetermined significance: human papillomavirus testing in adolescents. Obstet Gynecol 2005;105:741–6. (Level II-3)

86. Sherman ME, Solomon D, Schiffman M. Qualification of ASCUS. A comparison of equivocal LSIL and equivocal HSIL cervical cytology in the ASCUS LSIL Triage Study. ASCUS LSIL Triage Study Group. Am J Clin Pathol 2001;116:386–94. (Level II-2)

87. Sherman ME, Lorincz AT, Scott DR, Wacholder S, Castle PE, Glass AG, et al. Baseline cytology, human papillomavirus testing, and risk for cervical neoplasia: a 10-year cohort analysis. J Natl Cancer Inst 2003;95:46–52. (Level II-2)

88. Eltoum IA, Chhieng DC, Roberson J, McMillon D, Partridge EE. Reflex human papilloma virus infection testing detects the same proportion of cervical intraepithelial neoplasia grade 2-3 in young versus elderly women. Cancer 2005;105:194–8. (Level II-3)

89. Bruner KS, Davey DD. ASC-US and HPV testing in women aged 40 years and over. Diagn Cytopathol 2004; 31:358–61. (Level III)

90. Moscicki AB, Schiffman M, Kjaer S, Villa LL. Chapter 5: Updating the natural history of HPV and anogenital cancer. Vaccine 2006;24(suppl 3):S42–51. (Level III)

91. Liman AK, Giampoli EJ, Bonfiglio TA. Should women with atypical squamous cells, cannot exclude high-grade squamous intraepithelial lesion, receive reflex human papillomavirus-DNA testing? Cancer 2005;105:457–60. (Level II-3)

92. Srodon M, Parry Dilworth H, Ronnett BM. Atypical squamous cells, cannot exclude high-grade squamous intraepithelial lesion: diagnostic performance, human papillomavirus testing, and follow-up results. Cancer 2006;108:32–8. (Level II-3)

93. Sherman ME, Castle PE, Solomon D. Cervical cytology of atypical squamous cells-cannot exclude high-grade squamous intraepithelial lesion (ASC-H): characteristics and histologic outcomes. Cancer 2006;108:298–305. (Level I)

94. Sherman ME, Schiffman M, Cox JT. Effects of age and human papilloma viral load on colposcopy triage: data from the randomized Atypical Squamous Cells of Undetermined Significance/Low-Grade Squamous Intraepithelial Lesion Triage Study (ALTS). Atypical Squamous Cells of Undetermined Significance/Low-Grade Squamous Intraepithelial Lesion Triage Study Group. J Natl Cancer Inst 2002;94:102–7. (Level II-3)

95. Evans MF, Adamson CS, Papillo JL, St John TL, Leiman G, Cooper K. Distribution of human papillomavirus types in ThinPrep Papanicolaou tests classified according to the Bethesda 2001 terminology and correlations with patient age and biopsy outcomes. Cancer 2006;106: 1054–64. (Level II-3)

96. Dunn TS, Burke M, Shwayder J. A "see and treat" management for high-grade squamous intraepithelial lesion pap smears. J Low Genit Tract Dis 2003;7:104–6. (Level III)

97. Guido R, Schiffman M, Solomon D, Burke L. Post-colposcopy management strategies for women referred with low-grade squamous intraepithelial lesions or human papillomavirus DNA-positive atypical squamous cells of undetermined significance: a two-year prospective study. ASCUS LSIL Triage Study (ALTS) Group. Am J Obstet Gynecol 2003;188:1401–5. (Level II-2)

98. Davey DD, Neal MH, Wilbur DC, Colgan TJ, Styer PE, Mody DR. Bethesda 2001 implementation and reporting rates: 2003 practices of participants in the College of American Pathologists Interlaboratory Comparison Program in Cervicovaginal Cytology. Arch Pathol Lab Med 2004;128:1224–9. (Level III)

99. Alvarez RD, Wright TC. Effective cervical neoplasia detection with a novel optical detection system: a randomized trial. Optical Detection Group. Gynecol Oncol 2007;104:281–9. (Level I)

100. Massad LS, Collins YC, Meyer PM. Biopsy correlates of abnormal cervical cytology classified using the Bethesda system. Gynecol Oncol 2001;82:516–22. (Level II-3)

101. Kurman RJ, Henson DE, Herbst AL, Noller KL, Schiffman MH. Interim guidelines for management of abnormal cervical cytology. The 1992 National Cancer Institute Workshop. JAMA 1994;271:1866–9. (Level III)

102. Irvin WP Jr, Andersen WA, Taylor PT Jr, Stoler MH, Rice LW. "See-and-treat" loop electrosurgical excision. Has the time come for a reassessment? J Reprod Med 2002; 47:569–74. (Level III)

103. Numnum TM, Kirby TO, Leath CA 3rd, Huh WK, Alvarez RD, Straughn JM Jr. A prospective evaluation of "see and treat" in women with HSIL Pap smear results: is this an appropriate strategy? J Low Genit Tract Dis 2005;9:2–6. (Level III)

104. Ferris DG, Hainer BL, Pfenninger JL, Zuber TJ. 'See and treat' electrosurgical loop excision of the cervical transformation zone. J Fam Pract 1996;42:253–7. (Level III)

105. Shafi MI, Luesley DM, Jordan JA, Dunn JA, Rollason TP, Yates M. Randomised trial of immediate versus deferred treatment strategies for the management of minor cervical cytological abnormalities. Br J Obstet Gynaecol 1997;104:590–4. (Level I)

106. Tidbury P, Singer A, Jenkins D. CIN 3: the role of lesion size in invasion. Br J Obstet Gynaecol 1992;99:583–6. (Level III)

107. Trimble CL, Piantadosi S, Gravitt P, Ronnett B, Pizer E, Elko A, et al. Spontaneous regression of high-grade cervical dysplasia: effects of human papillomavirus type and HLA phenotype. Clin Cancer Res 2005;11:4717–23. (Level II-2)

108. McIndoe WA, McLean MR, Jones RW, Mullins PR. The invasive potential of carcinoma in situ of the cervix. Obstet Gynecol 1984;64:451–8. (Level II-3)

109. Milne DS, Wadehra V, Mennim D, Wagstaff TI. A prospective follow up study of women with colposcopically unconfirmed positive cervical smears. Br J Obstet Gynaecol 1999;106:38–41. (Level II-2)

110. Hellberg D, Nilsson S. 20-year experience of follow-up of the abnormal smear with colposcopy and histology and treatment by conization or cryosurgery. Gynecol Oncol 1990;38:166–9. (Level III)

111. Sharpless KE, Schnatz PF, Mandavilli S, Greene JF, Sorosky JI. Dysplasia associated with atypical glandular cells on cervical cytology [published erratum appears in Obstet Gynecol 2005;105:1495]. Obstet Gynecol 2005;105:494–500. (Level II-3)

112. DeSimone CP, Day ME, Tovar MM, Dietrich CS 3rd, Eastham ML, Modesitt SC. Rate of pathology from atypical glandular cell Pap tests classified by the Bethesda 2001 nomenclature. Obstet Gynecol 2006;107:1285–91. (Level II-3)

113. Tam KF, Cheung AN, Liu KL, Ng TY, Pun TC, Chan YM, et al. A retrospective review on atypical glandular cells of undetermined significance (AGUS) using the Bethesda 2001 classification. Gynecol Oncol 2003;91: 603–7. (Level II-3)

114. Derchain SF, Rabelo-Santos SH, Sarian LO, Zeferino LC, de Oliveira Zambeli ER, do Amaral Westin MC, et al. Human papillomavirus DNA detection and histological findings in women referred for atypical glandular cells or adenocarcinoma in situ in their Pap smears. Gynecol Oncol 2004;95:618–23. (Level III)

115. Krane JF, Lee KR, Sun D, Yuan L, Crum CP. Atypical glandular cells of undetermined significance. Outcome predictions based on human papillomavirus testing. Am J Clin Pathol 2004;121:87–92. (Level III)

116. Greenspan DL, Cardillo M, Davey DD, Heller DS, Moriarty AT. Endometrial cells in cervical cytology: review of cytological features and clinical assessment. J Low Genit Tract Dis 2006;10:111–22. (Level III)

117. Simsir A, Carter W, Elgert P, Cangiarella J. Reporting endometrial cells in women 40 years and older: assessing the clinical usefulness of Bethesda 2001. Am J Clin Pathol 2005;123:571–5. (Level III)

118. Solomon D, Stoler M, Jeronimo J, Khan M, Castle P, Schiffman M. Diagnostic utility of endocervical curettage in women undergoing colposcopy for equivocal or low-grade cytologic abnormalities. Obstet Gynecol 2007; 110:288–95. (Level II-3)

119. Sevin BU, Ford JH, Girtanner RD, Hoskins WJ, Ng AB, Nordqvist SR, et al. Invasive cancer of the cervix after cryosurgery. Pitfalls of conservative management. Obstet Gynecol 1979;53:465–71. (Level III)

120. Mitchell MF, Schottenfeld D, Tortolero-Luna G, Cantor SB, Richards-Kortum R. Colposcopy for the diagnosis of squamous intraepithelial lesions: a meta-analysis. Obstet Gynecol 1998;91:626–31. (Level III)

121. Mitchell MF, Tortolero-Luna G, Cook E, Whittaker L, Rhodes-Morris H, Silva E. A randomized clinical trial of cryotherapy, laser vaporization, and loop electrosurgical excision for treatment of squamous intraepithelial lesions of the cervix. Obstet Gynecol 1998;92:737–44. (Level I)

122. Alvarez RD, Helm CW, Edwards RP, Naumann RW, Partridge EE, Shingleton HM, et al. Prospective randomized trial of LLETZ versus laser ablation in patients with cervical intraepithelial neoplasia. Gynecol Oncol 1994;52:175–9. (Level I)

123. Duggan BD, Felix JC, Muderspach LI, Gebhardt JA, Groshen S, Morrow CP, et al. Cold-knife conization versus conization by the loop electrosurgical excision procedure: a randomized, prospective study. Am J Obstet Gynecol 1999;180:276–82. (Level I)

124. Townsend DE, Richart RM, Marks E, Nielsen J. Invasive cancer following outpatient evaluation and therapy for cervical disease. Obstet Gynecol 1981;57:145–9. (Level III)

125. Wright TC Jr, Richart RM, Ferenczy A, Koulos J. Comparison of specimens removed by CO2 laser conization and the loop electrosurgical excision procedure. Obstet Gynecol 1992;79:147–53. (Level II-3)

126. Messing MJ, Otken L, King LA, Gallup DG. Large loop excision of the transformation zone (LLETZ): a pathologic evaluation. Gynecol Oncol 1994;52:207–11. (Level III)

127. Nobbenhuis MA, Helmerhorst TJ, van den Brule AJ, Rozendaal L, Voorhorst FJ, Bezemer PD, et al. Cytological regression and clearance of high-risk human papillomavirus in women with an abnormal cervical smear. Lancet 2001;358:1782–3. (Level II-2)

128. Brewer CA, Wilczynski SP, Kurosaki T, Daood R, Berman ML. Colposcopic regression patterns in high-grade cervical intraepithelial neoplasia. Obstet Gynecol 1997;90:617–21. (Level II-2)

129. Kesic V, Dokic M, Atanackovic J, Milenkovic S, Kalezic I, Vukovic S. Hysterectomy for treatment of CIN. J Low Genit Tract Dis 2003;7:32–5. (Level III)

130. Ahdieh L, Munoz A, Vlahov D, Trimble CL, Timpson LA, Shah K. Cervical neoplasia and repeated positivity of human papillomavirus infection in human immunodeficiency virus-seropositive and -seronegative women. Am J Epidemiol 2000;151:1148–57. (Level II-3)

131. Maiman M, Fruchter RG, Serur E, Levine PA, Arrastia CD, Sedlis A. Recurrent cervical intraepithelial neoplasia in human immunodeficiency virus-seropositive women. Obstet Gynecol 1993;82:170–4. (Level II-2)

132. Maiman M, Watts DH, Andersen J, Clax P, Merino M, Kendall MA. Vaginal 5-fluorouracil for high-grade cervical dysplasia in human immunodeficiency virus infection: a randomized trial. Obstet Gynecol 1999;94: 954–61. (Level I)

133. Massad LS, Collins YC. Using history and colposcopy to select women for endocervical curettage. Results from 2,287 cases. J Reprod Med 2003;48:1–6. (Level II-3)

134. Tate DR, Anderson RJ. Recrudescence of cervical dysplasia among women who are infected with the human immunodeficiency virus: a case-control analysis. Am J Obstet Gynecol 2002;186:880–2. (Level II-2)

135. Adachi A, Fleming I, Burk RD, Ho GY, Klein RS. Women with human immunodeficiency virus infection and abnormal Papanicolaou smears: a prospective study

of colposcopy and clinical outcome. Obstet Gynecol 1993;81:372–7. (Level II-3)

136. Holcomb K, Matthews RP, Chapman JE, Abulafia O, Lee YC, Borges A, et al. The efficacy of cervical conization in the treatment of cervical intraepithelial neoplasia in HIV-positive women. Gynecol Oncol 1999;74:428–31. (Level II-3)

137. Fruchter RG, Maiman M, Sedlis A, Bartley L, Camilien L, Arrastia CD. Multiple recurrences of cervical intraepithelial neoplasia in women with the human immunodeficiency virus. Obstet Gynecol 1996;87:338–44. (Level II-2)

138. Wright TC Jr, Koulos J, Schnoll F, Swanbeck J, Ellerbrock TV, Chiasson MA, et al. Cervical intraepithelial neoplasia in women infected with the human immunodeficiency virus: outcome after loop electrosurgical excision. Gynecol Oncol 1994;55:253–8. (Level II-3)

139. Boardman LA, Peipert JF, Hogan JW, Cooper AS. Positive cone biopsy specimen margins in women infected with the human immunodeficiency virus. Am J Obstet Gynecol 1999;181:1395–9. (Level II-2)

140. Massad LS, Schneider MF, Watts DH, Strickler HD, Melnick S, Palefsky J, et al. HPV testing for triage of HIV-infected women with Papanicolaou smears read as atypical squamous cells of uncertain significance. J Womens Health 2004;13:147–53. (Level II-3)

141. Kirby TO, Allen ME, Alvarez RD, Hoesley CJ, Huh WK. High-risk human papillomavirus and cervical intraepithelial neoplasia at time of atypical squamous cells of undetermined significance cytologic results in a population with human immunodeficiency virus. J Low Genit Tract Dis 2004;8:298–303 (Level II-3).

142. Massad LS, Seaberg EC, Wright RL, Darragh T, Lee YC, Colie C, et al. Squamous cervical lesions in women with human immunodeficiency virus: long-term follow-up. Obstet Gynecol 2008.111:1388–93.

143. Heard I, Palefsky JM, Kazatchkine MD. The impact of HIV antiviral therapy on human papillomavirus (HPV) infections and HPV-related diseases. Antivir Ther 2004; 9:13–22. (Level II-2)

144. Wang SS, Sherman ME, Hildesheim A, Lacey JV Jr, Devesa S. Cervical adenocarcinoma and squamous cell carcinoma incidence trends among white women and black women in the United States for 1976-2000. Cancer 2004;100:1035–44. (Level II-3)

145. Soutter WP, Haidopoulos D, Gornall RJ, McIndoe GA, Fox J, Mason WP, et al. Is conservative treatment for adenocarcinoma in situ of the cervix safe? BJOG 2001;108: 1184–9. (Level III)

146. Lea JS, Shin CH, Sheets EE, Coleman RL, Gehrig PA, Duska LR, et al. Endocervical curettage at conization to predict residual cervical adenocarcinoma in situ. Gynecol Oncol 2002;87:129–32. (Level III)

147. Hwang DM, Lickrish GM, Chapman W, Colgan TJ. Long-term surveillance is required for all women treated for cervical adenocarcinoma in situ. J Low Genit Tract Dis 2004;8:125–31. (Level II-3)

148. Shin CH, Schorge JO, Lee KR, Sheets EE. Conservative management of adenocarcinoma in situ of the cervix. Gynecol Oncol 2000;79:6–10. (Level III)

149. McHale MT, Le TD, Burger RA, Gu M, Rutgers JL, Monk BJ. Fertility sparing treatment for in situ and early invasive adenocarcinoma of the cervix. Obstet Gynecol 2001;98:726–31. (Level III)

150. Orr JW Jr, Orr PJ. Cervical cancer: staging. In: Rubin SC, Hoskins WJ, editors. Cervical cancer and preinvasive neoplasia. Philadelphia (PA): Lippincott Raven; 1996. p. 171–82. (Level III)

151. Kalliala I, Anttila A, Pukkala E, Nieminen P. Risk of cervical and other cancers after treatment of cervical intraepithelial neoplasia: retrospective cohort study. BMJ 2005;331:1183–5. (Level II-2)

152. Hellberg D, Nilsson S, Valentin J. Positive cervical smear with subsequent normal colposcopy and histology—frequency of CIN in a long-term follow-up. Gynecol Oncol 1994;53:148–51. (Level II-3)

153. Soutter WP, Butler JS, Tipples M. The role of colposcopy in the follow up of women treated for cervical intraepithelial neoplasia. BJOG 2006;113:511–4. (Level II-3)

154. Kreimer AR, Guido RS, Solomon D, Schiffman M, Wacholder S, Jeronimo J, et al. Human papillomavirus testing following loop electrosurgical excision procedure identifies women at risk for posttreatment cervical intraepithelial neoplasia grade 2 or 3 disease. Cancer Epidemiol Biomarkers Prev 2006;15:908–14. (Level II-2)

155. Lu CH, Liu FS, Kuo CJ, Chang CC, Ho ES. Prediction of persistence or recurrence after conization for cervical intraepithelial neoplasia III. Obstet Gynecol 2006; 107:830–5. (Level II-3)

156. Moore BC, Higgins RV, Laurent SL, Marroum MC, Bellitt P. Predictive factors from cold knife conization for residual cervical intraepithelial neoplasia in subsequent hysterectomy. Am J Obstet Gynecol 1995;173: 361–6; discussion 366–8. (Level II-3)

157. Kalogirou D, Antoniou G, Karakitsos P, Botsis D, Kalogirou O, Giannikos L. Predictive factors used to justify hysterectomy after loop conization: increasing age and severity of disease. Eur J Gynaecol Oncol 1997;18: 113–6. (Level II-3)

158. Phelps JY 3rd, Ward JA, Szigeti J 2nd, Bowland CH, Mayer AR. Cervical cone margins as a predictor for residual dysplasia in post-cone hysterectomy specimens. Obstet Gynecol 1994;84:128–30. (Level II-3)

159. Chang DY, Cheng WF, Torng PL, Chen RJ, Huang SC. Prediction of residual neoplasia based on histopathology and margin status of conization specimens. Gynecol Oncol 1996;63:53–6. (Level II-3)

160. Kobak WH, Roman LD, Felix JC, Muderspach LI, Schlaerth JB, Morrow CP. The role of endocervical curettage at cervical conization for high-grade dysplasia. Obstet Gynecol 1995;85:197–201. (Level II-2)

161. Reich O, Pickel H, Lahousen M, Tamussino K, Winter R. Cervical intraepithelial neoplasia III: long-term outcome after cold-knife conization with clear margins. Obstet Gynecol 2001;97:428–30. (Level III)

162. Reich O, Lahousen M, Pickel H, Tamussino K, Winter R. Cervical intraepithelial neoplasia III: long-term follow-up after cold-knife conization with involved margins. Obstet Gynecol 2002;99:193–6. (Level II-3)

163. Ghaem-Maghami S, Sagi S, Majeed G, Soutter WP. Incomplete excision of cervical intraepithelial neoplasia and risk of treatment failure: a meta-analysis. Lancet Oncol 2007;8:985–93. (Level III)

164. Cristoforoni PM, Gerbaldo DL, Philipson J, Holshneider C, Palmieri A, Bovicelli A, et al. Management of the abnormal Papanicolaou smear during pregnancy: lessons for quality improvement. J Low Genit Tract Dis 1999; 3:225–30. (Level II-3)

165. Benedet JL, Selke PA, Nickerson KG. Colposcopic evaluation of abnormal Papanicolaou smears in pregnancy. Am J Obstet Gynecol 1987;157:932–7. (Level III)

166. Paraskevaidis E, Koliopoulos G, Kalantaridou S, Pappa L, Navrozoglou I, Zikopoulos K, et al. Management and evolution of cervical intraepithelial neoplasia during pregnancy and postpartum. Eur J Obstet Gynecol Reprod Biol 2002;104:67–9. (Level III)

167. Coppleson M, Reid BL. A colposcopic study of the cervix during pregnancy and the puerperium. J Obstet Gynaecol Br Commonw 1966;73:575–85. (Level III)

168. Roberts CH, Dinh TV, Hannigan EV, Yandell RB, Schnadig VJ. Management of cervical intraepithelial neoplasia during pregnancy: a simplified and cost-effective approach. J Low Genit Tract Dis 1998;2:67–70. (Level III)

169. Boardman LA, Goldman DL, Cooper AS, Heber WW, Weitzen S. CIN in pregnancy: antepartum and postpartum cytology and histology. J Reprod Med 2005;50: 13–8. (Level II-3)

The MEDLINE database, the Cochrane Library, and ACOG's own internal resources and documents were used to conduct a literature search to locate relevant articles published between January 1995 and November 2007. The search was restricted to articles published in the English language. Priority was given to articles reporting results of original research, although review articles and commentaries also were consulted. Abstracts of research presented at symposia and scientific conferences were not considered adequate for inclusion in this document. Guidelines published by organizations or institutions such as the National Institutes of Health and the American College of Obstetricians and Gynecologists were reviewed, and additional studies were located by reviewing bibliographies of identified articles. When reliable research was not available, expert opinions from obstetrician–gynecologists were used.

Studies were reviewed and evaluated for quality according to the method outlined by the U.S. Preventive Services Task Force:

I   Evidence obtained from at least one properly designed randomized controlled trial.

II-1 Evidence obtained from well-designed controlled trials without randomization.

II-2 Evidence obtained from well-designed cohort or case–control analytic studies, preferably from more than one center or research group.

II-3 Evidence obtained from multiple time series with or without the intervention. Dramatic results in uncontrolled experiments also could be regarded as this type of evidence.

III   Opinions of respected authorities, based on clinical experience, descriptive studies, or reports of expert committees.

Based on the highest level of evidence found in the data, recommendations are provided and graded according to the following categories:

Level A—Recommendations are based on good and consistent scientific evidence.

Level B—Recommendations are based on limited or inconsistent scientific evidence.

Level C—Recommendations are based primarily on consensus and expert opinion.

ISSN 1099-3630

The American College of Obstetricians and Gynecologists
409 12th Street, SW, PO Box 96920, Washington, DC 20090-6920

Management of abnormal cervical cytology and histology. ACOG Practice Bulletin No. 99. American College of Obstetricians and Gynecologists. Obstet Gynecol 2008;112:1419–44.

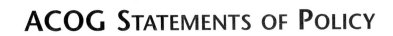

ACOG STATEMENTS OF POLICY

ACOG Statements of Policy

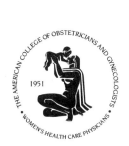

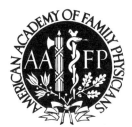

ACOG *Statement of Policy*
As issued by the ACOG Executive Board

This document was developed by a joint task force of the American Academy of Family Physicians and the American College of Obstetricians and Gynecologists.

AAFP—ACOG JOINT STATEMENT ON COOPERATIVE PRACTICE AND HOSPITAL PRIVILEGES

Access to maternity care is an important public health concern in the United States. Providing comprehensive perinatal services to a diverse population requires a cooperative relationship among a variety of health professionals, including social workers, health educators, nurses and physicians. Prenatal care, labor and delivery, and postpartum care have historically been provided by midwives, family physicians and obstetricians. All three remain the major caregivers today. A cooperative and collaborative relationship among obstetricians, family physicians and nurse midwives is essential for provision of consistent, high-quality care to pregnant women.

Regardless of specialty, there should be shared common standards of perinatal care. This requires a cooperative working environment and shared decision making. Clear guidelines for consultation and referral for complications should be developed jointly. When appropriate, early and ongoing consultation regarding a woman's care is necessary for the best possible outcome and is an important part of risk management and prevention of professional liability problems. All family physicians and obstetricians on the medical staff of the obstetric unit should agree to such guidelines and be willing to work together for the best care of patients. This includes a willingness on the part of obstetricians to provide consultation and back-up for family physicians who provide maternity care. The family physician should have knowledge, skills and judgment to determine when timely consultation and/or referral may be appropriate.

The most important objective of the physician must be the provision of the highest standards of care, regardless of specialty. Quality patient care requires that all providers should practice within their degree of ability as determined by training, experience and current competence. A joint practice committee with obstetricians and family physicians should be established in health care organizations to determine and monitor standards of care and to determine proctoring guidelines. A collegial working relationship between family physicians and obstetricians is essential if we are to provide access to quality care for pregnant women in this country.

The American College of Obstetricians and Gynecologists
409 12th Street, SW, PO Box 96920 • Washington, DC 20090-6920 Telephone 202-638-5577

A. Practice privileges

The assignment of hospital privileges is a local responsibility and privileges should be granted on the basis of training, experience and demonstrated current competence. All physicians should be held to thesame standards for granting of privileges, regardless of specialty, in order to assure the provision of high-quality patient care. Prearranged, collaborative relationships should be established to ensure ongoing consultations, as well as consultations needed for emergencies.

The standard of training should allow any physician who receives training in a cognitive or surgical skill to meet the criteria for privileges in that area of practice. Provisional privileges in primary care, obstetric care and cesarean delivery should be granted regardless of specialty as long as training criteria and experience are documented. All physicians should be subject to a proctorship period to allow demonstration of ability and current competence. These principles should apply to all health care systems.

B. Interdepartmental relationships

Privileges recommended by the department of family practice shall be the responsibility of the department of family practice. Similarly, privileges recommended by the department of obstetrics-gynecology shall be the responsibility of the department of obstetrics-gynecology. When privileges are recommended jointly by the departments of family practice and obstetrics-gynecology, they shall be the joint responsibility of the two departments.

Published July 1980
Reformatted July 1988
Revised and Retitled March 1998

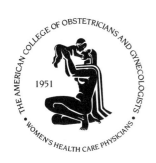

ACOG *Statement of Policy*

As issued by the ACOG Executive Board

ABORTION POLICY

The following statement is the American College of Obstetricians and Gynecologists' (ACOG) general policy related to abortion, with specific reference to the procedure referred to as "intact dilatation and extraction" (intact D & X).

1. The abortion debate in this country is marked by serious moral pluralism. Different positions in the debate represent different but important values. The diversity of beliefs should be respected.

2. ACOG recognizes that the issue of support of or opposition to abortion is a matter of profound moral conviction to its members. ACOG, therefore, respects the need and responsibility of its members to determine their individual positions based on personal values or beliefs.

3. Termination of pregnancy before viability is a medical matter between the patient and physician, subject to the physician's clinical judgment, the patient's informed consent and the availability of appropriate facilities.

4. The need for abortions, other than those indicated by serious fetal anomalies or conditions which threaten maternal welfare, represents failures in the social environment and the educational system.

The most effective way to reduce the number of abortions is to prevent unwanted and unintended pregnancies. This can be accomplished by open and honest education, beginning in the home, religious institutions and the primary schools. This education should stress the biology of reproduction and the responsibilities involved by boys, girls, men and women in creating life and the desirability of delaying pregnancies until circumstances are appropriate and pregnancies are planned.

In addition, everyone should be made aware of the dangers of sexually transmitted diseases and the means of protecting each other from their transmission. To accomplish these aims, support of the community and the school system is essential.

The medical curriculum should be expanded to include a focus on the components of reproductive biology which pertain to conception control. Physicians should be encouraged to apply these principles in their own practices and to support them at the community level.

Society also has a responsibility to support research leading to improved methods of contraception for men and women.

The American College of Obstetricians and Gynecologists
409 12th Street, SW, PO Box 96920 • Washington, DC 20090-6920 Telephone 202-638-5577

5. Informed consent is an expression of respect for the patient as a person; it particularly respects a patient's moral right to bodily integrity, to self- determination regarding sexuality and reproductive capacities, and to the support of the patient's freedom within caring relationships.

A pregnant woman should be fully informed in a balanced manner about all options, including raising the child herself, placing the child for adoption, and abortion. The information conveyed should be appropriate to the duration of the pregnancy. The professional should make every effort to avoid introducing personal bias.

6. ACOG supports access to care for all individuals, irrespective of financial status, and supports the availability of all reproductive options. ACOG opposes unnecessary regulations that limit or delay access to care.

7. If abortion is to be performed, it should be performed safely and as early as possible.

8. ACOG opposes the harassment of abortion providers and patients.

9. ACOG strongly supports those activities which prevent unintended pregnancy.

The College continues to affirm the legal right of a woman to obtain an abortion prior to fetal viability. ACOG is opposed to abortion of the healthy fetus that has attained viability in a healthy woman. Viability is the capacity of the fetus to survive outside the mother's uterus. Whether or not this capacity exists is a medical determination, may vary with each pregnancy and is a matter for the judgment of the responsible attending physician.

Intact Dilatation and Extraction

The debate regarding legislation to prohibit a method of abortion, such as the legislation banning "partial birth abortion," and "brain sucking abortions," has prompted questions regarding these procedures. It is difficult to respond to these questions because the descriptions are vague and do not delineate a specific procedure recognized in the medical literature. Moreover, the definitions could be interpreted to include elements of many recognized abortion and operative obstetric techniques.

ACOG believes the intent of such legislative proposals is to prohibit a procedure referred to as "intact dilatation and extraction" (Intact D & X). This procedure has been described as containing all of the following four elements:

1. deliberate dilatation of the cervix, usually over a sequence of days; 2. instrumental conversion of the fetus to a footling breech;
3. breech extraction of the body excepting the head; and
4. partial evacuation of the intracranial contents of a living fetus to effect vaginal delivery of a dead but otherwise intact fetus.

Because these elements are part of established obstetric techniques, it must be emphasized that unless all four elements are present in sequence, the procedure is not an intact D & X. Abortion intends to terminate a pregnancy while preserving the life and health of the mother. When abortion is performed after 16 weeks, intact D & X is one method of terminating a pregnancy.

The physician, in consultation with the patient, must choose the most appropriate method based upon the patient's individual circumstances.

According to the Centers for Disease Control and Prevention (CDC), only 5.3% of abortions performed in the United States in 1993, the most recent data available, were performed after the 16th week of pregnancy. A preliminary figure published by the CDC for 1994 is 5.6%. The CDC does not collect data on the specific method of abortion, so it is unknown how many of these were performed using intact D & X. Other data show that second trimester transvaginal instrumental abortion is a safe procedure.

Terminating a pregnancy is performed in some circumstances to save the life or preserve the health of the mother.

Intact D & X is one of the methods available in some of these situations. A select panel convened by ACOG could identify no circumstances under which this procedure, as defined above, would be the only option to save the life or preserve the health of the woman. An intact D & X, however, may be the best or most appropriate procedure in a particular circumstance to save the life or preserve the health of a woman, and only the doctor, in consultation with the patient, based upon the woman's particular circumstances can make this decision. The potential exists that legislation prohibiting specific medical practices, such as intact D & X, may outlaw techniques that are critical to the lives and health of American women. **The intervention of legislative bodies into medical decision making is inappropriate, ill advised, and dangerous.**

Approval by the Executive Board
General policy: January 1993
Reaffirmed and revised: July 1997
Intact D & X statement: January 1997
Combined and reaffirmed: September 2000
Reaffirmed: July 2004
Reaffirmed: July 2007

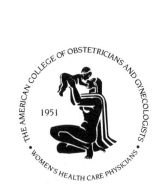

ACOG *Statement of Policy*

As issued by the ACOG Executive Board

ACCESS TO WOMEN'S HEALTH CARE

Excellence in women's health care is an essential element of the long-term physical, intellectual, social and economic well-being of any society. It is a basic determinant of the health of future generations.

The American College of Obstetricians and Gynecologists is the representative organization of physicians who are qualified specialists in providing health services unique to women. ACOG calls for quality health care appropriate to every woman's needs throughout her life and for assuring that a full array of clinical services be available to women without costly delays or the imposition of geographic, financial, attitudinal or legal barriers.

The College and its membership are committed to facilitating both access to and quality of women's health care. Fellows should exercise their responsibility to improve the health status of women and their offspring both in the traditional patient-physician relationships and by working within their community and at the state and national levels to assure access to high-quality programs meeting the health needs of all women. Fellows must not discriminate against patients based on race, color, national origin, religion, sexual orientation, or any other basis that would constitute illegal discrimination.

In addition, it is critical that all Americans be provided with adequate and affordable health coverage. There remains a considerable and increasing portion of the American population that does not have health insurance coverage. As a result, those individuals often defer obtaining preventive and medical services, jeopardizing the health and well being of themselves and their families. The College supports universal coverage that is designed to improve the individual and collective health of society. Expanding health coverage to all Americans must become a high priority.

Approved by the Executive Board July 1988
Amended September 1999
Amended and Reaffirmed July 2003
Amended and Reaffirmed July 2006

The American College of Obstetricians and Gynecologists
409 12th Street, SW, PO Box 96920 • Washington, DC 20090-6920 Telephone 202-638-5577

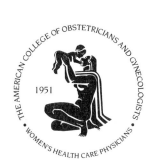

ACOG *Statement of Policy*
As issued by the ACOG Executive Board

CERTIFICATION AND PROCEDURAL CREDENTIALING

Resident training in obstetrics and gynecology incorporates the full spectrum of obstetric and gynecologic practice as defined in the special requirements promulgated by the Accreditation Council for Graduate Medical Education. These include diagnostic, therapeutic and operative procedures used in the practice of the specialty. The certification process of the American Board of Obstetrics and Gynecology Inc. (ABOG) evaluates medical knowledge and patient care skills of individual practitioners in the broad range of obstetrics, gynecology and women's health care. The Maintenance of Certification process, developed by ABOG, measures acquisition of new scientific knowledge and new practice guidelines as well as continuing proficiency in the range of practice in which the individual is currently engaged.

Subspecialty training in maternal-fetal medicine, reproductive endocrinology and infertility, gynecologic oncology, and female pelvic medicine and reconstructive surgery is also available through fellowship programs accredited by ABOG. Certification and maintenance of certification of special competence in maternal-fetal medicine, reproductive endocrinology and infertility, and gynecologic oncology are also available through ABOG. Through advanced training and certification of special competence, these subspecialists have demonstrated knowledge and skills in addition to those of general obstetrician-gynecologists.

ABOG certification (or active candidate for certification status) is an important factor considered by local institutions and organizations when credentialing obstetrician-gynecologists to provide in-patient care, and to perform in-patient or ambulatory procedures.

ACOG recognizes that ongoing education, training and experience are necessary to maintain competence and to assure development of competence in newly introduced procedures or technologies. To accomplish this, physicians should participate in continuing medical education programs, the ABOG Maintenance of Certification process as appropriate, and be familiar with current information and guidelines on patient care. In addition, physicians should review their individual patient outcome data, and participate in quality assurance programs that are relevant to the care they provide and to the procedures they perform. Obstetrician-gynecologists who desire to expand their procedural skills should participate in appropriate educational and training programs. Physicians will need to follow their institutional credentialing guidelines and requirements when applying for privileges to perform these procedures.

The American College of Obstetricians and Gynecologists
409 12th Street, SW, PO Box 96920 • Washington, DC 20090-6920 Telephone 202-638-5577

In conclusion, the American College of Obstetricians and Gynecologists reaffirms that current certification by ABOG and maintenance of certification of obstetrician-gynecologists is validation of the medical, surgical, imaging and laboratory knowledge and patient care skills relevant to the practice of the specialty. No additional certification should be required for credentialing for those procedures and care which fall within the scope of an individual's current ABOG certification.

Approved by the Executive Board February 2008

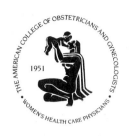

ACOG *Statement of Policy*
As issued by the ACOG Executive Board

A joint policy statement from the American College of Obstetricians and Gynecologists, the Society of Obstetricians and Gynaecologists of Canada, the Central American Federation of Associations and Societies of Obstetrics and Gynecology, the Gynaecologic Oncologists of Canada, the Society of Canadian Colposcopists, the Society of Gynecologic Oncologists, and the Royal College of Obstetricians and Gynaecologists.

CERVICAL CANCER PREVENTION IN LOW-RESOURCE SETTINGS

Cervical cancer is the third most common cancer in the world and the leading cause of cancer death among women in developing countries (1). Worldwide, an estimated 470,000 new cases occur and 233,000 women die annually from cervical cancer (2, 3). Eighty percent of these deaths occur where resources are the most limited (4).

Where organized comprehensive detection, treatment, and referral programs have been implemented, the incidence and mortality of this cancer have decreased dramatically (5). However, implementing programs characteristic of industrialized countries—including testing, treatment, quality assurance, follow-up, and information system components on a widespread basis—requires considerable resources and a high level of program coordination. These programs are impractical and unaffordable in low-resource settings. Yet, women deserve access to services that can safely, effectively, and affordably prevent cervical cancer.

Given the recognized obstacles to implementing cytology-based screening and the limited range of treatment methods available in low-resource settings, other program options are needed. Such options must be feasible and sustainable, and the optimal strategy for a particular setting will necessarily vary given local resource constraints; disease prevalence; and capacity for training, supervision, and infrastructure.

One evidence-based approach designed to prevent cervical cancer in low-resource settings is the "single-visit approach." This approach links a detection method with an immediate management option, such as an offer of treatment or referral, provided by appropriately trained and supervised personnel. There is growing evidence that a single-visit approach, incorporating visual inspection of the cervix with acetic acid wash (VIA), followed by an immediate offer of treatment with cryotherapy for eligible lesions, is a safe, acceptable, and cost-effective approach to cervical cancer prevention (6–9).

The American College of Obstetricians and Gynecologists, the Society of Obstetricians and Gynaecologists of Canada, the Central American Federation of Associations and Societies of Obstetrics and Gynecology, the Gynaecologic Oncologists of Canada, the Society of Canadian

The American College of Obstetricians and Gynecologists
409 12th Street, SW, PO Box 96920 • Washington, DC 20090-6920 Telephone 202 638 5577

Colposcopists, the Society of Gynecologic Oncologists, and the Royal College of Obstetricians and Gynaecologists recognize the value of VIA linked to immediate cryotherapy (or referral). It is a viable option for reducing over time the incidence of cervical cancer in settings where services are limited and where other approaches are considered impractical or too expensive.

The obstetric–gynecologic organizations supporting this statement have an important role to play in increasing the capacity of obstetric–gynecologic associations worldwide to include feasible and sustainable cervical cancer prevention programs as part of their national women's health strategies. In turn, national societies of obstetrics and gynecology have an important responsibility to educate both policy makers and the public about the importance of programs aimed at preventing cervical cancer in their countries.

Recognizing both the worldwide burden of this disease and the increasingly important role that women play in socioeconomic development, funding agencies should be aware of the public health importance of cervical cancer. They should be prepared to help underwrite cost-effective, resource-appropriate interventions to prevent unnecessary deaths caused by this disease.

References

1. World Health Organization. State of the art new vaccines: research and development. Initiative for Vaccine Research. Geneva: WHO; 2003. Available at: http://www.who.int/vaccine_research/documents/en/stateofart_excler.pdf. Retrieved November 21, 2003.
2. Program for Appropriate Technology in Health. Cervical cancer prevention. Reproductive Health Outlook. Seattle (WA): PATH; 2003. Available at: http://www.rho.org/assets/RHO_cxca_10-9-03.pdf. Retrieved November 21, 2003.
3. International Agency for Research on Cancer. GLOBOCAN 2000 database: cancer incidence, mortality, and prevalence worldwide. Lyons (FR): IARC; 2001.
4. Parkin DM, Pisani P, Ferlay J. Estimates of the worldwide incidence of eighteen major cancers in 1985. Int J Cancer 1993;54:594–606.
5. Sankaranarayanan R, Budukh AM, Rajkumar R. Effective screening programmes for cervical cancer in low- and middle-income developing countries. Bull World Health Organ 2001;79:954–62.
6. Gaffikin L, Blumenthal PD, Emerson M, Limpaphayom K; Royal Thai College of Obstetricians and Gynaecologists (RTCOG)/JHPIEGO Corporation Cervical Cancer Prevention Group [corrected]. Safety, acceptability, and feasibility of a single visit approach to cervical cancer prevention in rural Thailand: a demonstration project. Lancet 2003;361:814-20.
7. Mandelblatt J, Lawrence W, Gaffikin L, Limpaphayom KK, Lumbiganon P, Warakamin S, et al. Costs and benefits of different strategies to screen for cervical cancer in less-developed countries. J Natl Cancer Inst 2002;94:1469–83.
8. Goldie SJ, Kuhn L, Denny L, Pollack A, Wright TC. Policy analysis of cervical cancer screening strategies in low-resource settings: clinical benefits and cost effectiveness [published erratum appears in JAMA 2001;286:1026]. JAMA 2001;285:3107–15.
9. Martin-Hirsch PL, Paraskevaidis E, Kitchener H. Surgery for cervical intraepithelial neoplasia (Cochrane Review). In: The Cochrane Library, Issue 4, 2003. Chichester, UK: John Wiley & Sons, Ltd.

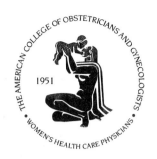

ACOG *Statement of Policy*

As issued by the ACOG Executive Board

HOME BIRTHS IN THE UNITED STATES

Labor and delivery is a physiologic process that most women experience without complications. Ongoing surveillance of the mother and fetus is essential because serious intrapartum complications may arise with little or no warning, even in low-risk pregnancies. In some of these instances, the availability of expertise and interventions on an urgent or emergent basis may be life-saving for the mother, the fetus or the newborn and may reduce the likelihood of an adverse outcome. For these reasons, the American College of Obstetricians and Gynecologists (ACOG) believes that the hospital, including a birthing center within a hospital complex, that meets the standards outlined by the American Academy of Pediatrics and ACOG,[1] or freestanding birthing centers that meet the standards of the Accreditation Association for Ambulatory Health Care or The Joint Commission or the American Association of Birth Centers,[2] is the safest setting for labor, delivery, and the immediate postpartum period. ACOG also strongly supports providing conditions that will improve the birthing experience for women and their families without compromising safety.

Studies comparing the safety and outcome of U.S. births in the hospital with those occurring in other settings are limited and have not been scientifically rigorous. The development of well-designed research studies of sufficient size, prepared in consultation with obstetric departments and approved by institutional review boards, might clarify the comparative safety of births in different settings. Until the results of such studies are convincing, ACOG strongly opposes home births. Although ACOG acknowledges a woman's right to make informed decisions regarding her delivery, ACOG does not support programs or individuals that advocate for or who provide home births.

[1] American Academy of Pediatrics and American College of Obstetricians and Gynecologists. Guidelines for Perinatal Care, 5th Edition. Elk Grove Village, IL, AAP/ACOG, 2002.

[2] American Association of Birth Centers, Standards for Birth Centers, Perkiomenville (PA), AABC, 2003.

Approved by the Executive Board May 4, 2007

The American College of Obstetricians and Gynecologists

409 12th Street, SW, PO Box 96920 • Washington, DC 20090-6920 Telephone 202-638-5577

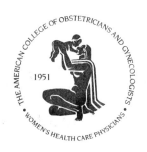

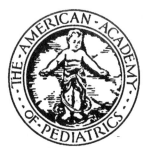

ACOG *Statement of Policy*

As issued by the ACOG Executive Board

This document was developed jointly by the
American Academy of Pediatrics and the
American College of Obstetricians and Gynecologists.

JOINT STATEMENT OF ACOG/AAP
ON HUMAN IMMUNODEFICIENCY VIRUS SCREENING

The problem of perinatal transmission of HIV infection was first appreciated in 1982. In 1991, the Institute of Medicine (IOM) recommended a policy of routine counseling and offering testing (with specific informed consent) for HIV infection to all pregnant women. Since 1991, there have been major advances in the treatment of HIV infection, including demonstration in 1994 of the efficacy of zidovudine to reduce perinatal transmission. The U.S. Public Health Service subsequently issued guidelines for use of zidovudine to reduce perinatal transmission and for counseling and voluntary testing for pregnant women. Dramatic declines in reported pediatric AIDS cases have been observed as a consequence of implementation of these guidelines. However, for a variety of reasons, screening pregnant women in the United States has been far from universal and infected babies continue to be born to undiagnosed infected women. Further reduction in the rate of perinatal HIV infection will require wider application of both screening to identify infected women, and treatments, which have demonstrated efficacy in reducing vertical transmission.

The IOM recently completed a study of interventions that would be helpful to further reduce the rate of perinatal HIV infection in the United States (Reducing the Odds). They have recommended that "the United States should adopt a national policy of universal HIV testing, with patient notification, as a routine component of prenatal care". Early diagnosis of HIV infection in pregnant women allows them to institute effective antiretroviral therapy for their own health and to reduce the risk of HIV transmission to their infants. The use of "patient notification" provides women the opportunity to decline to be tested but eliminates the obligation to provide extensive pretest counseling, which has been a barrier to testing in many settings. Care providers would be charged with responsibility for the details of how the notification would take place. The IOM has recommended universal testing for two reasons. First, attempts to identi-

The American College of Obstetricians and Gynecologists
409 12th Street, SW, PO Box 96920 • Washington, DC 20090-6920 Telephone 202-638-5577

fy those "at risk" for infection inevitably fail to identify some infected individuals. Second, universal testing of all pregnant women avoids stereotyping and stigmatizing any social or ethnic group. The IOM recognizes in its report that many states now have laws requiring a formal, and in many cases written informed consent process prior to testing. They recommend that the Federal government adopt policies that will encourage these states to change their laws.

The AAP and the ACOG strongly support efforts to further reduce the rate of perinatal transmission of HIV in the United States. We therefore support the recommendation of the IOM for universal HIV testing with patient notification as a routine component of prenatal care. If a patient declines testing, this should be noted in the medical record. We recognize that current laws in some states may prevent implementation of this recommendation at this time. We encourage our members and Fellows to include counseling as a routine part of care, but not as a prerequisite for, and barrier to, prenatal HIV testing.

Approved by the ACOG Executive Board, May 1999
Approved by the AAP Executive Board, May 1999
Reaffirmed by the AAP Executive Board, September 2005
Reaffirmed by the ACOG Executive Board, July 2006

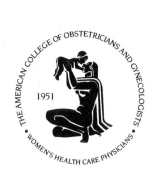

ACOG *Statement of Policy*

As issued by the ACOG Executive Board

JOINT STATEMENT OF PRACTICE RELATIONSHIPS BETWEEN OBSTETRICIAN-GYNECOLOGISTS AND CERTIFIED NURSE-MIDWIVES/CERTIFIED MIDWIVES*

The American College of Obstetricians and Gynecologists (ACOG) and the American College of Nurse-Midwives (ACNM) recognize that in those circumstances in which obstetrician-gynecologists and certified nurse-midwives/certified midwives collaborate in the care of women, the quality of those practices is enhanced by a working relationship characterized by mutual respect and trust as well as professional responsibility and accountability. When obstetrician-gynecologists and certified nurse-midwives/certified midwives collaborate, they should concur on a clear mechanism for consultation, collaboration and referral based on the individual needs of each patient.

Recognizing the high level of responsibility that obstetrician-gynecologists and certified nurse-midwives/certified midwives assume when providing care to women, ACOG and ACNM affirm their commitment to promote appropriate standards for education and certification of their respective members, to support appropriate practice guidelines, and to facilitate communication and collegial relationships between obstetrician-gynecologists and certified nurse-midwives/certified midwives.

*Certified nurse-midwives are registered nurses who have graduated from a midwifery education program accredited by the ACNM Division of Accreditation and have passed a national certification examination administered by the ACNM Certification Council, Inc. Certified midwives are graduates of a Division of Accreditation accredited, university-affiliated midwifery education program, have successfully completed the same science requirements and ACNM Certification Council, Inc., national certification examination as certified nurse-midwives and adhere to the same professional standards as certified nurse-midwives.

American College of Nurse-Midwives
American College of Obstetricians and Gynecologists
October 1, 2002

.

The American College of Obstetricians and Gynecologists
409 12th Street, SW, PO Box 96920 • Washington, DC 20090-6920 Telephone 202 638 5577

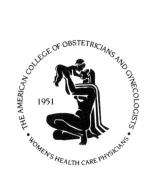

ACOG *Statement of Policy*
As issued by the ACOG Executive Board

MIDWIFERY EDUCATION AND CERTIFICATION

The American College of Obstetricians and Gynecologists (ACOG) is the representative organization of physicians who are qualified specialists in providing health services to women. ACOG is committed to facilitating access to women's health care that is both safe and high quality. One method of attaining this goal is to assure that providers of care meet educational and professional standards of a certification process. ACOG recognizes the educational and professional standards currently used by the American Midwifery Certification Board (AMCB)* to evaluate and certify midwives. While ACOG supports women having a choice in determining their providers of care, ACOG does not support the provision of care by lay midwives or other midwives who are not certified by the American College of Nurse-Midwives (ACNM) or AMCB.

*The American Midwifery Certification Board (AMCB), formerly known as the ACNM Certification Council (ACC), was incorporated in 1991. The AMCB develops and administers the national certification examination for Certified Nurse-Midwives (CNMs) and Certified Midwives (CMs). CNMs are registered nurses who have graduated from a midwifery education program accredited by the American College of Nurse-Midwives Division of Accreditation and have passed a national certification examination administered by AMCB. Certified midwives also have graduated from a midwifery education program accredited by the American College of Nurse-Midwives Division of Accreditation, have successfully completed the same requirements, have passed the same AMCB national certification examination as certified nurse-midwives and adhere to the same professional standards as certified nurse-midwives.

Approved by the Executive Board February 2006
Amended February 2007

The American College of Obstetricians and Gynecologists
409 12th Street, SW, PO Box 96920 • Washington, DC 20090-6920 Telephone 202 638 5577

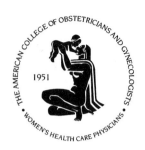

ACOG *Statement of Policy*
As issued by the ACOG Executive Board

THE ROLE OF THE OBSTETRICIAN-GYNECOLOGIST IN COSMETIC PROCEDURES

As cosmetic procedures receive increased attention from the media and patient requests for such procedures grow, there is a corresponding need to determine the proper role of obstetrician–gynecologists in this evolving field. A growing number of women are seeking service locations that provide "one-stop shopping" for both medical and aesthetic services. Some obstetrician–gynecologists have offered cosmetic services as an extension of providing gynecologic care, such as providing hair removal and acne treatment to patients with polycystic ovary syndrome.

The scope of obstetric–gynecologic practice includes more than reproductive health care. The specialty's broad focus on women's health may include cosmetic services and procedures, just as this broad focus includes a wide variety of primary and preventive care. The obstetrician–gynecologist may provide services that fill a need not adequately met in commercial sites, provide safer or more efficacious treatments than those available in nonmedical settings, or provide services as a convenience to patients. **Obstetrician–gynecologists who offer procedures typically provided by other specialists should possess an equivalent level of competence.**

For the physician offering cosmetic services, the health, well-being, and safety of the patient must be paramount, and the obstetrician–gynecologist must be knowledgeable of the ethics of patient counseling and informed consent. Inquiries regarding cosmetic products, services, and procedures must come from the patient, and the patient should feel no pressure or obligation to purchase or undergo any cosmetic services. As many patients look to their physicians, often particularly their obstetrician–gynecologists, to define "normal" anatomy, behavior, or function, any unsolicited comments or innuendo could create a perceived need for alteration when none was considered previously. It is the responsibility of the obstetrician–gynecologist to engage patients considering cosmetic services in dialogue that supports the individual's efforts to analyze and respond to societal or marketing pressures toward an often unattainable aesthetic ideal.

Special care must be taken when patients are considering procedures in an effort to enhance sexual appearance or function, as female sexual response has been shown to be an intricate process determined predominantly by brain function and psychosocial factors, not by genital appearance. Such procedures are not medically indicated, and their safety and effectiveness have not been documented.[1] Greater data acquisition and dissemination are needed regarding the safety and outcomes of cosmetic procedures. These will further improve efforts to obtain informed consent and strengthen decision-making.

A synopsis of the report authored by ACOG's Presidential Task Force on the Role of the Obstetrician–Gynecologist in Cosmetic Procedures is available upon request from the ACOG Resource Center.

[1]Vaginal "Rejuvenation" and Cosmetic Vaginal Procedures. ACOG Committee Opinion No. 378. American College of Obstetricians and Gynecologists. Obstet Gynecol 2007;110:737-8.

Approved by the Executive Board November 2008

The American College of Obstetricians and Gynecologists
409 12th Street, SW, PO Box 96920 • Washington, DC 20090-6920 Telephone 202-638-5577

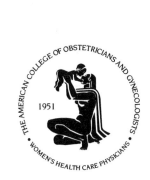

ACOG *Statement of Policy*
As issued by the ACOG Executive Board

TOBACCO ADVERTISING AIMED AT WOMEN AND ADOLESCENTS

The American College of Obstetricians and Gynecologists opposes the unconscionable targeting of women of all ages by the tobacco industry.

The health risks of tobacco use to women are well documented. It also is well known that smoking by a pregnant woman may be harmful to her fetus. It is unnecessary to catalogue all of these risks here. Because of these well-known dangers, it is irresponsible for tobacco companies to single out women, especially those who are young, educationally or otherwise disadvantaged women, and encourage them to smoke.

Specifically, tobacco companies must stop targeting their advertising to encourage adolescent women to smoke cigarettes. The health of all women and future generations demands that consideration.

Approved by the Executive Board July 1990
Reaffirmed July 2000
Revised and approved July 2004
Reaffirmed July 2007

The American College of Obstetricians and Gynecologists
409 12th Street, SW, PO Box 96920 • Washington, DC 20090-6920 Telephone 202-638-5577

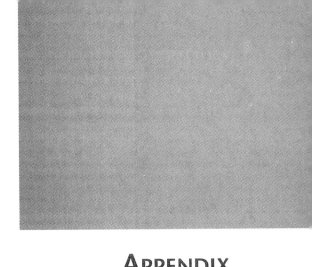

APPENDIX

APPENDIX

CONTENTS FROM OTHER ACOG RESOURCES*

ETHICS IN OBSTETRICS AND GYNECOLOGY, SECOND EDITION

*Page numbers refer to those in the original publication. ACOG members can view full text at www.acog.org.

GUIDELINES FOR PERINATAL CARE, SIXTH EDITION

GUIDELINES FOR WOMEN'S HEALTH CARE, THIRD EDITION

HEALTH CARE FOR ADOLESCENTS

SPECIAL ISSUES IN WOMEN'S HEALTH

ACOG COMMITTEE OPINIONS

LIST OF TITLES — DECEMBER 2008

Committee Opinions are intended to provide timely information on controversial issues, ethical concerns, and emerging approaches to clinical management. They represent the considered views of the sponsoring committee based on interpretation of published data in peer-reviewed journals. Committee Opinions are reviewed periodically for continued relevance or needed update. Also listed are Technology Assessments, which provide an overview of technology in obstetrics and gynecology.

The following titles have been withdrawn from circulation:

Committee Opinions

189 Advanced Paternal Age: Risks to the Fetus

291 Use of Progesterone to Reduce Preterm Birth *(Replaced by Committee Opinion No. 419)*

293 Uterine Artery Embolization *(Replaced by Practice Bulletin No. 96)*

294 At-Risk Drinking and Illicit Drug Use: Ethical Issues in Obstetric and Gynecologic Practice *(Replaced by Committee Opinion No. 422)*

304 Prenatal and Perinatal Human Immunodeficiency Virus Testing: Expanded Recommendations *(Replaced by Committee Opinion No. 418)*

308 The Uninsured *(Replaced by Committee Opinion No. 416)*

356 Routine Cancer Screening

Technology Assessment

3 Saline Infusion Sonohysterography *(Replaced by Technology Assessment No. 5)*

Number	Title	Publication Date	Reaffirmed Date
Committee on Adolescent Health Care			
300	Cervical Cancer Screening in Adolescents (Obstet Gynecol 2004;104:885–9)	October 2004	
301	Sexually Transmitted Diseases in Adolescents (Obstet Gynecol 2004;104:891–8)	October 2004	
302	Guidelines for Adolescent Health Research (Obstet Gynecol 2004;104:899–902)	October 2004	
310	Endometriosis in Adolescents (Obstet Gynecol 2005;105:921–7)	April 2005	
314	Meningococcal Vaccination for Adolescents (Obstet Gynecol 2005;106:667–9)	September 2005	
330	Evaluation and Management of Abnormal Cervical Cytology and Histology in the Adolescent (Obstet Gynecol 2006;107:963–8)	April 2006	
335	The Initial Reproductive Health Visit (Obstet Gynecol 2006;107:1215–9)	May 2006	
344	Human Papillomavirus Vaccination *(Joint with the ACOG Working Group on Immunization)* (Obstet Gynecol 2006;108:699–705)	September 2006	
349	Menstruation in Girls and Adolescents: Using the Menstrual Cycle as a Vital Sign *(Joint with American Academy of Pediatrics)* (Obstet Gynecol 2006;108:1323–8)	November 2006	
350	Breast Concerns in the Adolescent (Obstet Gynecol 2006;108:1329–36)	November 2006	
351	The Overweight Adolescent: Prevention, Treatment, and Obstetric–Gynecologic Implications (Obstet Gynecol 2006;108:1337–48)	November 2006	
355	Vaginal Agenesis: Diagnosis, Management, and Routine Care (Obstet Gynecol 2006;108:1605–9)	December 2006	
392	Intrauterine Device and Adolescents (Obstet Gynecol 2007;110:1493–5)	December 2007	
*415	Depot Medroxyprogesterone Acetate and Bone Effects *(Joint with Committee on Gynecologic Practice)* (Obstet Gynecol 2008;112:727–30)	September 2008	
*417	Addressing Health Risks of Noncoital Sexual Activity *(Joint with Committee on Gynecologic Practice)* (Obstet Gynecol 2008;112:735–7)	September 2008	
Committee on Coding and Nomenclature			
205	Tubal Ligation with Cesarean Delivery (Obstet Gynecol Vol. 92, No. 2)	August 1998	
249	Coding Responsibility (Obstet Gynecol Vol. 97, No. 1)	January 2001	2005

Number	Title	Publication Date	Reaffirmed Date
Committee on Coding and Nomenclature (continued)			
250	Inappropriate Reimbursement Practices by Third-Party Payers (Obstet Gynecol Vol. 97, No. 1)	January 2001	
Committee on Ethics† (see also *Ethics in Obstetrics and Gynecology,* **Second Edition**)			
297	Nonmedical Use of Obstetric Ultrasonography (Obstet Gynecol 2004;104:423–4)	August 2004	
321	Maternal Decision Making, Ethics, and the Law (Obstet Gynecol 2005;106:1127–37)	November 2005	
341	Ethical Ways for Physicians to Market a Practice (Obstet Gynecol 2006;108:239–42)	July 2006	2008
347	Using Preimplantation Embryos for Research (Obstet Gynecol 2006;108:1305–17)	November 2006	2008
352	Innovative Practice: Ethical Guidelines (Obstet Gynecol 2006;108:1589–95)	December 2006	
358	Professional Responsibilities in Obstetric–Gynecologic Education (Obstet Gynecol 2007;109:239–42)	January 2007	
359	Commercial Enterprises in Medical Practice (Obstet Gynecol 2007;109:243–5)	January 2007	2008
360	Sex Selection (Obstet Gynecol 2007;109:475–8)	February 2007	2008
362	Medical Futility (Obstet Gynecol 2007;109:791–4)	March 2007	2008
363	Patient Testing: Ethical Issues in Selection and Counseling (Obstet Gynecol 2007;109:1021–3)	April 2007	
364	Patents, Medicine, and the Interests of Patients *(Joint with Committee on Genetics)* (Obstet Gynecol 2007;109:1249–53)	May 2007	
365	Seeking and Giving Consultation (Obstet Gynecol 2007;109:1255–9)	May 2007	
368	Adoption (Obstet Gynecol 2007;109:1507–10)	June 2007	
369	Multifetal Pregnancy Reduction (Obstet Gynecol 2007;109:1511–5)	June 2007	
370	Institutional Responsibility to Provide Legal Representation (Obstet Gynecol 2007;110:215–6)	July 2007	
371	Sterilization of Women, Including Those With Mental Disabilities (Obstet Gynecol 2007;110:217–20)	July 2007	
373	Sexual Misconduct (Obstet Gynecol 2007;110:441–4)	August 2007	
374	Expert Testimony (Obstet Gynecol 2007;110:445–6)	August 2007	
377	Research Involving Women (Obstet Gynecol 2007;110:731–6)	September 2007	
385	The Limits of Conscientious Refusal in Reproductive Medicine (Obstet Gynecol 2007;110:1203–8)	November 2007	
389	Human Immunodeficiency Virus (Obstet Gynecol 2007;110:1473–8)	December 2007	
390	Ethical Decision Making in Obstetrics and Gynecology (Obstet Gynecol 2007;110:1479–87)	December 2007	
395	Surgery and Patient Choice (Obstet Gynecol 2008;111:243–7)	January 2008	
397	Surrogate Motherhood (Obstet Gynecol 2008;111:465–70)	February 2008	
401	Relationships With Industry (Obstet Gynecol 2008;111:799–804)	March 2008	
403	End-of-Life Decision Making (Obstet Gynecol 2008;111:1021–7)	April 2008	
409	Direct-to-Consumer Marketing of Genetic Testing *(Joint with Committee on Genetics)* (Obstet Gynecol 2008;111:1493–4)	June 2008	
410	Ethical Issues in Genetic Testing *(Joint with Committee on Genetics)* (Obstet Gynecol 2008;111:1495–502)	June 2008	
*422	At-Risk Drinking and Illicit Drug Use: Ethical Issues in Obstetric and Gynecologic Practice (Obstet Gynecol 2008;112:1449–60)	December 2008	
Committee on Genetics			
230	Maternal Phenylketonuria (Obstet Gynecol Vol. 95, No. 1)	January 2000	2004
298	Prenatal and Preconceptional Carrier Screening for Genetic Diseases in Individuals of Eastern European Jewish Descent (Obstet Gynecol 2004;104:425–8)	August 2004	2008
318	Screening for Tay–Sachs Disease (Obstet Gynecol 2005;106:893–4)	October 2005	2007
324	Perinatal Risks Associated With Assisted Reproductive Technology *(Joint with Committees on Obstetric Practice and Gynecologic Practice)* (Obstet Gynecol 2005;106:1143–6)	November 2005	2008
325	Update on Carrier Screening for Cystic Fibrosis (Obstet Gynecol 2005;106:1465–8)	December 2005	2007
338	Screening for Fragile X Syndrome (Obstet Gynecol 2006;107:1483–5)	June 2006	
364	Patents, Medicine, and the Interests of Patients *(Joint with Committee on Ethics)* (Obstet Gynecol 2007;109:1249–53)	May 2007	
383	Evaluation of Stillbirths and Neonatal Deaths (Obstet Gynecol 2007;110:963–6)	October 2007	
393	Newborn Screening (Obstet Gynecol 2007;110:1497–500)	December 2007	
399	Umbilical Cord Blood Banking *(Joint with Committee on Obstetric Practice)* (Obstet Gynecol 2008;111:475–7)	February 2008	

Number	Title	Publication Date	Reaffirmed Date
Committee on Genetics (continued)			
409	Direct-to-Consumer Marketing of Genetic Testing *(Joint with Committee on Ethics)* (Obstet Gynecol 2008;111:1493–4)	June 2008	
410	Ethical Issues in Genetic Testing *(Joint with Committee on Ethics)* (Obstet Gynecol 2008;111:1495–502)	June 2008	
1	Genetics and Molecular Diagnostic Testing (Obstet Gynecol 2002;100:193–211)	July 2002	2006
Committee on Gynecologic Practice			
240	Statement on Surgical Assistants (Obstet Gynecol Vol. 96, No. 2) *(Joint with Committee on Obstetric Practice)*	August 2000	2008
243	Performance and Interpretation of Imaging Studies by Obstetrician–Gynecologists (Obstet Gynecol Vol. 96, No. 5)	November 2000	2007
253	Nongynecologic Procedures (Obstet Gynecol Vol. 97, No. 3)	March 2001	2008
278	Avoiding Inappropriate Clinical Decisions Based on False-Positive Human Chorionic Gonadotropin Test Results (Obstet Gynecol 2002;100:1057–9)	November 2002	2007
280	The Role of the Generalist Obstetrician–Gynecologist in the Early Detection of Ovarian Cancer *(Joint with Society of Gynecologic Oncologists)* (Obstet Gynecol 2002;100:1413–6)	December 2002	2005
285	Induced Abortion and Breast Cancer Risk (Obstet Gynecol 2003;102:433–5)	August 2003	2005
311	Appropriate Use of Laparoscopically Assisted Vaginal Hysterectomy (Obstet Gynecol 2005;105:929–30)	April 2005	2007
313	The Importance of Preconception Care in the Continuum of Women's Health Care (Obstet Gynecol 2005;106:665–6)	September 2005	2007
319	The Role of the Obstetrician–Gynecologist in the Assessment and Management of Obesity (Obstet Gynecol 2005;106:895–9)	October 2005	
322	Compounded Bioidentical Hormones (Obstet Gynecol 2005;106:1139–40)	November 2005	2007
323	Elective Coincidental Appendectomy (Obstet Gynecol 2005;106:1141–2)	November 2005	2007
324	Perinatal Risks Associated With Assisted Reproductive Technology *(Joint with Committees on Obstetric Practice and Genetics)* (Obstet Gynecol 2005;106:1143–6)	November 2005	2008
332	Hepatitis B and Hepatitis C Virus Infections in Obstetrician–Gynecologists (Obstet Gynecol 2006;107:1207–8)	May 2006	2008
334	Role of the Obstetrician–Gynecologist in the Screening and Diagnosis of Breast Masses (Obstet Gynecol 2006;107:1213–4)	May 2006	2008
336	Tamoxifen and Uterine Cancer (Obstet Gynecol 2006;107:1475–8)	June 2006	2008
337	Noncontraceptive Uses of the Levonorgestrel Intrauterine System (Obstet Gynecol 2006;107:1479–82)	June 2006	2008
345	Vulvodynia *(Joint with the American Society for Colposcopy and Cervical Pathology)* (Obstet Gynecol 2006;108:1049–52)	October 2006	2008
357	Primary and Preventive Care: Periodic Assessments (Obstet Gynecol 2006;108:1615–22)	December 2006	
372	The Role of Cystourethroscopy in the Generalist Obstetrician–Gynecologist Practice (Obstet Gynecol 2007;110:221–4)	July 2007	
375	Brand Versus Generic Oral Contraceptives (Obstet Gynecol 2007;110:447–8)	August 2007	
378	Vaginal "Rejuvenation" and Cosmetic Vaginal Procedures (Obstet Gynecol 2007;110:737–8)	September 2007	
384	Colonoscopy and Colorectal Cancer Screening and Prevention (Obstet Gynecol 2007;110:1199–1202)	November 2007	
387	Pharmaceutical Compounding (Obstet Gynecol 2007;110:1213–4)	November 2007	
388	Supracervical Hysterectomy (Obstet Gynecol 2007;110:1215–7)	November 2007	
396	Intraperitoneal Chemotherapy for Ovarian Cancer (Obstet Gynecol 2008;111:249–51)	January 2008	
405	Ovarian Tissue and Oocyte Cryopreservation (Obstet Gynecol 2008;111:1255–6)	May 2008	
407	Low Bone Mass (Osteopenia) and Fracture Risk (Obstet Gynecol 2008;111:1259–61)	May 2008	
408	Professional Liability and Gynecology-Only Practice *(Joint with Committees on Obstetric Practice and Professional Liability)* (Obstet Gynecol 2008;111:1491)	June 2008	
*411	Routine Human Immunodeficiency Virus Screening (Obstet Gynecol 2008;112:401–3)	August 2008	
*412	Aromatase Inhibitors in Gynecologic Practice (Obstet Gynecol 2008;112:405–7)	August 2008	
*413	Age-Related Fertility Decline *(Joint with American Society for Reproductive Medicine)* (Obstet Gynecol 2008;112:409–11)	August 2008	

Number	Title	Publication Date	Reaffirmed Date
Committee on Gynecologic Practice (continued)			
*415	Depot Medroxyprogesterone Acetate and Bone Effects *(Joint with Committee on Adolescent Health Care)* (Obstet Gynecol 2008;112:727–30)	September 2008	
*417	Addressing Health Risks of Noncoital Sexual Activity *(Joint with Committee on Adolescent Health Care)* (Obstet Gynecol 2008;112:735–7)	September 2008	
*420	Hormone Therapy and Heart Disease (Obstet Gynecol 2008;112:1189–92)	November 2008	
4	Hysteroscopy (Obstet Gynecol 2005;106:439–42)	August 2005	2007
*5	Sonohysterography (Obstet Gynecol 2008;112:1467–9)	December 2008	
Committee on Health Care for Underserved Women			
307	Partner Consent for Participation in Women's Reproductive Health Research (Obstet Gynecol 2004;104:1467–9)	December 2004	2008
312	Health Care for Homeless Women (Obstet Gynecol 2005;106:429–34)	August 2005	
316	Smoking Cessation During Pregnancy *(Joint with Committee on Obstetric Practice)* (Obstet Gynecol 2005;106:883–8)	October 2005	
317	Racial and Ethnic Disparities in Women's Health (Obstet Gynecol 2005;106:889–92)	October 2005	
343	Psychosocial Risk Factors: Perinatal Screening and Intervention (Obstet Gynecol 2006;108:469–77)	August 2006	
361	Breastfeeding: Maternal and Infant Aspects *(Joint with Committee on Obstetric Practice)* (Obstet Gynecol 2007;109:479–80)	February 2007	
391	Health Literacy (Obstet Gynecol 2007;110:1489–91)	December 2007	
*414	Human Immunodeficiency Virus and Acquired Immunodeficiency Syndrome and Women of Color (Obstet Gynecol 2008;112:413–6)	August 2008	
*416	The Uninsured (Obstet Gynecol 2008;112:731–4)	September 2008	
Committee on Obstetric Practice			
125	Placental Pathology	July 1993	2006
228	Induction of Labor with Misoprostol (Obstet Gynecol Vol. 94, No. 5)	November 1999	2008
234	Scheduled Cesarean Delivery and the Prevention of Vertical Transmission of HIV Infection (Obstet Gynecol Vol. 95, No. 5)	May 2000	2008
240	Statement on Surgical Assistants *(Joint with Committee on Gynecologic Practice)* (Obstet Gynecol Vol. 96, No. 2)	August 2000	2008
248	Response to Searle's Drug Warning on Misoprostol (Obstet Gynecol Vol. 96, No. 6)	December 2000	2008
256	Optimal Goals for Anesthesia Care in Obstetrics *(Joint with American Society of Anesthesiologists)* (Obstet Gynecol Vol. 97, No. 5)	May 2001	2006
260	Circumcision (Obstet Gynecol 2001;98:707–708)	October 2001	2007
264	Air Travel During Pregnancy (Obstet Gynecol 2001;98:1187–1188)	December 2001	2006
267	Exercise During Pregnancy and the Postpartum Period (Obstet Gynecol 2002;99:171–173)	January 2002	2007
268	Management of Asymptomatic Pregnant or Lactating Women Exposed to Anthrax (Obstet Gynecol 2002;99:366–368)	February 2002	2007
275	Obstetric Management of Patients with Spinal Cord Injuries (Obstet Gynecol 2002;100:625–7)	September 2002	2005
276	Safety of Lovenox in Pregnancy (Obstet Gynecol 2002;100:845–6)	October 2002	2008
279	Prevention of Early-Onset Group B Streptococcal Disease in Newborns (Obstet Gynecol 2002;100:1405–12)	December 2002	2007
281	Rubella Vaccination (Obstet Gynecol 2002;100:1417)	December 2002	2008
282	Immunization During Pregnancy (Obstet Gynecol 2003;101:207–12)	January 2003	2005
283	New U.S. Food and Drug Administration Labeling on Cytotec (Misoprostol) Use and Pregnancy (Obstet Gynecol 2003;101:1049–50)	May 2003	2008
284	Nonobstetric Surgery in Pregnancy (Obstet Gynecol 2003;102:431)	August 2003	2006
295	Pain Relief During Labor *(Joint with American Society of Anesthesiologists)* (Obstet Gynecol 2004;104:213)	July 2004	2007
299	Guidelines for Diagnostic Imaging During Pregnancy (Obstet Gynecol 2004;104:647–51)	September 2004	2006
305	Influenza Vaccination and Treatment During Pregnancy (Obstet Gynecol 2004;104:1125–6)	November 2004	2006
315	Obesity in Pregnancy (Obstet Gynecol 2005;106:671–5)	September 2005	2008
316	Smoking Cessation During Pregnancy *(Joint with Committee on Health Care for Underserved Women)* (Obstet Gynecol 2005;106:883–8)	October 2005	

Number	Title	Publication Date	Reaffirmed Date
Committee on Obstetric Practice (continued)			
324	Perinatal Risks Associated With Assisted Reproductive Technology *(Joint with Committees on Genetics and Gynecologic Practice)* (Obstet Gynecol 2005;106:1143–6)	November 2005	2008
326	Inappropriate Use of the Terms Fetal Distress and Birth Asphyxia (Obstet Gynecol 2005;106:1469–70)	December 2005	
333	The Apgar Score *(Joint with American Academy of Pediatrics)* (Obstet Gynecol 2006;107:1209–12)	May 2006	
339	Analgesia and Cesarean Delivery Rates (Obstet Gynecol 2006;107:1487–8)	June 2006	
340	Mode of Term Singleton Breech Delivery (Obstet Gynecol 2006;108:235–7)	July 2006	
342	Induction of Labor for Vaginal Birth After Cesarean Delivery (Obstet Gynecol 2006;108:465–7)	August 2006	
346	Amnioinfusion Does Not Prevent Meconium Aspiration Syndrome (Obstet Gynecol 2006;108:1053–5)	October 2006	
348	Umbilical Cord Blood Gas and Acid–Base Analysis (Obstet Gynecol 2006;108:1319–22)	November 2006	
361	Breastfeeding: Maternal and Infant Aspects *(Joint with Committee on Health Care for Underserved Women)* (Obstet Gynecol 2007;109:479–80)	February 2007	
376	Nalbuphine Hydrochloride Use for Intrapartum Analgesia (Obstet Gynecol 2007;110:449)	August 2007	
379	Management of Delivery of a Newborn With Meconium-Stained Amniotic Fluid (Obstet Gynecol 2007;110:739)	September 2007	
381	Subclinical Hypothyroidism in Pregnancy (Obstet Gynecol 2007;110:959–60)	October 2007	
382	Fetal Monitoring Prior to Scheduled Cesarean Delivery (Obstet Gynecol 2007;110:961)	October 2007	
394	Cesarean Delivery on Maternal Request (Obstet Gynecol 2007;110:1501–4)	December 2007	
399	Umbilical Cord Blood Banking *(Joint with Committee on Genetics)* (Obstet Gynecol 2008;111:475–7)	February 2008	
402	Antenatal Corticosteroid Therapy for Fetal Maturation (Obstet Gynecol 2008;111:805–7)	March 2008	
404	Late-Preterm Infants (Obstet Gynecol 2008;111:1029–32)	April 2008	
408	Professional Liability and Gynecology-Only Practice *(Joint with Committees on Gynecologic Practice and Professional Liability)* (Obstet Gynecol 2008;111:1491)	June 2008	
*418	Prenatal and Perinatal Human Immunodeficiency Virus Testing: Expanded Recommendations (Obstet Gynecol 2008;112:739–42)	September 2008	
*419	Use of Progesterone to Reduce Preterm Birth *(Joint with the Society for Maternal–Fetal Medicine)* (Obstet Gynecol 2008;112:963–5)	October 2008	
*421	Antibiotic Prophylaxis for Infective Endocarditis (Obstet Gynecol 2008;112:1193–4)	November 2008	
Committee on Professional Liability			
380	Disclosure and Discussion of Adverse Events *(Joint with Committee on Patient Safety and Quality Improvement)* (Obstet Gynecol 2007;110:957–8)	October 2007	
406	Coping With the Stress of Medical Professional Liability Litigation (Obstet Gynecol 2008;111:1257–8)	May 2008	
408	Professional Liability and Gynecology-Only Practice *(Joint with Committees on Gynecologic Practice and Obstetric Practice)* (Obstet Gynecol 2008;111:1491)	June 2008	
Committee on Patient Safety and Quality Improvement			
286	Patient Safety in Obstetrics and Gynecology (Obstet Gynecol 2003;102:883–5)	October 2003	2006
320	Partnering With Patients to Improve Safety (Obstet Gynecol 2005;106:1123–5)	November 2005	2007
327	"Do Not Use" Abbreviations (Obstet Gynecol 2006;107:213–4)	January 2006	2007
328	Patient Safety in the Surgical Environment (Obstet Gynecol 2006;107:429–33)	February 2006	2007
329	Tracking and Reminder Systems (Obstet Gynecol 2006;107:745–7)	March 2006	2007
331	Safe Use of Medication (Obstet Gynecol 2006;107:969–72)	April 2006	2007
353	Medical Emergency Preparedness (Obstet Gynecol 2006;108:1597–9)	December 2006	
366	Disruptive Behavior (Obstet Gynecol 2007;109:1261–2)	May 2007	
367	Communication Strategies for Patient Handoffs (Obstet Gynecol 2007;109:1503–5)	June 2007	
380	Disclosure and Discussion of Adverse Events *(Joint with Committee on Professional Liability)* (Obstet Gynecol 2007;110:957–8)	October 2007	
398	Fatigue and Patient Safety (Obstet Gynecol 2008;111:471–3)	February 2008	
400	Technologic Advances to Reduce Medication-Related Errors (Obstet Gynecol 2008;111:795–8)	March 2008	

Current Committee Opinions and Technology Assessments

■ 1	■ 4	■ 5	125	205	228	230	234	240	243	248	249	250	253	256	260	264	267	268	275	276	278
279	280	281	282	283	284	285	286	295	297	298	299	300	301	302	305	307	310	311	312	313	314
315	316	317	318	319	320	321	322	323	324	325	326	327	328	329	330	331	332	333	334	335	336
337	338	339	340	341	342	343	344	345	346	347	348	349	350	351	352	353	355	357	358	359	360
361	362	363	364	365	366	367	368	369	370	371	372	373	374	375	376	377	378	379	380	381	382
383	384	385	387	388	389	390	391	392	393	394	395	396	397	398	399	400	401	402	403	404	405
406	407	408	409	410	411	412	413	414	415	416	417	418	419	420	421	422					

For ordering information, contact the ACOG Distribution Center at 800-762-2264, or order online at sales.acog.org.

*Title issued since publication of last index
†Title issued since publication of *Ethics in Obstetrics and Gynecology*, Second Edition

AC002

■ Technology Assessment

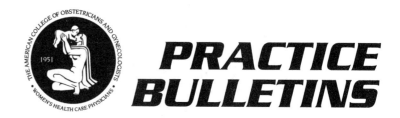

LIST OF TITLES — DECEMBER 2008

Practice Bulletins provide obstetricians and gynecologists with current information on established techniques and clinical management guidelines. ACOG continuously surveys the field for advances to be incorporated in these series and monitors existing bulletins to ensure they are current. Individual bulletins are withdrawn from and added to the series on a continuing basis and reaffirmed periodically.

The following titles have been withdrawn from circulation:

Practice Bulletins

   16 Surgical Alternatives to Hysterectomy in the Management of Leiomyomas
       (Replaced by Practice Bulletin No. 96)

   47 Prophylactic Antibiotics in Labor and Delivery *(Replaced by Committee Opinion No. 421)*

   58 Ultrasonography in Pregnancy *(Replaced by Practice Bulletin No. 98)*

   66 Management of Abnormal Cervical Cytology and Histology *(Replaced by Practice Bulletin No. 99)*

   98 Ultrasonography in Pregnancy

Educational Bulletin

  230 Assessment of Fetal Lung Maturity *(Replaced by Practice Bulletin No. 97)*

Number	Title	Publication Date	Reaffirmed Date
Committee on Practice Bulletins—Obstetrics			
4	Prevention of Rh D Alloimmunization (Obstet Gynecol Vol. 93, No. 5)	May 1999	2007
6	Thrombocytopenia in Pregnancy (Obstet Gynecol Vol. 94, No. 3)	September 1999	2007
9	Antepartum Fetal Surveillance (Obstet Gynecol Vol. 94, No. 4)	October 1999	2007
10	Induction of Labor (Obstet Gynecol Vol. 94, No. 5)	November 1999	2006
12	Intrauterine Growth Restriction (Obstet Gynecol Vol. 95, No. 1)	January 2000	2008
13	External Cephalic Version (Obstet Gynecol Vol. 95, No. 2)	February 2000	2008
17	Operative Vaginal Delivery (Obstet Gynecol Vol. 95, No. 6)	June 2000	2008
19	Thromboembolism in Pregnancy (Obstet Gynecol Vol. 96, No. 2)	August 2000	2008
20	Perinatal Viral and Parasitic Infections (Obstet Gynecol Vol. 96, No. 3)	September 2000	2008
22	Fetal Macrosomia (Obstet Gynecol Vol. 96, No. 5)	November 2000	2008
24	Management of Recurrent Early Pregnancy Loss (Obstet Gynecol Vol. 97, No. 2)	February 2001	2008
29	Chronic Hypertension in Pregnancy (Obstet Gynecol 2001;98:177–185)	July 2001	2008
30	Gestational Diabetes (Obstet Gynecol 2001;98:525–538)	September 2001	2008
31	Assessment of Risk Factors for Preterm Birth (Obstet Gynecol 2001;98:709–716)	October 2001	2008
33	Diagnosis and Management of Preeclampsia and Eclampsia (Obstet Gynecol 2002;99:159–167)	January 2002	2008
36	Obstetric Analgesia and Anesthesia (Obstet Gynecol 2002;100:177–191)	July 2002	2008
37	Thyroid Disease in Pregnancy (Obstet Gynecol 2002;100:387–396)	August 2002	2008

Number	Title	Publication Date	Reaffirmed Date
Committee on Practice Bulletins—Obstetrics (continued)			
38	Perinatal Care at the Threshold of Viability (Obstet Gynecol 2002;100:617–24)	September 2002	2008
40	Shoulder Dystocia (Obstet Gynecol 2002;100:1045–50)	November 2002	2008
43	Management of Preterm Labor (Obstet Gynecol 2003;101:1039–47)	May 2003	2008
44	Neural Tube Defects (Obstet Gynecol 2003;102:203–13)	July 2003	2008
48	Cervical Insufficiency (Obstet Gynecol 2003;102:1091–9)	November 2003	2008
49	Dystocia and Augmentation of Labor (Obstet Gynecol 2003;102:1445–54)	December 2003	2007
52	Nausea and Vomiting of Pregnancy (Obstet Gynecol 2004;103:803–15)	April 2004	2007
54	Vaginal Birth After Previous Cesarean Delivery (Obstet Gynecol 2004;104:203–12)	July 2004	2007
55	Management of Postterm Pregnancy (Obstet Gynecol 2004;104:639–46)	September 2004	2007
56	Multiple Gestation: Complicated Twin, Triplet, and High-Order Multifetal Pregnancy *(Joint with the Society for Maternal–Fetal Medicine)* (Obstet Gynecol 2004;104:869–83)	October 2004	2007
60	Pregestational Diabetes Mellitus (Obstet Gynecol 2005;105:675–85)	March 2005	2007
68	Antiphospholipid Syndrome (Obstet Gynecol 2005;106:1113–21)	November 2005	2007
70	Intrapartum Fetal Heart Rate Monitoring (Obstet Gynecol 2005;106:1453–61)	December 2005	2007
71	Episiotomy (Obstet Gynecol 2006;107:957–62)	April 2006	2008
75	Management of Alloimmunization During Pregnancy (Obstet Gynecol 2006;108:457–64)	August 2006	2008
76	Postpartum Hemorrhage (Obstet Gynecol 2006;108:1039–47)	October 2006	2008
77	Screening for Fetal Chromosomal Abnormalities *(Joint with the Society for Maternal–Fetal Medicine)* (Obstet Gynecol 2007;109:217–27)	January 2007	2008
78	Hemoglobinopathies in Pregnancy (Obstet Gynecol 2007;109:229–37)	January 2007	2008
80	Premature Rupture of Membranes (Obstet Gynecol 2007;109:1007–19)	April 2007	
82	Management of Herpes in Pregnancy (Obstet Gynecol 2007;109:1489–98)	June 2007	
86	Viral Hepatitis in Pregnancy (Obstet Gynecol 2007;110:941–55)	October 2007	
88	Invasive Prenatal Testing for Aneuploidy (Obstet Gynecol 2007;110:1459–67)	December 2007	
90	Asthma in Pregnancy (Obstet Gynecol 2008;111:457–64)	February 2008	
92	Use of Psychiatric Medications During Pregnancy and Lactation (Obstet Gynecol 2008;111:1001–20)	April 2008	
*95	Anemia in Pregnancy (Obstet Gynecol 2008;112:201–7)	July 2008	
*97	Fetal Lung Maturity (Obstet Gynecol 2008;112:717–26)	September 2008	
251	Obstetric Aspects of Trauma Management (Obstet Gynecol Vol. 92, No. 3)	September 1998	2006
Committee on Practice Bulletins—Gynecology			
11	Medical Management of Endometriosis (Obstet Gynecol Vol. 94, No. 6)	December 1999	2007
14	Management of Anovulatory Bleeding (Obstet Gynecol Vol. 95, No. 3)	March 2000	2007
15	Premenstrual Syndrome (Obstet Gynecol Vol. 95, No. 4)	April 2000	2008
28	Use of Botanicals for Management of Menopausal Symptoms (Obstet Gynecol Vol. 97, No. 6)	June 2001	2008
34	Management of Infertility Caused by Ovulatory Dysfunction (Obstet Gynecol 2002;99:347–358)	February 2002	2008
35	Diagnosis and Treatment of Cervical Carcinomas (Obstet Gynecol 2002;99:855–867)	May 2002	2008
39	Selective Estrogen Receptor Modulators (Obstet Gynecol 2002;100:835–44)	October 2002	2008
41	Polycystic Ovary Syndrome (Obstet Gynecol 2002;100:1389–402)	December 2002	2006

Number	Title	Publication Date	Reaffirmed Date

Committee on Practice Bulletins—Gynecology (continued)

42	Breast Cancer Screening (Obstet Gynecol 2003;101:821–32)	April 2003	2006
45	Cervical Cytology Screening (Obstet Gynecol 2003;102:417–27)	August 2003	2007
46	Benefits and Risks of Sterilization (Obstet Gynecol 2003;102:647–58)	September 2003	2008
50	Osteoporosis (Obstet Gynecol 2004;103:203–16)	January 2004	2008
51	Chronic Pelvic Pain (Obstet Gynecol 2004;103:589–605)	March 2004	2008
53	Diagnosis and Treatment of Gestational Trophoblastic Disease *(Joint with the Society of Gynecologic Oncologists)* (Obstet Gynecol 2004;103:1365–77)	June 2004	2008
57	Gynecologic Herpes Simplex Virus Infections (Obstet Gynecol 2004;104:1111–7)	November 2004	2006
59	Intrauterine Device (Obstet Gynecol 2005;105:223–32)	January 2005	2007
61	Human Papillomavirus (Obstet Gynecol 2005;105:905–18)	April 2005	2007
63	Urinary Incontinence in Women (Obstet Gynecol 2005;105:1533–45)	June 2005	2007
65	Management of Endometrial Cancer *(Joint with the Society of Gynecologic Oncologists)* (Obstet Gynecol 2005;106:413–25)	August 2005	2007
67	Medical Management of Abortion (Obstet Gynecol 2005;106:871–82)	October 2005	2007
69	Emergency Contraception (Obstet Gynecol 2005;106:1443–52)	December 2005	2007
72	Vaginitis (Obstet Gynecol 2006;107:1195–1206)	May 2006	2008
73	Use of Hormonal Contraception in Women With Coexisting Medical Conditions (Obstet Gynecol 2006;107:1453–72)	June 2006	2008
74	Antibiotic Prophylaxis for Gynecologic Procedures (Obstet Gynecol 2006;108:225–34)	July 2006	
81	Endometrial Ablation (Obstet Gynecol 2007;109:1233–48)	May 2007	
83	Management of Adnexal Masses (Obstet Gynecol 2007;110:201–14)	July 2007	
84	Prevention of Deep Vein Thrombosis and Pulmonary Embolism (Obstet Gynecol 2007;110:429–40)	August 2007	
85	Pelvic Organ Prolapse (Obstet Gynecol 2007;110:717–29)	September 2007	
89	Elective and Risk-Reducing Salpingo-oophorectomy (Obstet Gynecol 2008;111:231–41)	January 2008	
91	Treatment of Urinary Tract Infections in Nonpregnant Women (Obstet Gynecol 2008;111:785–94)	March 2008	
93	Diagnosis and Management of Vulvar Skin Disorders (Obstet Gynecol 2008;111:1243–53)	May 2008	
94	Medical Management of Ectopic Pregnancy (Obstet Gynecol 2008;111:1479–85)	June 2008	
*96	Alternatives to Hysterectomy in the Management of Leiomyomas (Obstet Gynecol 2008;112:387–400)	August 2008	
*99	Management of Abnormal Cervical Cytology and Histology (Obstet Gynecol 2008;112:1419–44)	December 2008	

Current Bulletins

4	6	9	10	11	12	13	14	15	17	19	20	22	24	28	29	30	31	33	34	35	36
37	38	39	40	41	42	43	44	45	46	48	49	50	51	52	53	54	55	56	57	59	60
61	63	65	67	68	69	70	71	72	73	74	75	76	77	78	80	81	82	83	84	85	86
88	89	90	91	92	93	94	95	96	97	99	251										

For ordering information, contact the ACOG Distribution Center at 800-762-2264, or order online at sales.acog.org.

*Title issued since publication of last listing

Index